CAMBRIDGE LIBRARY COLLECTION

Books of enduring scholarly value

History of Medicine

It is sobering to realise that as recently as the year in which On the Origin of Species was published, learned opinion was that diseases such as typhus and cholera were spread by a ,Äòmiasma,Äô, and suggestions that doctors should wash their hands before examining patients were greeted with mockery by the profession. The Cambridge Library Collection reissues milestone publications in the history of Western medicine as well as studies of other medical traditions. Its coverage ranges from Galen on anatomical procedures to Florence Nightingale,Äôs common-sense advice to nurses, and includes early research into genetics and mental health, colonial reports on tropical diseases, documents on public health and military medicine, and publications on spa culture and medicinal plants.

On Some of the More Important Diseases of the Army

Born in Cornwall, John Davy (1790–1868) physiologist and anatomist, and the younger brother of the distinguished chemist Sir Humphry Davy (1778–1829), was one of the most prolific medical experts of his day. After taking a medical degree from Edinburgh in 1814 he became an army surgeon. He later became a hospital inspector and spent time living in overseas territories including India, Sri Lanka, and Barbados. First published in 1862, Davy's book discusses the prominence of fever, dysentery, cholera, liver disease, pneumonia, and other diseases common to the army, estimating that 45% of deaths in the British army serving abroad were caused by disease rather than by conflict. Davy also records his observations on putrefaction of bodies, particularly the vital organs, emphasising the need to determine the normal condition of human organs so that abnormal, diseased organs can be easily identified.

Cambridge University Press has long been a pioneer in the reissuing of out-of-print titles from its own backlist, producing digital reprints of books that are still sought after by scholars and students but could not be reprinted economically using traditional technology. The Cambridge Library Collection extends this activity to a wider range of books which are still of importance to researchers and professionals, either for the source material they contain, or as landmarks in the history of their academic discipline.

Drawing from the world-renowned collections in the Cambridge University Library, and guided by the advice of experts in each subject area, Cambridge University Press is using state-of-the-art scanning machines in its own Printing House to capture the content of each book selected for inclusion. The files are processed to give a consistently clear, crisp image, and the books finished to the high quality standard for which the Press is recognised around the world. The latest print-on-demand technology ensures that the books will remain available indefinitely, and that orders for single or multiple copies can quickly be supplied.

The Cambridge Library Collection will bring back to life books of enduring scholarly value (including out-of-copyright works originally issued by other publishers) across a wide range of disciplines in the humanities and social sciences and in science and technology.

On Some of the More Important Diseases of the Army

With Contributions to Pathology

JOHN DAVY

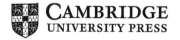

CAMBRIDGE
UNIVERSITY PRESS

CAMBRIDGE UNIVERSITY PRESS

Cambridge, New York, Melbourne, Madrid, Cape Town,
Singapore, São Paolo, Delhi, Tokyo, Mexico City

Published in the United States of America by Cambridge University Press, New York

www.cambridge.org
Information on this title: www.cambridge.org/9781108037655

This edition first published 1862
This digitally printed version 2011

ISBN 978-1-108-03765-5 Paperback

DISEASES OF THE ARMY.

ON

SOME OF THE MORE IMPORTANT

DISEASES OF THE ARMY,

WITH

CONTRIBUTIONS TO PATHOLOGY

BY

JOHN DAVY, M.D., F.R.S.,

LONDON AND EDINBURGH, ETC.; INSPECTOR GENERAL OF ARMY HOSPITALS H.P.

WILLIAMS AND NORGATE,

14, HENRIETTA STREET, COVENT GARDEN, LONDON

AND

20, SOUTH FREDERICK STREET, EDINBURGH.

1862.

"Vehementer certe optandum foret, ut medicus, casus in artis exercitio occurrentes, præsertim notabiliores, plenissimæ consignare, atque hoc facto, artis medicæ incrementum promovere anniteretur."—F. HOFFMAN.

PREFACE.

THE title of this work, I trust, will be found to be warranted by its contents. When I first formed the idea of engaging in it, the name proposed for it was Contributions to Pathology. A friendly critic to whom I submitted the MS. in part, held the designation to be too limited, and not sufficiently characteristic. I have yielded to his judgment.

The materials of which it is formed have been collected during the course of my professional life—reaching now nearly to half a century—of which the best portion has been passed in the public service. During the greater part of this period I was in the habit of making notes of every fatal case that came under my observation, of which a *post mortem* examination was instituted. My method was, immediately after the examination to describe the morbid appearances, refer when available to the Medical Register in which the case was recorded, make an abstract of the symptoms and treatment, and end with some brief remarks on what seemed most peculiar in each.

With the exception of about two years—viz., from 1821 to 1823—that I was in charge, as Surgeon to the Forces, of the Medical Division of the General Hospital

at Fort Pitt, Chatham, my duties were principally those
of an inspectorial and superintending kind, in the per-
formance of which I had to visit the hospitals frequently,
commonly daily, and was called into consultation by the
officiating Medical Officers in every case of more than
ordinary severity.

The stations at which my experience was largest were
Ceylon, the Ionian Islands, Malta, Fort Pitt Chatham,
and the West Indies. The number of fatal cases of
which I have notes, amounting altogether to 1,060,
may aid in showing the extent of that experience. I
am induced to make use of these materials now, having
more than ordinary leisure, and sensible that a longer
delay must, from advancing age, soon put it out of my
power to engage in the task. The plan which I proposed to myself, and which I have followed out, was to
make a selection of the cases of the like kind, leading
as much as possible to definite conclusions of practical
import. I have not attempted to strengthen these
conclusions by reference to medical authors, neither
space nor time, irrespective of other considerations, permitting. Whatever value may belong to my contributions will lie in the facts adduced.

I shall first treat of fevers, and some other of the more
important diseases to which troops are liable; next of
certain others, and of allied subjects respecting which I
have found most to offer, deferring to another occasion,
should life with health be spared, and this volume have
a welcome from my professional brethren, any further
contributions to pathology, which the means at my disposal may allow of.

The Introduction—a part distinct from the body of the work, though I trust it will not be considered foreign to it—is given with the hope that it may be of use to the young pathologist.

In stating briefly the statistics of some of the more serious diseases to which the soldier is subject, I have availed myself of the important Statistical Reports on the sickness and mortality in the British army at home and on foreign service, for which we are indebted to the industry and ability of Sir Alexander Tulloch and the late Mr. Marshall, and to his successor, Dr. Balfour.

Reflecting on the progress that has been made in medicine during the period of my professional experience—a period that has witnessed the introduction of the stethoscope, the improvement of the microscope, and its application to pathology, and, moreover, the vast advance of physiology and of organic chemistry—I am very sensible how very defective are many of the details in the following pages. Allowances, however, I trust, will be made for their imperfection, considering the circumstances under which they were made, "inter tœdia atque labores," and the few aids which were then supplied by the Medical Department of the army for the prosecution of scientific research, a Medical Officer having to provide himself then, at his own cost, with all the instruments needed, if he wished to attempt anything more than his mere duties of routine.

Now that a Medical School, so long a desideratum, and so often suggested, is established at Chatham, with, though somewhat stinted, most of the appliances required, both for instruction and research, with an able staff of professors,* a better time I would fain hope is opening, and warranting, without being too sanguine, the expectation that larger contributions than heretofore will be made by Army Medical Officers in the good cause of science, and especially of medical science; and, further, to encourage such exertion, that those Officers who so distinguish themselves will not be passed over without honour and substantial reward.

* This, the "Practical Army Medical School" (such is its name), is under the Secretary for War, and is governed by a senate consisting of the Director-General of the Army Medical Department, the Physician to the Council of India, the Professors, and the Principal Medical Officer of the station *ex officio.* It was first opened at the General Hospital, Fort Pitt, in October, 1860, under the auspices of that great benefactor of the army, Mr. Sidney Herbert—the late Lord Herbert. The Professors are :—Thomas Longmore, Esq., Deputy Inspector-General of Hospitals, Professor of Surgery; E. F. Parkes, M.D., Professor of Hygiene; Wm. Aitkin, M.D., Professor of Pathology; Wm. C. MacLean, M.D., Deputy Inspector-General of Hospitals, Professor of Military Medicine.

Fort Pitt, now a spot of so much interest, not quite fifty years ago was the quarter of a regiment of militia—the building now the hospital then a barrack, and another, now holding the library, then a canteen. The museum, dissecting and lecture-rooms, model-room, chemical laboratory, lunatic asylum, mess-house, etc., are comparatively recent additions.

LESKETH HOW, NEAR AMBLESIDE,

July 5th, 1862.

CONTENTS.

PREFACE.

PAGE

INTRODUCTION.—Preliminary remarks.—Observations on the average weight of organs; on the discoloration of parts; on the softening of textures and on putrefaction; on the temperature of the body after death; on air in the vessels and effused fluids; on the *post mortem* condition of the blood and rigor mortis; on the situation of organs 1

CHAPTER I.

ON FEVERS.—Intermittent, remittent and continued fever.—Remarks on.—Their statistics.—Cases illustrative of the several kinds, including yellow fever.—Their etiology in connection with climate and temperature.—Observations on malaria.—Precautions against.—Remarks on the pathology of fevers and their treatment 17

CHAPTER II.

ON DYSENTERY.—Observations on as to climate and causes.—Illustrative cases of the acute and chronic kind.—Description of symptoms.—Suggestions as to the prevention of the disease.—Remarks on its treatment 66

CHAPTER III.

ON CHOLERA MORBUS.—Remarks on the two kinds, the epidemic and common.—Special report on the former, as it occurred in Ceylon in 1819.—Observations on common cholera, as sporadic and endemic, with cases.—On the pathology of the disease and its treatment 111

CHAPTER IV.

ON DISEASES OF THE LIVER.—Remarks on.—Their statistics.—Causes of, with reference to climate, diet, etc.—Illustrative cases.—Difficulty of diagnosis.—Tendency to complication.—Treatment of 129

CHAPTER V.

ON PULMONARY CONSUMPTION.—Remarks on its importance in connection with
its prevalency, especially in the army.—Statistics of the disease.—Reasons for
writing on it.—Division into sections, with illustrative cases; 1st, Of latent
tubercles, without appreciable diseased action; 2ndly, Of the disguising
influence of insanity; 3rdly, Of a like influence of other diseases; 4thly, Of
ordinary consumption, acute and chronic.—Etiological and pathological
remarks.—Effects of ignorance and maladministration.—Hopeful prospective
views.—Treatment and prevention 157

CHAPTER VI.

ON PNEUMATHORAX.—Remarks on it viewed as an epiphenomenon of tubercles.
—Detailed cases of.—Observations regarding its semeiology, pathology and
treatment 218

CHAPTER VII.

ON EMPYEMA, HYDROTHORAX AND PERICARDITIS.—Remarks on their unfrequency.—Connection of empyema and hydrothorax with tubercles.—
Peculiarities from complications.—Illustrative cases with comments.—Statistics of pericarditis.—Cases of.—Some general remarks on these several
diseases, their origin, pathology and treatment 245

CHAPTER VIII.

ON THE COAGULATION OF THE BLOOD IN THE VESSELS DURING LIFE, AND THE
SOFTENING OF ITS FIBRIN.—Connection of the phenomena with some of the
preceding diseases and analogy to tubercle.—Our knowledge of it recent.—
Importance of the subject pathologically.—Instances of, with the diseases with
which associated.—Specification of vessels the seat of the coagulation.—Brief
description of cases.—Remarks on the coagulation and softening of fibrin in
these cases and the product.—Their pathology reverted to, as probably
explanatory of certain sudden deaths, etc. 267

CHAPTER IX.

ON PNEUMONIA.—Statistics of.—Influence of climate and of other causes productive of it.—Varieties and complications of the disease.—Illustrative cases
with comments; 1st, Of the least complicated; 2ndly, Of those complicated
with inflammation of the mediastina and cellular tissue; 3rdly, With hypertrophy of heart, etc.; 4thly, With cerebral disease; 5thly, With peritoneal
inflammation; 6thly, With anomalous symptoms; 7thly, With rheumatic
inflammation and deposition of lithic acid; 8thly, With tubercles; 9thly, Of
chronic pneumonia.—Remarks on the foregoing, as to predisposition, symptoms,
duration and treatment, and especially on blood-letting, and the constitution of
man present and past 291

CHAPTER X.

PAGE

ON PERITONITIS.—A comparatively rare disease in the army.—Its statistics.—
Most commonly, like pneumathorax, an epiphenomenon, the result of perforation of some one of the abdominal viscera.—Examples.—Diathesis.—Illustrative cases with comments.—Remarks on its pathology, semeiology and
treatment 331

CHAPTER XI.

ON CELLULAR INFLAMMATION.—Reasons for using the term.—Statistics of the
disease in connection with climate.—Habit of body favorable to its production.
—A certain periodicity belonging to it.—Detailed cases, with comments; two
especially remarkable, one for solution of a large portion of stomach and diaphragm, one for high temperature after death.—Remarks on its pathology,
symptoms, and treatment.—Notice of experiments on the effects of pus on
animals injected into the pleura 354

CHAPTER XII.

ON ANEURISM AND THE DILATATION AND OCCLUSION OF ARTERIES.—These
lesions in a manner cognate.—Statistics of aneurism in the cavalry and
infantry, and in different climates.—Varieties of, and their localities.—Cases
illustrative, with comments.—The constitution most prone to suffer from the
disease.—Remarks on its pathology and symptoms, and the dependency of the
latter on the site of the lesion.—Example of spontaneous cure.................... 372

CHAPTER XIII.

ON DEATHS FROM ALCOHOLIC INTOXICATION.—The subject still open for inquiry.
—Evils of intemperance.—Statistics of delirium tremens.—Suggestions for
checking drunkenness in the army.—Fatal cases of alcoholic poisoning.—
Remarks on the action of alcohol, and on its morbid effects.—Pneumonia one
of its most common sequences.—The lungs the chief emunctory of alcohol ... 396

CHAPTER XIV.

CASES OF SUICIDE, AND OF DEATHS FROM ACCIDENTS.—Motives for introducing
such cases.—Suggestion for recording them in the public service.—Detailed
cases; one of which remarkable for extensive solution of the stomach and
diaphragm.—Remarks on the tendency to suicide from *ennui* in the instance
of the soldier.—Expression of hope of the opprobrium ceasing with increased
attention to the comforts and health of the men.—Suggestive remarks as to
how the *post mortem* appearances of organs suddenly arrested in action by
death may serve as checks in necroscopic research, and be of service in
medical jurisprudence 406

CHAPTER XV.

PAGE

ON URINARY AND BILIARY CALCULI, AND ON ENTOZOA.—Unfrequency of urinary and biliary calculi in the army.—Conjectures why so.—Cases in which found noticed.—Instances given of calculi in brute-animals.—A peculiar kind of biliary calculus (indigo and copper detected in it) described.— Remarks on entozoa.—Their unfrequency in the army —Frequency of them, owing to peculiar circumstances, amongst the inhabitants of Malta 417

CHAPTER XVI.

ON PECULIARITIES OF ORGANS AS TO FORM AND POSITION.—Notice restricted to such peculiarities as were met with in ordinary *post mortem* examinations. —Examples described: 1st, of the alimentary canal; 2ndly, of the liver, spleen, and pancreas; 3rdly, of the kidneys and generative organs; 4thly, of the lungs and some adjoining parts; 5thly, of the mammæ; 6thly, of the heart and blood-vessels; 7thly, of the brain and nerves.—Questions as to the correlation of the abnormal; of their influence in relation to health, and their approximation to the normal in other animals 424

INTRODUCTION.

Preliminary remarks—Observations on the average weight of organs—On the discoloration of parts—On the softening of textures, and on putrefaction—On the temperature of the body after death—On air in the vessels, and effused fluids—On the post-mortem condition of the blood, and rigor mortis—On the situation of organs.

THE importance of distinguishing between the normal and abnormal, between the sound or healthy and the unsound or diseased, can hardly be too much insisted on in pathological enquiry. Under this impression the following preliminary remarks are offered, and with a double object: one, that of showing the cautions which have more or less been kept in view in conducting the post-mortem examinations—an account of which will form a considerable part of the following work; the other, with the hope of affording some aid to the young medical officer in his necroscopical labours.

The subject in its greatest generality, it must be confessed, is a difficult one. Normal forms pass by almost insensible gradations into the abnormal, sound structure as insensibly into the unsound: so too as regards functions; in these likewise there is that insensible gradation from the most perfect health to a high state of disease. And what specially adds to the difficulty is the complexity of organization and its subtilty as regards structure, and, as regards function, the more or less dependence of one organ or part on another, giving rise to that exquisite sympathy which is characteristic of animal life.

1. *Of the Weight of Organs.*—The knowledge of this in their healthy state must of course be ascertained before we can be prepared to draw any conclusion from what it may be found to be in cases of fatal disease. Average weight is that which it is the desideratum to have determined, as we cannot doubt that, in individuals in health the most perfect, it—the weight of a part—will vary within certain limits, according to age, size, condition of body, and even idiosyncrasy. Further, I think it may reason-

ably be inferred that, even within the range of health, some organs will be found more subject to variation than others, from the nature of their function and position, and *à fortiori*, still more so from the effects of disease.

Of all of them, it may be presumed that the brain, both from its nature and the manner in which it is confined in an unyielding case, will be least subject to fluctuating increase and decrease of volume or weight. In the adult man its weight has been estimated at 3 lbs. 2 oz. 3 drms.* The results of the trials I have made in nineteen instances accord very nearly with this, the average obtained having been 3 lbs. 2 oz. 2 drms. The individuals whose brains were weighed were soldiers, all of average height, or rather exceeding a little the average; men who had died of different diseases, chiefly phthisis, and who varied in age from 18 to 40 years. The heaviest brain of the whole number weighed 3 lbs. 7 oz. 4 drms. and the lightest 2 lbs. 11 oz.—both from men who had died of pulmonary consumption, the former 19 years of age, the latter 28.†

The lungs situated so differently, so subject to expansion and contraction and the influx of variable quantities of blood, might *à priori*, even irrespective of differences in the capacity of the chest, be expected to vary more in weight than the brain. The lighter they are, may they not be considered the healthier? From such trials as I have made, I am disposed to place the average weight of these organs at 2 lbs., or even under. The lungs of a Maltese boy ætat. 14 years, killed when in good health by an explosion of gunpowder, weighed 1 lb., that of each was 8 oz. They were in a state of collapse. Those of a private soldier ætat. 46, shot by a comrade through the head when in perfect health, weighed 1 lb. 11 oz. Those of a private ætat. 26, who when apparently in good health shot himself, weighed only 17½ oz.; the left lung 8½ oz., the right 9 oz. The wound was immediately fatal and was attended with much hæmorrhage. The lungs of another private who committed suicide in the same way, ætat. 30, also in apparently good health at the time, weighed 1¼ lb.: the

* Quain's Anat. by Sharpey and Ellis, ii. p. 434. According to another estimate, the average weight is less than the above, viz. 49½ oz. See Dunglison's Human Physiology," vol. i. p. 328.
† The lightest brain I ever weighed, was that of an old woman, in Malta, ætat. 98; it was 2 lbs. 4 oz. 48 grs. 44 oz. is stated to be the average weight of the female brain (op. cit.).

left, in which was some blood, ¾ lb.; the right, ½ lb. There was little hæmorrhage in this instance; and he lived an hour after the infliction of the wound. Those of a private ætat. 35, who had died of chronic dysentery, weighed 1 lb. 6 oz.; of another private who had died of the same disease, and whose lungs like those of the last seemed quite sound, the left weighed 10 oz., the right 9 oz.; of another, who died of ascites, the right lung weighed not quite half a pound; it was so collapsed, so small in volume in consequence, that it might have been covered almost by both hands. The left lung was heavier, but it was diseased; it contained three masses (the largest of which was about the size of a filbert) of curd-like scrofulous matter: even in the right, on careful examination, a few small clustered granular tubercles were detected. Of another, ætat. 28, who died labouring under a complication of disease —one of the lesions, effusion into the right pleura to the large amount of seven pints—the lung of that side weighed 8 oz.; of the opposite, 1 lb. 4 oz.: the volume of the former was equal to that of a pint of water, it displaced so much; of the latter to 23 oz. of water. The right lung contained a few granular tubercles; the left was similarly diseased, and to a greater extent. Of another, ætat. 29, who died labouring under chronic dysentery, the left lung weighed 11 oz., the right 14 oz.; both were healthy, with the exception of some superficial bronchial branches which were much dilated and, with the exception of some vesicles (probably air cells enlarged), filled with air, immediately under the pleura pulmonalis.* When the weight of the lungs has exceeded 2 lbs., I have always found them more or less diseased: thus in the instance of a private who died of inflammation of the pleura, with copious sero-purulent effusion, though each lung weighed only 1 lb. 1 oz., the right contained numerous tubercles and a few small vomicæ; the left, though fewer tubercles, pretty much effused serum.

The liver, though less subject to sudden variations of volume than the lungs, yet probably is more variable in weight, at least without manifestations of disease: this partly owing to its more mixed composition chemically considered, partly to the

---

* Before opening into the chest a ligature had been applied to the trachea: one vesicle contained ·03 cubic inches of air, which was found to consist of 2·5 oxygen, 5·5 carbonic acid, 92·0 azote. Air collected from one of the large bronchial tubes was composed of 4·0 oxygen, 3·1 carbonic acid, 92·9 azote.

elaborate and large venous system belonging to it, and partly to
the little sensibility that its substance possesses. Its average
weight deducible from the trials of which I have a note is about
3 lbs. 6 oz. * These trials were sixty in number. The ages of
the defunct varied from 18 to 46 years. The fatal diseases were
very various, many of them pulmonary consumption. The
heaviest of the whole number was 6 lbs., the lightest 2 lbs. 4 oz.;
the former from a private ætat. 32, the latter from one ætat. 35;
the former had died of peritonitis, the latter of paralysis from a
softening of the brain : in neither did the organ appear to be
diseased. As an indication of disease, I am inclined to attach less
importance to weight in the instance of this viscus than in that of
any other, excepting perhaps the spleen; and for the reasons
already assigned when adverting to the circumstances likely to
conduce to variations in its weight even in health, or to speak
more correctly, without recognised disease. Even corpulency,
or the opposite state, may have a marked effect. Proof of this is
afforded in the two following columns : No. 1, of the weight of the
liver in seven instances, of men who had died of aneurism;
No. 2 of seven others, who had died of wasting diseases, chiefly
phthisis, and were much emaciated.

No. 1.	No. 2.
6 lbs.	2 lbs. 8 oz.
4 lbs.	2 lbs. 12 oz.
5 lbs.	4 lbs.
3 lbs. 3 oz.	3 lbs. 8 oz.
4 lbs. 12 oz.	3 lbs. 12 oz.
4 lbs. 8 oz.	5 lbs.
4 lbs.	3 lbs. 8 oz.

Of the spleen, the average weight, judging from the trials I
have recorded, these fifteen in number, is 7 oz.† The heaviest
of these was 12 oz.; the lightest, 2 oz. 4 drs.; the former from
a private who had died of otitis, with suppuration extending to

* Haller (Element. Physiol. vi. 455) gives the weight of the liver, in health, as
about 45 oz. : this the average of ten; but of the ten specified, three weighed only
1 lb. Now, omitting these three, the average of the seven would be nearly the same
as that I have assigned, viz., 3 lbs. 7 oz. Dr. John Reid found the average of sixty
male livers to be 52 oz. 12½ drms.—Dunglison's Physiol. ii. 302.

† Haller (Element. Physiol. vi. 394) states " Solent lienies pondus in sano homine
inter sex uncias et semisse et decem, duodecem et quatuurdecem, demum sedecem
uncias definire."

the brain; the latter from one ætat. 33, who had died of paralysis. The liver of this man weighed 4 lbs. 5 oz.; of that 3 lbs. 8 oz. Most of the fatal cases from which the organ weighed was obtained, were of pulmonary consumption; and, in all, with the exception of a variable degree of softness, it had a tolerably healthy appearance.

Of all the glandular organs, so far as my experience allows me to form an opinion, the kidneys are least liable to variation in weight. Their accordance, too, comparing the one with the other in the same body, is remarkable, implying a degree of harmony we do not witness in the lungs, especially under the influence of morbid action. The average weight of the right kidney, deduced from sixteen trials, is 5 oz. 3 drms.; of the left, from fifteen trials, 5 oz. 3 drms. The heaviest of the whole number, 7 oz. 5 drms.; the lightest, 3 oz. 5½ drms. The greatest difference between the left and right kidney was 1 oz. 3 drms.; only in three instances was the weight of each in the same individual exactly the same. The bodies affording the specimens tried, had mostly died of pulmonary consumption; the organs in question were all of them apparently free from disease.*

The only other organ, the average weight of which I shall attempt to give, is that of the heart. It is obtained from seven examples only. The subjects of four of these had died of pulmonary consumption, three of other diseases. In all the organs appeared to be sound. In each instance it had been emptied of blood before being put into the balance. The average weight was 8 oz. 4 drms.; the heaviest, was 9 oz. 4 drms.; the lightest, 8 oz. The ages varied from 21 to 40 years.† Considering the function this organ performs, it may be presumed, as in the instance of the lungs, that the lighter it is commonly, the healthier it is, especially as the tendency of muscle from exercise is to increase not diminish in volume; and under morbific influences to suffer from hypertrophy rather than from atrophy.

2. *Of the Discoloration of Parts.*—Color is one of the qualities that first attracts the eye; and is, perhaps, that which

---

* From 65 trials, Dr. John Reid has deduced the average weight of the left male kidney to be 5 oz. 11½ drms.; of the right, 5 oz. 7 drms. Op. cit. ii. 326.

† M. Bouillaud estimates the average of the male heart 8 oz. 3 drms., the result of 13 trials. Op. cit. ii. 82.

is least to be depended on. I make the remark reflecting on the
difficulty often experienced in distinguishing between the redness
the result of inflammation, and the redness the result of staining
or dyeing effected on the white tissues of the body by the coloring matter of the blood with which they may happen to come
in contact. The similarity of appearance is sometimes so deceptive, that, judging from mere sight, the most experienced
may, I believe, be led astray. The staining in question is chiefly
witnessed in warm weather, and when the *post mortem* examination has been delayed, and putrefaction has in some degree
commenced. It is well exemplified by immersing white tissues,
such as the blood-vessels, in cruor which has been kept some
time, and which, on the addition of hydrate of lime or potash,
emits ammonia. The higher the temperature of the air at the
time of making the experiment, the more rapidly will the dyeing
effect be produced : so, in the same manner in the cadaver, the
warmer the weather, so much sooner may the discoloration be
expected ; and, as excess of blood in the body favors acceleration of putrefaction, the greater that abundance, the readier
also will the staining appear. Here, it may be remarked, that
owing to the many circumstances which either promote or retard
the effect, it is necessarily uncertain, indeed so uncertain, that
no exact rule as to time or temperature can be fixed for its
occurrence, there being an unknown quality in the problem, that
is, the degree of proclivity in the dead body to change,* that

---

* I find it noted in a case of phthisis which occurred in Malta in August, when
the temperature of the room in which the body was kept was between 82° and 83°,
that no appearance of staining was seen in the vessels, where the blood was in contact
with them, although 22 hours had elapsed between the time of death and the
autopsy : the cadaver was greatly emaciated. This may be considered an extreme
instance of exemption, and it is given as such, in support of the remark in the text.
I may mention another extreme case of the contrary kind, in which the vessels
containing blood were stained of a "bright red," though only 16½ hours had intervened between the death and the examination of the body. The case was also one
of phthisis, that of a soldier ætat. 26, at home, the time April, the temperature of
the room 56.° In this instance, the blood, the cruor which did not coagulate, mixed
with quick lime gave off a strong smell of ammonia. Further, it may be remarked that
the staining was confined to the deep seated vessels of the trunk; the temperature
under the liver was 70° : there was no trace of it in the vessels of the colder extremities : in the aorta, in which there was no blood, the inner coat was colorless. I
shall give a third case, that also an extreme one. It occurred in Malta, the death also
was from phthisis of a chronic kind, and the body was greatly emaciated. The
examination was made 39 hours after death ; the temperature of the air at the time
(the middle of August) was between 80° and 86°; the wind, the south-east, the
moist sirocco. The cadaver emitted an offensive smell and was livid; the abdomen
was distended and tympanitic; on opening into its cavity, the intestines were found

varying according to the nature of the fatal disease, and the condition of the individual, so as to baffle all precise calculation : but yet, with due consideration of what aids and what retards putrefaction, allowing of inference at least approaching the truth. It might, perhaps, be supposed that the difference between a stained part and an inflamed part, would be distinguishable by subjecting them to the process of washing ; but on trial I have been disappointed ; the color of the one not being more readily removed by water than the other. In cases of extreme doubt, as when the *post mortem* examination has been unduly deferred, the only conclusive evidence, I am disposed to think, is the presence of effused lymph.

Other cases of discoloration may be deserving of some attention. I shall mention two or three ; there may be more than I can now call to mind, or am acquainted with. In the brain, a yellow ochery stain is sometimes met with, sometimes diffused, sometimes limited to a small circumscribed spot. Wherever it occurs, I believe it to be owing to blood that has been effused and afterwards absorbed with the exception of the iron belonging to the coloring matter of the corpuscles, which has remained in the state of peroxide. In the few instances I have tested this stain, I have found this oxide present; and mostly, in the appearance of the texture of the part, there has been corroborative proof of blood having been at a former period extravasated. After dysentery, after the ulcers have healed, and death has resulted from some other disease, or from gradual exhaustion the effect of the former, dark bluish stains, or stains approaching to this color, may be seen marking the cicatrices in the large intestines. I have watched their formation, if I may so speak, in the progress of the ulcers to healing in individuals who have died in different stages of the disease ; and hence the identification of the stain and the cicatrix, which latter otherwise might not be recognized. The color I am disposed to refer also to residual iron, but in the state of the black oxide or sulphuret

very much distended with gas; and both in this cavity and in the chest, the blood in the vessels was frothy, disengaging air ; and the same was observed in the substance of the liver and of the other viscera, and in the cellular tissue, and even in the thoracic duct. All the membranes and vessels were more or less colored by the coloring matter of the blood. Notwithstanding this rapid and advanced putrefaction, the temperature of the body, it is worthy of remark, differed very little from that of the air; there was no indication of the production of heat ; a thermometer under the lobulus Spigelii was 83° ; in the air of the room 82·5.°

so rendered in consequence of the action of the gases in the intestines. This, however, is only conjecture, for I have never examined the parts chemically. We have a striking example of the permanency of a metallic stain in the discoloration of the skin, which occasionally appears from the long-continued use of the nitrate of silver taken internally. In confirmation of the durability of such a stain, I may mention that so long as fifty years ago, when engaged in a chemical experiment, I received a wound from the explosion of some fulminating silver: after its healing a grey mark was left, made by a minute portion of the metal having been injected into the cutis. That mark still remains, without the least fading of its intensity.

Further, I need hardly observe, that in judging of the color of parts after death, the medicines used, the treatment previously employed, should not be lost sight of. The application of a blister, as is well known, is apt to produce strangury, —an affection owing to the action of the cantharides on the bladder, producing a state of phlogosis, often of ecchymosis of the mucous membrane of that organ, and also not unfrequently of the ureters and pelvis of the kidneys.* Now, without making allowance for this effect, the appearance would be referred to the disease existing at the time, so leading to an erroneous conclusion of a morbid complication. In like manner, if an irritant medicine be given, such as colchicum, its administration ought to be taken into account in estimating the redness of the stomach, if inflammation of that organ be a question. Even a mechanical cause may have an influence on the coloration of a part, such as the pressure of air or of fluid distending the cavities of the thorax and abdomen. For instance, if the latter be much inflated by gas disengaged in the stomach and intestines, and, in the *post mortem* examination, the brain be the first part laid open, the tendency of the inflation by pressing on the great vessels, in case they contained any liquid blood, will be to drive it towards the part where there is least resistance, viz., the brain, the confining skull-cap being removed, and so occasion the injection of the cerebral vessels, which, without reference to the cause producing it, might be pronounced to be morbid.

* The strangury from this cause, I may remark, I have always found relieved by introducing a catheter into the bladder; how it acts, I am ignorant; rarely more than a few drops of urine are obtained.

Relative to the effect of gravitation on the blood in producing discoloration, sugillation of the integuments of the decumbent parts, and engorgement of certain deep seated parts, especially the lungs, it is nowise necessary to insist, it being so well known and thoroughly understood. And much the same remark applies to the staining effect of bile, exuding from the gall-bladder after death, it being so very obvious. However, being so conspicuous and unquestionable, it affords a good illustration of the pervious quality of the tissues, after the extinction of life, and how it proceeds in an increasing degree with the length of interval between death and the observation, and, under the influence of the other circumstances before adverted to favoring putrefaction.

3. *Of the Softening of Parts.*—By this expression, I wish to imply a diminution of cohesive power, so that a part is more easily torn, or more easily broken under the pressure of the nail or fingers, in contradistinction to that softness which may belong to the same in health,—a softness distinguished by toughness, or power of resistance. The morbid condition in question is difficult of appreciation, is one specially requiring the *tactus eruditus*, that tact gained by experience, sharpened by science. The pathologist is oftenest called on to exercise it on mucous membranes and on the glandular organs; of the former, most of all on the stomach; of the latter most frequently on the brain,* the spleen, and the liver. The stomach, perhaps of all organs, offers the greatest difficulty, in consequence of the peculiarity belonging to it, its liability to be softened and even dissolved by its own gastric juice. Instances of this kind, as is well-known, were first described by John Hunter. Amongst my collection of cases, I find two remarkable ones, which will hereafter be given, in both of which, in the *post mortem* examination, not only was a portion of the stomach, its great arch, dissolved, but also the diaphragm adjoining, and yet the residue, even the nearest portion, had not in either instance become unusually

---

* The circumstance of the brain being incased, and more than any other organ protected from the influence of external air after death, should be kept in mind. This remark is made reflecting that it is sometimes found firm after putrefaction has commenced in other parts, and they have become softened thereby. In fifteen cases of men who died in Malta and Corfu (6 in the warmer, 9 in the colder months) of pneumonia, peritonitis, and aneurism,—cases in which there was no reason to believe that the brain was affected, this organ was found of its normal consistence after an average interval of 24 hours between the death and the examination.

soft. The softening from the action of the gastric juice, or to speak more correctly, in connexion with the presence of that juice in the stomach at the time of death, seems to be most uncertain, and this even in instances of death from accidents. In many cases of such deaths, though the persons previously were in vigorous health, I have not been able to detect any traces of it. As regards the softening of organs generally, considered as a *post mortem* change, and nowise to be taken into account as the effect of fore-existing disease,—length of time reckoning from the death, and the temperature of the air at the time, may be held to be the two circumstances most deserving of attention; to which may be added, the condition of the body as regards its tendency to putrefaction,—this hardly of less importance for the purpose of arriving at a just conclusion. These circumstances scarcely require comment. It is well-known to every one, how rapidly meat becomes tender, and how very short a time it will keep during the warm weather of summer, and how the contrary is noticeable in winter. Within the tropics, at a temperature of 80° and higher, so great is the proclivity to putrefy, that meat cannot be salted with a chance of its preservation, unless immersed in brine as quickly as possible after the slaughtering of the animal; indeed the pieces should be immersed whilst still warm. This aptness to putrescence necessitates in hot climates the speedy funeral of the deceased, a service commonly performed on the day of the fatal event, or at the farthest not beyond the following. The same reason is assignable for the examination of the body very soon after death, many instances of which will be found specified in the following pages. In addition to the preceding circumstances, as regards the stomach and the parts immediately adjoining it, I am disposed to think another should be taken into account, viz., the contents of the organ. In one instance in which the putrefaction had commenced and much gas was disengaged, the stomach, which contained a good deal of fermenting chyme, was not at all softened, nor was the spleen adjoining. Might not the carbonic acid disengaged have preserved the stomach? The case was one of death from an accident; the examination was made 23 hours after death. Blood abounded in the body; the temperature of the air of the room was 74°. In this instance, air-bubbles were found even in the anterior chamber of the eye,—a very unusual occurrence, even in very advanced putrefaction. Even the direction of the wind and the state of the atmosphere as to moisture and electricity are important in relation to the change in question. It is well known how rapidly milk sours during a thunder-storm, and how difficult it is to keep meat in damp muggy weather. During the war of freedom in Greece, the little and flourishing island of Ipsara was invaded by an overwhelming force of Turks; after a hard fight, most of the inhabitants were slaughtered, and the island was made a desert. Visiting it three years later, on one side, that exposed to the moist and warm sirocco, bleached bones only met the eye: this was at the tower and castle. On the other side, exposed to the cool and dry north-east, the Etesian wind, the fallen were lying where they fell, and in the attitudes in which they expired; their clothes were still on them, and so little were they changed that our guide, the only solitary inhabitant, was able to designate each man by name: this was at a battery called Fitellio, where between three and four hundred men were slain, resisting to the last.

4. *Of the Temperature of the Body after Death.*—This, like the coloring of parts, may sometimes become a question needing consideration. The observer may be in doubt, if the temperature of the cadaver be higher than that of the atmosphere, whether it be owing to retained heat from slow cooling, or to heat generated after death. The data, I presume, for the solution of the doubt are the temperature of the body at the instant of expiring, the interval between the death and the observation, and the temperature of the surrounding air during the interval; and, further, if putrefaction have taken place, the degree of heat that may be referred to that process: one or more of these particulars are not likely to be available unless special attention may have been given to the matter as a subject for inquiry. From such trials as I have made, I am induced to conclude that no heat is generated in the body after death, till putrefaction sets in, and that the degree of heat so produced is so small as hardly to be appreciable; and, consequently, any unduly high temperature, or any supposed to be such, is owing to the temperature existing at the moment of death.* If the question be what has the

* See my Research. Anat. and Physiol. i. 228, where the subject is discussed. The conclusion arrived at, as stated in the text, does not accord with that of Dr.

interval been between the time of the decease and the trial of the
temperature of the body—sometimes a matter of legal importance,—I apprehend the conclusion can only be an approximate
one, and to arrive at that, much the same data are required as
those just mentioned.

  5. *Of Effused Fluids.*—In examining the body, it may sometimes be a question, whether the fluid in a part, in a closed
cavity, was effused during life, or was a *post mortem* effect, the
result of exudation from an adjoining collection. From such
observations and experiments as I have made, the conclusion
arrived at is, that so long as the tissues of the body are free
from putrefaction, exudation does not take place in an appreciable
degree,—I speak of quantity : and that when the change alluded
to is in progress and advanced, the weakened power of retension
or that of impermeability differs so little, as possessed by the
several textures, as to warrant the same conclusion regarding the
result. I may refer for the data on which this view is founded
to a former work.* To that work also I would beg to refer for
the conclusion, that the degree of strength of adhesions formed
of coagulable lymph morbidly connecting serous surfaces is
hardly a just criterion of their age, as is sometimes asserted,—
except, indeed, the matter of them is very soft, hardly offering
any resistance when touched.†

  6. *Of the Presence of Air in the Vessels.*—That air is sometimes
found in the vessels on a *post mortem* examination is certain ;
but there is commonly much uncertainty as to its source, whether
it may have had entrance after the use of the scalpel or before ;
and, if before, whether before or after death. I believe, it may
be stated as a fact, the result of the most careful inquiries, that
the blood vessels in health contain no free air, or any free elastic

Bennet Dowler, of New Orleans, who from his observations on bodies dead of yellow
fever, infers that the temperature of the cadaver may rise many degrees after respiration and the heart's action have ceased. These observations are so contrary to the
experience of others, and are so difficult to reconcile with any well-established facts,
that I hardly know how to receive them, except in the way of doubt. I may briefly
mention, that in no instance of death from yellow fever have I ever witnessed any
increase of temperature in the cadaver; and the experience of my friend, the late
Dr. Blair, of British Guiana, who studied the disease very carefully in two endemic
invasions, of which he has published an account, is equally negative. The only
notice I have seen of Dr. Dowler's observations, is that in Professor Dunglison's
Human Physiology (ii. 718), who refers to the "Western Journal of Medicine and
Surgery" for June and October, 1844.
  * Res. Anat. and Physiol. vol. ii. 242.
  † Opus cit. ii. 237.

vapor, such as has been imagined by some authors; and, also as
a fact, that in a great majority of cases, when due care has been
taken to prevent the admission of air *ab externo*, none will be
found in the arteries or veins after death. For evidence in proof
of this, I may refer to the work already quoted.* If air, however, should be found, then its source becomes a question, and if
putrefaction have nowise advanced, the inference seems unavoidable that it is not a *post mortem* occurrence, and that its presence
may be viewed as an effect of diseased action, and may have
been concerned in the production of the fatal event,—a conclusion that will be confirmed should the air, on analysis, be found
to differ from atmospheric air and that which results from putrefaction. The same remarks are for the most part applicable to
air found after death in any of the serous cavities.

7. *Of the Condition of the Blood after Death.*—This is a
subject which I am disposed to think has not had that attention
paid to it which its importance deserves. In the following
pages, many observations will be found respecting it; all, however, more imperfect than I could wish. Were it duly investigated, results probably would be obtained interesting both to
physiology and pathology, conducing it may be, in the one instance, if not to the forming of a correct theory of the coagulation of the fluid, at least to the checking of erroneous views of
that phenomenon; and, in the other instance, it may be to the
explanation and the better understanding of certain diseases and
the causes of death. At present, it seems to be a question
whether blood circulating in the system in its healthiest state
contains ammonia. It has been maintained, and that in a very
laboured manner, and with much ingenuity, not only that the
alkali is essential to its healthy composition, to the solution of
its fibrine, but likewise that its escape is the cause of the coagulation of the blood.† My researches do not accord with this
view, but are contrary to it.‡ Further, they tend to prove that
though ammonia does not exist in the blood in an appreciable
quantity during healthy life, it begins to be formed with the
extinction of life, as a *post mortem* change, and as such is one of

* Res. Anat. and Physiol. vol. ii. 183.
† The cause of the Coagulation of the Blood, etc. By W. B. Richardson, M.D.,
8vo., London, 1858.
‡ Some Observations on the Coagulation of the Blood. Trans. Roy. Soc. of Ed.
vol. xxii. part i.

the first signs of incipient putrefaction;* and, also, that in some diseases with a putrid tendency, the production of the same alkali in the blood may precede death.

8. *Of the Condition of the Brain.*—When we consider the part performed by this great nervous centre in health, it is difficult to avoid the conclusion that its condition is more or less concerned, either directly or indirectly, in most diseases : and, if so, the slightest appreciable lesions should be recorded in *post mortem* descriptions. Such lesions, it is easy to conceive, though not indicated by any well marked symptoms, yet may have had an important influence on the course of the malady,—to compare things hardly comparable, like the thinning by wear, or thickening by incrustation, of a boiler, in the production of its steam. I advert to this, having in many of the dissection reports which follow, noticed morbid appearances of the encephalon often so slight, that to some persons they may seem altogether undeserving of attention.

9. *Of the Situation of Parts.*—That this is a matter requiring special attention, when abnormal, has only to be announced to be admitted. Perfect health, it may be laid down, can hardly be expected unless every part of the complex frame is in its right place; and may it not with equal probability be stated that any deviation from the proper position of an organ must according to its *error loci* have more or less a morbid influence? The displacement of the intestines may be mentioned as one of the most common. Who can say (the subject I apprehend not having been sufficiently studied) what are its various effects; first, as connected with the action of the bowels,—disposing them to irregularity; and next, that irregularity as a disposing cause of more serious diseases, mental and bodily?

10. *Of the post mortem Rigidity of the Muscles, "rigor mortis."*—This obscure phenomenon I shall here barely glance at. No doubt it is deserving of attention in every case, and it

* One example I will give here:—An hour after death from phthisis, the carotid and jugular vein were laid bare, and no air was found in either. A little blood was obtained from the vein; it speedily coagulated: mixed with kali purum, there was no indication of the presence of ammonia,—no fume on the approach of muriatic acid reduced by dilution to the non-fuming point. 22 hours after, at the autopsy, tried in the same way, a small portion from the right ventricle of the heart, the result was the same. Another portion from the same ventricle, exposed to the air about an hour, gave a different result; fume was produced on the approach of the muriatic acid. This blood, which was liquid 22 hours after death, coagulated when taken out of the body and confined in a bottle closed by a glass stopper.

might be well to record it when specially observed ; that is, carefully and minutely in the way of research, with attention to collateral circumstances of temperature, time, state of the blood, etc. In looking over my collection of cases, I find it mentioned in a large number of instances ; in some as occurring in the lower extremities when absent in the upper ; in some, the majority, accompanied by the presence of coagulated blood in the heart; in others, a comparative few, with liquid blood in that organ ; in others, in which at the time of examination it was altogether absent, the limbs flexible. In the subjoined note, the results are numerically given.* These, in the following cases, I have omitted mention of individually, not having made the subject a special study. I am induced to give them as below, thinking that they may be suggestive to inquirers, who may wish to have the opportunity to engage in it after what has been already done for its elucidation by the very interesting researches of Dr. Brown Séquard.†

In introducing the foregoing remarks, I have adverted to the connexion of physiology and pathology. Life may be regarded as a perpetual struggle, and in one point of view, almost as a perpetual miracle,—particles of dead matter at the same moment of time starting into life, derived from sustaining food taken in ; whilst others, too, at the same time, particles endowed with life,

* 1. In 62 cases, the limbs were found rigid in both extremities from four hours after death, the shortest time observed, to three days the longest,—the average of the whole being 19 hours.
2. In 15 cases, the upper extremities were found flexible, the lower rigid, from 12 hours after death the shortest time, to 37 hours the longest,—the average being 24 hours.
3. In 11 cases, both the upper and lower extremities were found flexible, from 4 hours the shortest, to 42 hours the longest,—the average being the same as the last, viz., 24 hours.
In cases No. 1, the blood was found coagulated in the heart in 16 instances; in 1 liquid (this death from drowning) ; in the remainder, the quality of the blood in the heart was not specified.
In cases No. 2, the blood in the heart was more or less coagulated ; in 2, liquid; in 3 not specified.
In cases No. 3, in 6 the blood was coagulated in the heart; in 2 it was partially coagulated, partially liquid ; in 3, not specified.
The diseases of which the subjects of the observations had died, were principally pulmonary consumption, dysentery, aneurism, apoplexy, and small-pox.
In one instance, of death from lightning, the limbs were found rigid after putrefaction had taken place. It will be found described in the chapter on suicides and deaths from accidents.
In several instances one extremity has been found flexible and the other rigid ; and not unfrequently the inferior extremities have exhibited the rigor mortis, before the superior.
† See Proceedings of Roy. Soc. vol. xi. 204.

are dropping into decay and death to be thrown off from the system as excrementitious. As the one predominates, so life is vigorous, and the vital powers are energetic ; as the other has the mastery, so the chemical and ordinary physical agencies take the lead, conducing ultimately to death and dissolution. This intermixture of actions, of vital and non-vital, always in progress, constitute, I cannot but think, a great part of the problem of life itself, and, in subordination, much of the problem of health and disease.

ON SOME OF THE MORE IMPORTANT

DISEASES OF THE ARMY.

CHAPTER I.

ON FEVERS.

Intermittent, Remittent and continued Fever; remarks on.—Their Statistics.—Cases Illustrative of the several kinds.—Their etiology in connection with climate and temperature.—Observations on Malaria.—Precautions against.—Remarks on the Pathology of Fevers and their treatment.

IT is not necessary to comment on the importance of these diseases in military life, that and their fatality being so well known. It may suffice to state that of the total mortality of the British army serving in various climates, so large a proportion as 45 per cent. has been owing to this class of diseases alone ; and that at the majority of foreign stations it has exceeded this, even in the high ratio of 57 in the Ionian Islands, and the still higher of 83 and 84 per cent. in Jamaica and Sierra Leone.*

In the army medical returns, until recently altered, the nomenclature adopted to denote the several kinds of fever was the following :—Intermittent, remittent, common continued fever, synochus, typhus, and typhus icterodes. The manner in which they were employed was far from uniform, partly from the difficulty of distinguishing the kinds of fever, if we consider them distinct species, and partly from the circumstance that medical officers educated in no common school, may have taken different views of their nature, and have designated them accordingly.

The time seems to be past that diseases, and especially fevers, are to be received as distinct entities, as pure species, according to the old natural history principle. It seems more philosophical to consider them as varieties, morbid phenomena occurring in groups more or less well marked, but rarely so strongly as to be unmistakable, and often so graduating one into the other as to

* These results are deduced from the army medical statistics comprised in the reports published between 1838 and 1840.

2

render it doubtful to which group the disease should be assigned when a name is to be given to it.

The etiology of fever is an obscure part of the subject, and is open in a remarkable manner to doubt. We seem to know little more than that their causes, whatever they may be, vary in character in different countries, following climatic conditions, in themselves seldom well defined ; fevers of the intermittent kind, which have been called marsh-fevers, often occurring where the country is dry ; malignant typhus, which has been called jail-fever, though commonly connected with crowding and filth, not being invariably so ; whilst yellow fever in its unmistakable intensity, has been witnessed only in certain regions of the globe ; but why in them and not in others of an apparently like climate, is a problem as yet unsolved.

If the etiology is obscure, the pathology of these diseases is not less so ; and this after their study from the time of Hippocrates downwards by men who in the cultivation of the exact sciences have contributed so largely to their advancement.

Using the terms as we find them, the following table drawn up from the army statistical reports, before referred to, is well adapted to show the habitats, if the expression may be employed, of the different forms of fever, and also their severity, taking the mortality as a criterion. It has this advantage to recommend it, viz., that the subjects were men, nearly all, if not of kindred race, of nearly allied races, similarly clad, having nearly the same ration of food, and as soldiers similarly occupied ; occasionally, however, as when employed in an active campaign, undergoing great bodily exertion, and exposed to privations of the most telling kind, singularly contrasted with their ordinary, monotonous kind of life. I have said nearly all of the same race ; the exceptions, though few and numerically small in amount, were well marked, such as African negroes, comprising chiefly the West India Regiments, Malays, forming the 1st Ceylon Rifle Regiment, and Hottentots and Singalese—the latter of little account, numerically —all of them serving associated with white troops, all of them in their native climate or in climates similar thereto, and thus well adapted by comparison to show the influence of race in resisting or modifying disease.

For the sake of greater distinctness I shall first give the proportionate prevalency of the several fevers in each country separately, stating the admissions into hospital, and deaths—these calculated for 10,000 of aggregate strength, during the term in years specified for each station. I may further premise that the troops were all infantry with the exception of the Dragoon Guards and Dragoons selected as an example of the army at home for an unbroken period :—

1.—United Kingdom. From 1837 to 1847, both included.

	Admitted.	Died.
Febris intermittens	5·5	—
„ remittens	2·2	0·36
„ com. cont.	503·1	8·40
„ typhus	16·1	5·1
All other diseases	9,271·0	110·5

2.—Gibraltar. From 1837 to 1847 :—

Febris intermittens	39·5	—
„ remittens	15·3	0·9
„ com. cont.	737·6	12.3
„ typhus	16·9	6·3
All other diseases	8571·0	91·0

3.—Malta. From 1837 to 1847 :—

Febris intermittens	21·7	—
„ remittens	6·6	2·8
„ com. cont.	2025·0	14·6
All other diseases	9098·0	145·0

4.—Ionian Islands. From 1837 to 1847 :—

Febris intermittens, quot.	308·8	2·5
„ tertian.	134·6	0·0
„ quart.	5·7	0·0
„ remittens	262·9	20·2
„ com. cont.	752.9	34·7
All other diseases	8838·0	135·0

5.—Bermudas. From 1837 to 1847 :—

Febris intermittens	12·2	—
„ remittens	3·5	0·88
„ com. cont.	892·6	17·8
„ icterodes*	504·0	124.7
„ synochus*	245·0	23.1
All other diseases	10218·0	138·0

6.—West Indies. Windward and Leeward Islands command. From 1817 to 1836 :—

Febris intermittens	3082	18·6
„ remittens	2520	226·0
„ com. cont.	1942	83·8
„ icterodes	89	39·0

* Year 1843.

	Admitted.		Died.
Febris synochus and typhus ...	6.4	... ...	1·2
All other diseases	...11859	... ...	428·0

Black Troops.

	Admitted.		Died.
Febris intermittens	243	... ...	3.4
„ remittens	346	... ..	18·0
„ com. cont.	1082	... ...	22.0
„ icterodes	6.3	... ...	1.7
All other diseases	6522	.. ...	344.0

7.—Jamaica. From 1817 to 1836 :—

Febris intermittens	1181	... ...	7·0
„ remittens	7445	... ...	991·0
„ com. cont.	382	... ...	12·4
„ icterodes	3.8	... ...	2·9
„ synochus	5·5	... ...	0.19
All other diseases	...90023.0	... ...	194.0

Black Troops.

Febris intermittens	211	... ...	3·5
„ remittens	848	... ...	77·0
„ com. cont.	48	... ...	1·8
All other diseases	2260	... ...	218·0

8.—Ceylon. From 1817 to 1836 :—

Febris intermittens	1218	... ...	24·2
„ remittens	1080	... ..	202·0
„ com cont.	2554	... ...	19·0
All other diseases	9599	... ...	452·0

Malay Rifles.

Febris intermittens ...	...10171	... ...	101·0
„ remittens	792	... ...	54·0
„ com. cont.	356	... ...	15
All other diseases	4294	... ...	182·0

Pioneer Corps—chiefly Singalese. From 1821 to 1833.

Febris intermittens ...	·3876	... ...	42
„ remittens	650	... ...	55
„ com. cont.	1906	... ...	12
All other diseases	9061	... ...	288

9.—Mauritius. From 1818 to 1836 :—

Febris intermittens	4	... ...	0·3
„ remittens	1·8	... ...	0·3
„ com. cont.	1531·0	... ...	16·0
„ typhus and synochus ..	5·0	... ...	—
All other diseases	...10945·0	... ...	256·0

10.—Sierra Leone. From 1819 to 1836 :—

Febris intermittens	5143	... ...	59
„ remittens	8686	... ...	4009
„ com. cont.	192	... ...	13
All other diseases	...15620	... ...	727

Black Troops.

	Admitted.	Died.
Febris intermittens	142	1·3
„ remittens	186	9·3
„ com. cont.	192	13·1
All other diseases	7574	277·0

11.—Cape of Good Hope. From 1818 to 1836 :—

Febris intermittens	5·0	—
„ remittens	6·6	0·4
„ com. cont.	847·0	18·0
„ typhus and synochus	18·0	0·4
All other diseases	9030	118·0

12.—Canada. From 1837 to 1847 :—

Febris intermittens, quot...	89	0.44
„ „ tert.	183	0·63
„ remittens	17	1.3
„ com. cont.	716	15.2
„ icterodes	0.44	0 11
„ typhus	6·8	3·52

13.—Nova Scotia and New Brunswick. From 1837 to 1847 :—

Febris intermittens	159·3	1.1
„ com. cont.	405·1	6.3
„ typhus	10·4	3.3
All other diseases	8430·0	119·0

These statistics are not a little instructive. To comment on them fully would require a volume apart. They tolerably tell their own tale, showing how the amount of febrile disease, cæteris paribus, increases with temperature ; how certain forms of fever are more prevalent in one climate than another; and how, also, even where there is *apparent* similarity of climate, there are different forms of the disease ; also, under like circumstances how in the same climate, different races of men, the European, the African, the Malay, the Singalese, are liable to suffer variously. I refrain from further remarks at present; after giving a selection of cases I may have occasion to offer a few more.

1.—OF INTERMITTENT FEVERS.—These fevers in their simple, least complicated form are remarkable for the small mortality attending them ; indeed, it seems probable, that *per se* they would never prove fatal. The statistics of the disease are favorable to this conclusion ; thus, at those stations where there is least tendency to such complications, and least danger of the intermittent passing into the remittent, the fatal issue is small indeed, compared with what it is at other stations where the contrary tendency prevails. The following table, formed from the preceding, shows this in a striking manner; it also shows that though the colored races are not exempt from intermittent fever, they are subject to it in a less degree than the white; and what is remarkable, the nearer their approach to the white in hue the greater seems to be their liability to contract it and suffer from it.

	Admitted.		Died.
Nova Scotia and New Brunswick ...	159·3	..	1·1
Canada	272	...	1·07
Mauritius	4	...	0·3
Cape of Good Hope	5	...	—
Bermudas	12·2	...	—
Malta	21.7	...	—
Ionian Islands	449	...	2·5
Gibraltar	39·5	...	—
Great Britain	5·5	...	—
	967·9		4.97
Sierra Leone	5143	...	59·0
Ceylon	1218	...	24·2
West Indies	3082	...	18.6
Jamaica	1181	...	7·0
	10,624		108·8
Malays—Ceylon	10,171	...	101
Singalese ,, ...	3,876	...	42
Negroes—West Indies	240	...	3·4
,, Jamaica	211	...	3·4
,, Sierra Leone	142	...	1·3
	14,640		151·1

The same conclusion as to complication, is further confirmed by the very few fatal cases of which I have a record. These are the following :—

Case I.—J. Smith, ætat. 38 ; 51st Regiment ; admitted into hospital at Corfu, 7th Feb., 1828; died 14th February. "*Febris* intermittens tertiana."—This man when working on the roads had, it is stated, a fit of ague on the 5th February. On the 7th there was a recurrence of the attack, followed by loss of sense and motion ; the eyes were fixed, the pupils dilated ; mouth frothing ; pulse small and rapid ; breathing short and hurried ; skin warm, with profuse sweating ; slight convulsions ; an involuntary start in bed ; copious V.S., without apparent relief at the time ; has passed some detached joints of tape-worm ; about two hours after the blood-letting consciousness returned ; he experienced no pain of any part ; purgative medicine. On the 9th there were chills in the morning, followed by heats, with a throbbing pain shooting across the forehead ; the countenance was flushed, its expression wild ; he answered questions rationally ; pulse 100 full ; much thirst ; leeches to temples ; mercury in alterative doses, with fever mixture. 10th—Relieved by leeches ; feels better ; has voided a large tapeworm ; sulphate of quinine. 11th—A restless night ; morning chills followed by heat and pain and throbbing of temples; blister to temples; cold applications to head; mercury and fever mixture; an anodyne diaphoretic draught at night. 12th—A bad night; febrile symptoms not abated; mouth tender; mercury omitted; fever medicines continued; purgative repeated. 13th—A bad night; some delirium; chills in the morning; pulse 135, weak; floccitatio; blister to nape of neck; bark and wine. 14th—He died this morning.

Autopsy 30 hours after death. Body very little emaciated. The vessels of the brain rather large; not much fluid in the ventricles or at the base of the brain. A good deal of blood, and some large fibrinous concretions in the cavities of the heart and the great vessels. The lungs rather distended with air; redder, perhaps, and containing more blood than natural. The stomach, duodenum and small intestines generally distended with air; the two first very much so and also the cœcum and the ascending and transverse colon; the descending colon contracted. Parts of the small intestines more vascular than usual. No appearance of ulceration in either the large or small intestines. The spleen large and very soft, like a mass of stale crassamentum.

Was this a case of ague modified by undue cerebral action and becoming remittent?

The individual was of robust make, had a large head, a short neck, and was of intemperate habits.

The distended state from flatulency of stomach and intestines is a note-worthy circumstance.

Case II.—R Walsh, ætat. 21; 33rd Regiment; admitted into hospital at Corfu, May 27th, 1827; died June 24th. "Febris intermittens."—This man was admitted with symptoms of intermittent fever, for which since November he had been twice in hospital before this his last attack. The day after admission he complained of pain of chest and troublesome cough; bowels costive; V.S. 36 oz.; aperients. On the 29th May had a severe paroxysm of ague, with vomiting; purgatives and sulphate of quinine. 30th—Urticaria; is free from ague; quinine and calomel. June 1st—No return of ague; nausea and uneasiness of stomach; stools dark and fetid; the same medicine. On the 2nd he suddenly experienced severe pain in stomach, attended with cough and nausea; V.S. 50 oz.; relief; the blood was cupped and buffed. On the 14th it was reported that he had been improving until the 12th, when at noon the lower extremities became cold, the coldness spreading over the body, followed by pyrexia, ending in sweating towards evening. The mouth had become affected by mercury; the ptyalism had now ceased; the bowels were open; the stools dark; aperients with sulphate of quinine. On the 17th he complained of tormina, the pain increased by pressure; tenesmus; stools bloody; pulse 100 hard; omit the quinine; 36 leeches to abdomen; castor oil. 18th—Some relief; calomel 2 grains, with ½ grain of opium, thrice daily. Towards evening all the symptoms were aggravated; V.S. 32 oz.; an anodyne draught. 19th—Some relief; calomel gr. iij. thrice daily; a blister to abdomen. 21st—Much the same; the vomiting, which was distressing, is subsiding; castor oil; an anodyne at bed time. 22nd—The vomiting has returned; the other symptoms much the same. It is added, he daily became worse, expiring on the 24th.

Autopsy 18 hours after death. Body rather emaciated. The chest sounded well on percussion. Some fluid was found in the tissues of the pia mater and at the base of the brain, and in the spinal canal. The left lung was generally adhering. Its parenchyma was redder than natural and yet very little gorged with blood, nor anywise hepatized. The right lung was sound. The bronchia, especially in the left lung, were redder than natural. The bronchial and œsophagial glands were very much enlarged and very vascular. There was no appearance of inflammation of the stomach or of abrasion about the cardiac orifice to account for the vomiting and hiccough which in the advanced stage of the disease were distressing. The liver externally was of natural appearance; but its substance was very tender and easily broken. The gall-bladder was distended with bile. The spleen was rather larger than usual and firmer. The lower part of the ileum was unduly red, and its villous coat, chiefly in the situation of the glandulæ aggregatæ, was slightly ulcerated. The cœcum was nearly sound. The colon was inflamed and ulcerated throughout. The ulcers were generally small, little larger than the flat surface of a split pea; in most places they were red, in some grey—altogether they were not unlike the eruption of small-pox when declining. The intestines contained no scybala, only a small quantity of reddish fluid, of an offensive smell. The abdominal glands were enlarged, but in a less degree than the thoracic.

Was there phlogois in this case of the lung, as well as disease of the lower ileum and colon?

Was the vomiting owing to the state of the intestines, or to the loss of blood; and was not the blood-letting, if indicated at all, carried too far, and so might it not have conduced to the fatal termination?

Case III.—G. Davis, ætat. 26; 28th Regiment; admitted into hospital at Corfu, 19th May, 1826; died 23rd June. Feb. intermittens.—This man on admission had been ill seven days; his illness set in after getting wet at night. Daily he experienced a rigor which was followed by pyrexia, ending in cold sweat. Pulse 74; some debility; little headache; thirst; bark and aperients, and blue pill. On the 29th May mercurial ointment was rubbed into the thigh. On the 31st the mouth was affected; the pulse was 60 and rebounding; no perspiration. From the 1st June to the 7th there was little change; pulse 84; breathing short and laborious; some cough; urgent thirst; bowels irregular; a blister to chest; a purgative enema. From the 7th to the 15th there was sometimes profuse sweating; other times a hot and dry skin; the bowels irregular; tonics and aperients. On the 16th petechiæ appeared. On the 20th he became insensible, and remained so till he expired on the 23rd.

Autopsy 6 hours after death. Body considerably emaciated; skin very thickly spotted with petechiæ, like flea-bites. A little fluid was found effused between the membranes of the brain; a good deal in the ventricles and at the base of brain. Very many red points appeared on sections of the cerebral substance. The chest sounded well. The left pleura contained a small quantity of serum. On the pulmonary pleura of the same side, towards the root of the lung, there was a thickening from deposition of lymph, and the parenchyma of the adjoining lung was to some extent partially hepatized. The right lung was pretty sound. The liver was very generally adhering to the adjoining parts, especially to the diaphragm and colon. Its substance was apparently sound. The spleen was larger than natural. It contained three soft cheese-like tubercles, the largest about the size of an almond. The colon was distended with air. The mesenteric glands were rather enlarged. The viscera not mentioned were apparently sound.

In this instance there appeared to have co-existed with the intermittent some partial disease of lung and spleen, with a typhoid or putrid tendency.

It was asked at the time, as I find noted down, " were not the petechiæ connected with the tonic regimen, and rather stimulating treatment ;" and might not the antiphlogistic with venesection have had a better effect ?"

Case IV.—W. Dixon, ætat. 32; 32nd Regiment; died in hospital at Corfu, 1st August, 1825. Febris intermittens.—This man for several months had been laboring under complicated disease, which began in Santa Maura with intermittent fever. He has had a tumor in the left hypochondrium and frequent pain there. On the 19th July he was attacked with diarrhœa, with tormina and tenesmus; the stools were bloody. Latterly his feet became œdematous, and there was a fluctuation perceived in the abdomen; the pulse full, strong, and bounding. The dysenteric symptoms continued almost to the last, as did also the dropsical, with some pain in both hypochondria.. No mention is made in my notes of the treatment.

Autopsy 13 hours after death. The body was very much emaciated; the hands, feet and scrotum œdematous. About a drachm and a half of serum at the base of brain; the cerebral substance rather softer than usual. About a pint and a half of serum in each pleura. The right lung was adhering by long *transparent* bands of false membrane. Both lungs contained more blood than usual. The bronchia were redder than natural. The pericardium contained 4 oz. of serum. The spleen was very large; its weight about 2lbs; it was very generally adhering to the adjoining parts. It contained several masses of irregular forms; these were yellow superficially— internally, as exposed by section, either yellowish or light pinkish; they were of firm consistence, slightly fibrous, very much resembling the udder of a cow. The substance of the spleen generally was firmer than usual. The pancreas was harder than common. The liver was firm, yellowish and granular, more like the substance of the pancreas. The glands bordering the aorta were enlarged and red. There were about 6 oz. of serum in the abdominal cavity. The large intestines throughout their whole course were studded with minute ulcers and bluish spots, the cicatrices of healed ulcers, and were unusually vascular. The left testicle was wasted; hardly a vestige of it remained.

In this instance, in the hardened state of the pancreas, spleen and liver, we have indications of obstructed circulation ; and, in the fluid effused in its several cavities, of its effects.

These few cases may suffice to show how death may result in cases of intermittent fever from their complications and sequelæ : these latter, commonly various morbid states of some of the most important viscera, especially the chylopoietic, productive often of a cachetic condition of the system, marked by a low inflammatory action, by wasting, debility and dropsical effusions. It is worthy of remark that in those countries in which agues are most prevalent, and their recurrence in the same individuals most frequent, there these sequelæ are most witnessed, and the mortality from them is greatest, as is illustrated in the preceding table. This tendency to recur is one of their striking features, and is often witnessed even in countries to

which persons who have had the disease may have removed,
though these, their new places of abode, may be altogether
exempt from that malaria which is presumed to be their first
exciting cause; as if from a first attack a taint were left in the
system, a germ, ever ready to become active under any circumstances of a favoring kind. Very striking examples of the
kind were witnessed amongst our troops on their return home
after the disastrous Walcheren expedition; and in Malta they
have been observed in an unmistakable manner in regiments
coming there after having been exposed to malaria in the Ionian
Islands.

2.—OF REMITTENT FEVER.—This fever seems to be more or
less allied to the other forms of fever, in its mildest kind differing
but little from the ephemeral; in its severest, having a certain
resemblance to yellow fever; and in its tendency to pass into the
intermittent, and of intermittent to pass into it, exhibiting somewhat of a common nature. And yet the remittent has more or
less of a distinctive character, its habitat not being always
identical either with intermittent fever or yellow fever. Thus it
has occurred frequently in Malta, where agues seldom originate,
and also in Barbadoes where they are almost equally rare; and it
is prevalent in Ceylon and in India, where yellow fever as an epidemic disease, is unknown.

The following tabular statement, drawn up from the preceding
more general one, will bring more distinctly into view the stations
in their degree of productiveness of the disease and its severity,
as marked by its fatality :—

				Admitted.		Died.
United Kingdom ...	...	...	...	2·2	...	0.36
Gibraltar ...	...	...	...	15·3	...	0·9
Malta ...	...	...	...	6·6	...	2·8
Ionian Islands	...	...	...	262·9	...	20·8
Bermudas ...	...	...	...	3·5	...	0·88
West Indies	...	...	...	2520·0	...	226·0
Negroes ...	...	...	...	240·0	...	34·0
Jamaica ...	...	...	...	7445·0	...	991·0
Ceylon ...	...	...	...	1080	...	202·0
Malays ...	...	...	...	792	...	54·0
Singalese ...	...	...	...	3876	...	42·0
Mauritius ...	...	...	...	1.8	...	.3
Sierra Leone	...	...	...	8686	...	4009
Negroes ...	...	...	...	142	...	1·3

I shall give some account of the disease as I witnessed it in the Ionian Islands and Malta, in the former between the years 1824-27, in the latter between 1828 and 1834, both included. Its symptoms as there observed tolerably accorded even in their varieties with those which I had before witnessed in the disease in Ceylon and afterwards in the West Indies.

First, of the fever of the Ionian Islands. It commonly commenced with sudden prostration of strength and apparent diminution of all the vital energies. The pulse was almost invariably quick and feeble ; the respiration quick and short; the temperature either below the natural standard, or only a little above it, accompanied with a sensation of chilliness, sometimes amounting to rigor. There was generally headache, though not severe ; or a sensation of weight of head, with pains of back and limbs. Often there was nausea ; occasionally vomiting ; occasionally yellowness of the skin ; often flatulent distension of the abdomen ; occasionally relaxation of the bowels.

The remittent type of this disease was commonly well marked in its progress. The exacerbation was in most cases of irregular occurrence and of uncertain duration, often many times in the course of the twenty-four hours, with stages of apyrexia intervening. Some cases approached the confines of fever of the intermittent type, others of the continued. Most commonly the exacerbation was not preceded by chilliness nor followed by sweating. It was not unfrequently accompanied with delirium.

The danger was almost always greater than the symptoms would indicate to the inexperienced. With the exception of flatulent distension of abdomen, a common occurrence, all the symptoms the least distressing were easily relieved, especially pain, but without diminution of danger, which was chiefly indicated by feebleness and rapidity of pulse and by prostration of strength. When I reflect on the severe cases, no other disease occurs to me, with the exception of spasmodic cholera and yellow fever, that gave such an idea of the energies of the constitution being overpowered, as if a subtle active poison had been administered, paralysing the nervous system and endangering life. The course of the fever accordingly was commonly rapid ; when fatal, generally before the ninth day, often on the third or fourth.

In the fatal cases the appearances on dissection were very various. They may conveniently be divided into three classes :—

1st—Those belonging to the disease when pure, or not distinctly complicated; 2ndly—When complicated; 3rdly—When misnamed. I shall give the results of the examinations of thirty-eight bodies returned as having died of the disease. The cases were all treated in our regimental hospitals under the care of their respective medical officers. I saw most of them in progress, and was present at each *post mortem* examination, and immediately made notes of the principal morbid appearances:—

CLASS I.—1.—Ætat. 25; admitted August 4th; died August 10th; autopsy 6 hours after. Much fluid in the lateral ventricles and at base of brain; spleen large, not unlike the crassamentum of blood, but less dark; lower portion of colon dark red, as if from ecchymosis; partial undue redness of stomach and intestines.

2.—Ætat. 22; admitted August 5th; died August 8th; autopsy 13 hours after.— Lower part of the ileum redder than natural; glandulæ aggregatæ enlarged; cœcum red and rough, as if from the deposition of a little lymph; the spleen about twice its natural size, soft like the clot of blood.

3.—Ætat. 24; admitted July 24th; died July 31st; autopsy 8 hours after.—Pretty much fluid in the ventricles and at base of brain; red spots in the lower portion of the ileum; a few minute ulcers where the colon passes into the rectum; the spleen about twice its natural size, and like the preceding.

4.—Ætat. 36; admitted July 19th; died July 26th; autopsy 13 hours after.—The spleen about thrice its natural size, and very soft.

5. Admitted October 25th; died Nov. 4th; autopsy 7 hours after.—Skin yellow; gall-bladder distended with thick viscid bile; common gall duct pervious; omentum reflected over and adhering to gall-bladder and stomach; stomach and intestines partially red; the spleen large, dark, red and firm.

6.—Ætat. 28; admitted June 15th; died June 23rd; autopsy 18 hours after.— Portions of dura and pia mater more vascular than usual; pretty much fluid in the ventricles and at the base of the brain; red patches on mucous coat of stomach and ileum; spleen large and soft.

7.—Ætat. 29; admitted July 26th; died August 1st; autopsy 18 hours after.— Stomach and duodenum redder than natural; spleen large, dark and soft.

8.—Ætat. 36; admitted July 25; died July 31st; autopsy 18 hours after.—Inner coat of stomach in part dark red, in part brown; much bile in the gall-bladder; liver voluminous and rather soft. Death occurred suddenly, unexpectedly, the symptoms having been mild,—an event not uncommon in cases of this disease.

9.—Ætat. 28; admitted July 16; died July 20; autopsy 24 hours after.—Two ounces of fluid in the ventricles and at the base of brain; spleen large and very soft; weight about 2 lbs.; a little coagulable lymph on surface of liver. The blood-vessels, the air and alimentary passages were more or less red, probably from staining; putrefaction had commenced.

10.—Ætat. 25; admitted July 19; died July 24; autopsy 12 hours after.—Much fluid in the tissue of pia mater, in ventricles and at base of brain; the spleen large and exceedingly soft, of the color of burnt umber.

11.—Ætat. 30; admitted August 22; died August 30; autopsy 24 hours after.— Three ounces of serum in pericardium; the heart large; the aorta diseased throughout, its inner coats irregularly thickened; its middle atrophied irregularly; the spleen large, little softer than natural.

12.—Ætat. 20; admitted September 30; died October 5th; autopsy 12 ·hours after; deep-seated parts still warm. The trachea unduly red; the solitary glands of colon unusually large; many of the follicles of the rectum the seat of small ulcers; the spleen large, of pultaceous consistence, of low specific gravity, extremely fetid; putrefaction far advanced in it; its smell was so offensive as to be almost intolerable; it required some resolution to make the examination; it excited nausea and a peculiar acrid sensation in the pharynx; the right side of heart and the larger veins tinged with blood, mostly liquid; excepting in the spleen, nowhere were there marks of even incipient putrefaction.*

13.—Ætat. 47; admitted Oct. 15th; died Oct. 23rd; autopsy 8 hours after.—A good deal of fluid in the pia mater, the ventricles, and at base of brain; three and a half ounces of serum in the pericardium; large fibrinous concretion in right ventricle, with a little clot; spleen large and soft.

All these cases occurred in Corfu with the exception of the last, which was in Paxo:—

14.—Ætat. 34; admitted August 31st; died September 6th; autopsy 14 hours after.—The surface of lungs studded with vesicles full of air, from the size of a pin's head to that of a pea; diaphragm unusually vascular; a little lymph on adjoining surface of liver; red patches towards the cardiac portion of stomach, from which a slight oozing of blood; a blackish fluid in stomach like coffee-grounds (had hiccough and vomited a similar fluid); duodenum redder than natural; the spleen unusually large and soft.

15.—Ætat. 30; admitted Sept. 11; died Sept. 20th; autopsy 16 hours after.—Dura mater very vascular; much fluid at base of brain; two ounces of yellow serum in the pericardium; the spleen large, about 2 lbs., like crassamentum.

16.—Ætat 30; admitted Sept 12; died September 23; autopsy 19 hours after.—(The wife of a soldier).—Inner surface of intestines very red; spleen large and extremely soft; liver, pancreas, and kidneys soft.

17.—Ætat 30; admitted September 21; died October 2; autopsy 14 hours after.—Dura and pia mater unduly red; much fluid in the latter, in the ventricles and at base of brain; aspera arteria of a dark red throughout; rough transverse stripes of warty appearance covering in many instances ulcers in cœcum, ascending colon, and upper part of rectum.

18.—Ætat. 29; admitted Sept. 30; died Oct. 5; autopsy 21 hours after.—The membranes of the brain, the air-passages, the alimentary canal unusually red, pro-bably the effect of staining; the spleen large and soft.

19.—Ætat. 32; admitted Sept. 4; died Sept. 13; autopsy 6 hours after.—The trachea unduly red; partial abrasion of epithelium of lower portion of œsophagus, with redness of its mucous coat; slight œdema of posterior mediastinum; spleen large and soft.

20.—Ætat. 25; admitted Oct. 22; died Oct. 27; autopsy 10 hours after.—Much fluid in pia mater; about an ounce and a half in the ventricles and at base of brain; bubbles of air in the thoracic duct; the lower part of ileum unduly red, also the lower parts of rectum, its glands enlarged; the descending colon dark red, smeared with thin bloody mucus, in one spot slightly ulcerated; gall-bladder distended with bile, spots of ecchymosis on its inner coats; spleen large, its weight about 3 lbs., very soft.

21.—Ætat. 24; admitted Oct. 24; died Oct. 28; autopsy 9 hours after.—A good deal of fluid in the pia mater; spleen large, not unusually soft, but friable.

* This case was treated chiefly on the tonic plan; bark and quinine having been administered. He was blooded once (24 oz.) on account of oppressed breathing.

22.—Ætat. 31; admitted Sept. 16; died Sept. 18; autopsy 14 hours after.—Much fluid in the ventricles and at base of brain; spleen very soft; its weight between 2 and 3 lbs.

23.—Ætat. 18; admitted Sept. 17; died Sept 21; autopsy 18 hours after.—Lower parts of œsophagus and cardiac orifice of stomach unusually red; spleen large and soft.

24.—Ætat. 28.; admitted Sept. 17; died Sept. 21; autopsy 18 hours after.— Much serum in the ventricles and at base of brain; an ounce and a half in peri-cardium; two pints in cavity of abdomen; inner coat of stomach unduly red; the liver firmer than natural, its surface rough; spleen large and soft.

These latter cases occurred in Zante.

Besides the morbid appearances noticed, others were common. The vessels of the dura and pia mater were frequently much injected with blood; but whether from what is commonly con-sidered inflammatory action, or a *post mortem* effect from pressure on the great vessels from flatulent distension of the stomach and intestines, which, as already observed, was of common occurrence, it may be difficult to decide. The right cavities of the heart, the venæ cavæ, the vena azyzgos and the depending parts of the lungs, were in most instances more or less gorged with blood, and the blood generally was either liquid or only softly coagulated; it seldom showed a buffy coat, or, what is equivalent, fibrinous concretions.

CLASS II.—1.—Ætat 32; admitted Oct. 28; died Oct. 31; autopsy 18 hours after.— Much fluid in the pia mater, the ventricles and at the base of brain; the upper portion of the corpora striata were softer than natural; the inferior trachea and the bronchial tubes dark and spotted with lymph, producing an appearance like that of minute tubercles; the lungs loaded with dark blood, especially their inferior portion; red patches in jejunum; the spleen about twice its natural size, unusually soft.

2.—Ætat. 28; admitted July 21; died August 1; autopsy 22 hours after.—Two ounces of fluid at base of brain; left lung extensively hepatized, and in parts œdematous; the right in a less degree similar; the spleen large, dark and soft; the liver soft; the gall-bladder distended with viscid bile and a curd-like substance.

3.—Ætat. 23; admitted Dec. 2; died Dec. 7; autopsy 6 hours after.—The intestines and other abdominal viscera unduly red, as if from vascular fulness; lower part of ileum dark red, studded with deep ulcers, the largest one of about an inch and three-fourths long, with elevated edges; the valve of colon ulcerated and partially destroyed; the colon and rectum unduly red; the spleen large, dark and soft.

4. Ætat. 23; admitted Sept. 13; died Sept. 25; autopsy 15 hours after.—The pia mater infiltrated with serum; about 2 oz. in the ventricles and at base of brain; the great sympathetic nerve rather red; portions of stomach and of small intestines redder than usual; upper portion of colon thickened from œdema of its cellular coat; its mucous membrane rough, red, and here and there green, with ulcerated streaks and spots; like spots in its descending portion; the rectum unduly red.

5.—Ætat. 31; admitted Oct. 1st; died Oct. 11; autopsy 18 hours after.— Slight œdema of cellular tissue of right side of neck; second ganglion of pneumo-gastric nerve unusually vascular; aspera arteria unduly red; the inferior portion of both lungs hepatized; that of left lung very soft; spleen very soft.

Of these cases, three occurred in Corfu, two in Zante. In neither of them were there any symptoms noticed indicative of the unusual lesions discovered after death, except in the second, in which the pulmonary affection might be considered as connected with cough, slight at first, before death troublesome. In this last-mentioned instance the general character of remittent fever was sustained in the well-marked exacerbations and remissions of the disease. Such a masking of lesions in relation to symptoms is not uncommon, nor more than might be expected from experience in fever generally, especially when accompanied with delirium, or a tendency to it. Under excitation of brain, or the reverse, whether in mania or amentia, in furious or in low, muttering delirium, diseased states of the important organs are commonly latent, and advance often to a fatal issue without materially affecting their functional actions, at least under ordinary observation, unassisted by the best methods of medical examination.

CLASS III.—1.—Ætat. 39; admitted Sept. 5; died Nov. 13; autopsy 7 hours after.—Much fluid in pia mater and at base of brain; 2 oz. in pericardium; the lungs abounded in minute tubercles in different stages of softening; the superior lobe of each contained an excavation; there were small ulcerated spots in the bronchia; dark patches, as it were gangrenous, in the lower portion of the œsophagus; the epithelium for most part abraded; slight ulceration of the lower parts of ileum; severe ulceration of large intestines, as in chronic dysentery.

2.—Ætat. 25; admitted Nov. 18; died Nov. 23; autopsy 24 hours after.—Both lungs unusually red, even their upper surface; in them were spots, some dark, others of a florid hue; the air-passages throughout were very red, as was also the epiglottis; gelatinous mucus in the large bronchial tubes; patches and stripes of ecchymosis, interspersed with elongated lines, as of coagulable lymph, throughout the whole of the large intestines; the spleen of natural size, appearance and consistence.

3.—Ætat. 30; admitted Sept. 1; died Sept. 20; autopsy 18 hours after.—A few hydatids, the largest about the size of a hazel-nut adhering to the posterior part of the left pleura; several melanotic tubercles in both lungs; small vomicæ in the left; a large one in its inferior lobe; a few small cavities in middle and inferior lobe of right lung; a deep ulcerated cavity penetrating to the cartilage under the border of left sacculus laryngis; the aspera arteria of a livid hue, with purplish spots, as if becoming gangrenous; the spleen and pancreas harder than natural.

4.—Ætat. 26; admitted September 20; died September 27; autopsy 19 hours after —Much fluid in the pia mater and at base of brain; the bronchia very red; the gall-bladder distended with a black fluid of slightly putrid odor, without viscidity; the inner coat of gall-bladder stained by it, also the cystic and common duct, and a portion of the duodenum; the hepatic duct contained some orange-colored bile; the liver seemed healthy; the spleen small and firm; the epithelium of œsophagus very thick, like a false membrane; and the subjacent surface unusually red.

5.—Ætat 47; admitted Sept. 8; died Sept. 19; autopsy 10 hours after.—Much fluid in pia mater, the ventricles, and at base of brain; a hemispherical mass about the size of a walnut attached to the dura mater beneath the left parietal bone; the portion of cerebrum on which it pressed not apparently diseased; the stomach very red, with bright streaks of a vermilion hue, of raw appearance, without any adhering mucus; the spleen firm, of ordinary size.

6.—Ætat. 27; admitted August 30; died September 13; autopsy 8 hours after.— A considerable quantity of fetid serum, with some pus and coagulable lymph in the abdominal and pelvic cavities; a live round worm in right iliac fossa, close to a per- foration in the lower part of the ileum; numerous large ulcers in the same part, in some the muscular coat laid bare, in some the peritoneal; similar ulcers but smaller in its upper portion; a few in the jejunum; the folds of intestines glued together by lymph.

7.—Ætat. 27; admitted Dec. 11; died Dec. 21; autopsy 31 hours after.—Much fetid sero-purulent fluid, mixed with a little fecal matter and oil in the cavity of the abdomen; the intestines adhering together; a small perforation in the upper portion of the ileum, communicating with an ulcer in the mucous coat; in the lower portion of the same intestine several deep ulcers, two of which had nearly penetrated through the peritoneal coat; Peyer's glands enlarged; the spleen large and rather soft.

8.—Ætat. 22; admitted August 3; died August 28; autopsy, 6 hours after.— Much fluid in the ventricles and at base of brain; two ounces of purulent fluid in cavity of pelvis; the lower part of ileum studded with ulcers, two of which had penetrated through all the coats of the intestine; the spleen of natural firmness, very little larger than usual.

9.—Ætat. 34; admitted Sept. 8; died Sept. 10; autopsy 16 hours after.—Vessels of dura and pia mater very turgid; a considerable quantity of blood effused between those membranes over the cerebrum, especially of right hemisphere; a good deal of fluid in the ventricles; the cerebral substance apparently natural; a slight abrasion here and there of epithelium of œsophagus; its mucous coat dusky red; the spleen firm, of moderate size.

In these cases, seven of which occurred in Corfu, one in Zante, and one in Cephalonia, the symptoms in the beginning were those of remittent fever; the name of the disease was then given; the after symptoms were of a different description, and accorded more or less with the principal organic lesions discovered at the *post mortem* inspection.

I shall next speak of the disease as I witnessed it in Malta. During the years 1832, '33, '34, remittent fever was unusually prevalent there, not amongst the inhabitants, nor amongst the troops generally, but confined to one or two localities, and the regiment or regiments quartered there. In the year 1832 it was principally confined to the 42nd Regiment, stationed in Florian, a suburb of Valetta. The disease, though distinctly of the remit- tent kind, was mild, of short duration, almost ephemeral, and hardly needing any medical treatment. In 1833, the cases of fever which occurred were in the same regiment, and also in the 7th, the one quartered in Cottonera, another suburb, the other in Florian. These two were of a mild character,—all that were severe and fatal, proving, on *post mortem* examination, to have been complicated with local phlegmasiæ. In the following year the disease broke out in the regiments stationed in Lower St. Elmo, in Valetta, the extreme point of the city towards the sea. The fever was unusually severe and fatal, strongly marked and in some respects peculiar. On account of its peculiarities, I shall give a small number of the cases in detail.

The total, returned as this disease, which came under treatment were 150; of these 10 proved fatal; 107 belonged to the 42nd, of whom 3 died; 42 to the 53rd, of whom 6 died;—these two regiments were in Lower St. Elmo;—1, and that fatal, to the 73rd, which, till its departure for Corfu in April, occupied the same quarters.

Case 1.—T. Neary, ætat. 30; 73rd Regiment; admitted into hospital 10th March; died 27th March.—This man of temperate habits and of a good constitution, was admitted from the Marino Guard, complaining of headache, pain along the spine, with prostration of strength and a languid pulse. An emetic, with effect. On the 11th the symptoms were nearly the same. The bowels had been frequently opened by saline and antimonial purgatives. In the morning of 12th, after some sleep during the night, he appeared somewhat better. The skin and conjunctivæ of eyes had become yellow; calomel and James' powder. On the 13th the conjunctivæ were more turgid; there was an increase of debility with a languid pulse and a clammy surface; the calomel and antimony stopped; mild tonics; ale during the night. On the 14th there was no improvement; irritability of stomach (which had come on yesterday with vomiting and purging, and which seemed to be checked by the bitter ale) has returned; what has been vomited is described as "dark matter;" hæmorrhage from gums; the tongue is blackish with fetor of breath; the stools offensive; great debility; tonics, with nitric acid and T. opii; a blister to pit of stomach and nape of neck; the vomiting of dark matter continued, with retention of urine; low delirium set in and never left him; before death there was great vascularity of conjunctiva of one eye. He expired on the morning of the 17th.

Autopsy 25 hours after death. Body stout; the eyes flaccid from deficiency of fluid; the left conjunctiva very red; the cornea of left eye slightly ulcerated; the dura mater very yellow, the pia mater not distinctly so, nor the cerebral substance; when the brain was incised blood oozed from the minute vessels, followed by a yellow stain, as if from colored serum; there was a good deal of yellow serosity in the lateral ventricles, and their walls were stained yellow; the pericardium was yellow and lubricated with a yellow viscid serum. The heart was large; its valves were stained yellow, as was also the aorta, and in a less degree the veins; the right auricle and ventricle were distended with blood and with a little fibrinous concretion; on the outer surface of the heart there were slight spots of ecchymosis or petechiæ. The pleuræ were injected, especially their inferior portion. The left lung, its inferior part, contained much coagulated blood; its superior portion was pale and crepitous. In the right lung there was even more coagulum—more than could be well attributed to gravitation. The bronchia and lower trachea were red. The liver was rather soft. The gall-bladder contained a little thin slightly viscid bile of natural color. A probe was easily passed from the common duct into the duodenum; the inner surface of this duct was redder than natural, and the mucous glands near its termination were unusually large. The spleen was rather large and firm. There was a slight abrasion of the epithelium of the œsophagus near its termination. The cardiac portion of stomach was unduly soft; a thick mucus encrusted its lining membranes, and was not confined to its cardia. There was no well-marked lesion of the small or large intestines, except near the end of the colon, where its mucous coat was unusually red. A portion of the great sympathetic close to the ductus communis choledochus was of a brown hue and apparently swollen. By maceration for twenty-four hours it became still darker, and when torn longitudinally, its membrane seemed distended with coagulable lymph, discolored by blood. The portion of nerve thus affected was rather thicker than the eighth nerve in the neck. Neither the urinary bladder, nor pelvis of kidney, nor common gall duct, nor the intestines were stained yellow.

This case is remarkable in having a certain resemblance to yellow fever, and this both in the symptoms and *post mortem* appearances; indeed the surgeon of the 73rd, who had witnessed yellow fever at Gibraltar, spoke of it as " exactly like that disease." In relation to this similarity, the hæmorrhagic tendency, the spots of ecchymosis on heart, the injected conjunctivæ, the ulcerated cornea, the ichteric discolorations are very noteworthy.

Case 2.—J. Macdonald, ætat 35; 42nd Regiment; admitted June 9th; died June 22nd.—This man since he had epidemic yellow fever at Gibraltar in 1828, had been in good health until the day of his admission. He then complained of headache and severe pains in loins and legs; had a quick pulse, thirst; his skin was hot and dry; the tongue white. There was an exacerbation at noon, and again in the evening, without remission until the following morning, when he perspired freely. On the 10th the fever ran the same course. On the 11th gastric irritability set in; the pulse quick and soft; the stools clay-colored. Purgatives had previously been given: now calomel, with a little opium and effervescing draughts were ordered. On the 12th there was the usual morning remission and mid-day exacerbation; the treatment the same. On the 13th the skin had become jaundiced; the febrile exacerbation was less; headache and pains of extremities had ceased, the gastric irritability continuing. On the 14th "the fever" was moderate; the skin more deeply jaundiced. On the 15th the gastric irritability was reported to be excessive, nothing remaining on the stomach; there was suppression of urine; he complained only of a sense of "sinking;" the pulse quick, not feeble; heat of skin not above the natural; the tongue white and dry; bowels open; stools watery and light-colored; mercurial friction to hypochondria. On the 16th the vomiting was almost continued; a small quantity of highly-colored urine was passed; pulse very weak; no undue heat of skin; iced wine and water was now used; the vomiting was immediately checked. From this time to the 20th there was no distinct change of symptoms; the stomach continued tranquil, the secretion of urine tolerably abundant; there was no febrile exacerbation; the skin never above the natural temperature; he complained only of extreme exhaustion and thirst; the tongue now was dry and black; the pulse of good strength; he was "constantly dozing;" the mercurial treatment had been discontinued since the 16th; since had a liberal allowance of wine and bottled porter, and a pint of strong beef-tea daily, and camphor mixture. On the 21st he was worse; vomiting had recurred, with distressing hiccough; the urine scanty; bowels loose;

stools of a brownish red color. On the 22nd there was extreme exhaustion after an attack of syncope; during the night a large quantity of dark green fluid was vomited, and in the morning fluid of a reddish color; the stools were of like description. He expired at 5 p.m.

Autopsy 15 hours after death. Body muscular; not emaciated; skin of intensely saffron color; the dura mater of the same hue; the arachnoid and walls of the ventricles slightly yellow; on the former, over the pons Varolii, a little coagulable lymph was effused; the pia mater unduly red; some fluid under the arachnoid, and in tissue of pia mater; a good deal of yellow fluid in the ventricles and at base of brain; the cerebral substance natural; the pericardium very yellow and lubricated with a yellow viscid serum; the right cavities of heart contained a good deal of blood and fibrinous concretion, the left cavities very little; the inferior portions of both lungs were very red and seemed gorged with coagulated blood; in other portions of them there was pretty much serosity; the aspera arteria throughout was unduly red, and especially the rima glottidis; the pharynx was dark red; most of the œsophagus was redder than natural, and here and there whitish matter, like coagulable lymph, was found deposited on it; there were dark red streaks on the mucous coat of stomach, which was unduly soft; on the lower part of ileum, which was redder than natural, there were on its villous coat a few red granulations; the large intestines were of a dark red, their mucous and submucous tissue œdematous; here and there were small ulcers and patches of a dusky white color, as it were in the act of ulcerating; the gall-bladder contained a small quantity of dilute yellow bile; without more pressure than that employed in opening the body, some bile had flowed into the duodenum; other portions of the gut were free from bile-stain; the papilla of the common duct was red and rather turgid, and the angular fold of the villous coat beneath it was œdematous; the liver, spleen and pancreas were natural; there was some dark fluid blood in the vena portœ; some urine in the urinary bladder; perhaps the ganglia of the sympathetic were slightly œdematous; the thoracic duct contained a little transparent fluid.

In this case what seem most noteworthy in relation to the symptoms, are the lymph on the arachnoid, the fluid in the ventricles of the brain, the state of the air-passages and of portions of the alimentary canal, seeming to denote a low phlogosis, and the state of the common biliary duct, especially its papilla.

Case 3.—W. Kitchen, ætat. 25; 42nd Regiment; admitted 11th Jan.; died 18th Jan.—This man, previously healthy, on admission had headache, severe aching pains in loins and lower extremities; thirst, cool skin, pulse quick and soft, tongue white. Yesterday he had a rigor followed by increased heat through the night and sweating. At noon to-day there was an exacerbation, which lasted till evening, ending in perspiration at night. On the following day, the 12th, there was a morning remission, and a noon-day accession of fever. On the 13th there was no distinct remission; the headache continued intense; the skin hot and dry; the tongue dry and loaded; the pulse quick and soft; the eyes suffused; the treatment hitherto chiefly purgative; the stools dark, highly offensive; the urine natural; calomel 3 gr., opium ⅛ gr., every fourth hour; a draught of liq. ammon. acetat. and vin. antimonii at night; a blister to nape of neck. On the 14th, in the morning, there was a remission; now he complained of pain in right hypochondrium, which was increased by inspiration and pressure; the skin had become jaundiced; the stools were dark and watery; the tongue dry and brown in centre; the same medicine; 12 leeches to epigastrium. At noon, again an exacerbation; in the evening pyrexia was urgent; the pain of side had abated; there was constant gastric irritability; urine suppressed. On the 15th there was no morning remission; irritability of stomach continues; is dull and oppressed; about 2 oz. of urine voided; the skin deeply jaundiced; the pulse small and intermitting; blue pill and mercurial friction to hypochondrium; wine or porter. In the evening there was no improvement; troubled with hiccough all day and frequent vomiting; no urine, or stool; says "he feels better;" pulse small and intermitting; a purgative enema; effervescing saline draughts. On the 16th the urine was still suppressed; though an enema was thrice repeated during the night, it had no effect; the vomiting continues, throwing up what he drinks and nothing more; the tongue dry and black; a turpentine injection; iced wine and water. In the evening he seemed better; the vomiting had ceased; he had passed a small quantity of urine; says "he feels quite well;" the turpentine enema to be repeated. On the 17th it is stated that he makes no complaint of any kind, and that he had voided during the night about two gills of urine; no stool; pulse of better strength, and intermitting less; the stomach tranquil; the tongue the same; is inclined to doze; the iced wine continued and turpentine enema; at noon profuse epistaxis, followed by delirium at 4 p.m., ending in death at 1 a.m., of the 18th.

Autopsy 9 hours after death. Body well formed; not emaciated; skin intensely yellow; air of room 72°; temperature under liver 92°; under heart 91°; the dura mater rather less yellow than the skin; a little fluid effused under the arachnoid and in the tissues of pia mater; the vessels of the latter much injected; very little fluid in the lateral ventricles, and not yellow; pretty much at base of brain; the cineritious portion of a pinkish hue; the cerebral substance of natural consistence. The spinal chord was examined; in the lumbar portion of the canal there was a good deal of fluid; the thoracic portion of the chord, especially its central part, was softer and greyer than usual; the sympathetic nerves and ganglia were unduly red, as if injected with blood, with the exception of the semilunar ganglia and solar plexus, which were pale; the pericardium contained some thick, viscid fluid like synovia; the right side of the heart and the venous trunks were turgid with blood; some blood from the latter, put aside liquid, coagulated; there was a large fibrinous concretion adhering to the right ventricle; the structure of heart was tender and easily broken; the right pleura contained a little viscid serum; the greater portion of the superior lobe of the right lung was distended with coagulated blood, resembling crassamentum; as were also the lower portions of the middle and inferior lobes; the left lung, partially adhering, presented nearly the same appearance; the consistence of the impervious portions was even greater and more suggestive of hepatization; the bronchia and lower part of trachea were very red; the œsophagus in some places had lost its epithelium, especially towards the cardia; its mucous coat was unusually red, and here and there its surface was rough and grey, as if from a deposition of lymph; the stomach, somewhat redder than natural, contained a considerable quantity of blackish matter, like coffee-grounds, which rubbed on white linen left a brown stain; the gall-bladder contained about 1 oz. of very viscid, dark, almost black bile, which imparted a green stain; the inner surface of the bladder was very dark, as if stained; that of the common duct was nearly of its natural hue; before the gall-bladder was opened, pressure was applied to it, at first gentle, without effect; when increased, a small quantity flowed into the duodenum, preceded by a little whitish matter, probably mucus, which might have obstructed it, otherwise the duct was pervious; the margin of the papilla was slightly red, so also was the inner coat of the duodenum in streaks; the small intestines contained a good deal of brownish matter, not differing much from that in the stomach; the glandulæ aggregatæ were unusually red and large, and close to them in the lower portion of the ileum, there were some slight granulations as if from effusion of lymph ; the large intestines were flabby ; the inner coat of the cœcum was red and thickened in transverse ridges from œdema of its submucous tissue; the liver, spleen and pancreas presented nothing morbid ; the kidneys were large and pale.

As in the preceding case, so in this, the state of the primæ viæ and of the lungs is noteworthy, and especially the contents of the stomach and ileum so much resembling the " black vomit" of yellow fever.

The condition of the spinal chord and of the great sympathetic may claim some consideration, and the more so as in the preceding cases there was some appearance of lesion of the latter.

Case 4.—J. Rhodes, ætat. 30 ; 53rd Regiment; admitted Jan. 18 ; died Jan. 24.— After experiencing rigors he was admitted in the afternoon of the 13th, complaining of headache and general pains of limbs, accompanied with some nausea ; the pulse 90, full ; no undue heat of skin; bowels open ; an emetic of ipecacuanha and tartarized antimony, followed by calomel and salts. On the 19th the symptoms were much the same ; the medicines had had full effect ; calomel, 4 grs., James' powder, 6 grs. On the 20th the report was that he had had no sleep during the night, and that he felt languid and weak ; pulse 100, feeble ; pungent heat of skin ; urgent thirst ; bowels open ; abdomen·tympanitic ; a laxative enema ; aperients ; a blister to nape of neck. On the 21st, languor and prostration of strength had increased ; thirst continues; heat moderate ; pulse feeble, fluttering, intermitting ; tongue dry and red ; pains in lower extremities ; skin slightly yellow ; carbonate of soda 10 grs. thrice daily ; mercurial friction to thighs; wine, a gill. On the 22nd, delirium was reported during the night; no improvement; skin more yellow, warm ; the same medicine with effervescing draughts. On the 23rd the symptoms but little changed ; tongue hard and dry ; skin of a deep yellow color ; suppression of urine ; pulse 100, feeble ; heat of surface moderate ; passes his fœces involuntarily ; a turpentine enema ; wine. Died at half-past 2 a.m. of the following day. Some few hours previously a little urine was voided.

Autopsy 8 hours after death. Body not emaciated; skin yellow ; the pia mater more vascular than usual; some fluid between the dura mater and arachnoid, and between the latter and pia mater ; a small quantity in the lateral ventricles ; about 2 oz. at base of brain; the pericardium contained about an ounce of yellow serum ; the muscular substance of the heart soft, its right cavities contained some blood and fibrinous concretion ; the aorta was very yellow, and yet partially stained red ;—" the red was spread as it were over the yellow ;" both lungs were partially collapsed ; their inferior portions resembled crassamentum, as if blood had stagnated there and had coagulated either shortly before or soon after death ; the bronchia contained a frothy fluid and were very red, as were also the trachea and larynx, and pharynx ; the œsophagus, except at its junction with the pharynx, had lost its epithelium, and was unduly red; the great arch of stomach was dark red ; portions of the ileum were redder than usual, and the solitary mucous glands towards its termination were more than usually large; in the colon there were a few small dark streaks, and in one or two spots, a whitish incrustation, as of coagulable lymph ; the gall-bladder contained a small quantity of olive green bile, which was forced with difficulty by pressure through the common duct into the duodenum ; a little whitish mucus was driven before it;

there was a good deal of mucus of the same kind adhering to the intestines; a portion of blood taken from the heart and great vessels was found to contain a notable quantity of urea and a little of the coloring matter of bile.

This case is interesting on account of its obscurity, and may well give rise to reflection. How many queries may it not suggest?

Case 5.—G. Dunn, ætat. 35; 53rd Regiment; admitted 29th May, 1834; died 3rd June.—On admission, in addition to ordinary symptoms of fever, rigors, and cramps were experienced in the lower extremities; calomel 10 grs., opium 1 gr. On the 30th it was reported that headache and nausea continue, and that the medicine ordered and repeated had been thrown up; the bowels loose; heat of surface irregularly diffused; thirst urgent; pulse 86, full and strong; a blister to epigastrium; V.S. 20 oz.; the same medicine. 31st—Was delirious during the night; the vomiting and purging continue; face flushed; heat of skin pungent; a blister to nape of neck; calomel and opium as before. June 1st—The medicine rejected; passed the night in wild delirium; tongue dry and brown; pulse 100, feeble; is with difficulty kept in bed; camphor mixture every second hour. On the 2nd the report was, "is sinking fast;" no pulse at either wrist; extremities cold; delirious during the night; no vomiting since the evening visit. He expired at 4 a.m. of the 3rd.

Autopsy 6 hours after death. Body stout; skin yellowish; pretty much fluid was found between the arachnoid and pia mater, and at base of brain; the cerebral vessels turgid; the posterior part of the left lung was in "the first stage of hepatization;" and this lung generally, and also the right, was unduly gorged with blood; the bronchia were very red; the omentum and intestines were "injected" with blood; the stomach and duodenum contained grey pultaceous matter; on the mucous coat of the former there were red patches; there was a good deal of dark green bile in the gall-bladder and common duct; it colored water very slightly greenish yellow; before the bladder was opened, when pressure was made on the distended common duct, the bile flowed readily into the duodenum, showing that the obstruction was slight, and probably owing to mucus at the mouth of the papilla; there was a good deal of dark fluid blood in the vena portæ; in the mesenteric vein, towards its junction with the vena portæ, there was a pretty firm fibrinous concretion; granulated patches were found in the lower portion of the ileum, and red streaks with slight ulceration in the cœcum and upper portion of colon; the spleen was of ordinary size, rather soft, when incised and pressed there was an exudation from it of a pultaceous matter.

This case is noteworthy for rapidity of progress, and for the little relation distinctly apparent between the symptoms and the organic lesions.

These cases are chiefly interesting for their resemblance to yellow fever; and thus, as it were, establishing a link between the two.

Yellow fever hitherto in its aggravated form and unmistakable, such as it had appeared at Gibraltar, Cadiz and Lisbon, had never occurred in Malta. Of all places in the garrison where it was most likely to occur was St. Elmo, from its low situation, and other circumstances of an unsanitary kind. And yet, its condition this year was little different from that of ordinary years. The only particular in which it differed was, that, previous to the outbreak, the great tank which supplied it with water was cleaned out, and the sediment that had collected (it contained very little vegetable matter) was spread over a small portion of the adjoining ditch.

3. OF CONTINUED FEVER.—This form of fever being most prevalent in the Ionian Islands and Malta and the countries bordering the Mediterranean, has been called the summer fever of the Mediterranean. Elsewhere, whether in temperate or tropical climates, the disease returned as Febris communis continens, seems very analogous to it, at least in its purest form.

The following table, extracted from the more general table, shows its prevalency at one view at different stations, and its *apparent* fatality.

	Admitted.	Died.
Great Britain	503 ...	8·4
Gibraltar	737 ...	12·3
Malta	2025 ...	14·6
Ionian Islands	1752 ...	34·7
Bermudas	892 ...	17·8
West Indies	1942 ...	83·8
Jamaica	382 ...	12·4
Ceylon	2254 ...	19
Malays	356 ...	15
Singalese	1906 ...	12
Mauritius	1531 ...	16
Sierra Leone	·192 ...	13·2
Blacks	142 ...	1·3
Cape of Good Hope	847 ...	18
Canada	716 ...	15·2
Nova Scotia and New Brunswick ...	405 ...	6·3

In character this summer fever approaches the ephemeral, and in many instances is purely ephemeral. It commonly terminates in health in three or four days. If protracted beyond these limits local internal inflammation is to be apprehended.

Of its ordinary symptoms a brief notice may suffice. Its invasion is sudden. It generally commences with some severity of symptoms, especially headache, not a little alarming to those who have had no experience of the disease. Besides headache there is usually pain in the back and limbs. The pulse is commonly much accelerated, small and hard, the skin hot, the tongue foul, with urgent thirst and anorexia. The attack is sometimes ushered in with a rigor.

When the disease terminates fatally, it is, I believe, invariably in consequence of some local inflammation, or complication of organic lesion, and this generally with little distinction as to climate, except, indeed, when there has been an error of diagnosis, as has too frequently happened,—and other forms of fever, such as the remittent, have been returned as this. In illustration I shall give a few fatal cases out of the many which have come under my own observation in the Ionian Islands, Malta and the West Indies :—

1.—Ætat. 27; admitted May 3rd; died May 5th, of inflammation within the cavity of the cranium.—Pus (tried by the optical test) was found in small quantity in the posterior cornea of the lateral ventricles, and at the base of the brain, mixed with lymph; the disease commenced with a rigor on the 2nd May, after exposure to the sun and excess in drinking, followed by severe headache and nausea, and on the 4th by violent delirium, which was not relieved by copious blood-letting.

2.—Ætat. 23; admitted December 5th; died December 10th; also it is probable of inflammation within the cavity of the cranium.—Fluid was found under the arachnoid membrane, about 1½ oz. at base of brain, and a small quantity of lymph and puriloid fluid in 'one of the convolutions. The ordinary febrile symptoms were accompanied with severe delirium.

3.—Ætat. 28; admitted May 2nd; died May 9th, of inflammation of the lungs, complicated with inflammation within the cavity of the cranium.—The lungs were found gorged with blood and serum, and the bronchia unusually red; the choroid plexus in the inferior portion of each lateral ventricle was covered with lymph, and there was a pretty thick pellicle of lymph on the pons Varolii and medulla oblongata. At the onset of the attack the febrile symptoms were accompanied by some pain of chest, and towards its end by deafness and delirium.

4.—Ætat. 35; admitted August 28th; died October 15th, of chronic dysentery, following inflammation of lung.—The inferior part of superior lobe of right lung was found densely hepatized, of a light color; the colon was studded with chronic ulcers. No symptoms of pneumonia were observed during the progress of the disease; in its early stage the febrile symptoms were accompanied by jaundice.

5.—Ætat. 25; admitted July 16th; died July 23rd; the cause of death doubtful. —The epithelium of œsophagus was partially abraded; the stomach and intestines were distended with air and contained a dark grumous matter, which became red on dilution with water, as if colored by blood; there were no traces of inflammation in stomach or intestines. Jaundice preceded death, and nausea and vomiting, and a matter was thrown up not unlike coffee-grounds.

These cases occurred in the Ionian Islands.

6.—Ætat. 23; admitted August 30th; died September 8th; cause of death uncertain.—Some air was found in the cavities of heart;* the stomach and intestines

* The air contained in the heart was collected under water, after the great vessels had been tied. The portion obtained from the right side hardly amounted to a cubic inch, from the left, to about 1-hundredth merely of a cubic inch; 38 measures of

were much distended with air; the former contained much greenish fluid; its cellular coat was œdematous, especially towards the cardia, and was distended with bloody serum; the spleen was large and pultaceous. The symptoms were of the remittent kind, accompanied by vomiting of bilious matter, by vertigo, and muscæ volitantes, but without delirium.

7.—Ætat. 20; admitted August 19th; died 13th September, of pneumonia and ulcerated intestines.—Much of the inferior lobe of left lung was found hepatized, and a portion of the superior lobe œdematous, with purulent fluid in bronchia; small ulcers were found in the ileum, cœcum and colon; the spleen was large and soft. The early symptoms were those of continued fever, followed by slight cough, and finally by muttering delirium.

8.—Ætat. 26; admitted April 14th; died April 19th, of pleurisy and pneumonia.— The right pleura was found coated with lymph; the greater part of the superior lobe of right lung hepatized; its vessels filled with white fibrin; the middle lobe also was partially hepatized, and the inferior likewise in a less degree. The attack was ushered in with symptoms of continued fever; delirium soon followed, ending in coma; the thoracic disease was altogether latent.

9.—Ætat. 22; admitted July 1st, died July 4th; the death was sudden, as if from syncope.—The diaphragm continued to contract for a very short time after the heart had ceased to act; the lower portion of the ileum was found extensively ulcerated; the ulcers elliptical with raised spongy granulations; the glandulæ aggregatæ enlarged, presenting an appearance like the eruption of distinct small-pox; the spleen enlarged and soft. The febrile symptoms were at first smart; after blood-letting and the use of calomel and tartarized antimony, the prostration of strength was extreme; the fatal syncope took place after an alvine evacuation.

10.—Ætat. 48; admitted June 6th; died June 13th; cause of death uncertain.— Unusual redness of air-passages, œsophagus and stomach; the blood vessels, except of the liver, stained bright yellow;* the little fluid in the gall-bladder had no bitter taste, was brownish, and was rendered turbid by nitric acid. Stages of pyrexia and apyrexia occurred several times; the skin shortly before death became very yellow; the abdomen tympanitic.

11.—Ætat. 27; admitted October 18th; died November 24th, of complicated organic disease.—An ulcer was found in the margin of the epiglottis; granular tubercles in superior lobe of left lung; œdema of right lung; a small ulcer in œsophagus, near its termination; hypertrophy of the glandular structure of duodenum; numerous small ulcers scattered through the ileum; the spleen about thrice its natural size, of the firmness of liver; fine shreds, as it were of coagulable lymph, adhering to inner coat of vena portæ; numerous small abscesses in left kidney. The early symptoms were those of continued fever; the later were indicative of gastric and intestinal disturbance, such as bilious vomiting, hiccough, and pitch-like stools.

All these latter cases occurred in Malta.

12.—Ætat. 28; admitted Feb. 26th; died March 29th, of cerebral disease.—There was an appearance of flattening of the convolutions of the brain, as if from pressure; the lateral ventricles were much distended with turbid fluid; some lymph was found

the former by solution of potash were reduced to 37; by phosphorus to 35; the residue was azote. No air was found in the aorta, and there were no indications of putrefaction.

* In this case it was remarked that whilst no bile appeared to be secreted by the liver, it abounded in the blood.

in the third and fourth ventricle, and on the pons Varolii; in the ventricles it was accompan ed by a little pus; the superficial portion of the corpera striata was soft; the former and septum lucidum were almost pultaceous; the thoracic and abdominal viscera were sound. Rigors and severe headache, with a rapid pulse, were some of the early symptoms, accompanied by a very hot skin; delirium soon followed; after blood-letting and the use of mercury, there was an apparent improvement; shortly dullness followed and a disposition to heavy sleep; coma preceded death.

This case occurred in Barbadoes, at a time that yellow fever prevailed.

4. OF YELLOW FEVER.—The following table shows at one view the prevalency of this disease at different stations when most strongly marked and returned as *icterodes*, exclusive of the cases designated and returned as remittent fever and continued fever, a large proportion of which both in Jamaica and others of our West Indian colonies have unquestionably been of this disease.*

	Admitted.	Died.
Bermudas	504 ...	124
West Indies	89 ...	39
Jamaica	3·8 ...	2·9
Canada	0·44 ...	0·1

On this disease I shall be very brief, so much having been written on it, and my experience having been limited nearly to two outbreaks of it, those which occurred, following close upon each other in Barbadoes in 1847-48, when, in the short space of little more than one month, viz.—from the 15th December to the 24th January, the first proved fatal to 23 men and 1 officer; the number attacked being 97, out of a strength of 387 at headquarters of a single regiment—the 88th. In this its first outbreak, the disease was characterized by great irritability of stomach, a difficulty of retaining anything swallowed, a tendency to passive hæmorrhage in the mucous membrane of the primæ viæ, and in the aggravated cases, the expulsion by vomiting of a blackish fluid, containing blood corpuscles darkened and altered by the action of an acid in the stomach.† Yellowness of skin was an almost invariable accompaniment.

* There is a reason often acted on for not calling an endemic fever, yellow fever, that name creating alarm, and, where quarantine is in use, subjecting the station to all the annoyances and losses which the enforcing the quarantine system entails. The two invasions of fever, hereafter to be mentioned, which I witnessed in Barbadoes in 1847-8, both genuine yellow fever endemics, were returned, one as remittent, the other, the later, as continued fever.

† The acid, I believe, is commonly the muriatic. In a specimen of "black vomit"

The body in every fatal case was examined. In no tissue were there any marks found of inflammation; in no organ any well-marked visible lesion. The vessels of the mucous membranes, and more especially of the stomach and intestines, were turgid and discolored, often in patches and with dark blood. The lower parts of the lungs, and the integuments of the inferior parts of the body, were similarly discolored, and from the same cause. The vessels of the brain, too, were commonly loaded with blood. No effusion of lymph was observed in this organ, and but little more serosity than usual. The white parts, the skin, the serous membranes, and the coats of the arteries were in most instances more or less yellow. The liver, too, was generally yellow, the color nearly of unbleached wax. The bile was more or less viscid, and the common biliary duct, with the exception of its being often clogged with mucus, was pervious. The blood was generally thick as well as dark, coagulating either not at all, or imperfectly; and in several instances it was found acid by the test of litmus paper. The glandulæ aggregatæ, it may further be remarked, were nowise affected; and the spleen in most instances was found little enlarged or softened.

This outbreak of the disease in the 88th was shortly followed by a similar one in the 66th, a regiment recently arrived, and which occupied, after a certain interval, the same quarters. Out of an average strength of 384, it lost 34, the number that came under treatment being 197.

The symptoms in this instance, on the whole, were less strongly marked than in the preceding,—indeed in many cases they were rather those of continued fever. Even in the fatal cases their severity was less and the proportional mortality was less. Moreover, whilst in the fatal cases of the 88th, scarcely any instance of complicated organic disease was detected, in those of the 66th several examples of the kind occurred. The blood, too, was found in the cavities of the heart more frequently coagulated and accompanied by fibrinous concretion.

As at Malta in 1834, the disease was confined to one small locality, men in nearly adjoining barracks escaping the fever. Nor was there any obvious cause to which the endemic could rationally

sent me by Dr. Blair, from British Guiana, I found muriatic acid and muriate of ammonia, and the acid in no small quantity. I could detect no acetic or lactic acid in it, or lithic acid, which my friend supposed might have been present.

be referred. The locality was low and objectionable, like that of St. Elmo; but its sanitary condition was apparently neither better nor worse than usual. The only new circumstance associated with the outbreak was the breaking up a portion of ground hard by (that ground remarkably dry and destitute of organic matter) for the purpose of a road improvement. Further, no more than in the fever of Malta was there any, the least, proof of the disease being imported. In each instance, it was so asserted; and in each careful inquiry disproved it.*

I shall give a few of the fatal cases of which I have notes. Being myself an invalid at the time, the number is smaller than I could wish, and the details are less minute. Imperfect as they are, they may not be altogether useless for the purpose of comparison. My notes were made according to my constant practice, immediately after the autopsy.

Case 1.—H. M'Guire, ætat. 30; 88th Regiment; admitted 24th December, 1847; died 30th December.—A man of intemperate habits; from admission to time of death there was great irritability of stomach, with vomiting, whatever was swallowed being almost immediately rejected; "black vomit" occurred only a few hours before death; apart from this state of stomach, the symptoms were not alarming; I saw him on the 29th about 10 a.m.; then he seemed pretty well; the day before he had ate some fish with butter which had been secretly brought him; calomel and sulphate of quinine had been early prescribed; of the latter altogether 120 grs. had been taken, little of which probably had been retained; cinchonism was not produced; he had besides effervescing draughts, etc.

Autopsy 7 hours after death. Skin generally yellowish; integuments of back "ecchymosed."—The vessels of brain congested; much fluid acid blood in the lungs, especially in their inferior portions; some dark semi-fluid blood, with portions of soft crassamentum in the right cavities of heart; the blood from the lungs mixed with quicklime emitted an ammoniacal odor; the stomach contained some black acid matter, as did also the large and small intestines; the mucous coat of the stomach was injected; the liver was pale, soft and brittle; the gall-bladder contained some viscid greenish bile.

Case 2.—J. M'Guire, ætat. 34; 88th Regiment; admitted 15th December, 1847; died 19th December.—A man of intemperate habits; in the early part of the month he had been under treatment for delirium tremens; on admission his case was considered one of common continued fever; purgatives were administered, followed by calomel and opium. On the 17th there was vome vomiting. On the 19th, a few hours before death, there was black vomiting. On this day, after the "black vomit" had taken place, had sulphate of quinine and calomel (10 grs. of each) every second hour without effect,—indeed the case was then hopeless.

Autopsy 19 hours after death. The brain presented nothing remarkable; the lungs

* See a letter on the subject addressed to the author by Lieut.-General Berkeley, then commanding the Forces in the West Indies, appended to Dr. Blair's work on yellow fever.

were rather gorged with blood; the trachea and bronchia were stained red; a very small cluster of granular tubercles was found at the apex of each lung; the heart flaccid, it contained a little fibrin; in the stomach there was some black fluid, which reddened litmus; blood from the brain and heart did not; the great arch of stomach was of a suffused red; when pressed, a bloody fluid exuded from its mucous coat; the spleen was of natural size and consistence; the liver was rather pale and easily broken; a good deal of dark bile was found in the gall-bladder; the mucous coat of intestines was redder than natural.

Case 3.—Assistant-Surgeon Dr. C., ætat. about 24; died Feb. 4, 1848.—Of the symptoms in this case, I have no note. Dr. C., previous to his attack, was in robust and excellent health; the duration of the disease did not exceed a few days; the treatment was by calomel and quinine in large and frequently repeated doses.

Autopsy 5 hours after death. The cerebral vessels were turgid; the pia mater in some places was stained red to the extent of a quarter of an inch from the large veins; much blood flowed from the divided vessels on removing the skull-cap; it presently coagulated; the coagulum was soft, nearly of natural color; there was pretty much serous fluid in the tissue of the pia mater and at base of brain, and a little in the ventricles; the cerebral substance natural; the lungs were moderately collapsed; portions of them, chiefly, but not entirely their inferior, were solidified as if from pulmonary apoplexy; a good deal of dark blood flowed from them on the division of the large blood-vessels; in the right ventricle of heart there was a little soft clot; the muscular substance of the heart was firm,—nowise softened; the stomach contained a blackish semi-fluid, and there was a good deal of the same in the small and large intestines; there were streaks, as it were of ecchymosis, in the mucous coat of stomach, chiefly in its large curvature; the epithelium of œsophagus, near its termination, was slightly abraded; the spleen, of ordinary size, was softer than natural; the liver was friable.

Case 4.—G. Tonglin, ætat. 24; admitted 26th Feb., 1848; died 20th March.— This man was admitted an account of a bubo in groin, which suppurated and was healing slowly. On the 18th March febrile symptoms set in with vomiting of bilious matter; there was no headache; the tongue clean; pulse 96. On the 19th he was reported better; towards night the skin became hot. On the 20th, after a restless night, had frontal headache. During the morning he vomited some bilious fluid, and continued to do so at intervals until two hours before death, when be became semi-comatose; the treatment was by calomel and James' powder; later by quinine and calomel.

Autopsy 12 hours after death. Discoloration of shoulders; the brain rather soft; the lungs congested; portions of them heavy, and appearing when cut as if in the first stage of hepatization; bronchia and trachea red; a mass of fibrinous concretion in each cavity of heart, yellow and yielding a yellowish serum; the cardiac valves and lining membranes of aorta stained yellow; the blood did not redden litmus; the stomach contained a good deal of blackish fluid like "black vomit" and acid; its mucous coat generally was pale, in parts softened; nowhere bloodshot; the liver was very little paler than natural; the bile was of a greenish yellow hue, and only slightly viscid; the spleen was large and soft; there was no lesion of the intestines.

Case 5.—M. Gilmore, ætat. 23; admitted 5th March, 1848; died 9th March.— The symptoms in this case were those of continued rather than of yellow fever; coma preceded death; the treatment was by purgatives and antimonials.

Autopsy 7 hours after death. Some yellowness of skin and conjunctivæ without suggillation; the vessels of brain were congested; portions of the lungs were solidified from blood effused and firmly coagulated; similar coagula were found in muscular substance of right ventricle, especially towards its apex and near the entrance of the coronary vein ; and in the left in the substance of a columna carnea ; the right auricle and ventricle contained some fibrinous concretion; there was some dark colored fluid in stomach, not distinctly "black vomit;" no redness of the organ; its mucous coat to a considerable extent was raised and emphysematous from air in the cellular tissue; this portion was softened ; no other lesion was noticed.

Case 6.—D. Hanna, ætat. 28; admitted 24th Oct., 1845; died 4th Nov.—This man was " a free-liver," but seldom drunk. On admission he had the appearance of one who had been drinking; his hands and tongue were tremulous; he had nausea, with occasional bilious vomiting; an emetic, followed by an aperient; he continued in a precarious state until the morning of the 27th, when he complained chiefly of extreme debility and tinnitus aurium. On the following day he was considered almost convalescent. On the 29th symptoms of fever became manifest; skin hot, pulse quick; slight vertigo ; stools dark and feculent; from this time to the 3rd November he was in a state of low continued fever, with irregular slight exacerbations, without rigors; he seemed "slowly mending" till the morning of the 3rd, when he suddenly fell back as it were comatose; the left side of face was convulsed; the pulse small and quick; he remained comatose till death. After the 29th the treatment was chiefly by quinine and blue pill, wine, etc.

Autopsy 10 hours after death. Body robust; the minute cerebral vessels much injected; a good deal of sub-arachnoid effusion and effusion into the ventricles and at base of brain ; the substance of brain firm; the lungs partially collapsed; they contained a good deal of blood; there was a good deal of blood of natural color in right cavities of heart, with some fibrinous concretion; the blood mixed and triturated with quicklime did not emit any ammoniacal odor; the stomach was distended with air, and contained about a pint of blackish fluid, resembling "black vomit;"* on removal by washing of adhering mucus, the inner coat exhibited red spots, little larger than flea-punctures, and some diffused redness towards the cardia ; the mucous coat was softer than natural; the liver was rather large ; the bile thick, but of natural color; the spleen about thrice its natural size, was soft and most easily broken; triturated with lime, it yielded a distinct ammoniacal odor ; on removal of the capsules of the kidneys, red spots were seen on their surface; the emulgent veins were stained red; blackish spots, the largest about the size of the human nail, were found scattered here and there in the small intestines, and were equally visible as seen through the peritoneal and mucous coat, suggesting the idea of blood effused and partially absorbed ; the lower ileum was red, and the colon was speckled red like the stomach ; about 4 ozs. of serous fluid in the cavity of pelvis.

From the dates of these few cases it will be perceived that besides those of the endemic referred to, solitary ones had occurred during the two or three preceding years. And, it is worthy of being kept in recollection that the disease is not exclusively epidemic or endemic, being not unfrequently sporadic, instances of it more

---

* Seen under the microscope, it exhibited epithelium plates, numerous corpuscles, not unlike those of the blood, slightly altered by the action of water, and greyish clusters containing granules, which it may be inferred were of starch being rendered blue by iodine. The fluid evaporated and heated left a considerable carbonaceous residue, which was incinerated with difficulty. The ash was reddish and saline; acted on by muriatic acid, a brownish yellow solution was formed, which was pretty copiously precipitated by ammonia and ferro-cyanide of potassium, indicating the presence of iron.

or less well marked occurring from time to time, and even of an aggravated form and fatal issue.

I shall now offer some remarks on the etiology, pathology and treatment of fevers, passing by typhus, of which, having served chiefly in hot climates, I have had the least experience.

Speaking before of the obscurity of their etiology, I remarked that with the exception of elevation of atmospheric temperature there seems to be no one condition which can be mentioned, that can be received in any way in the relation of cause to effect. A comparatively low degree appears to favor the production of typhus, most commonly a disease of winter in temperate climates. A higher temperature is associated with the appearance of intermittents; and a higher still with fevers of the continued and remittent type, and with yellow fever. In all parts of the world subject to these diseases, with the exception of typhus and typhoid fever, and, in a less marked manner, yellow fever, the warmer months of the year are the feverish months, but not in exact proportion to the degree of temperature. This is illustrated by the following table, showing *per mensem* the number of cases of fever admitted into the hospital of one regiment, the 51st, in the Ionian Islands, from 1825 to 1832, both years included :—

	Feb. con. cont.	Remittens.	Intermittens.	Total.
January	20	28	36	84
February	30	17	26	67
March	32	11	34	77
April	51	18	44	113
May	69	14	37	120
June	113	80	33	226
July	145	69	32	246
August	144	128	27	199
September	64	100	24	188
October	61	63	22	146
November	32	45	20	97
December	14	30	28	72

From this it appears that whilst the total amount of these fevers rises and falls with tolerable regularity with the increasing and diminishing monthly temperature, July being about the hottest and February the coldest of the twelve, the particular fevers observe as to frequency a different ratio; thus, of intermittents, the greatest number occurred in April, of continued fevers in July, and of remittent in August. Yellow fever, at

least where it is most rife, as in the West Indies, seems even
more exceptional as regards high temperature than remittent fever.   This is shown by the following table, in which are
given the deaths from the disease monthly amongst the troops
in Barbadoes, exclusive of officers, for a period of 11 years—viz.,
from 1838 to 1848, both included, in the first six of which and
parts of the two last, yellow fever was the prevailing malady :—

January	...	34	May	...	5	September	...	22
February	...	20	June	...	16	October	...	30
March	...	30	July	...	9	November	...	90
April	...	17	August	...	18	December	...	77

The same order of frequency there is reason to believe, with
little difference, prevails through all the countries north of the
line within the fever range.   This is in accordance with the view
that whilst a high temperature is most conducive to continued
fever, something else is requisite for the production of remittent,
intermittent and yellow fever.   And, further, since all fevers prevail in the same countries in different years in the most inconstant
manner, not to be measured absolutely by the thermometric scale,
we are under the necessity of having recourse to other agencies, or
agent, for their production.   Every inquirer who has given close
attention to epidemic diseases, from Hippocrates to Sydenham,
and from Sydenham to our contemporaries, has been forced into
the acknowledgement of a hidden cause—a something known only
by its effects, a something impalpable, invisible, distinct from the
causes of ordinary diseases : according to Hippocrates a something divine; according to Sydenham a something emanating
from the bowels of the earth.   In the instance of fevers, in
modern times, it has been called malaria.

Now, what is malaria ?   I apprehend were it not for the effect
attributed to it, the production of certain fevers, the word would
not be in use.   The great obscurity of the subject is manifest
from this, that there is so little agreement amongst authors
respecting it.

Some have supposed that the substantial cause is principally
light carburetted hydrogen, the gas of marshes, generated by
the fermentation and decay of vegetable matter under water, or
at least in a moist state, at a certain temperature.   Others have
supposed that it is sulphuretted hydrogen produced by the
decomposition of salts containing sulphuric acid by the agency

of decomposing vegetable matter; others that it is aqueous vapor and a high temperature combined; and a fourth class of inquirers have attributed the effects to vicissitudes of temperature successively heating and chilling the animal body.

But these views appear to be partial and not sufficiently supported by facts, or, in brief, are not an induction from established facts.

That the light carburetted hydrogen of marshes is not the gas constituting malaria, seems to be well proved by the experience gained in our laboratories and collieries; and I am of opinion that a similar remark is applicable to sulphuretted hydrogen and all other known gases which have been made the subject of research, and have been breathed more or less in conducting experiments.*

The other views of the nature of the cause of these fevers are also opposed by strong negative evidence: no constant association of the presumed cause and effects can be traced. At a certain elevation in a mountainous region, even within the tropics, and in situations where the plains are extremely unwholesome, and intermittent and remittent fever of common occurrence, these diseases cease to appear, though the changes of temperature by day and night are great and sudden, very much more so than in the valleys beneath, or in the lower levels. And, at a certain distance from land in the tropical ocean there is a like exemption, though there moisture often abounds and the heat is great, as in the region of squalls, towards and under the equator, where the gusts of wind, followed by calms are usually accompanied by drenching rain.

* That sulphuretted hydrogen, in a certain quantity, is injurious to health, and even fatal to life, is well known; but I am not aware of any fact in proof of its being capable of producing either remittent or intermittent fever, as supposed by the late Mr. Daniel. How many watering-places may be mentioned where the atmosphere is partially tainted with this gas and yet exempt from the fevers in question! And how many other places might be named, subject occasionally to severe malaria-fevers, the atmosphere of which is not perceptibly contaminated with it! Mr. Daniel specially attributed the destructive fevers of the western coast of Africa to this cause. Now, we know that the worst parts of that coast are not constantly equally unhealthy; that occasionally, for months together there is an exemption from the destructive fever; but we cannot suppose that at the same time there is any cessation of the decomposition of vegetable matter or of its action on the salts of the brackish or salt water, or of the production of sulphuretted hydrogen as a consequence of that action. On such an obscure subject as malaria it is advisable that speculation should be conducted with extreme caution, especially with a view to practical results and the offering of suggestions with a hope of protection. If the hypothesis be false, the suggestions founded on it may not only be of no avail—as on one memorable Niger expedition,—but by imparting undue confidence, tempting to exposure and leading to the neglect of ordinary precautionary measures, may do vast harm.

4

It is far more easy to say what malaria is not than what it is.
All that relates to its production appears to be enveloped in pro-
found mystery. I am not, I repeat, aware of a single circumstance, excepting one, which with propriety can be called a
common one, always existing where there is malaria, or where
there are fevers attributable to it ; and this, as before said, is
warmth, or a certain temperature many degrees above the freezing
point ; its exact limit is not easily defined.

I shall mention some facts tending to show this mysterious
nature of malaria,—facts which have led me to the above conclusion.

1. The most striking fact, perhaps, in relation to this
mysterious origin of malaria, and which is unquestionable, is
the irregularity of its occurrence, and this even in situations
where it occasionally operates with extraordinary intensity and
violence, and in regions remarkable for equability of climate, as
in Sierra Leone, the West Indies, the interior of Ceylon and the
islands of the Mediterranean, and especially the Ionian Islands.
I have known a tract of country in the interior of Ceylon free
from fever for three or four years and peculiarly healthy, and
suddenly, without any apparent cause, becoming the reverse, the
weather being as before, and all the circumstances of life of the
inhabitants as before, so far as they were appreciable. For a
few months destructive remittent fever has scourged the population, converting a flourishing district almost into a desert ; and,
then, still without any apparent change of climate or other circumstance, its ravages have ceased and the country has recovered
its usual healthiness. Facts of the same kind have been witnessed in Malta, in all the Ionian Islands, especially in Santa
Maura, Zante and Cephalonia, and in all the West India Islands,
and in British Guiana.

2. Other striking facts bearing on the mysterious origin of
malaria, present themselves in connection with situation.

In some places, marshy grounds, as is well known, are the
seat of agues and of remittent fevers ; in other places this is not
the case. The Pontine marshes are a remarkable example of the
former ; the low and marshy grounds on the south-west coast of
Ceylon, between Negumbo and Galle, are not a less remarkable
example of the latter.

In some situations the production of malaria appears to be

associated with profusion of vegetable matter, undergoing decomposition, but not always. In the interior of Ceylon, in some of the hilly districts where forest is abundant, the smell of vegetable matter undergoing decomposition is strong and disagreeable, and yet the country is free from malaria-fever.

In other situations the reverse appears to be the case,—where there is no apparent source of malaria, no decomposing vegetable matter that is appreciable; where the air is free from any unpleasant smell; the climate so far as sensation is concerned agreeable, the country, like our English parks, abounding in herds of deer and in wild animals, and yet is most unwholesome, is without human inhabitants, and the passing traveller is often the victim of fever.* The reverse, too, is the case in a still more remarkable manner in some of the Ionian Islands. There it is not uncommon for remittent and intermittent fevers to break out in places remarkable for aridity and want of water and almost destitute of vegetation. Parts of the mountainous district of Zante are of this description; the little island of Meganisi is so in an extreme degree, as is also the still smaller island of Vido; these, the latter two, being almost barren rocks. And in the Ionian Islands, and in the islands and shores of the Mediterranean generally, and also in Ceylon, the severest form of fever, that of the remittent kind, is most rife towards the end of summer, when the ground is most parched and the circumstances are least favorable to the decay of vegetable matter.

3. Were particular instances collected of the prevalency of remittent and intermittent fever, limited to small spots, and the reverse—instances of partial and very limited exemption—the mystery of the origin of malaria would be increased. Of a party of men occupying two rooms in a small barrack-building divided by a narrow passage, in Vido, I have known the inmates of one room to have been attacked in a large proportion, whilst those in the other entirely escaped, although the aspect of the two rooms was similar:—the only difference between them that I could

---

* Many parts of Ceylon, between the mountains of the interior and the sea-coast, now desert, overgrown with jungle and forest, or, in some situations as above mentioned, only agreeably varied with clumps of trees, formerly were populous and cultivated, as is clearly proved by the works of man which are there to be met with, some of them of vast dimensions, as the tanks of Candelay and Minery,—the one about 20 miles in circumference, the other about 12 miles; and the ruins of great cities of proportional magnitude in the country adjoining.

ascertain was, a tank under the one, and not under the other; but this was a constant circumstance, whilst the occurrence of the fever was sudden and unexpected, and considered altogether extraordinary and inexplicable. Further, I have known a detachment stationed at the little fort Alexandria, in the midst of the brackish lagoon of Santa Maura, retain their health during the sickly season when fever was prevailing in the adjoining fort of Santa Maura, at the extremity of the lagoon and one side exposed to the sea-breezes. By reference to authors, there would be no difficulty in multiplying such instances; and, even from my own knowledge, I could mention other examples, especially in the West Indies, and of disappointment there in the selection of sites for forts and barracks, those making the choice having been guided by the promising healthy character of the situations, sadly disproved by experience.

From what has been stated, and from all the information I have been able to collect relative to malaria, it appears to me to be proved that we are entirely ignorant both of the nature of this agent, or agency, and of its causes. In relation to its causes or sources, I believe I am fully borne out by facts in expressing the following negative conclusions;—and this, confining the attention to the Ionian Islands solely, without having recourse to other supporting instances.

1st. That they are independent of luxuriant vegetation, which is proved by the instances of Meganisi, Cerigo, etc.

2ndly. That they are independent of the decomposition of vegetable matter, which is proved by the same islands and Paxo.

3dly. That they are not referrible to the sun's rays acting on a moist surface, or on underground moisture; the power of the sun being much the same every year; the underground moisture being in all the islands mentioned very scanty, and, there is reason to believe, very little subject to variation of quantity from year to year; and, further, there being no constant relation between hot summers and rainy winters and malaria, or *vice versâ*, which is a well-established fact.

Lastly. That they are independent of the mixing of fresh and salt water, and of the alternate inundation and exposure to the sun and air of muddy surfaces, there being hardly an appreciable tide in the Mediterranean, and the shores of the Ionian Islands being remarkably free from mud.

A conviction of our ignorance is a good preparatory state of mind for the discovery of truth. This, it seems to me, is the principal progress hitherto made in the investigation of malaria. We know not whether it is a ponderable or an etherial substance; simple or compound; whether generated in the atmosphere, or produced from the soil, or emanating from the bowels of the earth. That it is a substance *sui generis* can, I think, hardly be doubted; that it is extremely subtle; that if ponderable, it acts in extremely minute quantities; and if imponderable and etherial, it possesses properties peculiar to itself, and for their discovery may require new instruments and new methods of research. The progress of physical science in modern times holds out the highest encouragement. There are still a few living who remember the philosophers to whom we are indebted for pneumatic chemistry, previous to whose labors water was considered an element—atmospheric air was considered an element. Within a few years we have witnessed two new substances brought to light, possessed of energetic properties, iodine and bromine, which exist in excessively minute quantities in the waters of the ocean, and which, we may be sure, would never have been discovered except by processes of concentration. Could analogous processes be brought to the aid of atmospheric chemistry, it is impossible to say what new substances might not be discovered in the aerial ocean. That it must contain, in however minute quantity, portions of everything gaseous and volatile, is manifest to reason; but how few of them have been detected. And that it must contain also a variety of substances in the solid form, in impalpable powder, is highly probable: the matter of blight wafted by the wind, the spray of the sea carried inland very many miles by the storm, dust falling in showers over a vast extent of surface, are facts in favor of it, without taking into account meteoric stones, the history of which is not less mysterious than that of malaria, and the existence of which, though marked by properties so manifest and striking, was so long disbelieved, merely because in opposition to current ideas and common-place knowledge. The analogies of nature may be considered in favor of different species of malaria. Certain epidemic diseases, the probable effects of atmospheric influences, are also in favor of their existence, and especially what is known of that most remarkable and terrible of all diseases, cholera. This view of the subject it may be well to keep in mind, as it imparts to it a peculiar interest and importance, and gives additional motive to engage in the careful investigation of it.

I have dwelt so long on malaria on account of its vast importance in relation to the health of the soldier; and, for the same reason I shall venture to extend my remarks.

Although entirely ignorant, as I believe we are, of the true nature of malaria, we have learnt by experience many circumstances which prove its operation, and some of the best means of avoiding its effects. It seems to be principally active by night, or when the sun is below the horizon; those who are employed in the night air being most subject to the fevers which it produces. The evidence in proof of this is very strong. In the Ionian Islands and in most parts of the Mediterranean, where the hot dry weather of summer sets in after the snows have disappeared from the mountains, the inhabitants, especially the working class, are much in the habit of sleeping in the open air, partly for the sake of coolness and the avoiding the torment of insects which abound in their dirty dwellings, and partly for the purpose of protecting their garden and field-crops from nightly depredations. These people are particularly subject to the fevers under consideration, and in a much greater degree than the higher ranks who sleep in their beds under cover. And amongst our troops there is a similar difference between the common soldiers and the officers. From 1821 to 1834 inclusive, the 51st Regiment, serving in these islands, lost eighty-one men from remittent fever, and only one officer, who fell a victim to the disease the first summer. According to the returns in the statistical reports of our army, the mortality from fever amongst the soldiers during a period of twenty years on the same station, was thirteen yearly per 1,000, whilst amongst the officers during a period of seventeen years inclusive, estimating their aggregate strength at 2,506, the total mortality from fever was only ten.* The common soldiers, like the peasantry, are much exposed to the night air— the officers little; the former on duty or guard: and independent of this, which is unavoidable, many of them, from the crowded state of the barracks, and from the rooms being infested with

---

* That is about 5 per 1,000, instead of 13 amongst the men,—an estimate in which there can hardly be any fallacy, as the fevers which prove fatal are rapidly so, not giving time for removal and for return home on sick leave.

fleas and bugs, are tempted to come out and sleep in the open air. I am speaking of what the barracks *were*, and the habits of the soldiery during a *past* period! In Italy, especially in the Roman States and in the vicinity of Rome, the harvest is gathered in by laborers who come from a distance for the purpose, and who, during the period of harvest, sleep exposéd at night. Fever (*la periodica*) every year is more or less prevalent amongst them, and is often very destructive; whilst amongst the factors of the great landed proprietors, who live on the estates, we are assured that those who avoid exposure to the night air escape fever and enjoy good health.* In Ceylon, during the period of the rebellion which broke out in October, 1817, and was not subdued till October of the following year, our troops were tolerably exempt from fever so long as they were chiefly employed by day, and no longer; so soon as they were employed more by night than by day, particularly in convoys and the relieving of posts, fever became very prevalent and terribly destructive.† The natives of that island, no doubt warned by experience, carefully avoid the night air, and in the interior commonly have a fire in the sleeping-rooms. The temple of Kattragam, in Ceylon, is situated in one of the most unwholesome districts of that island, and which there is reason to believe has been converted into a desert by the destructive effects of fever. It is a place of pilgrimage, and a large number of pilgrims are reported to be swept off annually by the disease. Yet the officiating priest, a Brahmin, had resided there many years during the worst season, and with impunity. When I visited the temple, I found him in good health,

---

* Some interesting details on this subject are to be found in a treatise "Sull' origine delle intermittenti di Roma e sua Campagna," by the experienced Dr. Giacomo Folchi, senior physician to the great hospital S. Spirito.

† At one station in the outlying district of Welasse, every white soldier sent there was attacked with fever, with the exception of the officer commanding and the medical officer in charge, who were least exposed to the night air: the mortality was terrible; out of about 254 men, as many as 209 died, 45 only escaping alive. (See Stat. Report on Sickness among Troops in Ceylon, page 11, where details will be found.) The only special precaution taken by the two officers was to wash from head to foot daily with soap and water: this I learnt from the assistant-surgeon, and he laid stress on it; and they avoided exposure to the night air. I recollect another instance during the same rebellion almost on a par with the preceding: a party of about 70 strong was formed of picked men from the light companies of two or three regiments, at head-quarters in Kandy, for the purpose of relieving a post in danger of falling into the hands of the enemy. They had to fight their way there and back, sleeping one night in the open air. After their return every man was taken into hospital with fever, with the exception of the commanding officer, and very many of them died.

active and energetic, though of the sparest form. The only precaution, I could learn, which he took to guard against fever, was sleeping in an inner room, without windows, having a fire in the middle of it on the floor, behind which, on leopards' skins, he lay at night, so that the outer air before it could reach him must have passed through or over the fire.*

Dr. Allan in his account of the remittent fever of the African Islands—viz., Madagascar and the surrounding islands, including the Seychelle group, adduces some facts equally strong of exemption from this very destructive malady by avoiding the stopping on shore at night. " It is deserving of notice (he remarks) that all who slept on board ship escaped : every victim seen or heard of had passed one night on shore ; and no instance of recovery was known in those who were taken on board affected." He adds :—" The writer had a vessel of a hundred tons moored within the reef at Foul Point (on the east coast of Madagascar) under his charge, mainly for the purpose of protection from sickness. Such as remained in her all night were quite healthy ; but no one slept on shore with impunity. The same occurred everywhere else.† The natives there, like the Singalese, it would appear, endeavour to protect themselves from the fever by avoiding the night air and by having fires in their sleeping-rooms. Dr. Allan, speaking of the little faith the Madagascans have in their own remedies, remarks :—" Their grand object is, when compelled to domicile in the low countries, to prevent attack. For this purpose, believing that the cause of all the evil is a *Tanghuin* (an indigenous vegetable poison) in the atmosphere, and that this poison can only be destroyed by fire, as it rises from the earth during the night, every house has in the centre of each apartment a raised box of sand on which wood is kept smouldering after sunset."

Next to the avoidance of the night air in regard to prevention, the due attention to clothing, is perhaps most important,—indeed the two have frequently been coupled together in degree of importance. Thus, Dr. Folchi, in his treatise already quoted,

* When I visited this wild and beautiful part of Ceylon, it was in the dry season, that commonly the unhealthy season, as it proved to us, for we were soon under the necessity of breaking up our party and hastening to the hill-country, from fever attacking our followers.

† Observations on some of the Predominant Diseases of the African Islands. By J. B. Allan, M.D. Monthly Journal of Medical Science for August, 1811.

when comparing the condition of the peasantry engaged in the labor of the harvest, as a prey to fever from lying out and but thinly clad, with that of their superintendents, remarks :—" It is a well-known fact that some of the latter, inhabiting spots the most insalubrious that are in the Roman territory, have kept their health perfectly good for many years by the precaution of retiring to their houses in the early evening, closing the windows and warming the apartment; not going out in the morning until the sun is high, and then protected by a good cloak."

The imprudence of sleeping out is frequently combined with that of throwing off part of the clothing for the temporary gratification of coolness, without consideration of consequences, especially in the hottest weather. Our soldiers are particularly thoughtless in this respect. When heated and perspiring on fatigue or other duty, so soon as they are at liberty they are apt to throw off their coat and perhaps their shirt, and for the sake of coolness expose themselves to the wind ; and, often half-un-dressed they will quit the guard-room or the barrack, when they are unable to sleep on account of the close oppressive heat, and seek repose in the open air. The effect, it is easily conceived, may be injurious and favorable to the operation of malaria and other malefic causes. In the Ionian Islands, taking their climate as an example, the night air is commonly dry during the period of drought and heat; no dew forms ; the difference between the moist and dry thermometer according to my obser-vations, varies with the land winds from 12° to 20°, and conse-quently, the degree of evaporation is considerable, and the cool-ing effect proportional. In Malta, with a south-west wind,—a wind blowing from the African desert, I have seen the difference of the two even greater, as much as 30°, the dry bulb-thermo-meter exposed to the air in the shade rising to 105°, the wet bulb falling to 75°.

By many respectable authors flannel has been recommended as a means of protection against malaria ; and, I am disposed to think justly, inasmuch as in common with cotton, but in a more marked manner, it possesses the property, when worn next the skin of a perspiring person, of moderating heat : this by a double function—by the evaporation which it allows from its outer sur-face, and the absorption of the perspired fluid, the sweat, by its inner,—the one cooling, the other warming or evolving heat, thereby, jointly, producing a happy medium effect. The chief objection to flannel for the use of the common soldier is its greater cost than cotton, its less strength in wear, and its less fitness for washing. For these reasons, when not in active service in the field, cotton, coarse soft cotton shirts may be deserving of preference. When I have compared the health of corps in a warm climate, such as that of Malta, some wearing flannel, others cotton, I have not noticed any well marked difference,— but then these regiments had only light easy garrison duty to perform. It would be for the advantage of the service, I believe, on the score of health, were the soldier, as in the United States' army, provided with under clothing at the public expense.[*]

It is commonly supposed that persons fasting are most susceptible of the agency of malaria; and, from general observation, I am inclined to think that the opinion is well founded. Perhaps the comparative exemption of officers from fever may be partly owing to their fast being earlier broken than that of the men, and to the principal meal, dinner, being taken by them at a later hour. The meal hours of the common soldiers are indeed very unfavorable to health, especially where malaria prevails. They rise early, with the early dawn, are often exercised before sunrise without eating; they breakfast at seven or eight; dine at one, and till recently,[†] having had no regular meal after one, they—I am speaking of the past—commonly fasted until the following morning; so that both early and late they were exposed to the air, when it is unwholesome, with an empty stomach. It is a good practice, and generally followed by those who can command comforts in the East, to take a cup of strong coffee, or what may be better, a cup of good cocoa hot, with toasted bread, on rising, and breakfasting about two hours later, after taking exercise. And, were this practice followed in our army, and not merely an evening meal, but a good substantial one provided for the men (dinner then, luncheon at one p.m.,)

---

[*] At present the soldier on enlistment gets £1 bounty and a free kit, which includes all his clothing, upper and under—the latter 3 cotton shirts and socks. Afterwards his under-clothing is to be provided at his own expense.

[†] Now the evening meal is a regular and enforced meal, and not as before at the discretion of the commanding officer. In England 4d. a day is paid by each soldier for his commissariat ration (1lb. of meat and 1lb. of bread), and 4d. a day for improving the ration by vegetables, etc. The remaining 5d. the soldier has clear, unless under stoppage for under-clothing, etc.

it can hardly be doubted that the effects would be excellent both directly and indirectly,—directly by checking the disposition to be influenced by malaria, and indirectly by diminishing the temptation to resort of an evening to the canteen and wine and spirit shop and commit excess in drinking. Diet, too, in relation to prevention, as well as the time of eating, there is reason to believe, is of some importance; and that kind of diet is best adapted to enable the constitution to resist malaria, which is most conducive to general vigorous health, and of which animal food, fresh meat with good bread, forms a considerable part; living rather above than below par during any unhealthy season; and, if attainable, using sound wine after dinner or supper in moderation. Abstemiousness, perhaps, is even more injurious than slight excess in eating and drinking; but as there is little disposition to undue abstemiousness, it is sufficient to give the hint that when malaria is dreaded the drink should not be water alone, nor the diet poor. By some authors, I cannot but think that too much stress has been laid on intemperate habits in con- nection with the fatal effects of the remittent fever of hot climates. It is not uncommon to hear it said that in the West Indies and on the Western Coast of Africa, the dreadful mortality that occasionally occurs there is more owing to the intemperance of the sufferers than to the intensity of the malaria. The mere circumstance of the periodical nature of the disease, the habits of the individuals being the same, is a sufficient refutation of the allegation. That intemperance is injurious to the general health is most certain, and conducive to organic changes likely to ter- minate in serious disease, especially of the brain and liver; but experience does not seem to prove that it at all conduces to attacks of the fever in question. I am more disposed to the contrary conclusion, partly from witnessing that men of appa- rently the best constitutions, seem to be most susceptible of the malaria influence; and partly from observing in fatal cases, on *post mortem* examination, how comparatively rare are the organic complications, conveying to me the idea that the existence of tubercles of the lungs or of serious organic lesion of a chronic kind of any other viscus, may act as a protection against malaria and secure the constitution against its influence. Now that at length an earnest exertion is being made to improve the health of the army, it is to be hoped that the subject of the soldiers' rations will have due consideration, and that they will be regulated not by a uniform scale, but, as much as possible, according to circumstances of climate and duty. The inquiries recently made into prison dietaries have afforded very instructive results,* and may supply some good data to any Commission appointed to regulate the diet of the soldier. Two principles at least seem to be well established,—one, that of variety of food,—not the same day after day, as in the old ration ;—the other, the proportioning the supply to the waste, increasing the quantity of sustenance in some ratio with the exertion and fatigue to be undergone. Crimean war-experience, the early and the late, the disastrous and the prosperous, afford memorable, most impressive lessons on the subject of army-diet.

The choice of sites for barracks and their construction is another subject which it is to be hoped will now have due consideration on the same score—that of the health of our troops. Hitherto, unfortunately, medical officers have been little consulted in the matter; too frequently these buildings have been placed in low situations difficult to drain, and not unfrequently in notoriously unhealthy spots, and their construction has been such as no sanitary officer would approve. Considering the mystery of malaria as to its cause, I believe the only principle that can be followed with safety in selecting a site for a barrack, or hospital, or encampment is, when attainable, experience of its salubrity, as denoted by the healthy aspect of the inhabitants on or near the locality, and the assurance of the absence of miasmatic disease. When such experience is not procurable, then the judgment must be exercised as to the probable salubrity of the spot, and advice given accordingly.

In the naval service prophylactics have been employed with benefit on stations where malaria has been dreaded, as on the western coast of Africa, where the sulphate of quinine in wine has been the chief one used. In the army generally, or in any large force in the field, this would hardly be practicable; but occasionally, when small parties of troops are employed on special service at night in malarious situations, it might no doubt be had recourse to with practical ease and with great advantage.

* See report on Effect of Prison Diet and Discipline upon the Bodily Functions of Prisoners. By Dr. E. Smith, F.R.S.; and Mr. Milner, in Proceedings of the British Association for the Advancement of Science, for 1861.

As the range of malaria, it is ascertained, is often extremely limited, the most certain method to avoid its effects is by leaving the spot where it has shown itself. Sometimes removal to a few hundred yards may suffice to give security, as has been witnessed at Gibraltar, and so remarkably at Foul Point, on the coast of Madagascar, in the instance already referred to described by Dr. Allan,—and as has been witnessed in the West Indies, especially in Barbadoes. Commonly a situation can be found within a few miles, which either from difference of elevation, or of exposure, or separation by water, is likely to have an untainted atmosphere. The importance of change of place, when destructive fevers are prevalent, cannot be too much insisted on. Removal is the only measure that can be calculated on with any confidence; and officers in command on whom the distribution of large bodies of men may depend, whether in the field or in garrison, have much to answer for, who, under medical advice, do not carry into effect this principle of security to the utmost limit that prudence, based on military considerations, permits. How many thousands of lives have been sacrificed in our West Indian possessions to tenacity of position!

I have classed yellow fever with those associated with malaria, believing, as I do, that in the great majority, if not in all instances, it owes its origin to a certain something existing in the atmosphere.

Whether it be contagious or not is a difficult question to answer. I am disposed to think that it is not. Those who are interested in the question will find it discussed at some length in Dr. Blair's monograph on this disease and in the notes which I have added to it. They will find also much interesting and valuable information on the subject in the " Papers relating to Quarantine;" which have been communicated during the last two or three years, and printed by order of the House of Commons. The literature of the disease I need hardly remark is vast, and especially that part of it relating to the *questio vexata* of contagion.

On the pathology of fevers, that most obscure subject on which so much has been imagined and so much has been written, I have little to say, having extremely little information to give. The lesions discovered in the fatal cases in the several forms of these diseases seem inadequate in a strict manner to account

for the event, and much less for the phenomena of each, such
as the state of the spleen in intermittents, the state of the
mucous follicles in the ileum, Peyer's glands in typhoid fever
and the remittents of warm climates, or the state of the
vascular system and its capillaries in yellow fever.* And, as
to the fluids, I am not aware of any exact observations to justify
the conclusion that these are *primarily* affected. In the instance
of yellow fever, so far as the blood corpuscles were concerned, I
could not detect any change in their form whether examined
early or late.†

That the several kinds of fever are allied to each other, and
run into each other, seems to be pretty well established. Their
symptoms and the *post mortem* lesions are equally in favor of
this ; so much so, that it might be plausibly maintained that
they are not species distinct, but merely varieties,—typhus in
one climate passing into typhoid in another climate or temperature, and typhoid into remittent and remittent into continued
and yellow fever. Plausible, however, as this view may be,
there are not wanting arguments in favor of a certain distinctness of species, as, as before observed, the occurrence of remittents where agues are almost unknown, the occurrence of yellow
fever where remittents and agues are rare, and the prevalency of
continued fever at times and in countries when and where the
other forms of fever are little known. Further, distinctions are
observable in their progress and terminations and sequelæ. We
do not expect organic disease after ordinary continued fever,
nor after yellow fever ; but we are not surprised at meeting

---

* As described by Dr. Blair in his last essay on the disease, viz.—a loss of substance of the extreme vessels allowing the blood to escape. See Report of the Recent
Yellow Fever Epidemic of British Guiana. By D. Blair, M.D., etc. London, 1856,
and the Brit. and For. Med. Chir. Review of the same year. Microscopic preparations made by Dr. Blair, illustrative of this lesion, are now deposited in the Pathological Museum at Fort Pitt.

† The following are the few observations of which I have notes :—

Barbadoes, Jan. 20th, 1848.—Cummins, moribund of yellow fever. A few drops
of blood were taken by a puncture with a lancet in the arm, and received into a solution of common salt with which I had tried my own blood; seen with a $\frac{1}{8}$-inch
object glass an hour after, the definition of the corpuscles was distinct and normal,
varying in diameter from $\frac{1}{4000}$ to $\frac{1}{3000}$ of an inch in diameter.

Dooling, ill of the same disease since the 17th, the blood corpuscles similar.

Foolingham, ill since the 18th ; his blood the same.

Wall, ill since the 19th ; the corpuscles somewhat smaller ; few exceeded $\frac{1}{4000}$;
some were about $\frac{1}{5000}$ and they seemed somewhat thicker, than ordinary.

with them after agues and remittent fevers. Yellow fever, further, is in a marked manner different from remittent in rapidity of convalesence, in little tendency to relapse, or to occur more than once during life.

Whether any inference can be made relative to their nature from the races of men in their degree of liability to suffer from them, is doubtful. The African appears to be in a great measure exempt from yellow fever; but so also commonly, though not always, is the white acclimated creole of the West Indies. The African, too, is little liable to ague and remittent fever, from which the white creoles in the West Indies, the colored natives of Ceylon and India and the Malays, though not so liable as the white northern races, are far from altogether exempt, thus serving to show that acclimation as to exemption has a powerful modifying influence; and this seems confirmed by the fact that the African negro by residing in a cool climate acquires a susceptibility to contract these fevers little inferior to that of the white creole.*

One quality seems to be common to all fevers—a want of tonicity, a certain weakening of the organisation, and this apart from inflammatory action. And, amongst other circumstances, is not this indicated by the serous condition of the urine, which has been observed now so generally in this class of diseases?

On the medical treatment I have little to state. So long as their nature is obscure, their treatment can hardly be otherwise than empirical.

I may pass over, under this head, intermittents and common continued fever,—the one commonly so readily yielding to quinine and arsenic; the other mostly so mild, or at least attended with so little danger, that in the majority of cases, recovery would ensue even were no medicine used.

As regards the severe and more dangerous forms of fever,

* Dr. Blair writing from his experience of yellow fever in British Guiana, states that the negro cook on board Nova Scotia and United States' traders was susceptible of taking the disease, and the dusky South Sea Islander, if prepared by a previous northern residence. He adds—"The lower the isochiemal curve of his native country or home, the more virulent was the attack of the epidemic on the subject of it." Illustrating this as follows :—" Thus, while the per centage of mortality among West India Islanders, in the Seaman's Hospital (George Town, Demerara) was 6·9, that of French and Italians was 17·1, that of English, Irish and Scotch was 19·3 ; that of Germans and Dutch was 20, and that of Swedes, Norwegians and Russians was 27·7"—Blair on Yellow Fever, p. 159.

remittent and yellow fever, judging from such experience as I have had, witnessing the trials that have been made of various modes, anxiously and carefully observed, I cannot say that I have seen any happy general results, any tolerable uniform success, from any special method. At present it is more easy to point out what is injurious than what is beneficial, at least in the heroical way. It is proved, I believe, by extensive experience that blood-letting, except in small quantities and under peculiar circumstances, is decidedly injurious. Experience too, as far as I can learn, is against the use of calomel or of any form of mercury given with intent to produce ptyalism. Quinine in large doses has had its advocates, and in some endemics, especially in the West Indies, combined with calomel, it has occasionally been decidedly successful; whilst in other it has failed. Its success has been most marked at those stations in which intermittents are prevalent, such as British Guiana and Tobago, and least so, at stations most exempt from ague, such as Barbadoes.* Were I to speak from my own convictions, I should be disposed to recommend the mildest treatment, watching the symptoms and the attempting the relief of them, paying particular attention to the bowels and their evacuations, administering, when needed, the gentlest aperients, especially the oleaginous. Nursing in all fevers is of the first importance. When the disease is at all severe, the patient should be kept strictly in the horizontal posture; a bed-pan should be used: many instances have come to my knowledge of sudden and unexpected death, apparently from syncope produced by the change to an erect posture, especially after an alvine evacuation.

Dr. Jackson recommended gestation, locomotion, as a curative means, and proposed a carriage of a peculiar and suitable construction for the purpose. That it would be beneficial, I have little doubt—the difficulty would be to make it practicable.†

---

* In the "Statistical Report on the Sickness and Mortality in the Army of the United States from January, 1839, to January, 1855," is to be found much valuable information on the effects of quinine administered in large doses, especially in fevers, such as are prevalent in the Southern States and of malarious origin. See appendix from page 638 to 690. The results described are favorable to its free use in these maladies, and accord with the earlier experience of Dr. Blair.

† As confirmatory of this practice, I may mention that I have always found that carriage exercise has had a lowering effect on the temperature of the heart's action. The observations I have made on this subject may be found in two papers, one on the temperature of man in England; the other on the temperature of man within the tropics.—Phil. Trans. for 1845 and 1850.

Sustenance, the supplying of food and proper drink, is not the least important part of the treatment. The adage is now given up of starving a fever. The danger seems rather that too much food will be given and too much stimulus in drink. The regulating of these will test the ability of the practitioner.

In considering the subject of treatment, it should ever be kept in mind that not only in different situations and countries, but also in different years, these diseases, whatever the form of fever, may vary more or less, and if not in type and character, at least in intensity and complications, so that the remedial means which may have been found useful in one endemic may fail in another, each, it may be, having a constitution of its own. We are told by Sydenham how difficult he found it on the breaking out of an epidemic to determine on the best mode of practice to be pursued, and how he came to a decision only after " *ingenti adhibita cautela intentisque animi nervis,*"—an example this well deserving of being followed.

CHAPTER II.

ON DYSENTERY.

Observations as to Climate and Causes.—Illustrative Cases of the Acute and Chronic kind.—Description of Symptoms.—Suggestions as to the Prevention of the Disease.—Remarks on its treatment.

OF all the diseases to which troops are subject on active service, especially abroad, dysentery is one of the most formidable and important; and, this almost equally on account of its frequency, its severity, the difficulty of its treatment, and its proportionally great mortality.

The circumstances productive of it seem to be many and various, and are probably better ascertained, and are in part more under control, than the causes of most other diseases. The following are some of those respecting which there seems to be least doubt :—1. High temperature. 2. Food deficient in nutritive power. 3. Water, that used for drinking, of impure quality. These three, in a campaign, especially a protracted one, and in a warm climate, are commonly more or less associated. With them too frequently are associated other conditions, exercising a deleterious influence, such as great fatigue, exposure to the night air and to its chilling influence, lying on the damp ground, privation of adequate rest, often scanty supplies of food, as well as bad food, tending altogether to weaken the powers of the system and produce a cachetic state peculiarly prone to dysenteric attack.

The medical records of the British army afford ample examples in illustration of the circumstances enumerated.

As to temperature, it is very remarkable how much more frequent is the occurrence of the disease in hot than in temperate and cold climates, and how much more intractable and fatal it is in the former than in the latter. This is well shown in the following table, calculated for an aggregate strength of 10,000 men, deduced from these records, exhibiting the numbers of those attacked and of those who died at the different stations named, during the periods specified ; the first column of figures gives the admissions into hospital, the second the deaths from the disease, acute and chronic :—

United Kingdom, Dragoon Guards and Dragoons, from 1st Jan. 1830 to 31st March, 1837		... ...	14·8	...	1·5
Nova Scotia and New Brunswick, from	1817 to 1836		52·5	...	3·8
Canada	,,	ditto ,, ditto	151·6	...	5·9
Malta	,,	ditto ,, ditto	343·1	...	23·0
Ionian Islands	,,	ditto ,, ditto	534·6	...	24·3
Gibraltar	,,	1818 ,, 1836	440·1	...	10·6
Bermudas	,,	1817 ,, 1836	1494·7	...	30·7
Western Coast of Africa	,,	1819 ,, 1836	120·0	...	23·8
St. Helena...............................	,,	1818 ,, 1821	1271·1	...	116·8
Cape of Good Hope—Cape District	,,	1818 ,, 1836	583·3	...	14·9
,, Frontiers do.	,,	1822 ,, 1834	343·9	...	16·6
,, Hottentot Troops	,,	ditto ,, ditto	314·3	...	38·4
,, Mauritius	,,	1818 ,, 1836	1776·1	...	93·4
West Indies—Windward and Leeward Islands Command—					
	,,	1817 ,, 1836	2058·8	...	157·7
,, Black Troops	,,	ditto ,, ditto	386·7	...	48·9
Jamaica	,,	ditto ,, ditto	951·9	...	35·7
,, Black Troops	,,	ditto ,, ditto	164·0	...	19·0
Ceylon	,,	ditto ,, ditto	2210·1	...	231·0
Malays—1st Ceylon..................	,,	1818 ,, 1836	328·0	...	47·6
Moelmyne, in Tenasserim Provinces	,,	1827 ,, 1836	2141.4	...	200·9
Rangoon, in the Burmese Empire, from 21st April, 1824, to 20th March, 1825		... ...	11288	...	1960·7

That high temperature is concerned in the production of the disease seems to be sufficiently shown by this table, seeing the accord there is between the prevalency and fatality of the disease, and the degree of elevation of atmospheric temperature. The same is indicated by its greater prevalency in the hot months than in the cold in those countries possessing a hot and cold season ; or even a hot and cool season, such as, to instance the former, the British North American possessions : and the latter, such as Gibraltar, Malta and the Ionian Islands. At the same time it is equally clear from the same table that other circumstances besides atmospheric heat operate in generating the disease, the ratio of its amount not being strictly in accordance with the elevation of temperature. Ceylon affords an example, comparing it with our West Indian Colonies, and more especially with Ceylon itself, taking the victims of dysentery in that island at different times under different circumstances ; thus, during one triennial period—1817-18-19, the cases admitted into hospital per 10,000 of the aggregate strength, were 2,609, of whom 390 died; whilst during another equal period, 1834-35-36, the number from the same aggregate admitted was 1297; the deaths 177. The differences in the circumstances of the two periods were remarkable. During a great part of the first period rebellion prevailed in the Kandyan provinces, and the inadequate force employed in suppressing it was overworked, ill-fed and subjected to all kinds of privations,—in brief, was exposed to a complication of causes, which in their direct and indirect influences are generally admitted to be most operative in the production of the disease. During the second period there was peace throughout the country, salt meat no longer formed a part of the men's rations, they had no longer to perform night and forced marches,—in brief they were exempted from the agency of the many extra causes to which they were almost unavoidably exposed during the rebellion. The vast prevalency of the disease and its terrible fatality amongst the troops employed in the Burmese war, may be adduced in confirmation,—as might also the destruction from the disease amongst the troops during the greater portion of the period of the siege of Sebastopol,—especially compared with the happy change which took place in the health of the same army as soon as its wants as to diet, shelter, and clothing were properly attended to.

That the quality of diet and the quality of the water used for drink, apart from other causes, may be concerned in generating the disease, there are facts, and not a few, which are tolerably conclusive. One great fact is, that the officers of our army, who are provided with good and nourishing food, and who use commonly wine and beer, are in a great measure exempt from the disease. The army returns show this in a remarkable manner: even in Ceylon, during the three years of the rebellion, the loss of officers from dysentery was small; and at that time, some of them at distant outposts fared but little better as to diet and drink than the men. In the Mediterranean, at the several stations where the officers are well quartered, and have the best of food and wine at their luxurious mess-tables, dysentery amongst them is rare indeed; during the many years that I served there, I do not recollect a single fatal case. And, the same remark applies nearly to the officers in the West Indies; during the three years and a half that I was there, I remember only one fatal case, and that was of an officer who before had suffered severely from dysentery in Ceylon.

Whenever salt meat is used in excess and for a continuance, there all experience shows that dysentery will be more or less prevalent and of a bad character. In the West Indies, in the Windward and Leeward Command, at one time, early in this century, the troops were supplied with fresh meat, only twice a week. The salt meat ration, to which they were confined the other five days, of low nourishing powers, whilst it did not satisfy the healthy appetite, excited thirst, to allay which water, with little regard paid to its quality, if scanty, was drunk in excess, too often mixed with the unwholesome new rum of the country, productive of drunkenness, undermining the health and morals of the men. In the records of the Inspector's office in Barbadoes, by every successive officer from the time of Drs. Jackson and Ferguson, to the time I had charge, the evil effects of salt provisions are dwelt on, and the use of fresh meat and of a better quality than that supplied urged, but with partial success only, that of diminishing the evil,—the salt-rations from five times a week being curtailed to three times. In Jamaica, where the troops were better fed, having had whilst supplied at the expense of the colonial government from 1817 to 1833 a larger allowance of fresh meat, and I believe of a superior quality, there, as is shown by the table, the disease was far less frequent and greatly less fatal than in the other islands, notwithstanding the little difference of climate, the similarity of duties and of other circumstances likely to affect the health.

The evidence we have of the injurious action of impure water is not so strong as the foregoing, yet I think it is tolerably conclusive. I shall make mention of a few facts which have come to my knowledge. The troops stationed at Morne Bruce in the Island of Dominica, were at one time very subject to bowel complaints; they suffered much from dysentery: this was when the garrison was supplied with water conveyed in an open conduit, liable to be rendered impure by the washing of clothes in it, etc.; as soon as it was covered over, the impurities excluded, the occurrence of the disease was arrested; from that time at least it ceased to be endemic. In the Island of Antigua, where there are few springs, and rain water collected in tanks is much used, dysentery has always been of common occurrence during a period of drought. During a period of the kind, when the disease was prevalent in the principal town, St. John's, a vessel touching there took in a supply of water; all of the crew using it were, as I learnt from the master, attacked either with diarrhœa or dysentery. In 1845, a year of unusual drought, when during 51 days no rain fell, and during other 40 very little, four companies of the 71st Regiment, stationed at the "Ridge" barracks in the same island, and using tank water—its dregs— in less than twelve months lost 52 men from dysentery and diarrhœa.* I examined a portion of the water; I found it abounding in impurities, especially infusoria,—justifying the term dregs. The tanks, which had but little attention paid to them previously for a long while, were cleaned out, replenished as soon as the usual rains set in, and then yielding a purer water, the endemic subsided. In Barbadoes, ponds of standing water are common. These, when covered with a greenish scum, to which they are liable during an unusually dry season, are con- sidered by the natives unfit for drinking use; they are believed to be poisonous to cattle, horses and poultry. I examined the scum from one of them; amongst other impurities I found it too to abound in infusoria. It is right to keep in mind that during a period of drought in a hot climate, when water becomes scarce and men are put on a short allowance, they are tempted to get it from any source, however impure. Nor should it be for- gotten that during such a season there are other circumstances predominating of a nature to promote the production of the disease. Owing to the parched herbage, cattle are ill fed, and in consequence the ration-meat is often of a more than ordinarily objectionable quality. The vicissitudes of temperature then are commonly unusually great; high by day, comparatively low by night, and, in consequence, men going out of their close and hot barrack-rooms† to obey the calls of nature into open, exposed privies, such as those at the Ridge, were peculiarly subject to be chilled, to have their perspiration—their skin moist with

---

* During the quarter ending the 31st October, out of a strength of 390, there were 141 cases of dysentery in hospital, of which 21 proved fatal.

† The closeness and ill-ventilation of soldiers' barracks are now, since the inquiry following the war in the Crimea, known even to the public: the barracks in the West Indies were few of them an exception; in some of them the cubic space per man was under 500 feet. In 1820, at Barbadoes, the head-quarters of the command, at a time that hammocks were used, no more than a width of 7 feet was allowed for 4 hammocks.

sweat—suddenly checked ;—a cause this, by itself, that may be and has been considered adequate to the production of the malady.

These few remarks on the causes of dysentery are offered as an introduction to the cases which I am about to detail.

The fatal cases of which I have notes are 85 ; of these 35 were called acute, 50 chronic. The average age of the men, the subjects of the former, was 35 years ; of the youngest 18, of the oldest 45. Of the latter, the average was 38·6 years, of the youngest 22, of the oldest 57 :—differences these as to age which might reasonably be expected, reflecting on the character of the disease, in its acute and chronic form.

The duration of the disease in the acute cases, reckoning from the time of admission into hospital to the fatal event, was on an average 13 days, the shortest was 2 days, the longest 51 days ; when more prolonged, the disease, it may be inferred, had its designation changed to that of chronic dysentery.

Of the chronic kind, as to duration, an average can hardly be given : the cases, of which I have notes, varied in their persistence from two or three months to many years.

In a great majority of instances both of the acute and chronic kind, complications existed ; organic lesions, apart from those of the large intestines, were detected, and of various kinds. Complicated with acute dysentery, the following lesions were most worthy of note, classed according to the organs in which they occurred :—

Liver—Abscess 1
Lungs—Tubercles and vomicæ 2
        Other lesions 3
Small intestines, chiefly ileum—Ulceration 5
Omentum and peritoneum—Thickening with marks of inflammation 16
Mesenteric and lumbar glands—Enlargement 12

Complicated with chronic dysentery, the following were the principal lesions :—

Lungs—Tubercles 4
    Tubercles and vomicæ 9
    Other lesions, œdema, hepatization, etc. 18
Liver—Abscess 5
Ileum and jejunum—Ulceration 1
Ileum   ditto 11
Longitudinal sinus—Fibrinous concretion softening 4
Vena portæ   ditto 1
Mesenteric and lumbar glands—Enlargement 3
Brain—Softening, etc. 6

The main lesions, those which are characteristic of dysentery, the lesions of the large intestines, I have not thought it necessary to give in the preceding tabulated form. I may briefly remark here *in limine* that in every fatal case of the acute disease, they (the large intestines) were found more or less ulcerated and otherwise disorganized ; and the same also with few exceptions, were seen in cases of the chronic kind. Dysentery, true dysentery, without ulceration, I believe to be rare, and most rare after the disease is established and has made progress : often, very often, I am persuaded, that even at its beginning,—when the symptoms have become distressing so as to compel the soldier to report himself sick and come into hospital, the ulcerative process is in activity, especially in the worst kinds of dysentery,—such as are rife amongst troops in a protracted campaign. In a cool climate and in the mildest forms of the disease, I can readily admit that a merely phlogosed state of the mucous membrane may be the pathognomonic state of the intestines at the outbreak of the malady.

1.—Of ACUTE DYSENTERY.—I shall now give some cases as examples of this most formidable disease. In the heading of each case, the more remarkable complication or complications will be noticed, without mention there of the state of the large intestines :—

Case 1.—Of acute dysentery, with thickened omentum and perforated colon.—C. Ailfounder, ætat. 26; admitted* 11th September, 1822; died 19th September.— This man on the day above mentioned was transferred from the Surgical Division of the General Hospital at Fort Pitt, where he had been under treatment for ophthalmia, to the Medical Division, on account of bowel complaint of some days' duration. He complained of acute pain in the umbilical region, increased by pressure, with severe griping, purging and tenesmus ; his stools were watery and mixed with blood ; pulse quick and small ; tongue loaded ; considerable thirst ; skin hot ; no appetite ; general health not previously affected ; castor oil 1 oz., with one grain of opium ; V.S. to 24 oz. ; had been blooded yesterday, but with no marked relief. September 12th— Blood not buffed ; symptoms much the same ; pain of abdomen continues ; castor oil ; opium a grain every hour. On the 13th the tormina and tenesmus were less severe ; other symptoms much the same ; a starch enema with opium ; calomel and opium—10 grs. of the former, 15 of the latter in pills ; a blister to abdomen ; castor oil. 14th—Symptoms much the same ; the same medicine. 15th—Mouth slightly affected by the mercury ; no decided amendment or change of symptoms. 16th— Pain of abdomen more severe, with increased tormina and tenesmus ; 12 leeches to abdomen. 17th—No amendment. 18th—Evidently sinking ; respiration hurried ; gums slightly ulcerated. 19th—Died at 4 p.m.

* When the station is not specified, it is to be understood that it is Fort Pitt, Chatham, and the General Hospital there.

Autopsy 20 hours after death. Body little emaciated; limbs rigid; abdominal viscera still warm; the pleura of a light red hue and vascular as if injected; the lungs red, turgid with blood and serum; the bronchia dark red, covered with puruloid matter; the lower portion of omentum a little thickened and adhering to the beginning of rectum, the latter misplaced to the right side, as was also the descending colon;—the bladder distended with urine, projected on the left side; the peritoneal coat of the jejunum, ileum and colon very vascular; the large intestines were much distended with fluid and flatus. On moving the transverse colon an ulcerated opening was found in its inferior surface large enough to admit three fingers, and were it not for the nice adaptation of parts, the contents of the intestines must have passed into the cavity of the abdomen during life. The large intestines throughout were severely diseased, exhibiting thickening, ulceration and sloughing of the worse kind. The thickening was most about the rectum, the sloughing in the cœcum and transverse colon; in some places the muscular coat was laid bare, in others both the mucous and muscular were destroyed, the peritoneal only left; and in one (the transverse colon) even this coat was destroyed.

This case was from its beginning to its termination, note-worthy for its severity and intractable nature. The blood-letting weakened without affording relief. The opium so largely given, might have increased the thirst; it hardly allayed pain; it had no hypnotic effect;—the mercury affected the mouth, without any beneficial result. Till a few hours before death there were no indications of any disease of lungs.

Case 2.—Of acute dysentery, with infarcted state of small intestine from coagulated milk.—Sergeant C. Wray, ætat. 30; 7th R.F ; admitted into regt. hospital, Malta, 31st October, 1831; died 11th November.—This man had been addicted to the use of ardent spirits; for some days before admission he had been laboring under bowel complaint. Now, Oct. 31st, has an almost continued desire to go to stool; tenesmus; castor oil and T. opii. Nov. 1st—Much abdominal pain during the night; many frothy bloody stools; tongue dry, white at the edges, dark red at the centre; a pill of calomel, opium and ipecac. every 2nd hour. Nov. 2nd—No improvement; retention of urine; two pints drawn off by catheter; pulse 64; no tenderness of abdomen on pressure. Nov 3rd—Stools extremely frequent; catheter still needed; the same medicine. Nov. 4th—Gums slightly affected; tongue cleaner and more moist. 5th—Stools less frequent, still bloody; no pain on pressure; skin soft; of natural temperature; pulse about 60, weak; is able to void his urine. For two or three days he appeared to be doing well, taking two grains of opium every 2nd hour, and this without any narcotic effect. Whilst his mouth was affected by mercury he passed coagulated blood. Once or twice his stools were scybalous and clay-colored; before death the evacuations became most offensive. It is stated that no marked change of symptoms preceded the fatal event.

Autopsy 12 hours after death. Body not emaciated; brain natural, fibrinous concretions in right cavities of heart; lungs apparently sound, collapsed; the stomach distended with air and fluid; the small intestines generally much distended with curd of milk, colored by yellow bile; the colon and gall-bladder adhering; the latter compressed by the distended colon contained merely a little greenish mucus; the large intestines thickened, ulcerated and sloughing; much lymph was deposited between their coats; they contained a reddish fluid of horrid odor, giving the idea of acridity, and actually occasioning a painful sensation in the nostrils; mixed with this sanies were small globular masses of coagulated blood, of considerable firmness, enveloped in a thin semi-transparent coating of lymph, and varying in size from that of a pea to that of a cherry; some ecchymosis towards the neck of the urinary bladder; an exudation of a reddish mucous fluid from the caput galinaginis.

In this case the low state of the pulse, the little pyrexia, and the little suffering, are noteworthy. The clogged state of the small intestines is specially worthy of notice; the effect could not but be deleterious: the patient had incautiously been allowed as much milk, on milk-diet, as he liked to drink; one day he had seven pints!

Case 3.—Of acute dysentery, with air in the anterior mediastinum, and partial hepatization of lung.—M. G. Angus, ætat. 22; 7th R.F.; admitted into regimental hospital, Corfu, 2nd September, 1825; died 10th September.—This man on admission had been three days previously ill, without reporting himself. Is much purged; has frequent bloody slimy stools, with tormina and tenesmus; abdominal pain on pressure; skin hot, pulse quick, urgent thirst; an anodyne draught; fomentation. Sept. 3rd—Relief from the fomentation; less pain of abdomen; otherwise no better; castor oil, calomel and opium. 4th—No improvement; the same medicine and a starch enema, with T. opii. 7th—No change for the better; a restless night; the stools still bloody and slimy; much debility; pulse 96; urgent thirst; complains now of distressing dyspnœa; the same medicine; sago, wine, chicken-broth. 8th—Breathing more difficult; the evacuations the same; a blister to abdomen; 1 grain of opium every 2nd hour. 9th—Is much worse; is constantly at stool; great debility and increased dyspnœa; chalk mixture with laudanum. 10th—Died at 3 a.m.

Autopsy 8 hours after death. Body not much emaciated; still warm; the anterior mediastinum distended with air; the posterior in a less degree; the cellular membrane round the great vessels redder than natural; a portion of the middle lobe of right lung red and hepatized; small masses like tubercles, judging from the feel, in the inferior lobe, but when cut into they showed the hepatized character; much blood in the superior lobe; the bronchia of this lung and also of the left, of a dark red, and contained a good deal of thin puriform fluid; the substance of left lung very red and gorged with blood; the omentum and portions of the ileum both externally and internally unduly red; the large intestines very much diseased, and most of all the lower portion of the colon and rectum; of a dark red color, they exhibited lines and patches of ulceration, intermixed with wart-like granulations and with thickening of their coats; some ulcerated spots in the cœcum; some of the mesenteric glands enlarged; the gall-bladder turgid with bile; the abdominal viscera not mentioned apparently sound.

This case is remarkable for its complications, and to these probably the fatal event was mainly owing. Whether a different mode of treatment might not have led to a different result, is open to question, especially after symptoms of pulmonary disease set in.

Case 4.—Of acute dysentery, without any distinct complication.—T. Coleman, ætat. 27; 73rd Regiment; admitted into regimental hospital, Malta, 3rd December, 1831; died 6th December.—A man of delicate constitution; subject to bowel complaints. On admission from Fort Tigné (an outpost), his appearance indicated illness of several days, yet he had been doing duty uninterruptedly. There was much prostration of strength; stools very frequent, bloody and slimy; much tenesmus; a small, quick pulse; brown tongue; castor oil. Dec. 4th—Stools of the same character; no improvement; calomel and opium; a blister to abdomen. 5th—Small black stools; says he is now free from pain and has no tenesmus; pulse 120; Ol. Ricini; calomel and opium. 6th—No improvement; stools very frequent; much tenesmus; pulse languid; some hiccough; the same medicine; the "countenance dejected; the skin clammy; the pulse sunk;" wine and water; starch enema. He died at midnight.

Autopsy 10 hours after death. Not emaciated; brain not examined; a quantity of brownish fluid in the bronchia, probably from the stomach; the great arch of stomach very red; the colon adhering to the gall-bladder and spleen; the large intestines throughout very much diseased, very tender, so as to require very gentle handling; in places ulcerated, and very generally encrusted with coagulable lymph.

This is a good example of the insidious progress of the disease, which, it can hardly be doubted, was fully formed before admission into hospital. The non-commissioned officer in charge at Fort Tigné, when questioned about the man, and his detention out of hospital, said he was known as an ailing man, and not having complained, he did not consider him ill.

Case 5.—Of acute dysentery, without any well marked complication.—Wm. Henderson, ætat. 23; 73rd Regiment; admitted in regimental hospital, Malta, 10th June, 1830; died June 17th.—This man on admission had been laboring under the ordinary symptoms of acute dysentery—viz., bloody stools, tormina, tenesmus, of some days' duration; a purgative, followed by Dover's powder; some relief. 13th— Reported convalescent; no medicine. 14th—Severe pain of abdomen; V.S. 2½ lbs.; Ol. Ricini; some immediate relief; stools bloody and slimy; towards evening aggravation of pain; pulse very rapid; V.S. 10 oz.; no more abstracted, syncope threatening, followed by cold clammy sweat; blood buffed; calomel and antimonial pill, with 1 gr. of opium; blister to abdomen. 15th—A very disturbed night; almost every half hour a bloody stool; pulse 128; skin cold and clammy; pain continues; a starch enema with opium; Ol. Ricini; calomel and opium. 16th—No amendment; stools the same; tenesmus; less abdominal pain; pulse 120; some nausea; Ol. Ricini; pulv. Doveri. 17th—A bad night; some hiccough; constant pain of abdomen. Died at 9 p.m.; a few hours before was comatose.

Autopsy 16 hours after death. Body pretty muscular; the brain rather soft, especially the corpora striata; about three ounces of serum in the pericardium; some liquid and coagulated blood in the left cavities of the heart; the right auricle much distended; the foramen ovale, obliquely open, admitting the little finger; when pressure was made on the left auricle blood flowed through the foramen into the right auricle; a little serous fluid in the cavity of the abdomen; a little coagulable lymph on sigmoid flexure of colon; no perforation; no pus; no adhesion of intestines; their peritoneal coat unduly red; so too the peritoneum generally; vast disease of colon; extensive ulceration; the muscular coat in many places laid bare; in many places sloughs separating, consisting of inner coat thickened by deposition of coagulable lymph; in many great thickening, from coagulable lymph effused in the cellular coat and on the mucous coat, with puruloid infiltration, but without ulceration, presenting yellowish elevated ridges in a transverse direction; the lumbar glands much enlarged; the hæmorrhoidal vessels gorged with blood; some green fluid in the stomach; the organs not mentioned tolerably sound.

In this case the amount of pain remarkable, and its sudden invasion, and the little effect of V.S. in relieving it. The lull, "the convalesence" reported on the 13th, noteworthy.

Case 6.—Of acute dysentery, without well marked complication, treated by large blood-letting.—Rd. Williamson, ætat. 26 ; 85th Regiment ; admitted into regimental hospital, Malta, September 25th, 1830 ; died September 27th.—This man some days before coming into hospital had been subject to diarrhœa. On admission there was great pain on pressure along the course of the colon ; much tenesmus ; much pyrexia ; V.S. 32 oz. ; syncope ; the blood slightly buffed ; 50 leeches to abdomen ; warm fomentation ; calomel gr. x., ext. opii gr. i. ; during the day very many stools with blood. Sept. 25—An exacerbation of pyrexia ; tenderness of abdomen continues ; purging severe through the night ; V.S. 25 oz. ; leeches 50 ; no relief followed ; calomel gr. xx., opii gr. ij. ; mercurial friction inside of thigh ; Vesp. can bear pressure ; febrile symptoms less ; less purged ; less tenesmus ; blister to abdomen. 26th—Incessant purging with tenesmus ; pulse rapid and feeble ; hydrag. c creta gr. x., bis indie, suppositorium c opii. gr. iij. 27th—In a state of collapse ; vital energies sinking ; died at 7 a.m.

Autopsy 4½ hours after death. Well-formed ; not emaciated ; brain not examined ; temperature under lobulus Spigelii and in left ventricle 101° ; a little serum in the iliac fossa, and a little coagulable lymph. The colon greatly diseased throughout, thickened, ulcerated and sloughing ; where free from ulceration, there the mucous coat was covered with a granular false membrane, soft and easily abraded.

A striking example this of the inefficiency of large depletion, when the disease is fully formed, as I believe it was on admission.

Case 7.—Of acute dysentery, with peritoneal inflammation.—J. Knowles, ætat. 31 ; 73rd Regt. ; admitted into regimental hospital, Malta, July 20th ; died July 24th.— A man of dissipated habits, subject to bowel complaints. On admission he had been four days ill ; stools bloody ; much tormina and tenesmus ; much debility ; pulse small ; tongue clean ; calomel and opium. July 21st—Tenesmus increased ; pulse full ; large quantities of sanies discharged ; V.S. followed by some relief ; calomel and opium. 22nd, 23rd—Each day worse. Died on the 24th.

Autopsy 4 hours after death. Body thin, but muscular ; a little œdema in posterior mediastinum ; right cavities of heart distended with blood and fibrinous concretions ; some purulent fluid and coagulable lymph in the cavity of the abdomen, principally in the iliac fossa ; in removing the cœcum, it appeared ruptured, but whether perforated before uncertain ; it probably was, and the cause of the peritoneal inflammation ; the inner coat of the cœcum and of the appendicula sloughing and gangrenous ; along the ascending, transverse and descending colon ulceration with thickening from effusion of lymph and pus in the cellular tissue ; the valvula coli partially destroyed ; in the upper part of the rectum, to the extent of the hand's width, the inner coat detached, still partially adhering, the muscular coat bare ; small portions of the intestines thin, and of a greyish hue, indicating old ulcers healed ; greenish fluid in the stomach and gullet ; the former exhibited the hour-glass contraction ; a little greenish bile in the gall-bladder ; spleen of natural size, soft, almost as soft as the crassamentum of blood.

The rapidity of this case remarkable. The disease, it can hardly be doubted, was fully formed on admission. It is astonishing how much organic disease can be borne without complete or even considerable prostration of strength, especially in instances of men of drunken habits, and even still more in instances of insanity.

Case 8.—Of acute dysentery, with perforated intestine and peritoneal inflammation.—Wm. Browning, ætat. 33; 80th Regiment; admitted into regimental hospital Malta, 2nd July, 1828; died 16th July.—This man on admission complained of purging of some days' duration; stools bloody; V.S. lb. ij.; Ol. Ricini; calomel gr. iv., ipecac. gr. iij., opii. griss h.s. July 3rd—An easy night; pulse 84; skin cool; tongue white; stools less bloody; solutio magnes. sulphat. (iij. oz. aquæ lib. ij.) i. oz. omni hora; the same opiate pill at night. 4th—Less griping and tenesmus; dislikes the salts; Ol. Ricini iv. drms., ter indie and rep. pil. h.s. 5th—Appears much better; the same medicine. 6th—Feels better; the same. 7th—Freely purged; stools improved, but still tinged with blood; pulse 96; tense; pain in colon on pressure; still some griping and tenesmus; V.S. lib. iij.; solutio magnes. sulphat. as before. 8th—Great relief; no pain; stools frequent, but without blood; very little tormina or tenesmus; thirst; pulse 100 soft; complains most of weakness; the solution every 2nd hour; beef tea. 9th—Bowels easy; pulse 112; appetite good; the solution to be continued with pulv. Doveri, gr. x. h.s. 10th—A good night; three stools, more natural; pulv. Doveri gr. x. ter indie. 11th—Stools still frequent; neither griping nor tenesmus; the same medicine; milk diet. Free from pain; not much purged; very thirsty; skin cool; pulse 116; pressure occasions little uneasiness; emplast. lyttæ abdomen.; the same powder; Vesp.; at times incoherent; pulse 118; no pain; four stools. 13th—A restless night; some delirium; pulv. Dov. gr. v. ter indie; chicken-broth. 14th—A better night; feels better; pulse 112; the same medicine. 15th—Eight stools, without tormina or tenesmus; feels better; pulse 108; the same. 16th—Still rather purged; stools less red, rather dark; no pain; tongue cleaner; still thirsty; pulse frequent, but not so weak; omitt. pulv., capt. calomel gr. i., ext. opii gr. js. ter indie; about 2 p.m. he became suddenly worse, with laborious breathing and increased debility. Died at 6 p.m.

Autopsy 17 hours after death. Rather emaciated; eyes very much sunk, features collapsed; brain not examined; fibrinous concretions and blood in the cavities of heart; the lining membrane of the larger blood-vessels stained dark red; the lungs pale; fluid effused with some drops of oil in the cavity of abdomen, from a minute perforation in the transverse colon; the colon throughout excessively diseased; most of its mucous membrane destroyed, sloughed off, leaving the muscular coat bare; the few shreds remaining gangrenous and black as ink; the small intestines loaded with a pultaceous substance, in some places mixed with air and light yellow; in others whitish; low down almost clay-colored, with some fæcal smell; their peritoneal coat generally redder than natural; the other viscera tolerably healthy.

The latency of organic disease in this case, the perforation of the intestines, the comparative mildness of the symptoms, the suddenness of the death, the little permanent good effect of the large abstraction of blood, very noteworthy. Was death owing to fibrinous concretions in the heart? The paleness of the lungs favors the conjecture.

Case 9.—Of acute dysentery, with inflammation of lower ileum.—William Egan, 2nd Battalion Rifle Brigade; admitted into regimental hospital, Malta, January 1, 1829; died January 7th—A man of dissipated habits, yet his general health previously good. On his admission he had symptoms of dysentery, but little tenesmus; no obvious constitutional disturbance. An emetic; calomel and opium at bed time. January 2nd—All the symptoms worse; V.S. xvii. oz.; fotus; Ol. Ricini c T. opii; calomel and opium. 3rd—Symptoms milder; unguent Hydrag. infrican.; opii grs. ij.; Ol. Ricini. 4th—Symptoms more urgent and distressing; pulse 96; countenance flushed; tenderness of abdomen; stools very frequent, bloody and fetid; much tormina and tenesmus; Hirudines xxx. abdomen; fotus; mercurial friction; opii i. grain 2da. q. q. hora; anodyne enema; emplastrum lyttæ. 5th— Free from pain; stools more bloody and putrid; countenance flushed; tongue very foul; slight nausea; skin cold and clammy; no appearance of ptyalism. 6th—No abatement of symptoms; the stools have become like the washings of raw meat, and are most offensive; the abdomen tympanitic; the skin below the natural temperature. He died the following day.

Autopsy 16 hours after death. Well made; little emaciated; coagulated blood and strings of coagulated lymph in the large vessels of the brain; some coagulated blood and polypi in the cavities of the heart of unusual firmness; notwithstanding, a little liquid blood collected from the internal jugular vein coagulated on exposure to the air; the coagulum very tender; the blood vessels and bronchia stained red; much blood in the inferior part of lungs; the colon adhering; lymph effused around the cœcum and lower portion of ileum; the large intestines excessively diseased, exhibiting the worst appearances, such as extensive ulceration, sloughs, and thickening; the small intestines and stomach much distended with air; an appearance of ulceration in the lower portion of ileum; after maceration, what seemed an ulcerated surface proved to be a rough patch of coagulable lymph; it was easily rubbed off, and, excepting an abrasion, the mucous coat there was smooth.

In this case, it may be inferred that extensive ulceration of the large intestines existed before admission, and was to a great extent latent.

Case 10.—Of acute dysentery, with perforation of intestine, and peritoneal inflammation.—William Guardam, ætat 26; 7th Regiment of Foot; admitted into regimental hospital, Malta, 13th August, 1833; died 21st August.—A sober man; in 1829, had acute catarrh; in 1830, cynanche tonsillaris; in 1832, at different periods, had colica, cholera, and icterus; in April, 1833, had a sharp attack of cholera, and again in July; on 13th August, after being on guard-duty, was admitted into hospital, complaining of purging, with griping and straining; stools scanty, mucous, and bloody; pulse natural; tongue moist and tolerably clean; skin cool; Ol. Ricini i. oz., T. opii m. x. 14th—Stools numerous, green, gelatinous, with frothy mucus; calomel xx. grs. opii i. gr. 15th—No change of symptoms; the bolus of calomel and opium again night and morning; a cold enema every third hour. 16th—Says he feels relieved by the cold injection; a good night. 17th—Purging recurred; stools firm and feculent, without blood; some tenderness of gums. 18th— Purging increased; stools liquid, bloody, offensive; one about every five minutes; cold injections cease to give relief; a nauseous taste in mouth; disposition to vomit; a thick brown fur on tongue; insatiable thirst, pulse quick, easily compressed; skin covered with sweat; pulv. ipecac. xxx. grs.; about a quart of pure bile vomited, with relief; purging returned towards evening; iced injections with T. opii; ext. opii i. grain, c aq. menth. pip. omni hora; stools less frequent. 19th—A tolerably good night; woke with singultus; purging troublesome; stools exceedingly offensive, gelatinous, bloody, with shreds of mucous membrane; pulse rapid and very small; tongue dry in the centre, and brown; urine turbid, passed with difficulty; profuse cold, clammy sweats on upper part of body; "*restlessness;*" "*insatiable thirst;*" opii ij. grs.; solution of gum arabic for drink; hiccup checked; less purging. 20th—A quiet night; two hours of sound sleep; only three stools during the night; less bloody and offensive, with a little feculent matter; pulse 130, feeble; tongue dry; sweating profuse; intense thirst, great debility; iced drinks; iced injections to be discontinued, not being retained; a suppository of opium, from which relief for a time. 21st—All night frequent gelatinous stools, with portions of mucous membrane; is at times delirious; restlessness extreme; died at one p.m.

Autopsy 8 hours after death. Tall, of spare habit; vessels of brain turgid with blood, owing, it may have been, to the distended and very tense state of the abdomen; pericardium pretty generally and firmly adhering; the aorta large, becoming rough, as if from incipient disease; a slight redness of the margin of the omentum, and of the peritoneum generally, especially of that investing the intestines; a little coagulable lymph between some of their convolutions; the colon much distended; a perforation in it near the spleen, large enough to admit the ends of three fingers; some of the contents of the gut in the abdominal cavity; this intestine throughout extremely diseased; lymph between its coats, severe ulceration, extensive sloughing; in one small space, where no recent disease had been, there were marks of old ulcers healed; other viscera not mentioned tolerably sound.

This case, it may be inferred, was far advanced on admission, though the man was relieved off duty. His constitution was probably impaired by the former attacks of disease. Restlessness, profuse sweating, rapid and feeble pulse, dysuria, with stools as above described—the worst symptoms of dysentery.

Case 11.—Of acute dysentery, with partial inflammation of peritoneum.—D. Duggan, 85th Regiment. ætat 20; admitted into regimental hospital, Malta, August 2nd, 1829; died August 8th —This man, three days before admission, is stated to have had frequent and bloody stools. When admitted, the evacuations were the same, with some tormina and tenesmus; the only other symptom noticed in the abstract of the case was "much thirst;" V.S., 20 oz.; calomel and Dover's powder; a warm bath; castor oil; Vesp. Hirud. xviij.; fotus; emplastrum lyttæ. August 3rd—No tormina or tenesmus; stools frequent—some containing blood, some frothy; pulse soft; skin cool; blood drawn of natural appearance; starch injections with opium. 4th—Some feculent, scanty, bloody stools; thirst; cont. med. 5th—Much the same; V.S., 12 oz.; Suppositorium opii gr. iv. 6th—Frequent liquid, bloody stools; tongue less foul; Unguent. Hydrarg. infricr. femoribus. 7th—Some pain in the right iliac region, slightly increased by pressure; pulse full; slight singultus; contr. unguent; ext. opii i. gr. omni hora; at the evening visit he was moribund. 8th—Died at 3 a.m.

Autopsy 9 hours after death. Tall, well made; brain not examined; the lungs collapsed and free from disease, with the exception of a small grey tubercle in the left, close to the spine; the right cavities of the heart and the great vessels distended with grumous blood, and some fibrinous concretions; the omentum redder than natural; it adhered to the cœcum and sigmoid flexure of colon; some coagulable lymph in right iliac fossa; the colon extremely distended; its outer coat in many places black, as if gangrenous; in many places there was to be seen through it a deposition of coagulable lymph between the peritoneal and muscular coat; adhering very generally, the gut was dissected out with difficulty; in the act its coats were ruptured in three places; internally very few parts of it were free from ulceration, and no part, except the inner verge of the anus, was free from disease; where least diseased, its inner coat was covered with false membrane (coagulable lymph), which was easily peeled off; in some places lymph was deposited in a granular form; the most superficial ulcers merely penetrated the inner coat, the cellular constituting their basis, on which generally there was a deposition of lymph; these ulcers were mostly circular; there were other ulcers larger and more irregular, the bottom of which was the muscular coat, either bare or covered with lymph; there were also many sloughs, large, dark brown, or black, infiltrated with puruloid matter, in which all the membranes seemed to be included, and effusion into the abdominal cavity of the contents of the gut was only prevented by adhesion; in the rectum the degree of disease was less than in any other part, and had a chronic aspect; the coats firm and thickened, owing to a deposition of lymph between them; of the few ulcers in this portion, some were coated with lymph—some were healing and cicatrised; no ulceration or abrasion was found close to the verge of the anus, or any appearance of inflammation; there were two or three small nearly spherical piles under the cuticle at the anus, communicating with very minute veins, branches of the hæmorrhoidal, and the latter above the sphincter were much distended, and partially varicose; the small intestines were free from any well marked disease, with the exception of the lower part of the ileum, where, in the situation of the glandulæ aggregatæ, there was slight ulceration; the mesenteric glands were enlarged; some of them were red and soft, one was infiltrated with reddish matter; the bladder of urine was contracted; it contained a little turbid fluid, which was rendered more turbid by nitric acid; its inner coat exhibited towards the neck patches of ecchymosis of a brownish red; they were partially covered with a brown crust, firmly adhering, which I found to consist of lithic acid; the liver, spleen, and other organs not mentioned appeared healthy.

In this case we have a striking example of dysentery of a very severe form, but without distressing symptoms, especially tormina and tenesmus, owing to which it was considered at first as an attack of diarrhœa, and was so returned by the surgeon. I did not see the patient till the 7th, when the case was hopeless. I then anticipated disorganisation of the large intestines, with the exception of the lower part of the rectum, there having been little tenesmus. The ecchymosis of urinary bladder was probably owing to the blister; and the deposit of lithate of ammonia to the ecchymosis. Had he recovered, this deposit might have become the nucleus of a calculus.

Case 12.—Of acute dysentery, with adhesion of intestines and enlarged mesenteric glands.—M. Haycock, ætat. 28; 7th R. F.; admitted into regimental hospital, Malta, 10th Nov. 1831; died 21st Nov.—This man when admitted, was ascertained to have been ailing a considerable time; the bowel complaint gradually getting worse. He is now (Nov. 10th) laboring under decided dysentery. Nov. 12th—Had yesterday castor oil and T. opii with some little relief; many stools during the night with tenesmus; abdomen tender to the touch; countenance anxious; leeches to abdomen; calomel, ipecac. and opium every 3rd hour. 13th—A good night; easier; fewer stools and of better character; the same medicine. 8½ p.m.—Violent pain of abdomen; leeches repeated. 14th—A restless night; stools frothy, bloody, offensive; pulse 80; tongue dark; heat of skin increased; abdominal pain continues; leeches to abdomen; the bleeding was profuse, and there was difficulty in stopping it; a feeling of faintness; the same medicine; Ol. Ricini c ext. opii; emplast. lyttæ abdomini. 15th—Pulse 64; much thirst; abdomen still tender to the touch; the same medicine; 16th—Pulse 60; debility; purging continues; gums slightly affected. From this time till death on the 21st, he gradually sank; his appetite failed; the abdomen became tympanitic, the dysenteric symptoms continuing; he disliked taking medicine; anodyne injections and suppositories were used with the intent to assuage pain.

Autopsy 9 hours after death. Body rather emaciated; brain not examined; the œsophagus very much distended with fluid from the stomach, owing to flatulent distension of intestines; the cœcum and colon and some of the folds of the ileum adhering to the adjoining parts; the mesenteric glands much enlarged; the large intestines, extremely distended with air, were so very tender as hardly to bear handling —in two or three places they were of a black gangrenous hue; they were very much thickened by a deposition of lymph between their coats, and extensively ulcerated with sloughing.

This I must consider a good instance of the intractable nature of neglected dysentery, and also of the inefficiency of the mercurial treatment. The state of the pulse and the state of the intestines, and the degree of pain (if indicative of inflammatory action) how little congruous!

Case 13.—Of acute dysentery, with partial thickening of omentum and closure and altered state of the gall-bladder.—E. M'Carm, ætat. 26; 85th Regiment; admitted into regimental hospital, Malta, 23rd June, 1829; died 29th June.—This man had a slight attack of icterus of eleven days' duration in the summer of 1826. On admission the bowels were much relaxed; he complained of tormina and tenesmus; tongue foul and dry; skin moist; magnes. sulphat., pulv. Dover., a warm bath, 24th—Symptoms the same; V.S. 24 ounces; fotus; magnes. suphat. c. T. opii. 25th—Less pain; stools less frequent; tongue still dry; calomel, pulv. Dov. magnes. sulphat. 26th—Easier; the same medicine, omitting the salts. 27th—Increase of tenesmus; ischuria; the same medicine. 28th—Worse; numerous watery stools; some tenesmus and griping; pain of abdomen on pressure; much debility; skin cooler than natural; tongue moist and red; wine, opium, mixt. cretæ, etc. 29th—Died at 9 a.m.

Autopsy 24 hours after death. Body little emaciated; brain not examined; 2 oz. of reddish serum in the pericardium; heart empty; collapsed; 4 oz. of reddish serum in left pleura; the lower margin of omentum very much thickened and red; the small intestines externally very red, probably the effects of staining; the large in many places grey, in some black, as if from gangrene, here and there adhering from lymph effused; the inner coat of colon extensively ulcerated and in many places sloughing; in many places pus and lymph between the inner and muscular and the muscular and peritoneal coat; liver externally of a dull leaden hue; internally light red; substance rather flabby; the gall-bladder of very unusual appearance; opaque white; felt thick, as if almost cartilaginous; opened, it was found to be moderately distended with a colorless fluid in which were suspended minute scales of cholesterine; it contained also many small calculi of the same substance; its internal structure was quite changed; its surface had become smooth and firm; its subcellular tissue was in the same indurated state, as was also its peritoneal investment; in some places the several layers were not adhering, or very slightly so; in some, cholesterine was deposited between them; near the beginning of the cystic duct, in the cellular and fibrous tissue of the neck of the bladder, was a small closed cyst full of cholesterine; the cystic duct, where it issued from the bladder, and only there, was impervious; the hepatic and common duct were unobstructed; they were colored orange by bile; the omentum adhered to the gall-bladder; nothing distinctly morbid was observable in the other viscera.

This case is a good example of the obscure kind in which the relation between the symptoms and organic lesions is but feebly marked. During life there was no suspicion of the peculiar state of the gall-bladder, become a closed sac, analogous to a serous membrane. The colorless fluid it contained had a slight saline, not the least bitter taste, and was coagulated by heat and nitric acid, much in the same manner as the serum of the blood.

Case 14.—Of acute dysentery, with hepatic abscess and partial thickening of omentum.—W. Rutledge, ætat. 23; 2nd B. R. B.; admitted into regimental hospital, Malta, 20th July, 1829; died 2nd August.—This man's health, with the exception of having had a slight attack of acute rheumatism in the August preceding, had been almost constantly good until the 25th of June, when he had a slight attack of icterus which yielded in a few days to laxatives; the bowels at the same time were torpid. Discharged on the 1st July, he was re-admitted on the 20th, laboring under dysenteric symptoms, said to be of three days' duration, attended with debility, but without pain; tenderness on pressure; anorexia, foul tongue, pulse 98, weak; castor oil and opium; Dover's powder at bed-time, without benefit; the stools continued very frequent and bloody; having complained of a loaded stomach an emetic was given; a great quantity of bilious fluid was thrown up with relief; opium, xii. grs., was next given in divided doses, without good effect; next an astringent mixture and mercurial friction were tried; the former was soon omitted, owing to the nausea it occasioned; the friction was continued with renewed calomel and opium, and occasional doses of castor oil; the disease still making progress, cream of tartar, as described by Dr. Cheyne in Dublin Hospital reports, was employed and injections of white of egg. For two days there was some apparent good effect; nausea and severe griping then occurred; the cream of tartar was discontinued, substituting for it opium, sulphuric acid and sulphate of quinine. Without pain, the pulse between 120 and 130, the purging continuing, he gradually became weaker. A week before his death, he mentioned the day on which he should die. In the morning he took leave of all his comrades who came on purpose to see him, and died at 4 p.m.

Autopsy 19 hours after death. Body sub-emaciated; brain somewhat softer than natural, especially the corpora striata, the fornix and the walls of the lateral ventricles; the pericardium generally adhering; substance of right ventricle unduly thin, yet provided with a considerable layer of fat; the left without fat; very little blood in either of the heart's cavities; the lungs on each side adhering to the pericardium; they were collapsed and apparently sound; about 2 pints of serum in the cavity of the abdomen; the omentum unusually red, in some places thickened, adhered to the colon by its lower margin; the mesentery also was unduly red, its glands a little enlarged; the stomach adhered to the liver and gall-bladder. An abscess, about the size of a small orange, ruptured in the handling, was found situated between the liver and gall-bladder and stomach; the matter it contained had the appearance of thin yellowish pus. The gall-bladder contained a little yellowish fluid, not bitter, chiefly, I believe, mucus and serum: it was not tested. The inside of the gall-bladder was bright red, not unlike the conjunctivæ when inflamed; in one spot there was a little shreddy deposit as if of coagulable lymph; it was where the abscess had almost penetrated into the gall-bladder; all the ducts were pervious; the liver was generally adhering; its substance here and there exhibited the nutmeg-like section; the spleen was very soft, like blood-crassamentum; the colon throughout, including the rectum, with the exception of its anal termination, bore marks of serious disease; it contained a good deal of reddish thick mucus; dispersed through it were bluish rough citatrices, many ulcers healing and many covered with soft pale granulations of feeble resistance to the nail, and which in water had a delicate villous appearance; shreds of lymph were hanging from some of the ulcers; others were covered with a layer of lymph; the inferior portion of the rectum was free from disease; there was little thickening of any part of the large intestines.

This case is in many particulars remarkable, especially for the mildness of its symptoms and the variety and severity of the organic lesions, and for rapidity of progress,—having in relation to progress the character of an acute disease, in relation to organic changes the character of a chronic one. Neither softening of brain nor abscess or inflammation of gall-bladder was suspected during life.

Case 15.—Of acute dysentery, with tuberculated lungs and ulcerated ileum.—T. Smith, ætat. 26; 7th Regiment of Foot; admitted into regimental hospital, Malta, 7th August, 1831; died 6th September.—This man of delicate make had been six years at the station, and had acted for some time as mess-waiter; he had seldom been in hospital; on admission, complained of purging with griping; up to the 12th he was improving, after the use of castor oil and laudanum; then there was a recurrence of purging; about a dozen scanty, mucous, bloody stools during the night; no pain of abdomen; no tenesmus; skin moist; pulse natural; an enema with T. opii and pulv. ipecac., followed by relief; went on favourably till the 30th; then he experienced pain of abdomen, with tenderness on pressure; stools with tenesmus, frequent, scanty, mucous, and bloody; warm bath; leeches, both to abdomen and verge of anus; blister; continuing the calomel and opium which he had been taking. Sept. 2nd—Mouth slightly affected; retching; this relieved by effervescing draughts. On the 5th, some pain of head and chest, but no difficulty of breathing; stools latterly like white of egg, mixed with blood; tenesmus severe, neither relieved by the warm bath, nor by opium suppositories; died on the morning of the 6th.

Autopsy 18 hours after death. Body thin; not emaciated; brain not examined; the left lung firmly adhering; the right free; in the superior lobe of each there were numerous tubercles; the largest of them curd-like, little larger than a large pea; the smallest firm and granular; in the left were a few minute, empty cavities; portions of both lungs were slightly hepatized; grey patches and one small ulcer in the ileum, near its termination; the large intestines were little thickened; numerous ulcers in them; the ulcers were not deep; some were covered with a white incrustation, others were bare; none penetrated to the muscular coat; many seemed to be in progress of healing; in some places there were bluish grey patches, as if from cicatrisation after ulceration; the mesenteric glands considerably enlarged; no well marked disease in any of the other viscera.

In this instance the organic disease of lungs was quite latent;

during life it had never been suspected. His delicacy of constitution might have been connected with it, and the want of healthy reaction adequate to resist the bowel complaint.

These cases may help to give those who are not practically acquainted with dysentery some idea of this horrid disease,—a disease the cause of more concern and anxiety to the army medical officer than any other with which he has to contend, hardly excepting Asiatic cholera and yellow fever; this partly from the nature of the symptoms so distressing to the patient; partly from the uncertainty of effect of the remedial means at his disposal, conjoined with the difficulty during a campaign, too often the impossibility, of providing the diet and nursing specially needed. It is when the disease prevails endemically that it presents itself in its most afflicting and repulsive form— then it is that the nerve of the administrative power, and the humanity of the army surgeon are most subjected to trial. Of all the painful scenes I have ever witnessed, the most painful that I can call to mind, was that of a dysenteric ward of a general hospital, unduly crowded and shamefully neglected. That hospital, I am thankful to say, was not a British, but a Turkish. Every sense there, that could be offended, was, and that of smell not least. I shall spare my readers a description of the horrors of the scene.*

Before adverting to the treatment, it may be well to notice cursorily some of the symptoms of the acute disease. The premonitory are commonly merely relaxation of the bowels and evacuations either mucous or stained with blood. Till blood is seen in the stools there is seldom alarm; and, too often the soldier does not report himself, till in addition to a bloody discharge, he is distressed with tormina and tenesmus; in brief, not

---

* The hospital was at Constantinople, and one of the largest military hospitals of that city. At the time it was prepared to receive the visit of the Hakem Bashi, the chief of the Turkish medical department, who had made an appointment to meet me, which he did not keep. The passages had been newly washed, bouquets were distributed through them, the show-wards were in extra order and tolerably clean; but the unfortunate dysenteric ward, holding at least a hundred patients, which was to have been passed by, and to which I had some difficulty in getting admission, was what I have designated it above. This was in 1840, when I was sent with a party by Her Majesty's Government, for the purpose of attempting the organization of a medical staff for the Turkish army, and the putting in order the military hospitals—both without success, owing very much to the venality of the authorities, the abuses of administration being connected with the peculations and dishonest gains of the administrators.

until ulceration of the bowels has set in, and the disease is fully formed.

Though no disease is more easily diagnosticated, yet in no one perhaps are the symptoms, at least the epiphenomena, more various; much depending on the constitution of the individual attacked, his habit of body, the climate and other adventitious circumstances, and not least on its complications. Great is the contrast in its features, comparing it when attacking men in the vigor of health, fresh from a cool climate, and men in a warm or tropical climate after having been subjected to all the debilitating noxious influences of a protracted campaign. In the one instance the character of the malady is more or less sthenic, in the other in a high degree asthenic; in the one there may be a plethoric state of the vessels; in the other an anæmic state, or deficiency of quantity of the circulating fluid. In the one a phlogosed state may prevail for a time without ulceration of the large intestines; in the other ulceration of the worst kind seems to be *ab origine* established.

Respecting the condition of the tongue, of the stomach, of the pulse, the cutaneous surface, the temperature, the muscular power, the expression of countenance—these are so various as to admit of no brief description.

In the mildest cases, in those doing well and in which the diagnosis may be favorable, the tongue is moist and a little red; the pulse is moderate and soft; the skin is moist and warm; the bodily strength not greatly impaired; the countenance not dejected.

In the severer cases, and of doubtful result, the tongue is dry and often very red; there is total anorexia; a quick and feeble pulse, sometimes a slow pulse, but then very feeble; a great relaxation of the skin and tendency to profuse sweating, and this whether the temperature be above the natural, or, as in the worst cases, below it. Hiccough, tormina, tenesmus, dysuria are some of the common, and, when severe, most distressing accompaniments of the malady. Hiccough, I believe, rarely occurs unless there be irritation or abrasion about the cardia; tenesmus is the invariable accompaniment of ulceration or abrasion of the lower rectum and verge of the anus; tormina may be referred most commonly to flatulent distension; abdominal tenderness with pain on pressure, increasing with the degree of pressure, is commonly considered, and I believe justly, a sign of peritoneal inflammation.   I am doubtful whether the ulceration of the intestine *per se* is or is not the cause of pain.   Were an ulcer high up truly the seat of pain, should we witness, as we so often do, perforation of the gut occasioning peritonitis, without premonitory suffering—that is, pain before the rupture?*   Ischuria, if not arising from a blister, is most commonly the result of inflammation extending from the diseased intestine to the urinary bladder, or it may be, of reflex action.

Of the complications of the disease, in accordance with the statement already given, the most remarkable lesions are those of the parts contained in the abdomen, especially such as are the results of inflammation, as the injected state and thickening of the omentum, the enlargement of the lymphatic glands, and the effusion of lymph with adhesions amongst the viscera.   The rareness of disease of the villous coat of the small intestines, the dysenteric ulceration so often stopping at the cœcum, is very noteworthy, especially comparing this arrest with the diffusion of inflammatory effect, of such common occurrence in the serous, the peritoneal lining.   Whether peritonitis with purulent effusion in connection with dysentery, ever occurs without ulcerative perforation of the gut, is, I think, questionable.   In some endemics, abscess of the liver is associated with dysentery and not unfrequently ; but whether in the relation of a coincidence rather than of a cause, is open to question.†   The same remark is applicable to the other complications mentioned, such as disease of the lungs and of the brain.   Lesions of these organs in their chronic stage may favor an attack of dysentery by undermining the general health and the producing of a feeble state ripe for inflammatory action, and may also retard recovery, protracting

---

* The frequent occurrence of ulcers in the small and large intestines in cases of pulmonary consumption, without pain, and never suspected during life; the occurrence, also not unfrequent, of ulcers in the larynx in the same complaint, often, too, without suffering, may be mentioned in confirmation of the above opinion—that ulceration and painful sensation are not necessarily connected.   Even in the skin, how often do we witness ulceration with little or no pain.

† I am aware that the association is viewed with less hesitation by some pathologists, who consider the two decidedly in the relation of cause and effect—the abscess in the liver conducing to the ulceration of the large intestines, and *vice versâ*, the latter, when first occurring, conducing to suppuration in the liver; and this not by reflex action, but by impurity of blood—that, flowing from the veins of the intestines into the liver, there, it may be, either coagulating or yielding a morbid deposit—the *causa mali.*

the disease until it becomes chronic. Displacement, or abnormal position, of the large intestines interfering with an easy passage of their contents, I am inclined to think, may have a like influence : in several cases of dysentery I have witnessed such a peculiarity.

On the treatment I shall be brief. No positive rules can, I think, be laid down with safety. Every case ought to be specially considered, and more especially the prevailing character of every endemic. General blood-letting, I am of opinion, is rarely beneficial, except in the early stage of the disease and in the instance of the plethoric, and in the purely sthenic cases. The local abstraction of blood, by leeches to the verge of the anus, is less hazardous, and in moderation seems often to be useful. Calomel, combined with opium and ipecacuanha, appears to be one of the modes of treatment that in the majority of cases has stood best the test of experience ; the calomel not exceeding ten grains in the twenty-four hours, the opium from five to twenty grains. Of the mercurial plan of treatment by itself, I have but a poor opinion, having seen it so often fail, after affecting the system, and after witnessing so much bad effect from its abuse—as I shall have occasion more particularly to notice when I shall have to speak of chronic dysentery. In some of the worst endemics—as those associated with a protracted campaign with unavoidable harassment, and bad fare—opium, judging from my own experience, may be considered the *ancora sacra* or heroic remedy, given in grain doses hourly. The test of its efficacy is its exercising no hypnotic effect, but altogether a curative influence, acting, so to speak, like a charm, as if its powers were expended in checking the diseased action and in restoring healthy action. Injections are deserving of much consideration and of being more used than they commonly are, especially anodyne ones with the addition of nitrate of silver or sulphate of zinc. Where ice is procurable, iced water enemata are worthy of trial ; often repeated, I have witnessed from them excellent effect, and also from iced water for drink.* Ipecacuanha was used by Sir John Pringle in

---

* I was first led to recommend iced water from once experiencing its beneficial effect on myself. Travelling exposed to the sun in Sicily, I was seized with a severe purging ; at night, on arrival at Girgenti, finding iced water on the table at supper, I was tempted to drink of it, having insatiable thirst, with loss of appetite. I drank of it freely, slept well, and rose the next morning free of my bowel complaint.

scruple doses in the dysentery of his time : recently it has been given in larger doses, as much as a drachm, and has been favorably reported on. An interesting paper on the subject by Dr. Massey is to be found in the first volume of the new " Statistical, Sanitary and Medical Reports,"—that for 1859, a publication which is to be welcomed as a good omen for the public service and the Medical Department.*

The diet is of the first importance as well as the drinks. These must specially exercise the judgment of the medical officer. Great care should be taken not to overload the stomach, and if milk be allowed, to use it in moderation, for as it coagulates before it is digested, if not digested it will pass into the intestines in the form of curd, and may there be injuriously accumulated as in No. 2 of the foregoing cases. Chicken-broth, beef-tea, light bitter ale, rice-water, iced-water are, one or other, suitable to most cases. There is often a craving for some particular kind of food or drink : the patient, I believe, may generally in moderation be indulged in it with safety, and sometimes with manifest good effect.

Be the treatment what it may, acute dysentery is so dangerous a disease in its worst forms, that only a limited success can be calculated upon : a considerable mortality seems unavoidable. Two axioms may be laid down with some confidence in their accuracy : one that the treatment cannot be too soon begun when any symptoms of the disease appear, it being most easily checked in the beginning; the other, that the patient should be allowed ample time for convalescence, the perfect healing of the ulcerated surfaces being slow, and the tendency to re-open and produce a relapse great.

I do not hold it necessary here to discuss the question whether dysentery be contagious or not, or the distinction pathologically considered, between dysentery and diarrhœa. My belief is that dysentery is not contagious; and the same, to the best of my knowledge, is the belief of those medical officers who have had

* Dr. Massey says :—" In nearly every case of acute dysentery. when first seen, half-an-ounce of castor-oil is at once given, with a view of clearing out scybala and vitiated secretions. As soon as the oil has freely acted, say in from four to six ounces, a drachm of ipecacuanha is given in a little water, a mustard plaister having been applied to the stomach about half an hour previously, at which time likewise thirty drops of laudanum are given. When one dose is rejected, I usually give a second soon after ; this generally succeeds, but if not, by waiting a few hours, the object is often readily effected."

most experience of the disease. As regards merely symptoms it is often difficult to distinguish between dysentery and diarrhœa, and in consequence they are often confounded, a mild attack of the former being liable to be returned diarrhœa, and a severe attack of the latter as liable to be returned dysentery. The seat of the one is undeniably the large intestines; that of the other may be, and I believe often is, the small intestines or the small and large together, and depending more on functional derangement than on organic lesion. When dysentery is rife, it is a safe rule to view in every instance an attack of diarrhœa as the beginning of the more formidable disease, which it so often is, and to treat it accordingly.

2.—Of Chronic Dysentery.—In sequence I shall now give a selection of cases of chronic dysentery: the distinction between which and the acute is very much a matter of time, the one passing into the other almost insensibly; it may be sufficient to remark that if the malady be protracted beyond four or five weeks, it is mostly called chronic, and that the symptoms then, if not of a milder are commonly of a less distressing kind, rendered so often by a partial healing of the ulceration belonging to the disease in its earlier and acute stage.

1.—Case of chronic dysentery, with hepatic abscess, ruptured, and peritoneal inflammation.—J. Greenwood, ætat. 25; 7th R. F.; admitted into regimental hospital, Malta, 13th June, 1832; died 24th August.—This man before his arrival in Malta, nearly four years ago, had experienced intermittent and remittent fever and dysentery whilst serving with his regiment in the Ionian Islands. On admission on the 13th June, he was suffering from a return of the last-named disease; his stools were frequent, mucous and bloody, with some pain of abdomen and pyrexia. Under treatment, consisting of calomel, ipecac. and opium, with mercurial friction and fomentation, slight ptyalism was produced, and by the 18th " the bowel affection had ceased." He continued well, it is stated, until the 24th June, when after irregularity of diet, the dysenteric symptoms recurred; the treatment before used was renewed, but without any permanent good effect. He became worse; on the 18th July he seemed in imminent danger; stools frequent, watery and bloody; pulse very rapid, small and intermitting; tongue dark-colored and dry; profuse clammy perspiration; great debility; iced water was now given for drink, and iced water injections used. He expressed himself greatly relieved; the same were continued with good effect; the pulse diminished in frequency; blood ceased to appear in his stools; his appetite improved. On 1st August he was pronounced convalescent, and the iced injections were discontinued. On 10th August he experienced pains in the right side with a short dry cough and some pyrexia; leeches were applied to the pained part, followed by a blister; small doses of ipecacuanha were prescribed. He became rapidly worse, hectic symptoms setting in; pulse rapid and feeble; tongue red, dry, and shining; anorexia, profuse sweats, the bowels however remaining regular, even to his death on the 23rd.

Autopsy 11 hours after death. Body much emaciated; nothing morbid observed in the brain; some fibrinous concretions in the heart, especially the right auricle, where they were mixed with a good deal of blood of a brighter red than usual; the inferior portions of lungs gorged with blood; a considerable quantity of serum with coagulable lymph and some pus, altogether nearly three pints, in the cavity of the abdomen and in the pelvis; there were marks throughout of diffused peritoneal inflammation. On examining the liver an abscess in it was found to have burst and to have discharged part of its contents; it was situated in the right lobe, near its edge and close to the gall-bladder; its cavity was lined with a false membrane; in the same lobe two other abscesses were discovered, one in the convex part, contiguous to the diaphragm, which contained about a pint and a half of pultaceous matter; the other in the inferior part contiguous to the supra-renal gland which contained about half a pint of matter; the substance of the liver both internally and externally had a healthy appearance; the gall-bladder whiter and thicker than usual, contained some bile of natural appearance, and three concretions formed of cholesterine; the right side of abdomen was lined with a thick layer of coagulable lymph, which, where in contact with the liver, was in part stained yellow by bile, and in part red by blood; there was a large quantity of greenish fluid in the stomach; the small intestines exhibited no appearance of disease; the large intestines throughout bore marks of old ulceration, now in every place healed or nearly so by granulation; that which, it may be inferred, was most recent was red and flabby; that probably older was paler and firmer, and that still older was dark grey, covered with a new membrane; adhering to one of infundibula of the right kidney was a small crust of calculous matter; the matter of the abscesses by the optical test was not purulent; the matter contained in the cavity of the pelvis, by the same test was found to be purulent.

This case affords a striking example of the latency of abscesses in the liver; of the healing of ulcers in the large intestines; and, may I not add, of the beneficial effect of iced drinks and enemata under the most unpromising circumstances.

Case 2.—Of chronic dysentery, with hepatic abscesses (one ruptured) and peritoneal inflammation.—W. M'Kay, ætat. 42; 17th Foot; admitted into general hospital, 28th May, 1823; died 18th June.—This man whilst in India, where he served twelve years, had labored under ague and repeated attacks of dysentery. A return of this last disease he experienced about five months ago and is not yet recovered from it. His stools are now frequent and watery, but with little tormina or tenesmus; he has some pain in the right hypochondrium and tenderness of abdomen increased by pressure; he cannot lie, he says, on his left side; has some thirst, tongue clean, pulse regular; his appetite indifferent; is not without cough; is very feeble and emaciated; using Dover's powder, with ext. of gentian and rhubarb, he appeared to be improving till the 8th June; during the night he experienced slight rigors followed by increased heat. From this time, till he expired on the 18th, he almost daily became worse. His stomach was irritable, rejecting food, and he was troubled with hiccough; had a dry cough and some pain, but not severe, of right side; debility, total loss of appetite, and a feeble pulse were the most marked symptoms of his last days. The treatment was entirely palliative.

Autopsy 12 hours after death. A good deal of serum in the ventricles of the brain; the left lung free from any well-marked disease; the upper surface of right lung of healthy appearance; the middle and inferior lobe of this lung were diseased; some portions were hepatized, some were emphysematous; the inferior portion of the superior lobe was œdematous; some of the air collected from the distended cells was not diminished by lime water; by phosphorus 11 measures were reduced to 10 ; the fluid from the œdematous portion was coagulated like serum by nitric acid ; the heart contained no blood; there was a very little fibrinous concretion in the right ventricle ; the omentum was thickened round its margin and adhering in several places to the colon ; the liver was of a light brownish hue, rough and granular, and very friable ; it contained several small abscesses full of viscid pus, and one pretty large abscess; this was situated in the upper part of the right lobe and held about three ounces; it appeared to be formed by a disorganising process, vessels more or less coroded crossing it ; the ascending colon adhered to the liver ; between them was a considerable sac of purulent matter; it communicated with a small abscess in the lobulus Spigelii, the rupture of which was probably connected with the formation of the purulent collection and the setting in of peritoneal inflammation; the lower portion of the ileum and the whole tract of the large intestines showed marks of disease ; in the former, of some small ulcers healed; in the latter, of ulcers in different stages of progress towards healing ; in some places the reparative process was only just beginning, the edges of the ulcers were pale and smooth, spots of granulations forming on their surface ; in others the ulcers had advanced farther, the granulations were almost covered with new epithelium ; in others the healing seemed to be complete ; in some, where probably the ulceration had been deep, there was considerable contraction from the cicitrisation ; the healed surfaces were of different shades of grey and dark bluish grey ; the appearances suggested forcibly the analogy of the healing of ulcers of the skin ; the kidneys were somewhat similar to the liver, they were rough, pale and very friable ; the spleen was large ; the gall-bladder was distended with bile.

This case is a good example of the complications of chronic dysentery, and of the healing of ulcers of the intestines. The air in the emphysematous portion of the lungs was probably entirely azote ; the little oxygen present in it may have been owing to exposure of the parts to the atmosphere ; whilst exposed, at least half-an-hour, it is easy to imagine that the oxygen found might have penetrated through the delicate pleura.

Case 3.—Of chronic dysentery, with vesicles in brain (cysticerci ?), hepatic abscesses and emphysematous and tuberculated lungs.—T. Williams, ætat. 41 ; 57th Regiment; admitted into general hospital, 4th October, 1836 ; died 7th October.—An old soldier of 23 years' service, the last four years in India, from whence he is just returned. He states that till about three weeks ago he never had any serious illness; then, when at sea, the complaint he still labors under, dysentery, began, for which he was blooded, blistered and fomented. Now the symptoms are severe ; there are thirty or forty stools in the twenty-four hours, bloody and very offensive; no tenderness ; no distension of abdomen ; has troublesome cough; pulse small and weak; a thick brown fur on tongue; great thirst; no appetite. During the 5th, and till the afternoon of the 6th, there was some alleviation of the purging and of the other symptoms ; towards the evening of the latter day he became much worse; the purging had returned and was violent ; vomiting now appeared for the first time. On the 7th, at the morning visit, he was excessively weak; facies Hippocratica ; he continued sinking during the day; at 11 p.m., in attempting to get out of bed, he suddenly expired. The treatment consisted in the use of mixt. cretæ with tinct. kino, confect. opii. and opium.

Autopsy 39 hours after death. Body sub-emaciated; the arachnoid partially opaque ;

under each opaque spot (there were two or three such spots over the upper surface of each hemisphere) there was a spherical vesicle, in size a little larger than a common pea; one of them was found situated between the arachnoid and pia mater, slightly adhering to the latter; its membrane was transparent, not sensibly vascular; when punctured a transparent fluid flowed out in which were suspended two or three flakes of lymph and of albuminous matter; within these was found a small, somewhat spherical mass, which was soft, almost gelatinous superficially and semi-transparent, but of increasing firmness and opacity towards its centre; on removal a complete hemispherical cavity was left in the cortical part of the cerebrum, lined with pia mater; most of the other vesicles were vascular, and were either attached to or had reflected over them the pia mater; when taken out a portion of cerebral substance was detached, adhering to each; one of the same kind was found in the substance of the right corpus striatum, apparently unconnected with the pia mater; all of these were very similar in structure. The substance of the brain generally had no abnormal appearance. Both lungs were more or less emphysematous, and in part œdematous; a small cluster of crude tubercles was detected in the upper part of the superior lobe of left lung, and some ecchymosis and hepatization, and a few tubercles, some of them softening, in the inferior lobe of the same lung; the liver adhering to the diaphragm contained two abscesses; one was situated superficially in the superior part of the right lobe; it (the largest) contained about a pint of matter; the smaller about half that quantity; the matter was thick, opaque and glairy; not purulent by the optical test; it was neither distinctly coagulated by nitric acid nor by boiling; a false membrane lined the cavities of the abscesses and bands crossed them in which were blood-vessels, some unobstructed, some obstructed by firm fibrinous concretion; the liver, after the emptying of the abscesses, weighed 4lbs.; its substance was rather pale and firm; the gall-bladder contained a little brownish bile, thick without being viscid; its lining membrane was very red, as if inflamed; the smaller abscess was contiguous to it, the gall-bladder forming part of its boundary; the colon was excessively diseased throughout, thickened, ulcerated and sloughing, as in the worst cases of the acute dysentery of India; the rectum was much less diseased; there the ulceration was slight; no well-marked disease in the other abdominal viscera; the lining cartilage of each patella was in part raised, softened and fissured; the synovia was scanty and thick.

In this instance during life there had been no suspicion of disease of liver, or of disease of brain, or of lungs. The complication might have conduced to the intractable nature of the dysenteric attack.

Case 4.—Of chronic dysentery, with hepatic abscess, peritoneal inflammation and obstructed vena portæ.—D. Buckley, ætat. 29; 94th Regiment; admitted into regimental hospital, Malta, 10th September, 1832; died 18th September.—This man had been under treatment for general febrile symptoms and pain of right hypochondrium extending to the shoulder, from the 29th March to the 9th April, when, after V.S., the use of antimon. tartar, calomel and a blister, he was discharged apparently well. According to his brother, though doing duty he had been ailing for some time. On the 9th July following he was re-admitted, laboring under dysenteric symptoms; the evacuations bloody, with slight pyrexia. On the 6th August, after V.S. and a course of calomel and opium, he was considered convalescent. In a few days there was a recurrence of the dysenteric symptoms of considerable severity, with tenderness of abdomen. Under similar treatment he again improved. On the 6th September he was discharged at his urgent request. In three days he was re-admitted with a return of his complaint in an aggravated state; stools frequent, bloody and frothy; severe tenesmus; tenderness of lower belly on pressure; small rapid pulse; dysuria; feeble and emaciated; small doses of castor oil were given with anodyne injections, from which no relief, nor from mercurial friction. Three days before his death, which was rather unexpected, he experienced relief of suffering from opium in large doses, with iced drinks and iced injections.

Autopsy 12 hours after death. Brain not examined; nothing morbid in the contents of the thorax; the right cavities of heart distended with coagulated blood; in the abdomen marks of peritoneal inflammation with effusion of lymph and serum; the omentum unusually red; it adhered to the cœcum and sigmoid flexure of colon; on separating it from the latter, a perforation of the gut was discovered; the adhesion retained the contents of the intestine; the lower portion of ileum, about half an inch from the valvula coli, was ulcerated; its mucous coat destroyed; the colon generally was very much diseased, ulcerated and sloughing; in places the muscular coat was laid bare; in the sigmoid flexure, the ulceration had penetrated even through the peritoneal coat and that largely where the adhesion already mentioned to the omentum occurred; in the rectum there were ulcers granulating, and dark cicatrices of old ulcers healed; an abscess was found in the liver, in the lower part of the right lobe, close to the supra-renal gland and ascending cava; its cavity lined with coagulable lymph was spherical, about the size of a large orange, and was full of thick, rather viscid cream-colored matter, not purulent by the optical test; the vena portæ was unusually distended and firm; it contained a blood-shot pultaceous matter, in color and general appearance not unlike cerebral substance; in the large branches the concretion had more the aspect of coagulated fibrin; there was no appearance of inflammation or of ulceration of the vein; the substance of the liver, of the spleen and pancreas was apparently normal; the gall-bladder and biliary ducts were distended with bile.

During the progress of this case no suspicion was entertained of the abscess in the liver or of the obstructed state of the vena portæ. During the last attack he passed a good deal of blood; this might have been owing to the obstructed state in question, and that state and the abscess might have prevented the healing of the ulcers and have conduced to the fatal termination. The substance occasioning the obstruction probably was fibrin of the blood undergoing softening. Thrice this patient was under the influence of mercury, and as regards the abscess in the liver, with what little effect!

Case 5.—Of chronic dysentery, with hepatic abscess.—H. Rowden, ætat 41; 70th Foot; admitted into general hospital, 18th February, 1837; died 25th February.— An old soldier of 23 years' service; the last two years and a half in Gibraltar and Malta, from whence (Malta), is just returned; has suffered much from rheumatism; about 18 months ago was attacked with purging, from which never since free; now, stools frequent, consisting chiefly of blood; has passed, he says, at different times, large coagula; does not complain of pain of abdomen on pressure, nor of tormina nor tenesmus; pulse 100, very feeble; tongue coated in the centre; skin cold and clammy; a large tumor occupies the left hypochondriac and epigastric regions, extending from the ensiform cartilage to the umbilicus; it is circumscribed, pulsates strongly, and fluctuation is distinct in it; he gives a very imperfect account of his ailments; is much debilitated; using astringents and opiates, the purging was arrested; his strength was supported by wine and nourishing food. On the 22nd he had apparently rallied considerably. On the 23rd, the tumor was much increased; as there seemed good ground to infer that it was not an aneurism, the pulsation of the femoral artery not being impaired, and the pulsation in the tumor, according to the patient, not having been felt till a few days before his landing, it was thought advisable to explore it; a small trocar was used; on its withdrawal, a limpid, greenish fluid was discharged, followed by a brownish fluid, less limpid and clear, and that by a puruloid thicker fluid, obstructing the canula; the quantity evacuated amounted to 14oz.; the thinner portion was of sp. gr. 1030, and was rendered turbid by heat; he felt immediate relief of the pain that was occasioned by the distension; could now change his position from the right side to decubitus on his back; he continued easier during the next 24 hours; during the night he sank rapidly and expired.

Autopsy 10 hours after death. Body sub-emaciated; much fluid effused between the arachnoid and pia mater, in the ventricles, and at base of the brain; both lungs, with the exception of adhesions, were free from disease; on opening into the cavity of the abdomen, the left lobe of the liver was found to be the seat of an abscess; it contained about four pints of curd-like fluid, so thick that its specific gravity could not be ascertained by the uranometer; though of uniform appearance, it had no effect in coloring light; the cavity was rough, lined with coagulable lymph; externally it adhered to the abdominal parietes; the liver weighed 5lbs.; its substance generally was pretty natural; a portion of it dried afforded no traces of fat; the abscess, it may be remarked, pressed on the stomach, especially the pylorus, and on the jejunum, the upper portion of which lay immediately over the aorta; the stomach and small intestines were empty and unusually contracted; the lower part of ileum was of about the thickness of the little finger; the large intestines, with the exception of the lower portion of the rectum, were much diseased; in the cœcum there were large ulcers, and also in the colon, with thickening and induration of the mucous and sub-mucous tissue; some of the ulcers were in progress of healing, and there were indications of others having healed.

The most interesting features of this case were the masked dysenteric symptoms—masked no doubt by the abscess, and the suspicious symptoms of aneurism, arising from the situation of the tumor, and the hæmorrhage, the latter probably owing to pressure on the venous trunks in connection with the ulcerated state of the large intestines.

Case 6.—Of chronic dysentery, with an excavating ulceration of liver.—Patrick Laffing, ætat. 42; 7th R. F.; admitted into regimental hospital, Malta, 22nd Aug., 1834; died 3rd October.—This man, of phlegmatic temperament and of intemperate habits, when on guard on the 22nd August, experienced bilious vomiting. On admission, the following were some of his symptoms: the tongue foul; thirst; skin hot and dry; pulse quick and soft; bowels constipated; some tenderness of epigastrium on pressure. On the 26th, after leeching and the use of aperients, he appeared to be convalescent. In the evening of the 26th he was found complaining of headache with nausea; the pulse soft and not of increased frequency; bowels regular. There was a feeling of restlessness with debility and confusion of mind; after leeches to the temples and cold applications to the shaved head, he slept well, and the following morning was free from any urgent symptom. On the evening of the 17th there was a recurrence of the paroxysm, but milder. On the evening of the 28th he escaped it.

About the same time on the 29th he vomited copiously green bilious matter; relief followed and a good night. On the 31st the bowels were irritable; there were frequent liquid yellow stools; pulse soft; tongue moist. After fomentation and the use of mucilaginous drinks, the diarrhœa soon ceased. On the 2nd September, he felt, he said, quite well. The following night there was a return of the purging, which was arrested by, or ceased after, the use of Dover's powder and Hydrag. c. Creta. On the 14th, after several slight changes of symptoms, he again seemed convalescent. Then though the tongue was preternaturally red, it was moist and clean, and his countenance good. For eleven days there were no urgent symptoms; the tongue became redder; he had little thirst; his appetite was good; "his spirits extraordinarily good;"—thus, till about the 26th, when the bowels became again "irritable;" the stools, thin, feculent, streaked with blood and offensive; no pain of abdomen, even under pressure; pulse small, regular; tongue glazed, red and dry; no urgent thirst; appetite good; using small doses of sulphate of quinine and Dover's powder, the stools became less mucous and less offensive; apthous spots appeared on the lining membrane of the mouth, yet he seemed improving until the 30th, when he voided about half a pint of dark coagulated blood; this, without pain, followed by several liquid scanty stools during the day without blood. On 2nd October, when his tongue seemed returning to a healthy state, and after a good night (pulse small, 110); he had three evacuations, chiefly of dark coagulated blood (about a pint and a half), after which he felt very weak, yet he was cheerful and his appetite good; there was no recurrence of the hæmorrhage; he slept at intervals during the early part of the night; at 2 a.m. singultus troubled him for about ten minutes, then he dozed and shortly after must have expired, as at 3 a.m. he was found dead.

Autopsy 8 hours after death. Body much emaciated; rather more serosity than natural in the ventricles of the brain and in the spinal canal; the walls of the fornix and of the lateral ventricles to the depth of a line abnormally soft; the lungs collapsed, pale and crepitous; 3 oz. of serum in the pericardium; the right cavities of the heart distended with coagulated blood; a good deal of coagulated blood in the aorta; the left cavities of heart empty; the blood which flowed out on dividing the great vessels in removing the lungs (before opening the heart) coagulated presently on exposure to the air; the tongue was red and raw; œsophagus here and there had lost its epithelium, was redder and more flabby than natural and smeared with purulent fluid, as tried by the optical test; about midway in its submucous tissue a small tumor was found of an eliptical form and of almost cartilaginous hardness; in the stomach there was a good deal of yellow bilious fluid; the mucous coat was generally softer than natural, as was also that of the duodenum in a less degree; the gall-bladder adhered to the duodenum; the common biliary duct before its entrance into the intestine was about thrice its natural size; it was distended with bile of healthy appearance; this distension might have been owing to the circumstance of the duct after penetrating the coats of the intestine, deviating and passing through a portion of the pancreas before coming out into the duodenum; the pancreas was firmer than natural, so also the spleen; the large intestines were very much diseased, with the exception of the lowest part of the rectum, where there was only slight excoriation about the verge of the anus; there had been no tenesmus; in the cœcum, the ascending and transverse colon, there was severe ulceration with sloughing, and the same in a less degree in the descending colon; the upper portion of the ascending colon adhered to the under concave surface of the liver, and there on examination it was found that the ulcerative process had entered into the substance of the viscus, forming a cup-like hollow rather larger than the hollow of the hand; the surface of the cavity was sloughing and shreddy, bounded by gangrenous black matter; the substance of the

liver generally seemed pretty sound; the coats of the intestine were generally more
or less thickened by infiltration of lymph and of a puruloid fluid; the mesenteric
glands were generally enlarged; the semi-lunar ganglia were enlarged, and of a more
waxy aspect than common.

This case is remarkable for its fluctuations and the little apparent relation between the symptoms and the severer organic
lesions.   Could this have been owing to the partial softening of
the brain, or to a peculiarity of brain which might have been
the cause of his phlegmatic temperament?   Was not the immediate cause of death syncope?

Case 7.—Of chronic dysentery, with fibrinous concretion softening in the longitudinal sinus.—J. Travers, ætat. 40; 36th Foot; admitted into general hospital, 12th
August, 1838; died 18th August.—This man, of 23 years' service, the last eight in
the West Indies, is just arrived from thence, and without any medical document,
having, though laboring under chronic dysentery, been sent home to join his depôt.
He states that when in the Mediterranean in 1814, he was attacked with epilepsy, to
which he has been subject ever since; and that whilst in the West Indies he experienced occasional attacks of dysentery, the last about three months ago, which
became more severe during the voyage, and still continues with unabated severity. His
evacuations now are very frequent, one about every half hour; they are watery, contain a good deal of blood, and are accompanied with much tenesmus; there is slight
pain in the lower part of the abdomen; the tongue is furred and dry; thirst; pulse
weak and intermitting; about 9 hours before death he was troubled with hiccough.
The treatment was palliative.

Autopsy 4½ hours after death.   Body sub-emaciated; limbs rigid;* a small mass
of fibrin, about the size of a lentil, was found adhering to the sides of the longitudinal
sinus, just over the pineal gland; cut into, minute portions of it appeared to be
softening.   It had all the character of having been formed during life; its surface
was smooth, and its adhesion on *one* side was firm; there was no clot or blood
adhering to it; the arachnoid over the upper portion of the cerebrum was partially
opaque; in the left lateral ventricle, attached to the plexus choroides was a small vesicle
very like a cysticercus; the substance of the brain generally was unusually firm; the
inferior portions of both lungs was more or less œdematous and contained coagulated
blood (perhaps extravasated) in patches; the bronchia were red and contained some
bloody fluid; a bloody fluid was found in the thoracic duct; the lymphatic glands
adjoining and between the receptaculum and brim of the pelvis were very red; with

* The following observations were made on the temperature of different parts,
rapidly in succession:—The temperature of the room at the time was 68°; thermometer in corpus callosum 85°; in lateral ventricle 86°; in upper part of spinal canal
87°; under lobulus Spigelii of liver 97°; in cavity of pelvis 97°; under the heart 93°;
in right ventricle, in which was some fibrinous concretion and a good deal of blood,
partly coagulated, partly liquid and many bubbles of air, which came out when a
puncture was made, 92°; in left ventricle, which was empty, 95°; in middle of thigh,
close to femoral artery, 82°; under integument of sole of foot 69°: the liquid blood
coagulated on exposure; put by in a stoppered bottle, after two hours it was found
coagulated; after twenty, covered with a slight buffy coat; broken up and agitated in
a pneumatic bottle, no air was disengaged; there was found to be a slight absorption
of air; the quantity of cruor was about 5oz.

the exception of a dark patch, like the cicatrice of an ulcer in the lower part of the ileum, there was nothing morbid in the small intestines; the large intestines were much diseased; their cellular coat thickened, their mucous ulcerated; in some places there were granulations, as of ulcers healing; in some the muscular coat was bare, or covered with a fine new membrane; in the lower portion of the rectum, the ulcers there were of so dark a color as to suggest the idea of gangrene; the viscera not mentioned had a tolerably healthy appearance; there was pretty much fluid in the vesiculæ seminales which was found to contain globules of various sizes and some spermatozoa.

The complications of organic lesions in this case are well deserving of notice, more especially the fibrinous concretion in the longitudinal sinus in connection with epilepsy, and the state of the large intestines in connection with dysentery. The condition of the blood is also noteworthy, especially in relation to coagulation; and also the quality of the fluid in the vesiculæ seminales; the latter as showing that even an exhausting disease, long protracted, does not prevent the production of spermatozoa.

Case 8.—Of chronic dysentery, with tuberculated lungs and ulcerated ileum.—John Neale, ætat. 38; 19th Foot; admitted into general hospital, September 18th, 1835; died 24th October.—This man, of 26 years' service, the last 8 in the West Indies, from whence just returned, is reported to have been suffering "from irritation of the digestive organs and derangement of the hepatic system." He is now extremely feeble and emaciated, in an almost hopeless state. The principal symptoms are a relaxed state of bowels, four or five stools daily without blood, but with tenesmus; slight cough, with expectoration of a greenish matter; difficult breathing; loss of appetite; the stethoscopic indications said to be very imperfect from his state not allowing of careful examination; the respiratory murmur was loud under the left clavicle with gurgling; on percussion the sound over the whole chest was clear. He never rallied. The treatment was merely palliative.

Autopsy 40 hours after death. Brain not examined; both lungs were generally and very firmly adhering; in the left lung, in its superior lobe was a large tubercular excavation lined with false membrane, freely communicating with the bronchia; the greater portion of this lobe was impervious to air, abounding in granular tubercles, a few small vomicæ intermixed; the inferior lobe was tolerably sound, yet was not entirely free from tubercles; the superior and middle lobe of right lung abounded in tubercles; the former contained two small excavations; the inferior lobe was without tubercles, and but little if at all diseased; there were some small pale ulcers in the sacculi laryngis, and the lining membrane of the trachea was more or less granular; the lower portion of the ileum was much ulcerated, and solitary ulcers were scattered through the whole of its course and in the inferior part of the jejunum; two pretty large and deep ulcers were found in the cœcum, several in the appendicula, one (an extensive one) in the upper part of the rectum, many in the descending colon; most of them were in process of healing and were mixed with cicatrices of old ulcers, marked by a depression and a dark grey color; the liver was of nutmeg-like section, it weighed 3lbs.; the mesenteric glands were much enlarged, distended with cheese-like matter.

In this instance we have a striking example of advanced tuber-

culosis of the lungs, with ulceration of the larynx and small
intestines, combined with the lesions distinctive of dysentery.
Did their existence at the same time tend to mask as it were the
severer symptoms of each ?

Case 9.—Of chronic dysentery, with cerebral and pulmonary disease.—W. Sharp,
ætat. 37 ; 74th Regiment; admitted into general hospital, 12th August, 1838; died
14th September.—This man, after 12 years' service, 4 in the West Indies, was sent
home from thence on account of chronic dysentery of about nine months' duration·
Just arrived, he is very feeble and greatly emaciated; has frequent watery stools
without blood; no tenderness of abdomen on pressure ; under treatment consisting of
anodynes, alteratives, cretaceus medicine and tonics, his evacuations became less
frequent and more consistent.   On the 24th August a rigor occurred followed by heat;
his hands and feet became œdematous; the œdema abated for a time, but it recurred
a few days before death ; ten days before this event the purging had ceased. He
gradually sank.

Autopsy 24 hours after death.   The feet and scrotum were œdematous; five hours
previously the jugular vein was carefully examined ; a good deal of air was found in
it ; where the vessel was not so distended or with coagulum, it was collapsed ; there
was much serosity between the membranes in the ventricles and at the base of the
brain ; its substance generally was soft, especially the walls of the ventricles, the
fornix and septum lucidum ; these were almost pultaceous ; the left pleura contained
12 oz. of serum, the right 3 oz., and the pericardium 1 oz.; the heart was small ;
the inferior portion of each lung was œdematous; the bronchia contained a good deal
of frothy fluid ; 56 oz. of slightly turbid serum were found in the cavity of the abdomen ; the liver weighed only 1½lb. ; the spleen was small and adhering to the diaphragm, its capsule where adhering was much thickened, its substance firm; the
pancreas and kidneys were apparently sound, as were also the small intestines and the
stomach ; the latter was small; the large intestines were free from ulceration, and
with the exception of the œdema of the sub-mucous tissue were exempt from any
well-marked lesion.   It is specially noted that there were no fibrinous concretions
found in the veins, or any staining of vessels or indications of putrefaction, or hepatization of lung or disease of liver.

The air in the jugular vein, the softening of the brain, the
serous effusions, the small size of liver, the indurated state of
spleen, are all noteworthy ; and yet how obscure the cause of
death ! Not the least remarkable circumstance is the absence of
ulcers or of cicatrices after chronic dysentery.

Case 10.—Of chronic dysentery, with tuberculated lungs and vomicæ.—Wm. Scott,
ætat. 35 ; 5th Foot; admitted into general hospital, 20th July, 1821; died 13th May,
1822.—This man just returned from the West Indies, has been laboring under chronic
dysentery, preceded by an attack of acute dysentery about a year and a half ago. He
is now feeble and much emaciated ; has about ten stools daily with tormina and tenesmus; his tongue is clean, his appetite good. Under palliative treatment, which with
modifications was continued, little change was noticeable until the beginning of
October, except that he was troubled with cough, with mucous expectoration and occasional pain of chest; his bowels remained much the same; a papular eruption of the
skin attended with much itching appeared, with œdema of feet, and persisted even to

his last hours. In October there was a mitigation of symptoms; the cough had left him; his stools were less frequent and more easy; his appetite better and he had gained strength a little. On the 10th November he was discharged "pretty well." On the 15th of the same month he was re-admitted with cough, referred to his taking "cold;" there was little uneasiness of bowels, about four stools daily; the skin and feet as before. In December his cough had become trifling; his bowels more open and uneasy; the other symptoms much the same. Through January and February there was some increase of cough with expectoration of thin mucus; his bowels were rather more uneasy, but his stools not more frequent; occasionally sweats; his emaciation continued and he lost strength. In March his bowels were sometimes constipated, sometimes loose; he had little uneasiness excepting what might be referred to flatulent distension; was almost free from cough, but was still wasting and losing strength. In April he had occasional cough and copious thin mucous expectoration; his stools were scanty, not very frequent, sometimes needing a laxative; is still deteriorating, without marked aggravation of any symptoms; his appetite is craving. From the 5th to the 13th of May, when he expired, his appetite gradually diminished and at last failed entirely; his pulse became very rapid and feeble; his voice so weak as to be scarcely audible; his body emitted a very offensive smell; his cough was short and troublesome; his bowels not much relaxed or uneasy; his debility and emaciation were extreme; he was sensible to the last.

Autopsy 8 hours after death. Body exceedingly emaciated; about 3 oz. of serum between the membranes, in the ventricles and at the base of the brain; the left costal pleura dotted with opaque spots, and a little thickened; both lungs partially adhering; the inferior lobes of both were gorged with blood, and a few indolent tubercles were scattered through them; their superior lobes contained two or three small vomicæ and numerous tubercles; these in different stages of softening; the bronchia were of ordinary appearance, with the exception of their minute branches, from which when divided there was a purulent exudation, and excepting those communicating with the vomicæ, where they terminated abruptly and were much ulcerated; the lower part of the trachea was slightly ulcerated; the larynx was free from ulceration; there were no distinct lesions either in the stomach or small intestines; the cœcum and colon were redder than natural and contained a few superficial ulcers, the largest not exceeding in size a sixpence; some of them healing; intermixed were a few red excrescences resembling warts, projecting from the mucous membrane; the rectum was even more diseased, especially its inferior portion; of a dark red color its surface was ulcerated in a singular manner, producing an appearance of reticulation; this arose from small sinuses and fistulæ extending from the mucous into the surrounding cellular tissue; the coats of this part were thickened, and the same wart-like excrescences were found in it as in the colon, some of them black, some excoriated. In connection with the extreme emaciation, it may be worth while to remark that though the heart was small, it was not deficient in fat; there was much about it; nor, whilst in other parts of the body, it was almost entirely absorbed, was there any deficiency of it about the colon and rectum. The liver of a light reddish brown was rather bulky, it weighed about 4lb. 6oz. and was rather soft and friable; the spleen was large; the glands of the groin, the mesenteric and lumbar glands were enlarged (the largest about the size of a pigeon's egg) and indurated; some of them when divided exhibited a cartilage-like appearance; one or two were undergoing softening; some contained a curd-like scrofulous matter.

One of the peculiarities of this case worthy of notice is that the diseased state of the rectum was not productive of more urgent symptoms; only now and then he complained of a distressing feeling in the lower part of the gut. The emaciation which was so remarkable in this instance was probably mainly owing to the altered state of the large intestines and to the diseased state of the abdominal glands, especially the mesenteric. The abdomen was always lank and very much contracted, as if the organic cause of the wasting was in that region.

Case 11.—Of chronic dysentery, with tuberculated and cavernous lungs and obstructed longitudinal sinus.—J. Leaper, ætat. 22; R. A.; admitted into ordnance hospital, Malta, 16th Nov., 1828; died 26th Feb., 1829.—The leading symptoms in this man's case were of a dysenteric kind with peculiarities, such as comparatively little pain, very little tenesmus, only occasionally tormina; his stools though frequent were generally copious; his appetite good; there was no hectic, little or no pyrexia; there was great debility and emaciation; his respiration was always easy; no complaint was made of chest; he had a slight cough a few days only before he died; various modes of treatment were employed on the idea that the disease was mainly of a dysenteric character; most relief was experienced from opium, of which, at one time, he took 24 grains daily.

Autopsy 17 hours after death. The chest sounded well on percussion; more fluid than usual was found under the arachnoid and at the base of the brain; a large fibrinous concretion, soft and in parts, almost pultaceous, was detected in the longitudinal sinus; a good deal of blood and fibrinous concretion in the right cavities of the heart and in the pulmonary artery and veins; both lungs viewed superficially were of pretty natural appearance; both were heavier than natural and redder; they contained a good deal of blood; the bronchia were very red and contained much purulent fluid, as ascertained by the optical test; there was an exudation of the same fluid from the minute branches when divided; in the superior lobe of each lung there were granular tubercles; in the left lung, both in its superior and inferior lobe there were small excavations and vomicæ; in the latter lobe there were also minute tubercles, with suppuration; these were apparently formed in the extreme bronchial branches; just anterior to each tubercle the branch was obstructed; the glandulæ concatenatæ were much enlarged; the lower part of the trachea was unduly red; the epiglottis was slightly ulcerated, and on its under surface there were minute tubercles; the ileum here and there was studded with tubercles and with small tubercular ulcers in different stages, the lowest most advanced; the large intestines throughout were much diseased, thickened and ulcerated; some of the ulcers had the appearance of healing and there were some cicatrices of old ulcers; the minute branches of the hæmorrhoidal veins towards the verge of the anus were varicose and distended with coagulated blood; the liver felt very greasy; its section somewhat nutmeg-like; a portion of it dried on paper was brittle; it left no oil-stain; another portion was boiled; no oil or fatty matter was obtained from it, so the appearance was deceptive; the gall-bladder was distended with bile of natural appearance as to color; the mesenteric, lumbar and sacral glands were enlarged; some contained a curd-like, some a puruloid matter; an unusual quantity of synovial fluid in each knee-joint; the cartilage of both patellæ rough, as if from interstitial absorption.

This case affords a striking instance of a complication of organic lesions, many of them, indeed all of them with the exception of the intestinal, of an undemonstrative kind. The state

of the lungs superficially crepitous, and the obstructed state of
the longitudinal sinus are peculiarly deserving of attention.
Some of the enlarged glands were immersed in boiling water;
they contracted very much; what was liquid in them coagulated
and the solid portion acquired increased firmness.

Case 12.—Of chronic dysentery, with œdema of lungs and gaseous distension of
intestines.—W. Watts, ætat. 53; 17th Foot; admitted into general hospital, 28th
May, 1823; died 18th June.—This man on admission had just returned from
India, where he had served the last five years. On the homeward voyage, in the
early part of it, about five months ago, he had an attack of dysentery, of which
there are still some slight remains. He now complained chiefly of debility and of
relaxation of bowels; there is no tormina or tenesmus; his appetite good, his
pulse regular; using Dover's powder with a bitter infusion and occasionally small doses
of Ol. Ricini and of Copaiva, with a milk-diet, his bowels became regular; he made no
complaint except of feebleness. He appeared to be gaining ground slowly till the
13th June, when he was unusually languid; there was a slight degree of pyrexia;
a small and quick pulse. On the 15th June, it was reported that he had a bad
night and was much exhausted; two watery stools; some pain in the lower part
of right breast, increased by pressure and inspiration, accompanied with cough.
Now he stated that he has been subject to frequent attacks of pain of chest with
cough; his pulse very quick and feeble; his appetite impaired From this time
till his death on the 18th the symptoms were much the same; extreme debility; a
relaxed state of bowels; slight pyrexia; cough, but little or no pain at chest;
tendency to delirium. The treatment was merely palliative.
Autopsy 4 hours after death. Cadaver greatly emaciated; limbs already rigid;
on dividing the abdominal muscles their fibres contracted; and on pricking them with
the scalpel the same action was produced; the body was still warm. With the
exception of about 3 oz. of serum in the ventricles of the brain, nothing unusual
was observed in that organ. The cellular membrane of the anterior mediastinum
was so distended with serous fluid as to be quite œdematous; in the right pleura
there were about 4 oz. of serous fluid; the lung on this side was partially adhering;
both its superior and inferior lobe were much consolidated; incised, a serous fluid
flowed out of them freely; their substance was pale; the middle lobe was red,
and crepitous; a remarkable difference in point of temperature was observable between the consolidated lobes and that free from this lesion; the latter was very
distinctly warmer than the former; in the right pleura there were about 3 oz.
of serum; no adhesions; the right lung was sound; the abdomen was distended
and sounded very tympanitic; owing, it was found, to air in the intestines; the
stomach was empty and unusually contracted, its parietes in contact and free
from any marks of disease. The duodenum and the upper part of the jejunum
were moderately contracted; they contained a little glairy mucus; the greater
part of the jejunum and the whole of the ileum, with the exception of a small
portion of its inferior extremity, were much distended with air; a portion of the
air from the former was collected for examination; the distended intestine was
here and there red; the end of the ileum and the cœcum were contracted; the latter
contained some bright yellow fæcal matter; a distinct cicatrix of an old ulcer was
found in the valvula coli; the villous coat of the contracted portion of ileum was
of a dark red; in the colon, just where it becomes ascending, there was a puckering
with contraction, the result, it may be inferred, of cicatrization, somewhat impeding a

free passage; beyond this the intestine was enormously distended with air; a portion of air was collected for examination from the sigmoid flexure; the rectum also
was much distended with air; in its upper part were small portions, they might
be called particles of fæcal matter, unusually dry, adhering to the mucous coat;
there was no air in the veins of the neck or of the abdomen; they were moderately
distended with blood; some bony matter was found in the inner coat of the aorta
just above the origin of the coronary arteries, and the semilunar valves below were
partially ossified; the viscera not named were apparently sound.   The air from the
intestines had very little smell, the odor could hardly be called fæcal; altogether
it must have amounted to 150 cubic inches at least; the air from the upper portion
of jejunum examined by means of lime-water and phosphorus appeared to consist
of 14 carbonic acid gas, 1 oxygen, 85 azote; that from the sigmoid flexure of 13
carbonic acid gas, 87 azote; neither inflamed and both extinguished flame.

In this instance was not death owing to the distension of the
intestines with air oppressing the feeble power of the constitution, debilitated by disease of lung and the preceding
dysenteric disease?   The source of the air may be a question.
There being no fermenting matter in the intestines would seem
to render it probable that it was derived from the blood, and
its composition, no more than the composition of the air in the
air-bladder of fishes, is contrary to this idea.   The irritable con-
tractile state of muscle witnessed four hours after death, and the
difference of temperature of the comparatively sound and diseased portion of right lung are specially noteworthy.

Case 13.—Of chronic dysentery, with tuberculated lungs and enlarged mesenteric
glands.—P. Kineally, ætat. 42; 58th Foot; admitted into general hospital, 8th
June, 1822; died 6th August.—This man during a service of three years in the
West Indies, from which he is just arrived, suffered much from repeated attacks of
fever, and of pectoral and abdominal disease.   The dysenteric complaint, a complaint
under which he still labors, commenced fourteen months ago; his pectoral several
months ago.   At present his principal symptoms are frequent alvine evacuations,
with tenesmus and griping; dyspnœa, cough, purulent expectoration.   There is great
debility and emaciation; pulse about 90, feeble; skin dry and harsh; tongue white
and smooth; feet œdematous.   Two or three times he seemed to rally and recover a
little, becoming worse with change of weather.   During the last month he gradually
more and more declined, losing strength and appetite, without suffering pain and
with little diarrhœa.   When questioned, his general reply was, that he was easy and
getting better.   A few hours before he died he experienced an acute pain at the
scrobiculus cordis.   The treatment was merely palliative with milk-diet and wine.
Autopsy 14 hours after death.   Body exceedingly emaciated; the right lung
firmly and very generally adhering; some serous effusion in its inferior lobe; in the
left lung, here and there a few tubercles, most of them in the superior lobe, and some
small vomicæ.   About 3 inches from the pylorus, the stomach was remarkably
contracted, the mucous membrane drawn into folds, resembling a second pylorus;
there was no apparent organic lesion, and no more thickening than might be
attributed to a spasmodic contraction; the cardiac and small pyloric portion were
both distended with air.   With the exception of a few red patches, chiefly in the

ileum, there was no marked disease in the small intestines; the large intestines bore marks of old disease, ulcers healed or healing with some thickening of their coats; the rectum was of a dark red color; the mesenteric glands were much enlarged; the viscera not mentioned seemed tolerably sound.

In this case there are some remarkable circumstances: the wasting, decline of power, the little suffering, the organic lesions; these so little severe. May not the contraction found in the stomach be attributed to spasm, and the acute pain experienced shortly before death to that cause? The limbs, it may be mentioned, at the time of the autopsy, showed the rigor mortis.

Case 14.—Of chronic dysentery, with hydrops pulmonum.—W. Sage, ætat 50; 39th Regiment; admitted into general hospital, Fort Pitt, 4th October, 1836; died 20th October.—An old soldier of 28 years' service, the last 12 in India, from whence he is just arrived. According to the document accompanying him, he was sent home on account of chronic rheumatism, and being weakly and worn out. No notice is taken in it of any bowel-complaint. He stated that he had a dysenteric attack a year ago from which he never recovered, and that it increased on the passage. His symptoms on admission were frequent slimy stools, occasionally bloody, with tormina and tenesmus; abdomen tender on pressure; appetite bad; tongue and mouth preternaturally red; skin dry; pulse small, feeble, irregular; very much emaciated; so weak as to be unable to leave his bed. At first there was some relief from treatment; stools were less frequent; there was less tenesmus and griping. On the 10th his hands became œdematous. On the 16th he was annoyed by hiccough, which ceased after the application of a blister; had pain at the same time at scrobiculus cordis and fulness of abdomen. On the 18th he complained of general soreness; had cough and expectorated a good deal of frothy fluid; stools more frequent; extremities cold. He rapidly became worse, dying on the 20th. Treatment—¼ grain acetate of lead, 1 grain of opium night and morning; chalk mixture with mucilage frequently. Afterwards opium with Hydrarg. c Cretâ.

Autopsy 42 hours after death. Body greatly emaciated; abdomen very lank; not in the slightest degree tympanitic; when a small opening was made into it, air rushed in as into a vacuum and the parietes became less tense. A good deal of serum under the arachnoid; pretty much in the ventricles; substance of brain firm and pale. Both lungs partially adhering; both more or less œdematous; no tubercles; a fluid (probably serous) in the bronchia. About 3 oz. serum in the pericardium; the band, the vestige of the ductus arteriosus, partially ossified; the heart natural. The stomach small; the small intestines nearly empty, and more or less contracted; both were without marks of disease; in the colon there were numerous ulcers healing and cicatrices of old ulcers; the latter of a bluish hue, the former pinkish with flabby granulations; the rectum was nearly free from ulceration; its surface was smeared with a thin purulent fluid. There were small hæmorrhoidal tumors at the verge of anus; liver of nutmeg-like section, weight 3¼lbs.; other abdominal viscera pretty natural; in one or two of the joints of the feet there was a softening of the cartilage; communicating with the vaginal sac of the left testicle was a small sinus, in which were many loose cartilage-like bodies about the size of snipe shot.

In this instance death probably was occasioned by effusion into the air-cells of the lungs and into the bronchia: not an uncommon termination of chronic dysentery, the dysenteric ulcers healing.

Case 15.—Of chronic dysentery, with œdema of lungs ; intestinal ulcers healed.— T. White, ætat. 32 ; 4th Foot ; admitted into general hospital, June 6th, 1840 ; died June 9th.—This man of 13 years' service, chiefly in New South Wales and India, from whence he has just returned, has, it would appear, labored under dysenteric symptoms about two years. He is now in a very exhausted state ; he fainted on removal to his room ; has no desire for food ; pulse 78, very compressible ; has frequent slimy stools tinged with blood ; no griping ; no tenesmus. The diarrhœa continuing, he rapidly sank. The treatment was palliative ; opiates and wine.

Autopsy 30 hours after death. Body but little emaciated ; pretty much fluid in the cellular tissue of the pia mater ; all the lobes of the right lung and the inferior lobe of the left were more or less œdematous, breaking readily on pressure ; no tubercles ; the liver weighed 5¼lbs. ; through the substance of both its lobes small white bodies were scattered ; they were nearly spherical and rather soft ; the spleen was rather large and soft. In the large intestines there were marks of numerous ulcers healed ; their coats were somewhat thickened and their mucous membrane variously discolored.

In this case two circumstances seem noteworthy : the healed or nearly healed state of the large intestines, and the effusion into, the œdema of, the lungs. The latter may account for the death. Was the œdema the result of debility occasioned by the dysenteric ailment, and the impaired functional state of the intestine.

Case 16.—Of chronic dysentery, with œdema of lungs and abdominal dropsy.— P. Byrne, ætat. 41 ; 25th Lt. D. ; admitted into general hospital 6th July, 1822 ; died 22nd August.—This old soldier is just returned from India, where he served thirteen years. He has had a bowel complaint for the last three months ; stools frequent without pain ; the abdomen is much distended ; there is distinct fluctuation ; is much troubled with flatulency ; his appetite bad ; is very feeble and much emaciated. Little change till the 15th ; he then complained of cough with dyspnœa, using ext. conii. and Ol. Terebinth ; no improvement took place. On the 28th July paracentesis abdomenis was performed ; 13 pints of serum were drawn off ; the feet œdematous ; relaxation of bowels the same ; appetite pretty good ; no improvement followed. On the 16th it was reported that his abdomen was again much distended ; his stools watery. On the 18th it is stated that for two days he has voided much urine, and as much as two quarts during the preceding night ; his debility increasing ; the abdomen much less in size ; the last medicine he took was T. cascarillæ with Decoct. cinchonæ and Vin. opii. He died on the evening of the 22nd.

Autopsy 35 hours after death. Body excessively emaciated ; adeps entirely wanting ; about 1 oz. of serum in the pericardium ; 4 oz. in the left pleura ; 2 oz. in the right ; both were vascular—i.e., had vessels carrying blood ; the right lung was bulky and œdematous, as was also the left in a less degree ; incised a fluid flowed from them copiously, of a light fawn color, which was coagulated by nitric acid like the serum of blood ; scattered through both lungs, in greatest number in the right, were cartilage-like tubercles varying in size from that of a pin's head to that of a pea ; they were contained in a semi-transparent vascular membrane ; within there was a brownish friable matter of different degrees of softness ; there was slight ulceration of the glottis and unusual redness of the bronchia; the bronchial glands were much enlarged; the peritoneal lining of the abdomen was unusually vascular; there were adhesions between it and the viscera in many places; the upper part of the colon and the cœcum contained a good deal of fæcal matter; the whole tract of the large intestines exhibited marks of old dysenteric disease, ulcers healed and a new coat formed, this of unequal surface and various color, mottled, grey, bluish, white, with a good deal of cartilage-like thickening of the colon, and of the rectum; there were no open ulcers; the mesenteric glands were enlarged; the spleen was rather large and firm; the liver was of a light color and firm; it contained many minute cartilage-like bodies of about the size of snipe-shot; no fluid remained in the cavity of the abdomen.

This case is noteworthy for many particulars—the great œdema of the lungs, the kind of tubercles scattered through them and the liver, the serous effusion into the abdomen, and its absorption shortly before death, and the cicatrised state of the large intestines.

Case 17.—Of chronic dysentery, with tuberculated lungs, hydrothorax and anæmia. —James Collins, ætat. 46; 16th L.; admitted into general hospital, June 8th, 1838; died 4th August.—An old soldier of 25 years' service, of these 24 in India. He was sent home to be invalided, being "worn out." On the voyage he experienced an attack of dysentery, under which he still labors; he is very feeble and emaciated, pulse 74; frequent stools. During the first few days he seemed to mend; his appetite became good; he slept well and had only three stools in the 24 hours; the bowels from that time became more relaxed; there was no mention made of tormina or tenesmus. On the 18th June it is stated that his evacuations had become involuntary, latterly they were eight in the 24 hours; his emaciation before death was extreme; he had little cough, made no complaint of his chest, he breathed easily. The treatment was palliative and various: ipecac. and opium, sulphate of copper and opium, etc.

Autopsy 29 hours after death. Though extremely emaciated, his nails were not curved; chest sounded well; a good deal of fluid between the membranes, in the ventricles and at the base of the brain; the cerebral substance generally soft, especially the fornix, septum lucidum, and walls of the ventricles; the right pleura contained 54 oz. of serum, in which were suspended flakes of lymph; the costal pleura of the same side and the diaphragmatic pleura partially were studded with granular elevations composed of lymph, or of tubercular matter; the left pleura contained 18 oz. of serum; in the right lung, in its superior lobe, there was a mass of tubercles nearly the size of a walnut, undergoing softening; here and there in the middle and inferior lobe were a few small clusters; a few clusters of the same kind were found in the inferior lobe of the left lung, and in its superior there was a bony concretion about the size of a hazel-nut; 5 oz. of serum in the pericardium; the heart was small and of a shrunken, shrivelled appearance; the little blood in its cavities was partly coagulated; an attempt was made to collect the blood from the heart and great vessels; the quantity obtained did not exceed 2 oz.; 33 oz. of serum in the cavity of the abdomen; the liver weighed 2¾ lbs.; its substance firm; the gall-bladder contained two concretions of the black kind about the size of cherries, and was distended with thin bile; the stomach was small; the small intestines were pale; the large were somewhat thickened and bore marks in many places of old ulceration; the only remaining ulcer that was found was situated near the verge of the anus; all the joints examined were more or less diseased, especially the patella; they were softening with atrophy; the body, though kept 29 hours, showed no signs of putrefaction, nor were there any marks of staining; it was conjectured at the time that if all the blood in the body could have been collected it would not have exceeded 4 oz., so anæmic was its appearance; the cruor from the heart was found coagulated the following day; the lens of eye was soft.

The emaciation, anæmia, the serous effusions, the softening of brain and of lens of eyes, and the generally healed state of the large intestines, are noteworthy circumstances.

Case 18.—Of chronic dysentery, with tuberculated lungs, hydrothorax and ascites.— J. Burrell, ætat. 28; 38th Regiment; admitted into general hospital, 20th September, 1835; died 12th December.—A man of intemperate habits, of 9 years' service in the Mediterranean and West Indies; from the latter he has just returned, laboring under "chronic dysentery and cough," said to be of 3 years' duration. He complains of pain in the course of the transverse and descending colon, increased on pressure and when at stool; bowels relaxed, stools slimy; is subject to tormina and tenesmus. Early in October the purging had diminished; but he did not gain strength; had cough with mucous expectoration; his chest sounded clear; the respiratory sound was louder in the right than the left side; in the latter it was rather indistinct. Towards the end of October his cough became worse, especially at night. Early in November he experienced griping pains in abdomen, tenderness on pressure, particularly on right side; his ankles and abdomen became swollen. Later in the month he complained of a "universal chilliness;" more pain of right side, with tightness of chest, and a very troublesome cough. In the beginning of December the fluid in the abdomen had increased; there was "gargouillement" in the upper and anterior part of the right lung, sibilant and sonorous râles pervading the right bronchia. The death was preceded by an increase of all the pectoral symptoms, with great emaciation and debility. The treatment in the first instance consisted chiefly of astringents and anodynes; latterly, when the pectoral ailments predominated, of tonics, expectorants, and blisters, etc.

Autopsy 48 hours after death. Brain not examined; the right pleura extended about 2 inches above the clavicle, it contained 7 pints of serum; the lung was very much compressed; it weighed 8 oz. and was equal in volume to a pint of water (so much it displaced when submerged); in its superior lobe there were two or three small vomicæ; in its middle lobe a few clusters of softening tubercles; its inferior lobe, with the exception of its condensation from pressure, was free from disease; the right pleura generally was coated with coagulable lymph and granules of tubercular matter; 6 oz. of serum in the pericardium; the heart was pressed towards the left ribs; the pericardium was partially adhering to the costal pleura; the lung was adhering very generally and firmly; it weighed 1¼lbs. and displaced 23 oz. of water; there was a small tubercular excavation in its superior lobe, and a few tubercles in both lobes; about 3 pints of fluid in the cavity of the abdomen; the liver weighed 3½lbs.; the gall-bladder contained five small concretions of the black kind; the cystic duct contained one which did not close the passage. There was no appearance of glandulæ aggregatæ in the ileum; there were very many solitary glands, these were enlarged, some of them were ulcerated; a small ulcer was found in the cœcum; throughout the large intestines there were patches of bluish discoloration, indicating the healing of old ulceration; the mesenteric glands were enlarged; in some of them there was a tubercular or cheese-like matter softening.

In this case we have an instance of one train of symptoms subsiding and of ulcers of the large intestines healing conjointly with the aggravation of another train of symptoms, and effusion into the pleura—an effusion that during life escaped detection, owing no doubt to the want of due examination. The tubercular granules, or granules like tubercles, on a false membrane, and the lymph effused on the right pleura, noteworthy. When the membranous lymph was peeled off, some of the granules remained adhering to the pleura as if that were their original seat; most of them, however, were removed with the false membrane.

Case 19.—Of chronic dysentery, with hydrops pulmonum, etc.—W. Moore, ætat. 46; 8th D.; admitted into general hospital, 7th May, 1823; died 8th May.—This old soldier was of 29 years' service, chiefly in India, from whence he has just returned, laboring under "chronic dysentery." His debility is extreme; is liable to syncope on the least exertion; pulse very small and feeble; bowels relaxed; evacuations brown and scanty. Wine with other stimulants were given, conjoined with Dover's powder; he never rallied; slight delirium preceded death.

Autopsy 12 hours after death. Body greatly emaciated; the right auricle and ventricle turgid with blood; the pericardium contained half-an-ounce of fluid; there was a good deal of serum in the lungs, especially in the left, almost amounting to hydrops pulmonis; the inferior lobe of right lung was unusually red and somewhat consolidated; it adhered very firmly and closely to the diaphragm; on dissecting it out, a mass of bony matter, about half the size of the hand, and of considerable thickness was detected, situated near the tendinous portion of the diaphragm; it consisted of two adhering plates—one apparently formed in the pulmonary, the other in the diaphragmatic pleura. The large intestines bore strong marks of old ulceration; there was some thickening of their coats; their mucous membrane was of a very mottled hue—bluish and greenish—indicative of old ulceration cicatrised; there were a very few ulcerated spots remaining. The liver and spleen were very friable.

This case seems chiefly interesting from want of accord between the organic lesions, the symptoms, and the fatal event. Was the debility mainly owing to the exhaustion, and the exhaustion to the deteriorated, cicatrised state of the large intestines? or more to the œdema of the lungs? Was the ossification which was detected in the diaphragm concerned in the tendency shown to syncope?

These cases may help to illustrate some of the peculiarities of chronic dysentery in connexion with its many complicated lesions. Judging from such experience as we have, I believe that chronic dysentery would rarely prove fatal in a cold or cool climate were it not for some one or other impeding complication, some lesion of the lungs, or liver, or other organs; or were it not for the permanent impairment of the functional action of the large intestines, and it may be of the mesenteric and other abdominal glands preventing due nourishment and repair of the waste of the system; that waste in its turn productive of gradual loss of power and of exhaustion ending in death. As instances of the kind, I would refer to some of the latter cases, in which, after the majority of the ulcers, the result of acute dysentery, had healed, and the whole or the greater portion of the tract of the intestine had its epithelium restored, yet the patient step by step, emaciated more and more, and with little or no suffering, and without any symptom of acute disease, gradually gave up the struggle of life. Such cases have made a strong impression on my mind; they seem to deserve particular attention, both on their own account, and, if I am right, as throwing light on the office of the large intestines as an absorbing surface. The accompaniments of this impaired state of the large intestines as described in the cases referred to, are many of them such as may be considered almost as the consequences of that state; for instance, the anæmic condition of the system, the wasting of the organs, the unusual quantity of serosity in the brain, the effusion into the cellular tissue and serous membranes, the fibrinous concretions in the vessels; these, all of them such as might result from want of due nourishment; and these, from effects, in their turn becoming causes of further prostration of vital power.

I do not consider it necessary to discuss in this place the treatment of chronic dysentery; it must vary more or less according to circumstances. Generally, when the disease has been formed in a warm climate, as is most commonly the case, removal to a cold or cool climate with attention to diet—that mild, nourishing, and strengthening—suffices for the recovery, aided by the simplest treatment. This remark of course does not apply to such cases as have been referred to, whether of a permanently injured state of the large intestines, or of complicated organic lesions. Such cases need special treatment and most careful attention.

When speaking of acute dysentery, I adverted to the evil effects of mercury given in excess, as it too often was in the treatment of the disease in India. I cannot forget the cases that used to be admitted into the general hospital at Fort Pitt coming from that country, men who had been dosed unremittingly with mercury before embarking, often continued at sea during the voyage, and who when they came into the cold and tempestuous latitudes of the Cape of Good Hope were attacked with periostitis in a severe form. On their landing many of them were in a most helpless, reduced, and suffering state; their bones (their periosteum) swollen and exquisitely painful; their limbs, especially the lower extremities, more resembling the knotted branches of the oak than anything human. One remarkable circumstance belonging to these cases was, that as the patients gained flesh and strength and their general health improved under a nourishing diet, ptyalism often to a troublesome amount took place, and this though not an additional particle of mercury had been administered, and though previously the mineral had no effect of the kind.

When we reflect on the tendency of dysentery to recur, especially in the country in which it originated, and its tendency there to become chronic and intractable, there can be no hesitation in laying it down as a principle or rule :—1. That every man severely attacked by dysentery, should, as soon as possible, be sent home for change of climate. 2. That no man who has suffered from the disease, whether acute or chronic, should, if kept in the service, be allowed to accompany his regiment abroad, except to a station where the disease is unknown as an endemic. Further, may it not be deserving of the consideration of Government, taking into account that colored troops, such as the Malays in Ceylon and the Africans in the West Indies, suffer less from this disease, as well as from all other tropical endemic diseases, whether white troops should not be withdrawn as much as possible from these and the like colonies and their place supplied by men who by constitution are better able to resist these diseases. It seems to be a well-established fact that foreigners and those least allied by blood and race to the natives of a country are always the greatest sufferers from the diseases of the country, and are subject to the highest rate of mortality, and that that is greatest, the greater the contrast of climate.

Comparing the exemption in a great measure of officers from this distressing and destructive disease with the great liability of privates and non-commissioned officers to contract it, is there not ground for hope that with improved sanitary measures tending more and more to approximate the condition of the common soldier to that of the officer, especially as regards diet, clothing, and shelter, the difference in question will disappear, and the disease will cease to be the scourge of our troops— "the fearful epidemic scourge," to use an expression of Sir James Emerson Tennent, in his elaborate and able work on Ceylon. As prophylactic means it would be conducive to this consummation and well for the health of the soldier, were the salt ration to be given up entirely; were the fresh meat to be supplied of a more varied kind and of a better quality than that commonly served out on foreign stations, contracted for at a low price; it would be well were the privies to be connected with the barracks by passages under cover; it would be well too were such alterations made in the dress as would adapt it to the wants of the climate, and were a warm sash* as a support and protection to the abdomen to form a part of the soldier's necessaries. It would be well too for the health of the troops were a wholesome beverage to form a part of their ration; besides coffee, cocoa, or tea for their morning and evening meal, were a portion of mild ale, or light sound wine, or light punch composed of rum (not new), of lemon-juice, and sugar, served out with their dinner. When we consider the high proportional mortality to which the army hitherto has been subject and the share that dysentery has had in producing that mortality, such improvements, whatever their cost might be, would, by the saving of life, eventually, it cannot be doubted, prove economical; and, great will be the merit, great the credit due to the Secretary for War who may have the resolution, and I would say the humanity, to effect the change.

---

* In most warm climates, especially in the South of Europe and in the warmer regions of Asia, a sash forms a part of the dress of the natives, and the swathing of the loins is a preparation for a journey. In the first voyage I made in the Mediterranean I had for a companion a London merchant, who occasionally visited Alexandria, where there was a branch of his business. He told me that he never left England for Egypt without adopting the Eastern precaution, and thereby, he believed he had always escaped bowel-complaint. I have followed his example with like good effect. A sash, I think, is preferable to a belt—such as the cholera belt— a knit sash of worsted, not more than two inches wide, and not less than twenty feet long. Its adaptability and elasticity recommend it. It may be worn in all climates with advantage: in a cold and moist climate it is no mean protection against lumbago; in the battle field, in case of bleeding from a wound, it would form an excellent bandage.

CHAPTER III.

ON CHOLERA MORBUS.

Remarks on the two kinds,—the Epidemic and Common.—Special Report on the former as it occurred in Ceylon in 1819.—Observations on Common Cholera, as Sporadic and Endemic, with Cases.—On the Pathology of the Disease and its Treatment.

On a disease which, during the better part of the last half century, has attracted so much attention and given rise to so much inquiry, I can hardly venture to hope that any contribution I can make will be of much value. However, as the malady is hardly yet divested of its obscurity, whether we look to its etiology or pathology, I shall venture to give my observations on the subject, restricting them nearly to the actual experience I have had of the disease.

In the statistical medical reports of the army a distinction is very properly made between ordinary cholera morbus and epidemic cholera.

The following table, extracted from these reports, showing the proportional mortality of each per 10,000, aggregate strength, is instructive. The description of troops is the same as that specified when treating of fevers and dysentery, the periods in part only differing.

			Admitted.	Died.
United Kingdom. Dragoon Guards and Dragoons, from Jan. 1830 to March, 1837, both included...	cholera morbus		55·1 ...	0·67
	cholera epidem.		83·3 ...	12·10
Gibraltar, from 1818 to 1836..........................	ch.	m.	204·1 ...	1·1
	ch.	ep.	76·1 ...	21.7
Malta, from 1818 to 1836...............................	ch.	m.	111·2 ...	1·2
	ch.	ep.	— ...	—
Ionian Islands, from 1817 to 1836....................	ch.	m.	182·9 ...	1·8
	ch.	ep.	— ...	—
Bermudas, from 1817 to 1836...........................	ch.	m.	329 ...	2·1
	ch.	ep.	— ...	—
Nova Scotia and New Brunswick, from 1817 to 1836...	ch.	m.	91·9 ...	0·6
	ch.	ep.	45·2 ...	12·7
Canada, from 1817 to 1836.............................	ch.	m.	71 ...	0.93
	ch.	ep.	53·7 ...	19·7
Sierra Leone, from 1819 to 1836.—White Troops.	ch.	m.	48·9 ...	10*
	ch.	ep.	— ...	—

* The actual aggregate strength of white troops was 1,843 ; in one year there were 5 cases of cholera and two deaths, altogether only 9 cases, which may account for the

		Admitted.	Died.
Cape of Good Hope, from 1822 to 1834............. }	cholera morbus	10·5 ...	1·5
	cholera epidemic	— ...	—
Mauritius, from 1818 to 1836......................... }	ch. m.	60 ...	1·3
	ch. ep.	87·8 ...	10.4
West Indies. Windward and Leeward Islands } Command, from 1817 to 1836...................... }	ch. m.	135·3 ...	2·7
	ch. ep.	— ...	—
Jamaica, from 1817 to 1836......... .... }	ch. m.	41·8 ...	0.59
	ch. ep.	— ...	—
Black Troops.. }	ch. m.	24·4 ...	1·7
Ceylon, from 1817 to 1836............................ }	ch. m.	95·1 ..	2.8
	ch. ep.	181·2 ...	57·4
1st Ceylon Rifles, Malays, from 1818 to 1836 ...... }	ch. m.	8 ...	0·29
	ch. ep.	60.3 ...	29·7

This table shows in a striking manner the difference in degree of mortality of the two diseases, taking a summary of the whole, exclusive of Sierra Leone, the deaths from the one being 1·2 per cent., of those attacked, of the other 27·7 per cent. It shows also how well the former deserves the popular name of common cholera, and the other of epidemic cholera. And further it shows, limited as are the data, that the colored races are not exempt from either form of the disease.

My experience of the more formidable disease—and what disease is more formidable than this and terrific in its intensity!—is confined to the epidemic which broke out in Ceylon in 1819, in which year out of 236 white troops attacked, it proved fatal to 89, and of 50 Malays of the 1st Ceylon Rifles attacked it proved fatal to 21. This outbreak was shortly after the great eruption of the disease in the army of the Marquis of Hastings in Upper Bengal, an eruption as sudden and unexpected as it was dreadful and destructive ; and what was equally marvellous was its arrest— that by the removal of the encampment to a short distance, less than a day's march ! I well remember a letter I received from a medical officer present descriptive of that march ; it reminded him of the flight of an army defeated, panic-stricken, followed by a relentless enemy, the road being strewed with dead and dying, the latter vastly exceeding any available means of relief, their numbers were so great, the medical officers present so few. I well too remember the consternation which the advent of the disease gave rise to in Ceylon amongst all classes of the people,

high mortality per 10,000 ; showing at the same time that estimates thus made are at best merely approximate. Amongst the black troops at this station, not one case of cholera was returned during the period.

the indescribable fear beyond all reasonable bounds in the families even of the best informed, the religious ceremonies and processions instituted by the Catholics, the extraordinary rites by the heathen sects with the hope of appeasing the wrath of their gods: a report even was spread and believed at the time that malignant demons had arrived and had been seen at night in the streets of the Pettah. And, what aggravated the individual alarm was, a general persuasion entertained that the dread of the disease increased the susceptibility to receive it. As soon as the epidemic had abated, as Acting Physician to the Forces, which I then was, I was called on by the Deputy-Inspector of Hospitals, in common with other medical officers, for a report of my experience. This I supplied in the following letter, written at the time on the spur of the occasion.

Colombo, August 1st, 1819.

SIR,—In compliance with the wishes expressed in your letter of the 26th May, I have now the honor to address you on the subject. of the epidemic cholera which lately prevailed in this island in common with a great part of India. I may premise that the opportunities I have had of observing the disease have not been numerous ; altogether I may have seen about 40 cases, of which the majority were amongst the natives.

1. In most instances the attack of the disease was sudden, not preceded by any warning ; a man has left his house in the morning to follow his usual occupation, apparently in robust health ; he has been attacked by cholera as if struck by lightning, has been carried home in an alarming state, and often before night he has expired.

2. Predisposition to the disease may exist in some habits—it is reasonable to suppose that it does ; but what the nature of the predisposition is, I am entirely ignorant. The feeble and ailing have been spared, while the healthy and robust have been struck down ; the temperate man has been attacked and the drunkard has been passed by. The indigent amongst the natives have apparently suffered most; but they form the great mass of the people ; and I am not aware of any document to prove that they have suffered in a greater proportion.

3. The symptoms of the disease in the cases which have come under my observation have exhibited some variations. They may perhaps be divided with advantage into those which have

occurred generally in every instance ; those of occasional occurrence, and those which have occurred in particular instances only.

The most general symptoms have been an extraordinary sinking of the pulse, diminution of muscular power and sudden cooling of the body. Without these symptoms I have not seen a single case of the disease ; indeed were the pulse natural, and much more were it strong, one would hesitate in allowing the case in which it occurred to be an instance of the epidemic.

The occasional symptoms were a slight purging, slight retching or vomiting and painful spasms of some of the muscles. Occasionally all these symptoms have been present at the commencement of the attack, but, with the exception of spasm, they have not been obstinate, and have readily yielded to opium, the disease continuing its progress ; and occasionally, viz., in two or three instances, neither purging nor vomiting has been observed during any period of the malady. The minor occasional symptoms which I have noted have been, at the commencement of the attack, restlessness, mental agitation, sensation of cold : in the advanced stage, confusion of intellect, diminished sensation, tendency to sleep, sometimes amounting to coma.

I shall detail a few cases as examples of the principal varieties I have met with, extracting them from my note-book :—

Case 1.—Daniel Vandort, ætat. about 35, a man of color, of the class commonly called Portuguese, of robust frame, a butcher, in very good circumstances inhabiting the Pettah (the suburb) of Colombo ; at 8 a.m. on the 27th of January last, when in perfect health he left his house and came into the Fort ; at 10 a.m. he suddenly became very weak, was seized with cramp in the calves of legs and with vomiting and purging. At 2 p.m., after he had been taken home, he was seen by assistant apothecary Mr. Kellert, who found him in a very alarming state ; no pulse at the wrist ; the action of heart imperceptible ; the skin cold covered with sweat ; spasms, and these severe, of various muscles, of legs, arms, and abdomen ; very restless ; neither purging nor vomiting urgent ; 40 drops of laudanum were administered. At 3 p.m. I visited him ; I could perceive no pulse of heart or arteries ; the extremities were cold and the whole surface of the body cool and bathed in sweat ; even the axilla felt cool ; a thermometer placed in it did not rise above 96°, and under the tongue it was stationary at 97°. I asked him if he felt any uneasiness about the chest ; he replied, "No ;" his breathing was quick, about 34 per minute, but not laborious. He said he had no fixed pain anywhere ; nor was pain produced by pressure on the abdomen ; cramps occurred frequently in different muscles, especially of the inferior and superior extremities, and of the abdomen ; and once, whilst I was present, the muscles of the face were severely affected as in trismus ; the spasms were of short duration and so painful were they that, under the agony they occasioned, he could not always refrain from crying aloud ; the tongue was clean ; he was rather thirsty and often called for water. Whilst I was with him—about an hour—he had no vomiting or retching or evacuation from the bowels. An enema that was prescribed and given was not retained. His expression of countenance was wild; the eyes a little sunk; the features not collapsed; his manner was agitated; his intellect clear. When I left him at 4 p.m. he seemed a very little better, more composed, and his pulse now and then was just perceptible. He expired at 8 p.m. Between this and my visit, I was assured that there had been little change of symptoms and no return of vomiting or purging, and that nearly to the last moment he retained his consciousness.

Case 2.—A palanqueen bearer, ætat. about 25, an active stout Singalese, was attacked at Colombo, on the 25th March, in the morning; in the afternoon he was brought to the Pettah Hospital, of which I had charge. On arrival the symptoms were severe; no pulse could be perceived; his debility was great; the extremities cold, the tongue warm; the surface of body was bedewed with a cold sweat, and he was suffering from cramps of the extremities, especially of the lower. Before admission he had vomited two or three times and had as many liquid stools. March 26th—No pulse has yet been felt—24 hours have elapsed—extremities still cold; has experienced no return of the cramps or vomiting; three liquid stools, resembling chyme and containing two round worms (Ascaris lumbicoides); is perfectly conscious. March 27th—Yesterday afternoon his pulse became perceptible; his skin warmer; now the pulse is distinct and not very rapid; has some little appetite; complains only of debility. April 3rd—He was discharged to-day perfectly recovered. During convalescence he experienced no febrile symptoms or undue heat of surface.

Case 3.—A native woman, ætat. about 20, of slender frame, previously in good health; in the middle of the night of the 20th February at Colombo, awoke with a feeling of indisposition; in the morning she found herself unable to walk, from extreme debility. In the course of the forenoon she vomited a little and had two or three liquid stools. At two p.m. she was brought to the Pettah Hospital; no pulse could then be felt; the skin was cold and covered with a cold sweat; no cramps, nor had she experienced any from the beginning of the attack, and it ended without any; she was conscious, and yet made no complaint of pain or suffering. At 4 p.m. she expired.

Case 4.—A native, a horsekeeper, ætat. about 25, a well-made active man, residing at Colombo; was quite well on the 16th February; on the 17th about 5 a.m. he suddenly became ill; between the hours of 5 and 7 he had vomited a little, had two or three liquid stools, and had experienced cramps in the legs; at the latter hour he was brought to my house; when called to see him I found him in the sitting posture, his back resting for support against the wall of the room; I could perceive no pulse; his breathing was a little quicker than natural; his extremities very cold, as was also the body, and he was covered with a cold sweat. He was perfectly conscious, made then no complaint of pain, or indeed complaint of any kind; after giving him a stimulating draught containing some opium, I ordered him to be taken to the Pettah Hospital; to my surprise he stood up and with a little assistance walked out, stopping at a distance of about 20 yards, where he sat down for a few minutes under the shade of a tree, whilst bearers were collecting to convey him. The hospital was little more than half a mile distant. He died by the way.

Case 5.—A Kandyan woman, ætat. about 17, of healthy constitution, in good circumstances, at Fort Macdonald, in the district of Ouva, where I saw her, in passing; was in perfect health on the 15th April; at night, on the 16th, she was seized with retching and vomiting and slight diarrhœa. On the following morning at 8 o'clock her pulse was very quick and feeble; there was much prostration of strength; the body was cool, the extremities almost cold; the retching, the vomiting and the diarrhœa were troublesome; there was no pain of abdomen; no cramps. In this state she continued the whole of the day. On the following day the symptoms had all abated and her recovery was rapid.

In describing these cases I have made mention of the expression of the countenance in one instance only. As I have observed it, it has commonly been wild, anxious and haggard, and the more so generally in proportion to the degree of danger; the features at the same time being collapsed, exhibiting frequently in a few hours very distinctly the *facies Hippocratica.*

The treatment employed in all of them was very much the same as that which I shall have to describe as I proceed.

4. The opportunities I have had to investigate the nature of the disease by dissection have been few, not exceeding four. I shall briefly describe what appeared most worthy of notice in each autopsy.

1.—Autopsy 12 hours after death. The vessels of the brain were unusually turgid, full of dark-colored blood; about 1 oz. of serosity in the ventricles and at the base of the brain; the stomach and intestines contained a good deal of air; the mucous coat of the former was of a pinkish hue; the peritoneal covering of the intestines, and especially of the small intestines, was redder and perhaps more vascular than usual; the liver was rather pale and soft; the gall-bladder contained about the usual quantity of bile and of natural appearance; the abdominal muscles, and indeed the muscles generally, were very red and tender.

2.—Autopsy 15 hours after death. The brain was not examined; the lungs were very full of liquid blood; the veins of the heart were distended with blood, and there was a good deal of blood in the auricles and ventricles and in the ascending aorta; the blood was of a dark color and very little of it was coagulated; the lining membrane of the heart and aorta where in contact with blood, was bright red, probably stained; the substance of the heart was remarkably soft, especially that of the left ventricle; it more resembled liver than muscle, not offering more resistance, breaking on pressure with as much facility; the muscles generally appeared to be softer but not redder than usual; the large intestines contained a whitish chyme-like fluid; the liver and spleen like the lungs were gorged with dark fluid blood; the bile in gall-bladder was natural both in appearance and quantity.

3.—Autopsy 14 hours after death. The pia mater was unusually vascular; there was a good deal of serosity between the membranes and in the ventricles, and at the base of the brain; the left lung was gorged with blood and serum; the substance of the left ventricle was unusually soft and friable; that of the left auricle rather less so, and that of the right ventricle still less; there was very little blood in the heart, but a good deal in the great vessels, and only slightly coagulated; the muscles of the chest and abdomen were red, and pretty firm; the peritoneal coat of the intestines was perhaps a little more vascular than usual; in the stomach there was some mucous fluid; on its inner coat, here and there, there were red spots, and similar spots were found on the villous coat of the small intestines; the urinary bladder was very much contracted and its mucous coat was somewhat vascular; the bile, and the viscera not mentioned exhibited no unusual appearance.

4. Autopsy 14 hours after death. The brain was not examined. The lungs were healthy, excepting perhaps that the left contained an undue quantity of blood

About half an ounce of serum was found in the pleura, and about two drachms in the pericardium. The substance of the heart, especially of the left ventricle, was unusually soft and friable. The stomach contained a considerable quantity of half digested food. There was a good deal of chyme or chyme-like fluid in the small intestines. In them and in the large intestines there were several round worms, and in the latter many ascarides (A. vermicularis). The abdominal viscera were healthy the bile natural.

Of these four autopsies, the subjects of the first and second were the bodies of soldiers, privates of the 83rd Regiment, who before the fatal attack had been in good health and were robust. The disease in both cases was of a few hours' duration. In the first there were violent spasms of the abdominal muscles and the muscles of the extremities ; some troublesome retching, but little purging. He was conscious to the last. In the second there was retching but not severe, and there were frequent calls to stool ; the stools liquid, but fæcal. There was no pain of abdomen, no uneasiness of chest, no cramps. Very early, no pulse could be felt.* The extremities and head were cold, and covered with cold sweat. He, too, retained consciousness to the last, expiring "without suffering." The subjects of the third and fourth were the bodies of natives; the third that of a woman, case 3; that of the fourth, of a man who was attacked after drinking largely of toddy (the fermented juice of the cocoa-nut palm), and died a few hours after. When brought to the Pettah hospital he was moribund. Just before he expired he experienced slight cramps : on admission there was no pulse ; he was restless, covered with cold sweat. No mention was made of vomiting in this case, or of purging.

In these few autopsies the most remarkable circumstance noticed seemed to have been the state of the heart and muscles, resembling the state in which they are said to be in animals hunted to death or killed by lightning. As many hours elapsed before the inspection of the bodies was made, it may be supposed that the weakness witnessed of the muscular fibre may have been owing to incipient decomposition, and that the same state of muscle would be observable in the bodies of persons dying of

* In my notes of this case, I find it remarked, referring to there being no pulse, no action of the heart perceptible, that it reminded me of the peculiar state in which John Hunter once found himself, walking about when the heart's action, judging from want of pulse, was suspended; for, like Hunter, this man had not lost the use of the voluntary muscles; he could turn in bed, and even with a little aid get out of bed (very improperly permitted) and go to the close stool. Though cold, I may add, he did not feel cold; and the eyes examined, the pupils appeared natural.

other and ordinary diseases after the same lapse of time.   The former supposition may be correct; it seems probable that the unusual weakness of the muscular fibre may be owing to or connected with incipient putrefaction.   But the latter inference I do not believe to be just, for in other instances, when the bodies of those who died of ordinary diseases had been kept as long or longer, I have not observed the same degree of softening of muscle ; and, as an experiment, at the season that cholera was prevailing I purposely deferred the inspection of the body of a native who had died of dysentery so long as 20 hours, when I found the substance of the heart firm and the muscles generally as they usually appear.   Were the heart and muscles discovered in every fatal case of the disease to be as above described, it would be, I need hardly remark, an important fact established. I have made inquiries of a few medical friends who have had a good deal of experience of cholera, what their observations have been on the subject, and their reply has been, that they have not accorded with mine.   Notwithstanding, I am far from certain that they would disagree were they made under the same conditions, and were the attention of the observers specially directed to the point in question.

5. The observations I have to offer on the state of the secretions in this epidemic are not nearly so numerous or minute as I could wish.

In no instance have I seen the bile vitiated ; nor am I aware of any proof of its being either deficient in quantity or excessive in quantity ; or that either it or its secreting organ is concerned in the disease.   In the evacuations both sursum and deorsum rather a deficiency than an excess of bile has commonly been observed. But as bile in its usual quantity has been found in the gallbladder after death, the deficiency in the evacuations cannot logically be connected with suppressed secretion.

In investigating the nature of the disease it appeared to me of some moment to attend not only to the appearance of the venous blood but to that also of the arterial, and to observe also at the same time the condition of the air expired.   The importance of this part of the inquiry occurred to me at Kandy in the latter end of April, when returning from a tour into some of the distant provinces of the interior.   I communicated my ideas on the subject to my very intelligent and worthy friend,

Mr. Finlayson, now Assistant Surgeon of the 8th Dragoons.*
He entered into my views with zeal and very kindly gave me
his assistance. During the few days I stopped at Kandy we
had an opportunity to make one experiment. The subject of
it was a negro who had been brought in from Matelè laboring
under cholera; he had experienced some vomiting and purging,
was conscious but could not speak; his extremities were cold,
his body cool; a thermometer introduced under the tongue was
stationary at 94°, in the axilla at 93°; the skin was dry; his
pulse very feeble and quick; the breathing not laborious. To
ascertain the effect of respiration on the air he expired, we made
him breathe into a collapsed bladder and tried the air by means
of a strong solution of potash. We made a similar experiment
on the air expired by a healthy negro. The latter was found
to contain four times more carbonic acid than the former. At
my desire Mr. Finlayson was so good as to continue the inquiry
at a time I had not an opportunity to follow it myself; the
result has been that in every instance, and he tried the experiments in several, he found the air expired very deficient in
carbonic acid; and he observed little or no difference in the
appearance of venous and arterial blood. Some observations
of his which he favoured me with in a letter dated Kandy, the
4th June, are very precise on this subject. I shall take the
liberty of quoting them. He writes: " I have repeated the
experiment in question on a pioneer with the following results :
He had been about six hours ill with cholera; temperature
under the tongue 91°; in the axilla 92°5; pulse small, feeble,
but distinct, in frequency 90; blood from the temporal artery
flowed feebly per saltum; it was received into a glass vessel;
it appeared of a very dark color; coagulated readily; contained
a small portion of whitish serum. Blood from a vein in the
arm, taken at the same time, flowed very slowly in a very
small stream; it coagulated readily; its color was very dark;
there was no separation of coagulable lymph, and only of a
very small quantity of serum. There was scarce any difference

---

* This my friend, a most promising medical officer, equally distinguished for
ability and acquirements, accompanied Mr. Crawford to Siam, as physician and
naturalist in 1820. Whilst on that service he contracted pulmonary disease, which
shortly proved fatal. He lived barely long enough to write an account of the
mission; the volume, and it is an interesting one, was published after his death,
edited by Dr. Somerville.

in the color of the arterial and venous blood; if any, the margin of the glass containing the arterial blood was of a lighter shade than that containing the venous; it was difficult to distinguish the one from the other. The air expired from the lungs was examined in the manner you suggested. Compared with that expired from the lungs of a healthy person of the same race and country the former seemed to contain only one-third the carbonic acid in the latter." In no instance that I have heard of has the blood taken from the vein of a person laboring under cholera exhibited a buffy coat.

6. Relative to the *lædentia* and *juvantia* in the treatment of this disease my own experience has also been very limited. I have never employed venesection; opium combined with calomel in large doses; gentle friction of the body with oil of turpentine; bottles of hot water to the extremities; hot fomentations to the abdomen, the warm bath; one or two enemata composed of castor oil, oil of turpentine, and laudanum at the commencement, and frequent injections of hot rice water through the course of the complaint have been the means most commonly had recourse to. This method of treatment in many instances appeared to do good; and in no instance that I am aware of were the symptoms aggravated by it. In the Pettah hospital, under my direction, it had a pretty fair trial. In that excellent charitable institution, there were admitted from the latter end of January to the latter end of May 21 cases of cholera, of whom 11 died, 10 recovered. Now, taking into consideration that three or four of the poor wretches were brought in moribund, and comparing this result with the general mortality in Ceylon, I think I may venture to draw a conclusion in favor of the practice followed.

The diminished action of the heart, often amounting to apparent cessation, seemed to indicate the use of electricity. In two instances I tried the effect of voltaic electricity passed through the chest from a small battery composed of thirty double plates, each 4 inches square. In one case it seemed to do some good, certainly the pulse rose under its influence. In the other it had no apparent effect, indeed any effect could hardly be expected, for before the apparatus was ready the patient was moribund. I regret much that I had not a greater electrical power, as I am much disposed to think it would have proved serviceable; at all events the result might have been of importance in the investigation of the nature of the disease.

After I had found by experiment that in respiration in this disease very little carbonic acid is formed, or evolved, it occurred to me that oxygen gas and stimulating vapors, as the vapor of ether and ammonia, might be inhaled into the lungs with a prospect of some advantage. I have yet had no opportunity to make trial of their effect. Mr. Finlayson, from the effect of the fumes of the sesqui-carbonate of ammonia in three cases, is inclined to think favorably of the method; two of the three recovered, and even in the fatal case the fumes seemed to be of some service.

7. I am not acquainted with any facts that throw the least light on this epidemic. During the months of January and June that it prevailed in the island I had opportunities of observing how very various the circumstances were under which it occurred, at the same place at different times, and in different places at the same time. It appeared to be quite unconnected with the direction of the wind, the dryness or moisture of the air, with heat or cold, with elevation or lowness of situation, with salubrity or unhealthiness of climate. Were it not that the details would occupy a great deal of space, I might mention facts which I collected in a tour I made into the interior of the island in the months of March and April, tending to prove that the cause of the disease is not any sensible, appreciable change in the state of the atmosphere; so much so, indeed, that were one guided by reasoning alone, like Sydenham in the instance of the fevers of his time, one might be led to conclude that its cause is either miasmata extricated from the bowels of the earth, the effect of an intestine motion, or emanating from above in consequence of some peculiar conjunction of the heavenly bodies. At present, perhaps, it is better to confess our ignorance. Yet, considering the progress of the disease, its epidemic character, the immense extent of country it has spread over, one can hardly hesitate in admitting the cause of it to exist in the atmosphere. It may be extricated from beneath the earth's surface; it may be generated in the atmosphere; like heat and light it may be capable of radiating through space independent of currents of air; like electricity it may be capable of passing from place to place in an imperceptible moment of time,—thus, we may throw

out conjecture after conjecture, and with Sydenham say :—" At vero quæ, qualisque sit illa aeris dispositio a quâ morbificus hic apparatus promanat nos pariter ac complura alia, circa quæ vecors et arrogans philosophantium turba nugatur plane ignoramus."

What is the seat of the disease, what its exact nature; whether the name cholera morbus is appropriate; whether it is to be classed with cholera or requires a distinct place in nosological arrangement, are important points for consideration which I must avoid as involving a general investigation of the subject foreign to my present object.

I have the honor to be, sir,
Your obedient humble servant,
J. DAVY.

To Dr. Farrell, Deputy Inspector
of Hospitals.

My experience of common cholera, I hardly need remark, has been more extensive than that of the epidemic disease, having witnessed it both at home, in Ceylon, in the Mediterranean, and the West Indies.

In certain features the two diseases have a close resemblance, so great indeed, that now comparing them as well as I can, I am disposed to say, as regards merely the symptoms, that the severer cases of the common kind are identical with the milder of the epidemic, and that the two are distinguished more by their termination than their phenomena—the common so rarely fatal, the epidemic so dreadfully fatal. In proof of the little mortality from common cholera I may refer to the table already given; further, I may mention that of 195 admissions in Malta from this disease from 1830 to 1834, both years included, 2 only proved fatal, and of these 1 owed its end to a different disease supervening on symptoms simulating those of cholera. Moreover, the two kinds are not unallied in the manner in which they occur; the common kind being occasionally epidemic or endemic, the severer kind occasionally sporadic. At Chatham in 1821 and 1822, when I was in charge of the Medical Division of the General Hospital at Fort Pitt, common cholera was prevalent there. Later, when between 1835 and 1839, I was at the same hospital in general charge, hardly a case of the disease occurred. In Ceylon there was a remarkable example of the severer form taking place sporadically. The surgeon of the naval hospital at Trincomalie, in perfect health in the morning, as he thought, was suddenly attacked with cholera and before night he was a corpse, and this at a time that the island was considered perfectly free from the disease. Writing from memory, I believe this solitary example occurred in 1820, after the epidemic visitation had entirely ceased. In illustration of the resemblance of the two kinds, I shall transcribe one case that occurred of the common kind at Fort Pitt in 1821, which, more than usually severe, recovered, and also the very few fatal cases I have witnessed of it, of which there was a *post mortem* examination. I shall preface them with extracts from my yearly reports in which they were described. The first is as follows :—

This disease, cholera, was unusually prevalent in September. The weather at the time was warm and showery, the wind mostly from the S.W. The cause of the complaint was commonly supposed to be the eating of bad fruit which then abounded; but as most of the men attacked declared that they had eaten little or no fruit; and when I reflect that several men in hospital laboring under other complaints were similarly affected in a slight degree, I am disposed to doubt the correctness of the popular opinion of its origin, and to infer that it depended on a peculiar state of the atmosphere.

The symptoms generally were slight and easily relieved; the most ordinary were frequent retching, vomiting, and diarrhœa; cramps of the muscles of the lower extremities; slight pyrexia indicated by increased heat of the trunk; accelerated pulse, but not much enfeebled; thirst. The countenance was little altered; the strength not much impaired. In most instances little bile was passed *sursum vel deorsum*. The alvine evacuations at the beginning of the attack were scanty and watery; towards its end in several cases fæcal and copious.

The treatment employed and which succeeded very well, was the exhibition of opium in conjunction with calomel and aperients.

The case that exceeded the others in severity was the following :—

John Cox, ætat. 25; of sanguine temperament, previously in good health, was seized last night, September 25th, with vomiting and purging; his stools watery;

had a feeling of oppression about the stomach with pain in the left hypochondrium like cramp; his extremities were cold, especially the feet; had cramps in the legs, thighs, and arms. These symptoms were preceded by loss of appetite and diarrhœa of two days' duration. Since his admission, about two hours ago, he has vomited a large quantity of fluid mixed with mucus and colored yellow by bile and he has had several watery stools without fæcal matter, containing a curd-like matter tinged greenish by bile. The symptoms now (9 a.m.) are great debility, countenance shrunk, extremities cold; heat of body rather increased; cramps in the extremities and stomach; pulse 120, small and feeble; tongue red and dry, its back part covered with yellow fur; thirst; complete anorexia. A bolus of 10 grs. of calomel, 2 of opium, and 3 drops of oil of peppermint. 3 p.m.—Has had three or four stools similar to the preceding; vomiting of the same kind of fluid; cramps severe; pulse exceedingly small and weak; extremities still cold. A warm bath of 101°; and whilst in it to have a bolus of calomel and compound colocynth extract, 10 grs. of each, with 1 gr. of opium and 2 drops of oil of peppermint, also a draught formed of 10 drops of liq. opii sedat. in 2 oz. of peppermint water. 9 p.m.—Was relieved by the bath; only a slight return of vomiting; two stools, differing little from the preceding, but with rather more fæcal odor; pulse 114, stronger; some diaphoresis; is easier in every respect, and inclined to sleep. Sept. 27.—Slept several hours during the night; three stools, these much the same as before; less nausea; tongue cleaner; pulse 110; extremities cold; still troubled with cramps, but less severe. The following draught to be taken immediately; and after it a warm bath at 100°. R. pulv. rhei xx. grs., T. rhei ii. drs.; magnes. ustæ xv. grs., liq. opii sedat. xv. gut., aq. cinnam i. oz. After the bath the same draught as that of yesterday and the same bolus. 9 p.m.—The first draught was thrown up; has vomited several times in the course of the day; two or three stools, not very fæcal; diaphoresis came on after the bath; has had some sleep; feels now pretty easy; pulse stronger; countenance flushed. A blister to epigastrium. September 28th.— Slept several hours during the night; no return of vomiting; three stools, the last more fæcal; pulse 104, soft; countenance flushed; increased heat of skin; tongue red; some thirst; only a slight return of cramps; on the whole feels better. To have the following draught: R. magnes. sulphat. ii. drs., infus. sennæ i. oz., infus. calumbæ iii. ozs. Vespere.—Has had six stools, the two last more copious and fæcal; pulse 92. September 29th.—A pretty good night; no return of vomiting; countenance flushed; tongue clean, of a bright red; the gums and lining membrane of mouth of the same color; the conjunctivæ slightly inflamed; some abatement of thirst; less heat of skin; pulse 90. September 30th.—Has passed a considerable quantity of natural fæces. No pain or cramps; pulse 82, soft; skin of moderate warmth; extremities nearly of natural heat; less thirst; tongue and fauces still red; gums slightly affected by the calomel. The following draught immediately: R. pulv. rhei, grs. xxiv., infus. calumbæ, ii. ozs. Vespere.—No effect from medicine. The following bolus to be taken: R. ext. colocynth compos. grs. viii., pulv. rhei, grs. vi. October 1st.—Two copious fæcal natural stools; tongue moist and clean; pyrexia has subsided; pulse good. October 2nd.—Six fæcal and consistent stools in the 24 hours; appetite improving; slight cough with mucous expectoration; no pain of chest, respiration easy. October 3rd.—Two stools since last night; slight cough; convalescent. October 6th.—Quite well; discharged.

The next extract is from my Report from Fort Pitt at the close of the following year, viz., 1822; I give it chiefly on account of the fatal case described in it.

The cases of cholera occurred in August, in the middle of which month without any assignable cause the disease was prevalent amongst the inhabitants of the adjoining towns, and attacked in a slight degree many men in hospital admitted with other diseases.

Commonly the spasms were severe, affecting chiefly the lower extremities, less frequently the muscles of the abdomen and thorax; the pulse and temperature were somewhat depressed; the vomiting and purging were not very urgent or bilious, indeed, what first came away, whether *sursum* or *deorsum*, was deficient in bile. The disease in most instances readily yielded to opium and purgatives combined. In one severe case, in which there was pain in the abdomen on pressure, the lancet was twice used with advantage. In this instance, after the purging and vomiting had been checked by opium, purgatives administered procured very copious fæcal evacuations; the stools previously were watery, light-colored, and scanty.

The one fatal case was an exception to some of the above remarks. On admission, the patient, an old soldier, ætat. 35, appeared to be in articulo mortis; his countenance was collapsed and cadaverous; the extremities cold; the surface generally covered with cold sweat; the pulse was imperceptible. After taking a stimulating draught he revived a little, and was just able in a faltering voice to answer the questions put to him. He had been attacked the preceding night; he expired in about forty-eight hours. The case reminded me of the cholera of India. It was remarkable for the symptoms above noticed, for the spasms, vomiting and purging not being distressing, for the loss of speech at the beginning of the attack, and for low delirium towards its close. The treatment tried had little effect; it consisted chiefly in the exhibition of diffusible stimuli, of purgative medicine and enemata with a little opium, and the application of heat through different media.

The autopsy was made 20 hours after. The body was not emaciated; the limbs were still rigid. Sanguineous congestion was very manifest in the membranes of the brain, of the spinal canal, in the coats of the intestines, and in most of the viscera. Some fluid was effused in the ventricles of the brain and in the spinal canal. The theca of the great sympathetic in the thorax and of the nerves which the sympathetic receives from the spine before its entering the abdomen, exhibited a similar vascular turgescence, as if inflamed. The substance of the heart and muscles was unusually soft, similar to what I had witnessed in Ceylon. In addition to the foregoing there were other morbid appearances, especially of the lungs and liver, the effects of former chronic disease contracted in Ceylon, for which he was sent home invalided, under the appellation of " general ill health."

Other two fatal cases I shall give, but with less detail than I could wish ; one occurred in Malta in 1831, the other in Barbadoes in 1845. Of the latter I have only my notes taken at the autopsy.

Case 1.—J. Chadwick, ætat. 43 ; 35th Regiment; admitted into regimental hospital 12th February; died 13th February.—A man of drunken habits; he stated on admission that during the preceding night he had experienced violent vomiting and purging; his countenance is shrunk; skin cold; pulse slow and feeble; a saline purgative with five drops of laudanum and a warm bath : vespere, stomach less irritable ; slight reaction ; one scanty watery stool; calomel 10 grs., extract of opium 2 grs. Feb. 12th—The vomiting returned at midnight with cramps of the muscles of abdomen and of the lower extremities; now vomits occasionally a watery fluid, slightly tinged with blood; pain at scrobiculus cordis; artificial heat to be applied and an enema to be given consisting of sulphat. of magnesia 1 oz., compound colocynth extract 10 grs., extract of opium 2 grs., warm water a pint : vespere, very slight reaction ; the stomach still rejects whatever is swallowed; pulse slow and feeble ; the enema to be repeated, and a pill of three grains of opium to be taken. 13th—The stomach now quiet; trunk of natural temperature and moist; extremities cold; pulse at wrist scarcely perceptible ; seems under the influence of opium ; to have hot brandy and water. Gradually becoming comatose, he died at 2 p.m.

Autopsy 22 hours after death. Body strongly formed and muscular; limbs very rigid; muscles hard; spots of ecchymosis like petechiæ on skin of legs; very little blood in the vessels of the extremities; the nails livid ; the feet and hands of shrunken appearance and skin in wrinkles, as if long macerated in water; the eyes very much sunk; the features sharp; the cerebral vessels moderately distended with blood ; the pia mater rather redder than common; a little fluid under the arachnoid and a little air ; a small quantity of fluid in the lateral ventricles; more than usual at base of brain and in the spinal canal; the brain itself of natural appearance; the pericardium contained 2 drs. of fluid and a few bubbles of air; the heart distended with blood of a dark color, coagulated, but soft; no separation of fibrin; the valves were stained reddish; the substance of heart more tender than usual and yielded readily to the pressure of finger and thumb, as did also the muscles of the legs and loins; the lungs were redder than usual from congestion of blood in their vessels; they collapsed only partially, which might have been owing to the fluid which was found in the larger bronchia—a bilious fluid probably derived from the stomach, and which may have entered the glottis in articulo mortis ; the thoracic duct was collapsed; there was pretty much fluid blood in the aorta; there were spots of ecchymosis on the costal pleura, especially its inferior portion; the great sympathetic nerve was examined; its appearance was natural; the vena portæ contained a little dark fluid blood; the liver was rather soft; the gall-bladder contained a good deal of thick bile, but of natural color; the outer coat of the small intestines was redder than natural; their inner coat was covered with adhering mucus, as was also the inner coat of the large; the cœcum and transverse colon were distended with air; the descending empty and contracted; the kidneys were very red; their vessels full of dark blood.

Case 2.—G. Reid; admitted into regimental hospital, July 24; died a few hours after. Autopsy 7 hours after death. Muscular, of spare habit; muscles rigid, generally hard, and contained a good deal of blood; the fingers firmly closed; the pia mater very red; the large cerebral vessels full of dark blood; the minute vessels injected; pretty much serosity at base of brain; the pericardium contained nearly an ounce of reddish serum; there was a good deal of blood in the great veins and in the right cavities of the heart; both lungs much collapsed; in the superior lobe of each there was some blackish consolidation, with granules; some of putty-like consistence, others firmer, and one gritty; some resembled miliary tubercles, and, where softened, exhibited very much the same character under the microscope; the stomach and small intestines contained a good deal of greyish fluid, like water-gruel, and their inner coat was covered with a soft thin layer of mucus; after having been washed, the villi of the small intestines appeared distinct and uninjured; the large intestines were partially contracted; they contained no fæcal matter; there was pretty much bile in the gall-bladder of natural color; the urinary bladder was empty and contracted; the other viscera were apparently sound; the fluid from the stomach and small intestines by boiling became more opaque, but there was no distinct coagulation; the appearance might have been owing to the effect of heat on the shreddy matter it contained, probably portions of epithelium.

In conclusion, I have little to state in the way of general remarks. As regards the epidemic disease, whatever its true nature may be, this seems certain, that rapidly in its progress the blood becomes surcharged with carbonic acid and more or less altered in consistence. The interesting researches of Dr. Brown Séquard on the qualities and functions of arterial and venous blood would lead to the inference that the painful cramps which are so common and so distressing a feature of the disease may in part be owing to the surcharge of carbonic acid.

In many instances after death from cholera the muscles have been seen to act; it is also reported that in some instances the temperature of the cadaver has been observed to increase, and that independent of putrefaction. The former phenomenon was witnessed in the epidemic in Ceylon in one or two examples by my friend Mr. Finlayson, and I could hear of no others. Of the rise of temperature in the dead body no example occurred.

I shall not here attempt the discussion of the question whether cholera of the epidemic kind be contagious or not. Every epidemic disease must necessarily have a good deal of the character of a contagious disease, and no one epidemic has yet escaped that charge. Were I to speak from my own experience I should be disposed to deny its having any infectious or contagious quality.   It is remarkable that during the whole of the epidemic in Ceylon, although no precautions whatever were taken of a preventative kind, not a single medical officer or attendant on the sick contracted the disease.

As to the treatment of cholera, the common and the epidemic, how different is the position of the medical officer!   Considering how rarely the former has a fatal termination, the great probability is, that were no medical aid given, recovery would take place in the great majority of cases.   On the other hand, considering how large is the mortality of the epidemic disease whatever the treatment employed, one can hardly avoid the conclusion that no reliance is to be placed on any remedial means yet tried, whether rational (if that term be applicable) or empirical.   It is true that under different modes of treatment there has been a difference in the ratio of deaths : but, may not this have been owing chiefly to different degrees of intensity of the disease in the several epidemics ?   In one may there not have been a larger proportion than in another of cases of mild cholera, differing but little from common cholera, and with a like tendency to terminate in health ?   A fair review of the facts will, I believe, warrant this inference.

CHAPTER IV.

ON DISEASES OF THE LIVER.

Remarks on hepatic diseases.—Their statistics.—Causes of with reference to climate, diet, etc.—Illustrative cases.—Difficulty of diagnosis.—Tendency to complication.—Treatment.

DISEASES of the liver though not of very frequent occurrence amongst troops, and far less frequent than is commonly supposed, yet are of no common interest to the medical officer, on account of their connexion with other diseases and the difficulties attending equally their diagnosis and treatment. The consideration of them may appropriately follow that of dysentery and cholera, with the former of which they are so often associated.

In the list of diseases in the medical statistical returns of the army, hepatitis, acute and chronic, and icterus are the only ones admitted; and, this probably in consequence of the obscure nature of other affections of the organ and the difficulty just alluded to of recognizing them by symptoms.

Like dysentery, hepatitis in the instance of the soldier varies in its frequency and severity in different countries and under different circumstances, and hardly in a less remarkable degree. The statistical reports above mentioned show this very clearly. Thus, the admissions and deaths at different stations from acute and chronic hepatitis and icterus, calculating on an aggregate strength of 10,000 are as follow during the periods specified:—

	Admitted.		Died.
Great Britain, from 1st January, 1830, to 31st March, 1837—Dragoons and Dragoon Guards	75	...	4·2
Gibraltar, from 1818 to 1836, both included	125	...	3·6
Malta, from 1817 to 1836	209	...	11·5
Ionian Islands do. do.	164	...	7·9
West Indies—Windward and Leeward Islands Command—from 1817 to 1836	225	...	18·6
Black Troops do. do.	73	...	9·0
Jamaica do. do.	104	...	9·8
Black Troops do. do.	24	...	1·2
Nova Scotia and New Brunswick do. do.	84	...	2·4
Canada do. do.	76	...	1·8

9

	Admitted.		Died.
Cape of Good Hope. Cape District from 1818 to 1836	214	...	11·0
Hottentot Corps, from 1822 to 1834	38	...	4·8
Mauritius, from 1818 to 1836	818	...	39·9
Ceylon, from 1817 to 1836	531	...	49·6
Malays—1st Ceylon Rifles—from 1818 to 1836	62	...	8·3

Here we see that there is a certain relation between the temperature of the climate of each station and the degree of frequency of occurrence and of fatality of the disease, both increasing with increase of atmospheric heat, but not in an exact ratio ; and thereby denoting, as before remarked when treating of fevers, that there are other circumstances which also must have an influence etiologically considered.   What these are is not very certain : I am disposed to refer them chiefly to two heads—the kind of diet, including drink, and the amount of exercise, especially in the open air. Taking the three Mediterranean stations, we see that the proportion of these diseases is considerably greater in Malta amongst the troops than at the other two, Gibraltar and the Ionian Islands. Now, at Malta the soldier leads a life of little activity, is chiefly confined to the town of Valetta, is not employed on the roads, as he was in the Ionian Islands, and from the nature of the barracks there, ill-ventilated and hot, the air he breathes is of higher temperature than ordinary even in that island so distinguished for heat as to be called the hot-house of the Mediterranean. Taking the three principal tropical stations, Ceylon, the Mauritius and the West Indies, we see how greatly these diseases preponderate in the two former.   Now in Ceylon, and I believe in the Mauritius, oily food is much more used by the soldier than in the West Indies.   In the Windward and Leeward Islands Command the meat ration of the troops is notoriously poor and lean, and the drink besides water is chiefly ardent spirits, new rum.   In Jamaica, though the meat may be of somewhat better quality, the kind of diet and drink is the same.   In Ceylon a taste for curries is acquired from the natives, and the cocoa-nut abounding in oil always enters into their composition.   Moreover, there, the favorite beverage of the soldier is toddy, the juice of the same palm, rich in sugar before it enters into fermentation, and containing also, I believe, a portion of oily matter. Further, if we compare the amount of these diseases at the different posts in Ceylon, the results would seem to be confirmatory, being greatest at those where the temperature is highest, as on the coast, and, where the cocoa-nut is most plentiful, and least, where the temperature is lowest, as in the interior, owing to increase of elevation, and where the cocoa-nut is less common. Thus, the mortality per 10,000 of aggregate strength, during a total period of sixteen years, was at Trincomalie 74·4, at Colombo 44·5 ; at Point de Galle 40; at Kandy and Kornegalle in the interior 31·2, and at Badulla and the Province of Ouva, still more elevated and cooler than either Kandy or Kornegalle, 27·2. That exercise in the open air is favorable to the prevention of hepatic disease, there seems little ground for doubt, or that indolence and little muscular exertion have a contrary tendency. During the rebellion in Ceylon, that of 1819, when the troops were engaged in the interior in a most harassing warfare, and at the same time were ill-fed, it was remarkable how with a great increase of sickness and mortality, hepatic disease, at least abscess of the liver, diminished—was proportionally much less than when the same regiments were leading an idle life in quietude in quarters, whether on the coast or in the interior. The little frequency of these diseases at Gibraltar may seem opposed to some of the foregoing remarks, especially as concerns the influence of high temperature. But I am inclined to attach little importance to the difference, keeping in mind the facility afforded there of sending invalids home, and that commonly regiments ordered for the Mediterranean commence their foreign service in that garrison. Whether the greater degree of exercise that the soldier there undergoes from the nature of the ground, " the rock," has a beneficial preventative influence, is a circumstance perhaps not undeserving of consideration.

Besides the causes I have hinted at, there may be many others in operation, of which we have no clear notion, causes of a special kind, somewhat akin, at least as regards their obscurity, to those productive of malaria-fever and cholera, those of the worst, the epidemic kind. The comparatively little liability of the negro and Malay soldier to affections of the liver, is rather favorable to the idea of such causes being in operation.

Having premised thus much, I shall now offer some cases selected from a large number; and I may state, not so much with any hope of making the diagnosis of these diseases more clear, as for the purpose of showing how often disease of the liver is in a manner latent and unsuspected during life, and this even

in some of its severest forms.   In bringing forward these cases,
I shall observe little order of arrangement, nor shall I keep back
the name of the disease which it had on admission.   In their
details I am well aware of their imperfections, yet, imperfect as
are the descriptions, I believe there was as much attention paid,
as much discrimination exercised, as in ordinary cases occurring
in civil life, not intended for publication.

Case 1.—Of abscess of liver, latent, penetrating through the diaphragm, returned
"Diarrhœa."—R. Clements, ætat. 41; 85th Regiment; admitted into hospital, at
Malta, 1st August, 1830; died August 24.—This man, of 19 years' service, had
commonly good health till within the last year or two, during which he had frequently been under treatment for dyspepsia and other symptoms of abdominal
derangement.   When admitted on the 1st August, there was severe bilious purging
with a feeling of uneasiness about the rectum ; one of the hæmorrhoidal veins was
considerably distended ; the tongue was furred ; the pulse was little disturbed ; the
skin natural; no thirst; no tenderness of abdomen.   A mild aperient, followed by a
copious evacuation of fæces ; leeches to anus; fomentations.   On the following day,
the distension of the vein had ceased ; the stools continued frequent and bilious.   A
warm bath ; small doses of castor oil.   On the 9th it is stated there was an uneasy
feeling in the situation of the ascending colon; the system tranquil ; the stools the
same ; 30 leeches to abdomen, followed by a blister ; calomel, chalk and opium in
small repeated doses; relief.   On the 11th and 12th little change; slight tenesmus ;
stools still bilious; a little blood in them ; mouth not affected.   On the 13th, 14th,
and 15th, much the same.   Unguentum hydrarg. to be rubbed into thighs night
and morning.   On the 17th, solution of chloride of mercury was substituted for the
calomel ; T. catechu and opium were given with it.   On the 19th the mouth became
affected by the mercury ; the purging continued ; the stools had become more green;
there was little general excitement ; pulvis hydrargyri. was now used with chalk.
From the 20th he began to emaciate; his pulse was more rapid and feeble ; the
surface cold and clammy.   Port wine, etc. were now ordered.   He lingered, gradually
sinking until he died.

Autopsy 3 hours after death.   Body greatly emaciated ; no œdema of any part.
A thermometer placed under the lobulus Spigelii rose to 99°.   The right lobe of the
liver was unusually large ; in its upper portion there was an abscess which contained
a considerable quantity of viscid thick ropy matter having an odor like that of malt;
the cavity was of an irregular form and was intersected by blood vessels; it communicated with the pleura by a small opening in the diaphragm, through which
a portion of its contents had passed into the pleural sac ; the liver and diaphragm
were otherwise generally adhering ; the parts of the liver not involved in the
abscess were tolerably healthy.   The right lung was much compressed ; its inferior
portion was destitute of air, and, as well as the diaphragmatic pleura, was lined with
coagulable lymph ; the left lung and heart were sound; the spleen generally adhering
was large and soft; the intestines were adhering together, as if from peritoneal
inflammation ; the small intestines internally were of natural appearance, excepting
that a good deal of greenish mucus adhered to them ; there were several small
ulcers in the cœcum and colon ; most of them were in a healing state; some were
covered with red granulations ; some with a new membrane, grey and puckered.
When the right kidney was incised, there was an escape of frothy blood from its
vessels.

The little relation existing between the symptoms and the disease of liver in this case was remarkable. No suspicion of the formation of an abscess was formed during life. There were no rigors, no dyspnœa, no acute pain; the attention was fixed on the bowel affection. The air in the blood of the renal vessels, without putrefaction, is a noteworthy circumstance.

Case 2.—Of abscess of liver, latent, penetrating into the lung with pectoral symptoms, returned "Abscessus pulmonis."—J. Ingham, ætat. 27; R. F.; admitted into hospital, Malta, 2nd November, 1830; died 22nd December.—This man previous to the 20th July was stout and healthy. Then he experienced a severe attack of acute dysentery. He was discharged convalescent on the 2nd September; on the 2nd November, when his health was considered re-established, on inspection, a considerable protuberance was observed, by the medical officer, of the right side, unaccompanied by pain or uneasy feeling. He then complained of nothing, except a slight tickling cough occasionally at night in bed. His bowels were regular; pulse 100; his appetite good. The tumor extended from the fourth to the last true rib externally, and was soft and rather elastic, pitting very little on pressure. The stethoscope gave no decided indications. He was placed under observation, using a mild diet without medicine. In the evening of the 8th November a violent fit of coughing occurred and he expectorated about a quart of a chocolate-colored fluid. Towards morning of the 9th he had some refreshing sleep, and afterwards said that he was quite well. From this time the cough returned in fits, commonly every third or fourth day, and from two to six ounces of fluid of the same character as before were expectorated; intermediately he felt pretty well. On the 20th he experienced slight diarrhœa and there was a little œdema of the face and feet; using small doses of rhubarb with opium and sulphate of quinine, he seemed to improve; the looseness of the bowels was checked, and there was less cough and less expectoration. On the 6th December he first complained of pain of side and that his breathing was difficult, especially in the recumbent posture, and that he was subject to night sweats. On the 12th there was a recurrence of diarrhœa, with increased œdema of extremities and some fluctuation of abdomen. His emaciation was now rapid; the cough and expectoration had nearly ceased. On the day following he experienced sudden debility; the surface becoming cold, the pulse not to be felt at the wrist or in the axilla, the respiration feeble but regular. Using warm stimulating drinks, aided by hot cloths and bottles of hot water to the trunk and extremities, the circulation and warmth were gradually restored. From this time his debility and emaciation continued to increase and the bowels relaxed. On the 20th he was nearly suffocated owing to difficulty in expectorating. The next day he experienced a similar paroxysm and seemed dying. The operation of paracentesis thoracis was now performed and three pints of healthy looking pus were discharged, followed by temporary relief. He died the following day without suffering; he was sensible to the last.

Autopsy 24 hours after death. Body extremely emaciated; there was a good deal of fluid between the convolutions of the brain; the lateral ventricles were distended with fluid; in the choroid plexus there were vesicles containing a transparent serosity nearly the size of peas; the substance of brain was generally softer than natural, and especially the fornix. The trachea and bronchia were unduly red and the former was granular; the heart was small and shrivelled; in the right ventricle there was a fibrinous concretion with smooth and rounded edges adhering by a peduncle to a columnea carnea; its appearance suggested the idea of its having been formed during life or in articulo mortis; in the aorta there was a strong solution of coloring matter (cruor) without any fibrin. The left pleura contained 4 oz. of bloody serum; the left lung was sound; the superior portion of the right lung was pretty healthy; its inferior was greatly diseased, the seat of several small abscesses which communicated with a large one in the liver through the diaphragm; its sac extended from the fourth rib to the last but one of the false ribs; it contained about two quarts of thick greyish viscid matter; it involved a portion of the lung and communicated with a large bronchial tube that had suffered ulceration; a considerable portion of the right lobe of the liver was destroyed; what remained seemed nearly sound; it generally adhered; the little bile that was in the gall-bladder was of healthy appearance; the mesenteric glands were enlarged; in the cœcum there were three or four ulcers of a pinkish hue and superficial; in the colon there were marks of old ulcers which had healed, as indicated by bluish discoloration and a puckered surface; the other abdominal viscera exhibited no marked lesion. About six ounces of serum were found in the cavity of the abdomen.

The insidious manner in which the hepatic abscess formed in this case was remarkable, and also the manner equally insidious that by the ulcerative process it found an outlet through the lung, occasioning for a long time so little suffering, or derangement of health, or bodily wasting. The state of the brain too may be mentioned as noteworthy, with the absence of any obvious morbid action. Had the pressure on it, from the fluid effused, the effect of blunting sensibility?

Case 3.—Of abscess of liver, latent, penetrating into the pleura, with pulmonary symptoms; returned " Phthisis pulmonalis."—T. Jones, ætat. 32; 73rd Regiment; admitted into hospital at Malta, 31st August; died 28th December.—This man, of intemperate habits, on the 8th August came under treatment for hepatitis, which seemed to yield to V.S., mercury and purging. He was discharged on the 17th to duty. On the 21st, after having been drunk, he was re-admitted, complaining of "a dull, heavy pain" in his right side. The bowels were regular, appetite indifferent; urgent thirst; tongue moist; pulse 90; V.S. 2 lbs.; the blood was highly buffed; purgative medicine. The pain having increased towards evening, V.S. was repeated to syncope with relief, followed by a blister and the use of small doses of calomel. On the 17th ptyalism was produced; the pain of side occurring, leeches were occasionally applied. On the 29th September he first complained of pain of chest and difficulty of breathing; the pulse was quick, but soft; the pain was supposed to be muscular, being aggravated by the slightest touch; bark was prescribed with hyoscyamus at bed-time, with apparent good effect for a few days; then the pain of chest recurred and with greater severity, and was accompanied with cough and expectoration, profuse sweating and emaciation. During the remaining period of his illness little change took place with the exception of an abatement, and finally a cessation of pain. It was also reported that latterly even pressure occasioned no pain, and that there was no fulness of the hypochondrium. His bowels were often irregular, and there was occasional diarrhœa.

Autopsy 17 hours after death. Body greatly emaciated; no œdema of feet or hands; slight puffiness of face; the pericardium contained 2 oz. of serum and "some bubbles of air;" in the anterior mediastinum there was an extensive sinus; it was lined with coagulable lymph and was full of a whey-like fluid, about a pint; the right pleura thickly coated with coagulable lymph, contained about two quarts of sero-purulent matter, a whey-like fluid holding in suspension flakes of lymph; there was an extensive opening through the diaphragm by which the pleural sac communicated freely with an abscess in the right lobe of the liver; the abscess contained rather more than two quarts of fluid, and was lined with coagulable lymph; the liver generally was adhering to the diaphragm; the sac of the abscess was bounded for most part by a cartilaginous layer, as if from an effort made to arrest the diseased action; in the remaining part of the right lobe there were some minute tubercles in a softening state; the left lobe was sound; the gall-bladder contained a moderate quantity of healthy bile; the right lung, owing to the fluid in the pleura, was compressed and greatly condensed; the inferior lobe of the left lung was œdematous; there were about two pints of serum in the cavity of the abdomen; the lower part of the ileum was unusually red, and its mucous coat was encrusted with what seemed a deposition of lymph, as was also the colon throughout; the stomach was apparently healthy; it was small, corrugated and nearly empty; the spleen was rather large and soft and had a fissured or ruptured appearance; the lacteals were distended with chyle, which flowed out copiously when these vessels were divided; there was a little limpid fluid in the thoracic duct, but no chyle.

That this case was mistaken for one of phthisis is not perhaps remarkable, considering how much its symptoms in its advanced stage resembled those of that disease. The great sensitiveness of the chest probably prevented a thorough examination by means of percussion and the stethoscope. It may be conjectured that an hydatid in the liver was the *origo mali.*

Case 4.—Of abscess of liver, communicating with the lung, with pulmonary following hepatic symptoms; returned "Hepatitis chronica."—W. Croucher, ætat. 26; 7th R. F.; admitted into hospital at Malta, 13th April, 1832; died 16th July.— This man, of sober habits, had remittent fever in the Ionian Islands in 1828, terminating in intermittent. In Malta, in the summer of 1829, he experienced an attack of continued fever. In the summer following he had a severe attack of dysentery. In 1831 he was twice treated for bowel affections. On the 10th April, 1832, when on duty at Gozo, he experienced "acute inflammation of the liver," for which he was transferred on the 13th of the same month to the regimental hospital in Valetta. He had then acute pain in the right side, a short cough, hot skin, white tongue, thirst, pulse quick and wiry; the body was bent forward, in which position only he could breathe with tolerable freedom; V.S. was employed with mercurial and saline purgatives. On the 18th he felt better; the mouth was slightly affected by the mercury. On the 24th there was a sudden recurrence of pain in the right side, extending towards the shoulder and increased heat of skin; V.S. was repeated, followed by a blister and saline aperients; he was much relieved. On the 26th a rigor occurred, ending in sweating; the same evening he had a fit of coughing, with copious mucous expectoration; tartar emetic and mercurial ointment were rubbed in on the skin over the liver and demulcents given. On the 1st May the system was slightly affected by the mercury; the cough was less. On the 4th he had a severe fit of coughing and expectorated muco-purulent matter; there was more pain in the region of the liver, with some difficulty of breathing; he was cupped and a blister was applied, which was kept open for a fortnight. On the 20th the cough was milder, there was less expectoration; he was considered convalescent. In June hectic symptoms set in with emaciation and night sweats; the lower extremities became œdematous; he was harassed by fits of coughing; the expectoration was purulent and streaked with blood. On the 10th June, an "abscess" was indicated by the stethoscope in the right side of the chest; the expectoration was copious and purulent and stained with blood; his appetite had failed and he was troubled with diarrhœa; using anodynes and astringents and a light nourishing diet there was rather an abatement of symptoms until the 6th July; then there was a great increase of dyspnœa and more copious expectoration. On the 8th he was more distressed; he appeared to be moribund; now a trocar was introduced between the fifth and sixth rib, and about ten pints of matter were discharged; he rallied. On the 14th severe purging set in which continued till he expired on the 16th.

Autopsy 14 hours after death. Body much emaciated; considerable œdema of the right hand and arm; the left side of the chest sounded well; the right dull, except towards the false ribs, where it was tympanitic; .and there, there was some discoloration of skin as if from incipient gangrene; the pericardium contained 8 oz. of serum; the left lung was free from adhesion and was sound; the right was very much diseased; an extensive abscess was found in it, reaching from the liver to the top of the lung, below bounded by the surface of the liver, above by that of the lung, of various thickness; the greater part of the diaphragm, corresponding to the convex surface of the right lobe of the liver, was completely destroyed; there was no communication between the abscess and the abdominal cavity, owing to the adhesion of the liver all round to the remaining portion of the diaphragm; the form of the abscess was irregular, branching variously into the substance of the lung, which was for the most part hepatized and adhering to the ribs; the substance of the liver not involved in the abscess seemed healthy, but when incised small tubercles were discovered in it in different stages of softening with suppuration; there was a small quantity of serum in the cavity of the abdomen; although there had been a troublesome diarrhœa during the last twenty-four hours of life, the cœcum was much distended with fæces of rather soft consistence; the rectum was very red and ulcerated; in the transverse and descending colon there were cicatrices of old ulcers.

The amount of painful and distressing suffering in this case is remarkable, especially comparing it with the preceding. Was it owing to the destructive process going on in the diaphragm? Considering the very extensive loss of substance of this organ, is it not surprising that life was so much prolonged?

Case 5.—Of abscesses in the liver, latent, with ulcerated intestines; returned "Diarrhœa."—G. Rey, ætat. 31; 18th Regiment; admitted into hospital, at Corfu, on the 27th October, 1825; died 7th November.—This man of bad character and dissolute habits, on admission complained of griping and purging of ten days' duration. His appearance was sickly; there was a fulness of epigastrium, but with very little pain on pressure, or in any part of the abdomen; the bowels were loose; the stools watery; the pulse small and regular; the skin cool; the tongue dry in centre; much thirst; no appetite. V.S., the blood drawn had a buffy coat. On the 31st there was an increase of swelling at epigastrium. On the 1st November it was called a tumor, and increasing, and painful on pressure; there was now great prostration of strength; the pulse hardly perceptible. From this time it is stated the tumor whilst increasing became more diffused; the purging continued without abatement up to his death. The treatment was mainly palliative.

Autopsy 14 hours after death. The body was not much emaciated. The cavity of the chest was unusually high, reaching to the lower margin of the thyroid gland; and the 1st rib loosely articulated was bent up in a very unusual manner; the right pleura contained about a pint of bloody serum in which were flakes of coagulable lymph; both lungs were much gorged with blood; there were about two pints of purulent reddish serum in the cavity of the abdomen; there were marks of general peritoneal inflammation; the intestines adhered together, the omentum to them and to the liver and spleen; the peritoneal surface was red and covered with coagulable lymph and purulent fluid; the liver superiorly was closely adhering by a thick layer of lymph to the diaphragm; when detached two large abscesses came into view; one was in the left hypochondrium and was situated partly in the left and partly in the right lobe; it contained about two pints of matter of unequal consistence; the other, little smaller, was in the superior part of the right lobe; it was full of a thick curd-like matter, and had almost penetrated into the chest; it had penetrated through the diaphragm at one point, and was only confined by the lung there adhering to the diaphragm. The liver was voluminous, it weighed between six and seven pounds; its appearance was nearly natural; there was very little bile in the gall-bladder; the stomach was rather contracted; it was strongly marked with red lines internally; portions of the villous coat of the small intestines were unduly red; in the colon there were numerous ulcers in different stages of healing and many cicatrices of ulcers that had healed; in the rectum there were none.

In this case we have an example of complicated lesions for the most part latent. And may it not be that they were latent in consequence of the complication? Another cause conducing to the latency was his intellect; there was delirium, or a tendency to it, during most of the time he was under treatment; and yet shortly before death his mind was clear.

Case 6.—Of abscess of liver, latent, communicating with lung, with ulcerated intestine, returned "Phthisis pulmonalis."—G. Slater, ætat. 35; 50th Regiment; admitted into general hospital, 24th November, 1835; died 30th December.—This man, a non-commissioned officer of 18 years' service at home, two months before his last admission into hospital had been under treatment on account of hæmoptysis with cough and purging, accompanied with night sweats. Discharged relieved on the 21st November, he was re-admitted on the 24th of the same month on account of a return of hæmoptysis, conjoined with severe cough and dyspnœa. On the 14th it is stated that he was greatly emaciated, that there was a slight œdema of the left side of the face, that the epigastrium was very tumid, and it was added that the stethoscopic signs were obscure. The debility was now extreme; the sputa copious and sanguineo-purulent; no abatement of the symptoms occurred; the bowels it is reported became irregular; the diarrhœa towards the end severe; the stools tinged with blood. Through the whole course of his illness he lay on his left side. The treatment was palliative.

Autopsy 49 hours after death. Body greatly emaciated; the pericardium contained two ounces of serum; on the right ventricle there was a large white patch, about a line thick and under it a thin layer of fat; the valves of the aorta were partially ossified, and in the centre of each there was a bony projection, preventing their normal action, viz., their collapse. The lungs were œdematous, but free from tubercles; in the right there was an abscess, communicating through the diaphragm witn an abscess in the liver; it extended from the inferior to the middle lobe; was capable of holding about a pint and a-half; a large bronchial tube ulcerated gave it exit; the abscess in the liver was nearly of the same capacity; it branched into sinuses, and contained a viscid opaque whitish matter, not globular by the optical test; the liver generally apart from the abscess was pretty natural; it weighed three pounds; the bile was thin, not viscid, and of a light brown color; the vena portæ was empty; the pancreas was unusually hard; the spleen was very small; there were about two quarts of serum in the abdominal cavity; the omentum was very short, of a dark grey hue and perforated as if from interstial absorption; the peritoneal coat of the colon was unusually vascular; this intestine throughout exhibited the worst effects of chronic dysentery; it was thickened, ulcerated, and sloughing; under some of the sloughs there was purulent matter; the valve of the colon was partially destroyed; the lower portion of the ileum was slightly ulcerated.

In this case during life there was no suspicion of abscess in the liver. The manner in which the disease simulated tubercular consumption is very noteworthy, as is also the little suffering—the absence of abdominal pains—considering the state of the contained viscera.

Case 7.—Of abscess in the liver communicating with the lung, not latent, operated on.—T. Taylor, ætat. 34; 2nd R. B.; admitted into hospital at Malta, 15th August, 1830; died 24th October.—This man, of dissipated habits, was often in hospital with slight febrile and ophthalmic attacks after being drunk. During the preceding three years he had passed many teniæ; one that he had voided was 21 feet in length. When last admitted he was supposed to be laboring under acute rheumatism. He was relieved of the pain, which was chiefly lumbar, by treatment—viz.: V.S., blistering and purging. On the 2nd September he experienced slight rigors and complained of a dull pain in the right hypochondrium, where there was some fulness, as if from enlargement of the liver. The disease was now returned chronic hepatitis. It continued to gain ground without material change of symptoms until the 30th of the same month, when, during a sudden fit of coughing, he expectorated about 8 oz. of sero-purulent matter tinged with blood. Daily afterwards he expectorated about 4 oz., with increasing debility and emaciation. On the 22nd October the swelling in hypochondrium having increased, and redness appearing over the 8th and 9th ribs, a trochar was there introduced; no fluid was discharged until a cupping glass was applied; then about 20 oz. of pus were extracted; it was very thick and mixed with blood; temporary relief, especially of breathing, followed; the abscess continued to discharge freely; he became gradually weaker and weaker, yet always in good spirits, till he died; the treatment was chiefly palliative; the bowels were always regular.

Autopsy 14 hours after death. Body considerably emaciated; the lungs were gorged with blood and muco-purulent fluid; in the inferior lobe of the right lung there was a cavity of an abscess, which communicated through the diaphragm with a like cavity in the convex portion of the liver; in each the cavity was lined with lymph; in the lung it had an exit through three bronchial tubes; in both it was nearly empty; there were some sloughs in it and little else; in the liver it was superficial, little more than an inch deep, but pretty widely spread, occupying a space equal to about the palm of the hand; the adjoining hepatic substance appeared healthy; the gall-bladder was large, distended with bile and adhering to the omentum; in the cœcum there were two or three ulcerated spots, the largest not exceeding a sixpence in size; in the transverse and descending colon there were bluish patches indicative of old ulcers healed; very many portions of tape-worm were found in the intestines.

It is noteworthy that though he had led a very intemperate life, the liver with the exception of the abscess was generally healthy. Another noteworthy circumstance is, that though the lungs had been subject long to irritation, no tubercles had formed in them.

Case 8.—Of abscess of liver, latent, communicating with the duodenum and abdominal cavity, productive of peritonitis; returned "Diarrhœa."—J. Burns, ætat. 26; R. F.; admitted into hospital at Malta, 27th July, 1833; died 19th August.—This man, of temperate habits, in 1831 was under treatment for pneumonia; in 1832 for fever; in June, 1833, for diarrhœa, and early in July of the same year for fever of a remittent kind. Discharged on the 17th of that month, he was re-admitted on the 27th, laboring under dysenteric symptoms—viz., frequent purging, stools thin, bloody and mucous, epigastric pain; pulse 90 and soft; skin cool. He was cupped and had a scruple of calomel with a grain of opium; relief of pain followed. Using cold drink, and having cold injections, the bowels became more regular. On the 4th August a sudden and severe pain was felt in the region of the right kidney, without pyrexia; he was again cupped; bottles of hot water were applied to the pained part; relief followed. On the 6th he was again cupped, the pain having recurred; the urine was scanty; pulse natural; some thirst; brown fur on tongue; bowels rather confined; rhubarb and magnesia. During the evening there was pain at epigastrium with vomiting; one stool; a scruple of calomel with half a grain of opium and a blister to the seat of pain, followed by a quiet night. Between the 6th and 10th he vomited twice a good deal of greenish, bilious fluid. Using carbonate of soda, with 30 drops of laudanum, at night he appeared to improve; the appetite was better and there was less pain. After this the bowels became more relaxed, the stools more offensive; without relief using blue pill and opium, with iced water for drink, and cold enemata. On the 17th blood appeared in the stools with shreds of membrane; laudanum added to the injections afforded temporary ease. On the 18th it was stated that he could not retain the enemata; a suppository of opium was substituted for them; the stools continued of the same bad character; the tongue had become dry and ulcerated; his thirst was insatiable; the pulse rapid and small; the trunk wet with a cold clammy sweat. Towards evening he suddenly became unable to speak, but was conscious and without apparent pain. He died the next morning.

Autopsy 9 hours after death. Body much emaciated; the contents of the thorax exhibited no marked lesion; on opening into the cavity of the abdomen a considerable quantity of brownish fluid gushed out; there were marks of general peritoneal inflammation; the intestines were glued together and the omentum was adhering to the pubes; an abscess was found in the liver in its right lobe, about the size of an orange; it was situated a little to the left of the vena portæ, and at the same time communicated with the duodenum by an ulcerated opening and with the cavity of the abdomen, the adhesion to the duodenum having there given way; in the same lobe, over the right kidney, there was the globular cyst of an hydatid, of cartilaginous firmness, partly imbedded, partly projecting; when incised a transparent fluid flowed out, the contents of the hydatid; a portion of the liver dried imparted to paper an oil-stain; with the exception of the ulcerated opening in the duodenum, the small intestines were free from disease, as was also the stomach; the large intestines were much diseased; there were many ulcers in them and extensive marks of old ulceration.

The lesions in this case were unusual and were unusually complicated; and the symptoms were proportionally obscure. At one time the kidney was suspected to be the seat of pain. There was little suspicion of disease of liver; in truth the bowel complaint arrested most attention. Dysentery prevailed at the time, and in the treatment of it iced enemata with iced water for drink, were found serviceable.

Case 9.—Of abscess of liver, of a scrofulous kind operated on; at first latent; returned "Diarrhœa."—C. Burns, ætat. 18; 80th Regiment; admitted into hospital at Malta, 19th June, 1828; died 16th August.—This man when admitted had dysenteric symptoms, with pain of right side. Between the 19th June and the 30th, V.S. was thrice performed, a blister applied and blue pill, with rhubarb and opium administered with occasional doses of castor oil. On the 30th it was reported that he had four or five stools daily without slime or blood, and that he had still a feeling of uneasiness hardly amounting to pain in the right hypochondrium, in which situation there was a little fulness and hardness; the same alterative medicine; the part to be fomented. On the 2nd July he was slightly salivated, without abatement of the uneasy feeling; bowels relaxed; a blister to the part; the medicine to be omitted. On the 21st July the swelling in hypochondrium was decided, having gradually increased, and fluctuation was distinct in it; he was unable to lie on the side affected; a trocar was now introduced and about 3 pints of purulent fluid were evacuated; for a few day he seemed to improve; but his appetite failing him, he emaciated rapidly with increasing debility; the discharge continued, slowly decreasing. On the 14th he was troubled with singultus and much difficulty of breathing. On the 16th he died. The fluid discharged, altogether amounting to about 14 pints, was free from viscidity and had suspended in it a curd-like substance in the form of particles and flakes; it was not coagulated by nitric acid. Daily, vinegar and water were injected into the sac of the abscess, washing out the matter and correcting the fetor; the acid was first diluted with five waters, afterwards with one.

Autopsy 8 hours after death. Body extremely emaciated; the deep-seated parts were almost cold; the substance of the brain was generally softer than natural, particularly the sides of the third ventricle and the corpora striata; the pericardium contained 3 oz. of yellow serum; the heart was small and had a shrivelled appearance; the left lung adhered to the pericardium and also to the costal pleura by long bands and fibres of coagulated lymph; the lung itself was sound; the right lung adhered closely to the spine; there was some extravasated blood in its substance, and patches of ecchymosis in the pulmonary and costal pleura; the œsophagus was very much on the left side of the median line; its mucous coat was red in places and slightly abraded; the greater portion of the convex surface of the liver was adhering; in the right lobe there was the sac of a large abscess, that which had been opened; it contained some thick, flaky matter; superior to it was another large abscess, which was bounded by the diaphragm above—the diaphragm confining its liquid contents—consisting of a limpid fluid and of a thick, scrofulous-like matter; in other parts of the organ there were softening tubercles, some of them almost reduced to a pultaceous state, especially a few which projected into the abscess; the left lobe was free from disease, whilst the substance of the right even where free from tubercles, was redder than natural and of unequal consistence, in some places abnormally soft, in others unduly hard; there was but little bile in the gall-bladder, its appearance natural; the valve of the colon was slightly ulcerated, as was also the cœcum; the ulcers in the latter were small and circular, and in process of healing; the vermiform appendix was distended with thick muco-purulent fluid, and was deeply and extensively ulcerated; the transverse colon was free from disease; the descending portion of a bright red internally, was thickened and spotted with small ulcers in process of healing and with marks of old ulcers healed.

The abscesses in this case seem to have been not of a phlegmoid but rather of a scrofulous origin and connected with the softening of tubercles of a peculiar kind. Neither V.S. nor mercury appears to have had any permanent beneficial effect. It is noteworthy that whilst the hepatic disease was making progress, the intestinal ulcers were healing.

Case 10.—Of abscesses in liver, latent, rupture of one of them into the abdominal cavity, followed by peritonitis; returned "Catarrhus chronicus."—W. Walker, ætat. 53; 85th Regiment; admitted into hospital, at Malta, January 6th, 1829; died January 10th.—This man, a serjeant-armorer, an old soldier, of 33 years' service, and of intemperate habits, had for many years been subject to paroxysms of asthmatic dyspnœa with excessive mucous expectoration. Before admission he had taken some saline purgative medicine; when brought to hospital he complained of pain of abdomen on each side of the umbilicus, which was increased by pressure; there was some thirst; tongue moist; bowels relaxed from medicine taken. Fomentation; a warm bath and 10 grs. of Dover's powder twice in the 24 hours. January 7th—Several stools; the pain continues; 12 leeches to the abdomen; again to be fomented; the same medicine. 8th—Three natural evacuations; pain the same; pulse small and weak; tongue cleaner; respiration easier. A blister to the abdomen. 9th—Last night his rest was better; less pain; pulse fuller; tongue moist and less furred; strangury; fæces passed without his knowledge. Mist. camphoræ. 10th—He expired at 7 a.m. this morning.

Autopsy 28 hours after death. Body nowise emaciated, but unusually fat; the temperature of the room was 58°; a thermometer placed under the lobulus Spigelii was 73°. The dura mater unusually vascular adhered firmly to the cranium; the ventricles were distended with transparent fluid; there was a great deal of fat in the anterior mediastinum and about the pericardium and heart; the heart was large; the aortic valves were thickened and partially ossified; the aorta between its origin and the innominata was considerably enlarged; there were white patches on its inner coat, and some calcarious matter deposited, which in one spot, was in the form of a sharp point projecting through the membrane; one of the coronary arteries was partially ossified; the abdominal aorta in parts was thickened, that is its inner coat, whilst in other parts this coat was almost entirely deficient; the inner coat of the vena cava ascendens was a little thickened, and was separated from the outer more easily than usual; the left lung was very generally and firmly adhering; there were no tubercles in either; both were much gorged with blood; the bronchia were very red, as were also the trachea and larynx. In the right lobe of the liver there were five abscesses, two or three of them were capable of holding a goose-egg; the others a hen's egg; they were all nearly spherical or oval; were lined with a thin layer of lymph, and were full of thick pus; one had penetrated through the peritoneal covering and there was a considerable collection of matter between it and the diaphragm; another lower down had nearly penetrated into the cavity of the abdomen; this one communicated with another abscess; in both lobes there were many small abscesses, varying in size from that of a pea to that of a hazel-nut; they were all similar, had a lining of lymph and contained thick matter; the substance of the liver was of pretty natural appearance, except contiguous to one or two of the abscesses, where it was unusually red; there were large ulcers in the cœcum, black and sloughing, which had laid bare the muscular coat. There were similar ulcers in the rectum, and many ulcers in the transverse and descending colon; the latter had the appearance of chancres, were well defined and about the size of a sixpence; more than one of them had nearly penetrated through all the coats; the spleen was pale and unusually soft; when pressed, a thick fawn-colored fluid, not in the least putrid, exuded from it, which, by the optical test, appeared to be purulent. There was an unusual quantity of fat about the omentum; there were adhesions between the liver and colon, and the colon and duodenum; lymph in a firm layer was deposited on the surface of the liver—its right lobe.

This case is chiefly remarkable for the variety and amount of latent organic disease, and the little apparent relation between the symptoms and lesions. There was no suspicion of the existence of either ulcers in the intestines or of abscesses in the liver. Habitual intemperance, somewhat after the manner of insanity, seems to have a remarkable effect in blunting healthy sensibility; and even more than insanity in impairing the *vis vitæ*.

Case 11.—Of abscesses in liver, numerous and small, with disease of the vena portæ; returned "Hepatitis acuta."—J. Jenkins, ætat. 28; 95th Regiment; admitted into hospital, at Malta, 23rd December, 1828; died 31st January, 1831.—This man, a non-commissioned officer, had been ailing three weeks before coming to hospital; on admission he had pain at epigastrium extending on each side as high as the clavicles, with a sense of fulness and an increase of uneasiness on pressure; the pulse was 92 and hard; heat moderate; tongue dry and rough; bowels irregular, inclined to costiveness; appetite impaired. From this time until the 7th January there were cessations and returns of pain; occasional sickness of stomach, and bilious vomiting; occasional pyrexia, as indicated by increased heat of skin, thirst and acceleration of pulse, and latterly rigor. From this time, it is stated, that his disease gradually advanced to its fatal termination. The symptoms assumed a hectic character and from time to time varied, rigors alternating with nausea, or bilious vomiting, headache and exacerbations of fever at night. His appetite, which before had improved a little, in a great measure failed him, his bowels continuing irregular. During the last eight or nine days he had "a stitch" in the right hypochondrium, relieved by a blister. He died rather suddenly, but apparently without pain; he was sensible to the last; his intellect clear. The treatment was varied, chiefly antiphlogistic and mercurial. Blood was abstracted by V.S. and leeches; calomel and blue pill were given till the mouth was affected and were repeated.

Autopsy 17 hours after death. Body small, rather emaciated.* The odor from it was peculiar and offensive; the fornix and corpora striata were rather softer than natural; there was pretty much fluid at the base of brain; about two ounces of

* Open air 60°; in centre of cerebrum immediately after removal of skull-cap, 70°; about half an hour after in right side of heart, 82°; under lobulus Spigelii, 82°. The body was covered merely with a sheet after death.

reddish serum in the pericardium; there was a good deal of blood and fibrinous concretions in the cavities of the heart; the lungs were unusually florid, and one more than the other, as if from the presence of arterial blood, and this throughout its substance; the liver was large; its surface was disfigured by red protuberances, denoting abscesses beneath. On attempting to introduce a thermometer under the lobulus Spigelii there was a gush of yellowish matter, which on examination was found to have come from the vena portæ; the part from which it issued was about thrice the ordinary size of that vessel; it adhered to all the surrounding surfaces; its coats were thin and easily broken, and lined with ragged coagulable lymph; the veins which terminated in it were closed at their entrance by coagulable lymph and beyond they were empty; this sinus of the vena portæ seemed to communicate with a large sinus in the liver; but the connexion was not traced in so satisfactory a manner as could be wished; the liver abounded in abscesses and sinuses; hardly any part of it was free from them; they communicated one with another and very much resembled the excavations which are met with in tubérculated lungs, and like them their sides were columnar and their cavities were crossed by blood vessels nearly bare and also by branches of the hepatic duct, which opened or hung loose, owing to ulceration in some of them; the hepatic substance adjoining them was redder and softer than natural; the fluid which they contained was thick, glairy, and yellowish; the gall-bladder was moderately distended with greenish bile; the spleen was a little larger than usual and unusually firm and hard; the splenic vein was empty; The other abdominal viscera appeared pretty natural; there was no ulceration of the intestines; the thoracic duct contained a small quantity of reddish fluid.

In this case many circumstances are remarkable; the obscurity of the symptoms, the peculiar abscesses and excavations in the liver, the sacculated state or abscess of vena portæ, the empty state of the veins communicating with it and their closure close to the sac; the state of the spleen. It is noteworthy that there was no jaundice, no ascites, no œdema, no hæmorrhage.

Case 12.—Of hydatid in liver, latent, with anomalous symptoms, returned "Febris communis."—J. Green, ætat. 28; 53rd Regiment; admitted into hospital at Malta, 12th May, 1834; died 19th May.—This man on admission had headache with thirst and heat of skin, preceded the day before by rigors; he had also some pain of throat, difficulty in swallowing, and pain at epigastrium; there was a yellow fur on the tongue; the bowels slow; an emetic followed by salts and senna. On the 13th the skin was pungently hot; thirst urgent; pulse 100; the bowels had been freely moved; V.S., followed by sulphate of soda and tartarized antimony. On the 14th the headache was less; still pain at epigastrium; the blood abstracted (20 oz.) was slightly buffed; six leeches to pit of stomach; rhubarb and magnesia. On the 15th it was reported that he had passed a sleepless night, that he coughed much and had pain of chest, with increased heat of skin; V.S. to 10 oz.; the blood was slightly buffed and cupped; solution of tartarized antimony. On the 16th the skin had acquired a deep yellow color; there was much debility; urgent thirst; bowels opened; 2 grs. of sulphate of quinine, with 3 grs. of blue pill thrice a day. On the 17th there was suppression of urine; no pain of any part; the surface warm; a fulness of abdomen; castor oil, camphor mixture; a starch injection. On the 18th there was still no flow of urine; the skin was very deeply colored yellow; he had no sleep at night; bowels were open and the fulness removed; pulse 100, feeble; no medicine but the camphor mixture. 19th.—Again a restless night; constant vomiting during the night; great prostration of strength; pulse feeble and irregular, about 100 ; the suppression of urine continues ; sitting up to take a draught he was seized with convulsions, which in a few minutes terminated in death ; the instant the convulsions occurred he became insensible; the jaws were firmly closed, there was grinding of the teeth and violent action of the muscles of the limbs; no pulse could be felt; the breathing was arrested ; the pupils immovable and dilated.

Autopsy 22 hours after death. Body not emaciated; deeply jaundiced and the skin of inferior surface, of a dark red, from gravitation of blood; the membranes of the brain were yellow, its substance white ; the lateral ventricles contained a moderate quantity of yellow fluid; the lungs contained a good deal of blood; the bronchia some frothy mucus; there was a little viscid yellow fluid in the pericardium; in the cavities of the heart there were some fibrinous concretions, without blood, suggestive of having been formed before death ; the cardiac valves were stained yellow; on the outer surface of the heart there were some spots of ecchymosis ; an hydatid about the size of an orange was found partly embedded in the right lobe of the liver and partly projecting close to the gall-bladder ; its outer coat was of cartilaginous hardness; its inner composed of two layers, was soft, almost pultaceous; its contents were a whitish fluid with a good deal of curd-like matter, and a matter resembling pus but not such, judging of it by the optical test; the substance of the liver seemed sound; there was pretty much thick bile in the gall-bladder and common duct ; the duodenum contained a brownish pultaceous matter, on the removal of which by the sponge, there was a flow of bile from the ductus communis, as if the mouth of the duct had been previously obstructed ; there was no appearance of bile in the stomach or in any part of the intestinal canal ; the pancreas was rather hard; in the pelvis of the kidneys there were some spots of ecchymosis ; the spleen was large and firm ; there was about an ounce of urine in the bladder ; there was no appearance of inflammation or of other disease in the stomach and intestines, and the examination of the spinal chord gave the same result ; 3 oz. of blood which had been obtained from the vena cava were tested for urea, and this substance in no inconsiderable proportion was found in it ; the fluid in the gall-bladder, with the exception of being slightly bitter, had not the character of bile ; it was coagulated by nitric acid, and its coloring matter appeared to be the coloring matter of the blood ; the cystic and common duct were stained brown.

This case appeared to me at the time altogether anomalous. Many conjectures may be made respecting it, especially its sudden and singular mode of termination. Was death owing to fibrinous concretions suddenly formed in the cavities of the heart, arresting the circulation of the blood; or, was it owing to an accumulation of urea in the blood acting as a poison? Probably the hydatid in the liver, excepting that it may have started a train of morbid actions, was little concerned in the event.

Case 13.—Of abscess of liver, not latent, operated on; returned " Hepatitis chronica."—J. Doolan, ætat. 42 ; 85th Regiment; admitted into hospital, at Malta, 4th July, 1829; died 25th July.—This man, of very intemperate habits, his favorite drink ardent spirits, had been known, it is said, to have drank 24 glasses of pure rum before breakfast. Notwithstanding his excesses, he had been twice in hospital only during the last 15 years; once for simple bubo in 1818; a second time for sprained ankle in 1827. He believed that his present complaint began in April last, when he was employed in the government yacht, and neglected reporting himself;

since then he has been subject to rigors. On admission on the 4th July he complained chiefly of pain at scrobiculus cordis extending to both hypochondria, not increased by pressure; his health generally seemed to be but little impaired. From this time to his death, the most prominent symptom was pain in the hypochondria, varying in intensity, never severe, relieved by treatment and recurring; there was occasionally nausea, occasionally relaxed bowels and bilious stools; latterly he was subject to profuse night sweats. On the 16th July there was distinct fulness in the left hypochondrium and a slight fluctuation was perceptible; a trochar was introduced into the tumor and about two pints of purulent fluid were discharged, with immediate relief; the discharge gradually decreased, its quality remaining the same until the 23rd, when it was chiefly "serous." With the exception of relief from pain, no improvement of health followed; he lost strength and emaciated; his appetite failed; the stools were sometimes bilious, sometimes of a bloody and coagulated appearance; he could lie on either side, and after the operation had no uneasiness of either side; the pulse varied from 96 to 146. He became delirious only a few hours before his death. The treatment was active and various; V.S. and leeches; calomel and opium; blisters, fomentation, etc. The matter discharged called purulent, by the optical test appeared to contain very few globules; a portion of it kept till the 31st July was seemingly unchanged; it had no putrid odor.

Autopsy 10 hours after death. Body much emaciated.* No well marked lesion of any of the contents of the thorax; the convex surface of the liver was generally adhering; the adhesions were soft and easily broken, especially round the spot which had been penetrated by the trochar; the left lobe was distended and larger than usual; there were several abscesses in it, and several also in the right lobe, which too was enlarged; the matter in them was puruloid; their form was irregular, internally they were rough, as if from erosion or absorption; the remains of vessels coated with lymph were seen in their sides; the adjoining hepatic substance was soft and red, indeed the greater part of the organ was in the same state; one of the largest abscesses was superficial, pressing on the gall-bladder, being situated between it and the lobulus Spigelii; it burst in the dissection; a collection of matter was found between the stomach, its great arch, and the concave surface of the left lobe, confined by adhesions; the gall-bladder contained a very little dilute yellow bile; the large intestines were studded throughout with ulcers, varying in size from a split pea to a sixpence; they were generally pale; some of them had penetrated to the muscular coat; the lower portion of the ileum exhibited marks of old ulceration; here and there the surface was without villi, or they were very indistinct, even when sought for in water; the aorta and left common iliac were partially diseased; their inner coat being in some places thickened, in others nearly absorbed.

In this instance no abscess was suspected but that which was opened; nor was there any serious disease of the intestines suspected. It is worthy of remark that there was no pain of shoulder, no effusion into the cavity of the abdomen, no œdema of feet, no jaundice. The stomach was retentive, it bore no marks of disease.

Case 14.—Of abscesses in liver, latent, with hæmatemisis; returned "Diarrhœa." —H. Rynor, ætat. 32; 85th Regiment; admitted into hospital, at Malta, December

---

* Thermometer in room 77°; in a deep abscess of liver 95°; under the heart 95°.

5th, 1828; died December 26th.—This man had on admission diarrhœa verging on dysentery, but without pain of abdomen even on pressure, and without tenesmus; the stools at first were copious, liquid, and feculent; afterwards they varied in character, sometimes scybalous, sometimes mucous and bloody or streaked with blood; tenesmus later was of frequent occurrence. Under a mild mercurial treatment with opium the bowels became more regular. After the 20th he was worse; on the 24th pain in the right hypochondrium was first noticed; it was increased by pressure; he had now become very feeble and emaciated. Before death much grumous blood was passed with his stools. Four days before that event his skin, it is stated, was below its natural temperature.

Autopsy 22 hours after death.* The pulmonary veins in the left lung were full of coagulated blood; in the branches of these veins there were concretions of fibrin, casts of these vessels; the pericardium contained one ounce of turbid serum; there was a partial deposition on it of coagulable lymph; the liver was large, its section nutmeg-like; in the right lobe, towards its convex surface, there was an abscess which contained about a pint of thick puruloid fluid; its cavity, nearly spherical, was lined with coagulable lymph; another abscess, a smaller one, was detected in the same lobe, situated more deeply; the hepatic substance adjoining the abscesses was congested with blood and redder than natural; there was some bile in the gall-bladder of healthy appearance. The œsophagus, stomach, and duodenum were very much distended with air and liquid; in the small curvature of the stomach there were spots about the size of pins'-heads, as if the mucous coat had been cut out, or its substance absorbed; there was no redness adjoining. The large intestines were ulcerated in many places; the ulcers were in different stages; to some coagula of blood adhered, others presented pale granulations, others were nearly healed, and there were cicatrices of some that had healed, which were covered with a bluish epithelium. In the transverse colon the ulceration was most severe; it had penetrated nearly to the peritoneal covering, and gave way when handled; there was least in the cœcum and near the extremity of the rectum.

The hepatic abscesses in this case were truly latent; they were nowise indicated during life. Even the bowel symptoms were mild compared with the lesions.

Case 15.—Of abscess of liver, latent; returned "Synochus;" treated by large blood-letting.—C. Taylor, ætat. 32; 80th Regiment; admitted into hospital at Malta, 5th July, 1828; died 13th July.—This man, previously in good health and tolerably robust, on admission had febrile symptoms with pain at epigastrium; it was most felt in the sitting posture; the day after coming into hospital he voided some tape-worm, and experienced rigors; he was blooded largely and blistered and ordered calomel and antimonial powder. On the 10th he complained of nothing but debility; pulse 76; he was pronounced convalescent. On the following day there was a recurrence of pain and of increased severity referred to the bowels; V.S. was again performed, and with relief from pain. In the night of the 12th there was a return of pain which was relieved by a blister; the pulse was 88. He was easy until 6 a.m. of the following morning, when he was seized with pain of stomach, shooting towards the loins and accompanied with bilious vomiting; leeches were applied to the lumbar regions, without much relief. He now complained of pain, not confined to one spot or region of the body, but widely, universally felt; in-

---

* The air of the room was 60°; thermometer under lobulus Spigelii, 82°.

spiration did not increase it; nausea continued with increasing debility. Towards evening his breathing became laborious and short; at 7 p.m. he expired; V.S. was performed four times, and as much as 130 oz. of blood were abstracted, besides what was drawn by the leeches.

Autopsy 16 hours after death. Body not much emaciated; both lungs were adhering; there was congestion of blood in their inferior portions; the liver was much enlarged; an abscess was found in the right lobe, deeply seated, which contained about 2 pints of purulent fluid; it was lined with a false membrane, about the thickness of the pleura; the adjoining hepatic substance was softer and redder than the more distant parts, and more gorged with blood; the little bile in the gall-bladder was of natural appearance; the other abdominal viscera appeared to be sound.

This case is remarkable for the rapidity of its progress to a fatal termination. What was the cause of death? Did the disease or the mode of treatment most conduce to it? I am disposed to think the latter, and that many of the symptoms might have been owing to loss of blood. No mention is made of diet, but I believe it was of the lowest kind. Chicken-broth was ordered the last day. Whatever the cause of death, it is certain that the severe antiphlogistic treatment, aided by mercury and antimony, had no effect on the hepatic abscess.

Case 16.—Of tuberculated liver, with vomicæ, latent, and ulcerated intestines; returned "Dysenteria."—T. Evans, ætat. 36; 66th Regiment; admitted into general hospital, August 14, 1821; died 22nd September.—This man had served in Spain and Portugal, and latterly in St. Helena, from whence he recently returned, and where he had suffered from dysentery. On landing he seemed strong and healthy. His present complaint, he states, began about a fortnight ago. His stools are frequent and slimy, and contain much blood, and are accompanied with tormina and tenesmus; there is much pyrexia. On the 6th September, after using calomel and opium, blue pill and opium, he felt much better. That day he had six natural stools; the tongue was clean. The day following he was worse, the dysenteric symptoms recurring, but with no great severity; occasionally he experienced nausea and vomiting; cholera was prevalent at the time. The same symptoms continued nearly to the end; leeches were once applied to the anus, and V.S. was once performed; 12 oz. of blood were taken. The treatment was otherwise various.

Autopsy 9 hours after death. No emaciation; the muscles were well developed, and there was an excess rather than a deficiency of fat; the lungs were nearly natural, their inferior portion rather gorged with blood; the omentum much diseased adhered to the cœcum, sigmoid flexure and urinary bladder; there it was thickened and unusually vascular; some coagulable lymph was effused on its surface; with the exception of a very few spots the whole tract of the large intestines was ulcerated and sloughing; in some places, particularly in the cœcum and rectum, the mucous and muscular coats were destroyed, the peritoneal only remaining; in other places there was much thickening of the coats; the cellular tissue had acquired a cartilaginous hardness; the mucous had become flabby and soft; the valvula coli was thickened and contracted; the duodenum and jejunum were unusually vascular; the ileum was pale, rough and granular; the liver, much enlarged, adhered to the diaphragm; it weighed 5½ lbs.; its appearance was peculiar, of a mottled hue, brown, with a tinge of purple and reddish brown, with yellowish spots interspersed; it was found to abound in tubercles, these ranging in size from a barley corn to a large pea; they were all of a light yellow color; a few of them were hard; the majority were softening; some had passed into vomicæ, their sacs being full of puruloid matter; their resemblance in their several stages to pthisical tubercle was remarkable.

In this case, during life, there was no suspicion entertained of the existence of hepatic disease. The state of the large intestines was sufficient to account for the fatal event. It is remarkable how rapid was the progress of the illness, also the want of rallying power, also the little or no emaciation, and with great severity of lesions comparative mildness of symptoms. Whether a cholera-taint was concerned, and may have had an effect, is open to question. Several cases of cholera occurred at that time in the garrison at Chatham, and one or two of them proved fatal. The state of the small intestines rather favored the idea of such an influence.

Case 17.—Of abscesses of liver, with ulcerated intestines; returned "Hepatitis acuta."—C. Russell, ætat. 26; 66th Regiment; admitted into general hospital, 14th August, 1821; died Sept. 6.—This man, recently returned from St. Helena, had been ill three weeks before admission. When admitted he was in a hopeless state; no detail of symptoms was given, it was barely mentioned that there had been no pain of shoulder, and that the bowels previous to death were not constipated; this in relation to the following entry that "a few hours before he expired he passed at stool a large quantity of purulent matter, suggestive of an abscess having burst into the intestine." It is added, "that after the discharge of blood and pus the pulse became indistinct, the extremities cold, denoting a moribund state." The time of the *post mortem* examination is not given; and in the account of it, only the following particulars:— The liver was adhering to the diaphragm; two large abscesses were found in its substance, one, the largest, was in the inferior part of the right lobe, and was so superficial that its lower portion was covered merely with the peritoneal lining of the liver, and where so covered there was an adhesion between it and the ascending and part of the transverse colon, but without any communication; it held about a pint of ill-conditioned thick matter; the other abscess was more deeply seated in the same lobe; it contained about half a pint of similar matter; there was some healthy bile in the gall-bladder; the cœcum and ascending colon were very red and severely ulcerated; some bloody matter, like that discharged at stool, was found in the latter.

What was most remarkable in this case was the quantity of purulent matter with blood, suddenly discharged per anum. Had there been no autopsy, or had it been carelessly conducted, the probable conclusion would have been that referred to above— viz.: its source a ruptured abscess which had opened into the intestine.

Case 18.—Of abscess in liver, latent, communicating with the lung; returned "Catarrhus chronicus."—E. Marr, ætat. 35; 20th F.; admitted into general hospital, May

10th, 1835; died May 25th.—This man was sent home to be invalided on account
of injury of the left knee from a gun-shot wound. When admitted he was in a very
feeble state, much emaciated, with a general appearance of hectic; he complained of
pain in the right side, increased by inspiration; had a troublesome cough with muco-
purulent expectoration and considerable dyspnœa; the same symptoms continued to
the last, with the addition of severe pain of abdomen, which came on suddenly on the
25th, and was increased by pressure, suggestive of peritoneal inflammation, from perforation of intestine; he was twice leeched. The day before he died this pain had
nearly ceased. The treatment was palliative.

Autopsy 30 hours after death. Body much emaciated; the left pleura contained 2
oz. of serum, the right about a pint, in which were flakes of coagulable lymph; the
left lung was free from disease, as also the superior lobe of the right; of this lung the
middle and inferior lobe were compressed and in part œdematous; the inferior lobe
adhered to the diaphragm, and through it communicated by an ulcerated passage,
capable of receiving the finger, with an enormous abscess in the liver. The liver was
unusually large, especially its right lobe, which partially adhered to the diaphragm;
its surface was very red; on percussion, fluctuation was distinct in it; cut into, a vast
cavity was found occupying the greater part of the right lobe; it was lined with a
thin layer of lymph, and was full of what appeared to be purulent fluid, with which
flakes of lymph were mixed, but its purulent character was not confirmed by the optical
test; the lymphatics on the surface of the liver were very large; the gall-bladder was
distended with bile; the spleen was large; a few ounces of serum with a little gelatinous lymph were lodged in the cavity of the abdomen.

Even in this case the disease of liver was not recognised during
life. The pectoral symptoms were most urgent; and latterly,
that is, only a few days before death, the abdominal pain (probably the result of incipient peritoneal inflammation, seemingly
indicated by the effusion) arrested most the attention. The state
of the injured knee was examined; the appearances may be
worth recording; some of the changes were well displayed by a
section of the joint. The thigh-bone and tibia were found united
by osseous matter, and the patella with each of them. No line
of separation was visible, as if all three were of the same formation, their structure being similar. The capsule of the joint was
nearly obliterated, as were also the synovial fringes; fatty
matter seemed to have taken their place; it surrounded, and in
no inconsiderable quantity, the ancylosed parts.

Case 19.—Of icterus, with no well marked lesions; returned "Icterus."—A. Mac-
pherson, ætat. 25; 2nd B. R. B.; admitted into hospital at Malta, 10th October,
1830; died 15th October.—This man on admission, previously in good health at duty,
had febrile symptoms of one day's duration. He complained of headache, lassitude,
and of frequent rigors; the tongue was furred, the breath fetid, bowels regular; pulse
100 and sharp; V.S. 16 oz.; a saline cathartic with tartar emetic; the blood was
buffed. At the evening visit, the symptoms the same; V.S. 12 oz.; calomel, with
antimonial powder and extract of hyoscyamus. October 11—No improvement; had
a restless night; headache continues with wandering pains; has a feeling of oppres-

sion at præcordia, much bilious vomiting and many bilious stools; thirst urgent,
anorexia; tartarized antimony gr. iii., followed by a saline purgative; a warm bath;
appeared rather better in the evening; the evacuations *sursum* and *deorsum* very
bilious; thirst excessive; the blood last drawn very slightly buffed. Calomel, pulv.
antimon. Hyoscym. of each 5 grs. at bed-time. On the 12th—Had a tolerable
night; the skin and conjunctivæ now deeply yellow; still occasional vomiting
of bilious matter and the stools bilious; pulse 102. Calomel, grs. x. and a saline
purgative after; at bed-time calomel, grs. x. with i. gr. of opium. 13th—Vomited
often during the night; many scanty watery stools without bile; jaundice more
intense; tongue cleaner, thirst urgent, abdomen rather tumid, without pain. Calomel
20 grs., opium, 1 gr.; a cathartic enema. Vespere, reaching during the day.
Calomel, 10 grs.; a saline draught with a scruple of T. opii; a purgative enema;
friction with mercurial ointment to thighs. 14th—Worse; stools frequent and very
bloody; no pain or tenderness of abdomen; thirst intolerable; pupils contracted, but
act freely; is quite sensible; jaundice intense; pulse 116, weak; 12 leeches to
temples, a large blister to abdomen Calomel, 5 grs., ext. Hyoscy. 3 grs., twice
during the day; mercurial friction, a warm bath, an anodyne enema. At 6 p.m., no
better; tenderness of abdomen on hard pressure; stools bloody, but less frequent;
occasional wandering of intellect. 24 leeches to abdomen; mercurial ointment,
anodyne enema, calomel 20 grs., opium 1 gr. 15th (When I saw him first)—He
is evidently sinking; no ptyalism; occasional delirium; stools dark without blood;
pulse 120. He died at 11 p.m.

Autopsy 10 hours after death. Body not emaciated, but fat; skin extremely
yellow; calves of legs and pendant parts slightly livid; much blood and fibrinous
concretions in the longitudinal sinus; the dura mater very yellow; the pia mater
and arachnoid slightly so; cerebral substance white; a little fluid in the lateral
ventricles, and more at base of brain slightly tinged yellow. In the choroid plexus
of each ventricle (the inferior, posterior cornu) a small gritty concretion about the
size of a garden pea; the pericardium contained about half-ounce of thick viscid
yellow serum; there was a good deal of blood and fibrinous concretions in the heart
and great vessels, the concretions very firmly adhering; no lesion of heart; the
lungs were generally and firmly adhering, their parenchyma was redder than usual;
their inferior portion had a hepatized appearance, but whether from morbid or *post
mortem* change, doubtful; the bronchia were redder than natural; the thoracic duct
contained a little yellowish fluid; the gall-bladder adhered to the pyloric portion of
the stomach; the inner coat of the latter was thicker than common and softer; some
flatus in intestines; these exhibited externally no marks of disease; there was no
appearance of bile in the intestines; the duodenum contained a good deal of brownish
mucus mixed with imperfectly formed chyme; the jejunum was pale; the ileum unusually red; its inner surface was in patches slightly granular, as if from deposition
of lymph, and most of all in its lower portion; there was the same appearance in the
large intestines, with bloody points or petechiæ; in some places the mucous coat exhibited fine flabby granulations, like those on an ulcerated surface, but there was no
breach of surface; the liver was of a yellowish tinge, otherwise apparently sound;
the hepatic and common duct were rather distended with bile; in the gall-bladder
there was little bile; it was moderately viscid and of a dark green hue; hard pressure
and continued was required to force any bile from the gall-bladder into the duodenum,
but when it once began to flow, it continued, less pressure being used; when the gall-
ducts were laid open, nothing morbid was found with the exception of some remaining
thick mucus at the extremity of the common duct, which might have closed its
mouth; there was no appearance of disease in the gall-bladder, or in the vena portæ

or hepatic artery, nor in any of the abdominal viscera not named; the ascending vena cava and vena portæ were empty.

The symptoms in this case and the treatment have been described with some minuteness on account of its obscurity. The treatment was energetic, according to common usage at that time. I thought it hazardous then; it will be condemned now. As neither the mercury nor antimony in large doses, nor the bloodletting often repeated had any good effect, they could hardly fail doing harm. Under such treatment there is unavoidably a difficulty in distinguishing between the phenomena of the disease and the epiphenomena, the results of the practice.

Case 20.—Of hydatid in liver, latent, with hydrops perircardii and hydrothorax, etc.; returned "Hepatitis chronica."—R. Simkin, ætat. 28; 2nd B. R. B.; admitted into hospital, at Malta, 26th December, 1830; died March 3rd.—This man, of a "strumous habit and weakly constitution," between the 20th August and the 19th October had two attacks of dysentery. Discharged relieved on the 8th November, he was re-admitted on the 26th December, complaining of a dull pain in the hepatic region extending to the right shoulder; the bowels were relaxed, but without tormina or tenesmus; he was weak, emaciated, and dejected, and had a presentiment that he should not recover. For some time under the use of blisters, the tepid bath, calomel and opium, etc., he appeared to improve; then the urine became scanty and high-colored with much sediment; the abdomen tumid and fluctuating, with œdema of feet and ankles, and in addition distressing dyspnœa. He could not lie easily on the left side; on the right side of chest no respiratory sound was distinguishable below the third rib. Using cream of tartar in half-ounce doses with infusion of juniper berries and gin, the urine increased, the dropsical symptoms nearly disappeared; he became cheerful and no longer hopeless of mending. The improvement was of short duration. On the 20th February the urine began to diminish and the dropsical symptoms to increase with occasional rigors, the dyspnœa becoming hourly more distressing until he expired, as if "from suffocation."

Autopsy 11 hours after death. Face tumid from œdema; general anasarca in a slight degree; the pericardium contained 6 oz. of serum; its upper portion presented a prominent tumor, from a cul de sac distended with serosity: this, being just over the great vessels and above the heart, during the action of the heart, might have pressed on the trachea at its bifurcation, and have been a cause of dyspnœa; the heart was large; its right cavities were thin and distended with soft coagulated blood; the left ventricle was thick; the right pleura contained 2 pints of serum and much gelatinous lymph; the left pleura contained less without any lymph; the lungs were partially adhering; their inferior portions were hepatized; there were no tubercles; the bronchia were very red and contained much frothy fluid; there was œdema of both mediastina; the thoracic duct was empty; the liver was unusually large, rather pale, of healthy consistence; in its right lobe, projecting slightly from the concave surface, was a large globular sac, resembling the sac of an hydatid; its coat was about a ¼ inch thick, and almost of cartilaginous firmness; it contained about 2 pints of thick, rather viscid matter; the hepatic substance adjoining was not apparently diseased; there was much dilute bile in the gall-bladder; the spleen was large and firm; the kidneys pale; there were some small ulcers in the cœcum, and very many cicatrices of ulcers in the rectum, and some in the colon; they were indicated by a dark color and being depressed; the mesenteric glands were considerably enlarged; about half a pint of serum in the cavity of the abdomen.

In this case the lesions tolerably accord with the symptoms and the progress of the disease. The sacculated state of a portion of the pericardium is noteworthy, especially in relation to the effects of its pressure on the contiguous parts. Another noteworthy circumstance is the change of feeling from despondency to hope. Whether the sac in the liver was an abscess or the remains of an hydatid, there can be little doubt that it was of long standing, gradually increasing, and that its pressure on the subjacent great vessels might have been one of the causes of the dropsical effusions, at least into the abdomen and lower extremities.

Case 21.—Of abscess in liver, communicating with hepatic duct, with abscess in brain, and ulcerated intestines; returned "Chronic Hepatitis."—G. Anghterson, ætat. 41; 45th Foot; admitted into general hospital, 13th September, 1823; died 26th September.—This man, of intemperate habits, had recently returned from Ceylon, where during the last year he had been under treatment for anasarca and hepatitis, leaving "a hardness and enlargement of the liver." After landing he was admitted into hospital, complaining of constant pain in the right hypochondrium, increased by pressure, and of inability to lie on the left side. There was slight dyspnœa, calm circulation, natural temperature, regular bowels, impaired appetite. After a few days, his health improving a little, and the weather being fine, he was discharged; this was on the 27th August. On the 13th September he was re-admitted, complaining of weakness, fainting, of pain at scrobiculus cordis and right hypochondrium; the bowels were regular; the tongue white; no appetite. On the following day the circulation was reported calm, and that, though he had had no sleep, he felt relieved. On the 15th it is stated that he slept pretty well, felt easy, and that the bowels were relaxed. On the 18th there were frequent watery stools, with occasional griping, apyrexia, great debility. On the 20th slight pyrexia; watery stools; a disposition to sleep; said he felt easy; tongue dryish; anorexia. On the 22nd increased disposition to sleep; skin cool, dry; pulse 86, feeble; bowels loose, stools passed involuntarily; still says he is easy. On the 23rd he was reported comatose; pupils rather contracted; breathing labored with slight stertor; pulse 90, full, easily compressed; temperature equable. In this state he remained until the 26th, when at 8 a.m. he died. In the comatose state he occasionally moaned; once or twice he was observed to move the left hand, but never the right. He now and then swallowed a little fluid poured into his mouth; the evening preceding his death his feet became swollen; the extremities were warm to the last. No mention is made of the treatment.

Autopsy 27 hours after death. Body much emaciated; limbs rigid; extremities cold; trunk still slightly warm; a thermometer introduced through a small incision at scrobiculis cordis rose from 60° (the temperature of the air of room) to 68°; on each frontal bone internally there was a depression of about the size of a silver-penny; there the bone was very thin and rough, as if from absorption, removing the inner table, and corroding the inner surface of the outer; the dura mater corresponding, and to a greater extent, was partly ossified and partly as it were absorbed, presenting a reticulated texture; underneath, the arachnoid had become thickened and opaque;

smaller cavities or depressions, as if from absorption, similar to the preceding in the frontal, were found in the parietal bones ; the anterior lobe of the right hemisphere of the cerebrum, almost throughout, was a mass of disease, being the seat of a large abscess, which was bounded above by the dura mater (the pia mater apparently destroyed), anteriorly by medullary substance softened, and so too posteriorly and inferiorly. On removing the dura mater a surface of semi-fluid pus, more or less tinged with blood, was brought into view ; the abscess had penetrated to a level with the corpus callosum, and by a small opening it communicated with the right lateral ventricle, in which there were rather more than 2 oz. of bloody sero-purulent fluid ; the parieties of this ventricle were very soft, especially the septum lucidum ; the choroid plexus was pale, and seemed as if macerated ; the foramen of Monro was unusually large ; the third ventricle was large, distended with fluid of the same kind, as was also the fourth ventricle ; the pineal gland was large ; there was about half an ounce of the like fluid in the left lateral ventricle, the parietes of which were less softened, and its plexus choroides of a more natural appearance ; the right hemisphere exhibited every degree of softening, from the slightest, where most distant from the abscess, to complete disorganization, where nearest ; the diseased cerebral substance had a yellow hue ; the left hemisphere, the base of the cerebrum generally, and the cerebellum appeared pretty natural ; the pericardium contained about 2 oz. of serum ; the right auricle and ventricle pretty much coagulated blood ; the aorta at its origin was a little dilated ; the walls of the heart were rather thin and soft ; the inferior lobe of the right lung adhered to the diaphragm ; it was of a dark red, partially hepatized, partially œdematous ; the left pleura contained about 3 oz. of serum ; the lung of the same side inferiorly was gorged with blood and serum ; the thyroid gland was of the color of unbleached wax, and more friable than natural ; the thoracic duct was quite empty and collapsed, and in consequence its surface was not rounded, as usual, but flat ; the liver was large, it weighed 8½ lbs. ; its right lobe adhered to the diaphragm ; its convex surface was dark red, soft and fluctuating, from an abscess beneath, in which were 3 pints of thick viscid matter ; the abscess was lined with coagulable lymph, was of an irregular form, and communicated by a small opening with the hepatic duct ; this duct and the cystic and common ducts were large and were distended with a light-colored bile mixed with pus ; the contents of the gall-bladder were similar ; its inner coat was much redder than natural ; the substance of the liver generally was pretty natural ; incised it exhibited slightly the nutmeg-like structure ; the stomach was nearly empty and much contracted ; it displayed the hour-glass contraction ; the small intestines were healthy ; the large intestines were very much ulcerated, most in the cœcum, less severely in the colon, and least in the rectum ; the ulcers were numerous, in size little exceeding a split pea, and were surrounded by a red margin ; they were in different stages ; in their advanced stage, the mucous membrane was destroyed ; in their early stage they resembled a small-pox pustule, being white in the centre, slightly elevated and having an inflamed areola ; there was an appearance of cicatrization (spots opaque and puckered) in portions of the mesentery where attached to the ileum and caput coli.

Amongst the noteworthy circumstances in this case not the least remarkable is the duration of life for so long a time, if it may be inferred, as I think it may, that both the hepatic and cerebral disease were of a chronic kind. It is singular that he never complained of headache. Is it not singular too, that after the occurrence of coma the right side appeared to be paralysed ? It may be mentioned that whilst in Ceylon he was repeatedly salivated; a treatment that might have conduced to disease of bone.

Case 22.—Jaundice with partial softening of brain and enlarged heart; returned "Hepatitis chronica."—P. Rawson, ætat. 35; 85th Regiment; admitted into hospital, Malta, 14th June, 1829; died 3rd July.—This man since April last had been thrice in hospital, twice for constipation, once for hepatitis, accompanied with pain in right hypochondrium. The treatment was leeches and V.S. and mercury. On the 10th June he was considered convalescent and was sent to Ricasoli to be under observation. On the 14th of same month he was brought back to hospital complaining of pain and heat at epigastrium; his breathing was quick; his pulse accelerated; there was some tenesmus with relaxed bowels. Up to the 20th he seemed to improve, using gentle aperients and "bitters;" on that day his countenance and the upper part of chest became partially livid; there was no pain, no cough. 3 grs. of blue pill and 3 of colchicum in powder twice daily. On the 21st there was diffused pain of chest, not increased by a full inspiration; his breathing was easier. Cream of tartar drink in addition and an aloetic pill. On the 23rd the œdema was less; frequent stools; some griping; skin of a yellow tinge; pulse strong. Cream of tartar omitted; V.S. 10 ounces. On the 28th there was less œdema; the skin was less yellow; his appetite and general feeling better; he complained chiefly of flatulency and a certain mal-aise. He was now ordered 2 grs. of sulphate of quinine twice daily, and 10 grs. of nitre, and 1½ grs. of extract of opium at night. On the 29th he was worse; much restlessness; had several bilious stools; pain at scrobiculus cordis; troublesome cough. On the 1st of July his breathing was quick and laborious; the pulse very quick; his appearance stupid, his answers confused. Very little respiratory sound could be perceived in the lower part of the left lung. There was after this date little change till he expired.

Autopsy 10 hours after death. The body rather large; the lower extremities œdematous; the face slightly so; much discoloration of the inferior parts from gravitation; the dura mater both externally and internally was bright yellow; the arachnoid was slightly opaque, but not so colored, neither was the pia mater. The cerebrum generally was softer than natural; the fornix and the parietes of ventricles and corpora striata were almost pultaceous; there was little serum in the ventricles or at base of brain; the cerebellum was nearly of its ordinary consistence; the pericardium contained about 4 ounces of serum; partially floating on it was a delicate yellowish-white membrane, formed, apparently of coagulable lymph, which had become vascular; about its middle it was contracted, surrounded by one or two fibres of a silky lustre, seemingly acting the part of a ligature; the vessels conveying red blood could not be traced further; its fixed portion was attached to the aorta; the heart was about twice or thrice its natural size; its cavities were enlarged, its parietes thickened; it was distended with black blood in the state of soft coagulum; the great blood vessels were similarly distended; the semilunar valves both of the aorta and pulmonary artery were rather rigid; the latter artery was large and very thin; the ascending aorta was unduly large and its coats were partially diseased, thickened in some places, wasted in others; with the exception of undue redness there was no marked disease of lungs. Like the principal arteries the venæ cavæ and the larger veins of the thorax and abdomen were distended with soft black coagulated blood; there were about 3 pints of orange-serum in the cavity of the abdomen; the omentum adhered to the right lobe of the liver; and the convex surface of the latter adhered to the adjoining parietes; the liver was rather firmer than usual; its section slightly nutmeg-like; its vessels full of blood; the gall-blader contained a moderate quantity of bile, apparently healthy; the spleen was very little larger than usual, but darker and firmer, probably from containing coagulated blood. The inner surface of the stomach was bright red, as if highly inflamed; the duodenum was less so, and the other intestines still less; there was some chyme in the former; the kidneys were large and abounded in blood; the mesenteric glands were unusually large and redder and softer than natural; the lymphatic vessels over the spine, just below the receptaculum chyli, were unusually large and distinct; the thoracic duct contained a little yellowish fluid.

It is noteworthy that during life in this case neither disease of brain or of heart was suspected. Whether the treatment was any wise concerned with the fatal result is open to question. The appearance of the stomach was very like that produced by a poisonous dose of colchicum; and sometimes we know that even a small dose of this medicine has an almost poisonous effect. The manner in which the heart and great vessels were distended with black soft coagulated blood is noteworthy; its condition, if the same during the latter part of life, might account for the termination.

The foregoing cases are only a portion of those of diseased states of the liver which I have by me; they may suffice to show how difficult is the diagnosis of hepatic disease, and the great liability there is in consequence to error; nor, when we consider the nature of the organ and its position, is such a liability at all surprising. Possessing little sensibility, even inflammation, even the formation of an abscess in it, is not necessarily productive of pain. And, placed as it is, contiguous to other organs, all of them of the first importance, in its morbid state it can hardly fail exercising a deranging influence on those nearest the seat of the lesion and producing epithenomena which may readily be mistaken for primary affections. The cases in which an abscess in the liver has penetrated through the diaphragm into the lung are striking examples of this, and their proportional frequency is remarkable.

Whether there be any true connection between disease of the liver, especially abscess, and ulceration of the large intestines, is open to question. I am disposed to adopt the affirmative opinion, and that the one exercises an influence on the other somewhat similar to that which pulmonary tuberculosis exercises on the ileum, especially productive of ulceration.

In some of the cases detailed a cachetic state of the system seems to have occurred in connection with hepatic disease, lowering the vital powers, and preventing healthy reaction, and in consequence occasioning death as it were by exhaustion. Many more instances of the same kind have been kept back.

The term abscess of liver, I have used, as it is commonly employed; yet it can hardly be doubted that what is so called is far from uniform, or of the same kind. Judging from its contents, in one instance it may have the character of a phlegmon; in another more the character of an excavation, as if formed from softening and softened tubercle; and in a third it may have a close resemblance to an hydatid sac, if not this in reality, in course of change after the death of the entozoon.

What are the effects of bile when absorbed after its secretion, or of its elements in the blood, if not eliminated by secretion, are curious questions for inquiry. That the effects, more or less, are toxical, seems probable.

On the treatment of hepatic disease I have little to offer, that little owing to my ignorance of any successful mode. When an abscess is once formed in the organ I am doubtful that any of the received modes of encountering it are efficacious, and this whatever may be the kind of abscess. Large blood-letting seems to exhaust the strength, without arresting the disease. Mercury used to salivation seems to have a similar weakening effect and no certain good effect. Both the lancet and mercury I feel pretty confident were abused in the old practice. I am inclined to think that kind of treatment is the safest which affords the best chance of the powers of nature, the vis medicatrix, being brought into action, consisting in the use of gentle means, mild medicines and regard to diet and exercise: life at least may thus probably be prolonged, if not a natural cure effected.

In no instance have I known recovery from an abscess in the liver, whether left to follow its own course and burst internally, or opened by the trocar of the surgeon. The operation, however, of paracentesis is unquestionably justifiable on the ground of affording a chance of recovery; almost invariably it affords relief, and often prolongation of life. Were it, in the most suitable cases, performed early, it is likely that the number of successful results on record would be greater; but unfortunately, the early stage is too often inappreciable; most commonly when the tumor is distinct, the abscess is advanced.

CHAPTER V.

ON PULMONARY CONSUMPTION.

Remarks on its importance in connection with its prevalency, especially in the army.—Statistics of the disease.—Reasons for writing on it.—Division into sections, with illustrative cases; 1st. Of latent tubercles, without appreciable diseased action; 2ndly. Of the disguising influence of Insanity; 3rdly. Of a like influence of other diseases; 4thly. Of ordinary consumption, acute and chronic.—Etiological and pathological remarks.—Effects of ignorance and of maladministration.—Hopeful prospective views.—Treatment and prevention.

THAT a disease which is so common and fatal as pulmonary consumption amongst the civil population not only of the United Kingdom, but of Europe generally, and of every country of which we have any statistical knowledge of a reliable kind, should be prevalent in the army and in a high degree, can hardly be considered surprising, keeping in mind the many circumstances peculiar to military life unfavorable to health, and which there is good reason to believe conduce to the formation of that morbid deposit, tubercle, which is the material cause and foundation of the disease.

Whilst the proportional mortality from phthisis pulmonalis of the people of the United Kingdom is estimated at about one-fourth of the whole, the deaths from this disease in the British army serving at home have exceeded one-half.

The following table, formed from the army medical reports, affords at least an approximate idea of this mortality both at home and at most of the principal stations where British troops are employed. The numbers, calculated per 10,000 of the aggregate force, will comprise the deaths returned under the head not only of phthisis pulmonalis, but also of hæmoptysis and catarrhus chronicus; the one commonly depending on a tubercular state of the lungs; the other, often latent phthisis, misnamed chronic catarrh from inattention, or from difficulty of diagnosis.

Dragoon Guards and Dragoons, from 1837 to 1847, serving at home	65·2
Infantry of the Line, do.	80·2
Foot Guards	125·3

Troops at Gibraltar .... 37·7
Troops at Malta .... 51·0
Fencible Corps, Maltese... 31·9
Troops—Ionian Islands.. 41·0
     „   Bermudas.. 63·2
Nova Scotia and New Brunswick .... 54·4
Canada.. 45·9
Newfoundland... 40·2
Sierra Leone (White Troops) from 1819 to 1836 .... 43·4
     „   (Black Troops)   „   .... 44·8
St. Helena from 1818 to 1821 .... 27·0
Cape of Good Hope, Cape District, from 1818 to 1836......... 26·8
          Do.   Frontiers,   from 1822 to 1834 .... 13·6
          Do.   Hottentot Troops .... 24·1
Mauritius (White) from 1818 to 1836............................... 39·6
     „   (Black) from 1825 to 1836................. .... 78·0
West Indies—Windward and Leeward Command (White)
     from 1817 to 1836.. 85·3
     „   „   „.   „   (Black) 115·8
Jamaica (White) .... 67·7
     „   (Black) .... 75·0
Ceylon (White) from 1817 to 1836 .... 31·6
     „   Malays, from 1818 to 1836 .... 15·6
     „   Armed Lascoryns, Natives of the Continent of India,
               from 1821 to 1835............... .... 12·1
     „   Black—Africans from 1816 to 1820 .... 72·1
Moelmyne (White) from 1827 to 1836 .... 5·9
N.B.—From all diseases of the lungs.............................. 20·5
Rangoon, from 1824 to 1826 .... 16·4
Interior of Burmese Empire from 1825 to 1826................. 6·1

Large as is the proportion shown of deaths from phthisis, with
a few exceptions, in the foregoing table, my belief is, that it is
below rather than above the mark, and that we should have proof
of its being so, could we have a true statement of the mortality
depending on tubercle, or, in other words, of the diseases with
which tubercle is connected and the probable cause of their fatal
issue.   This opinion is not a merely conjectural one ; it is mainly
founded on experience, that of the existence of tubercles as demonstrated by necroscopical research.   The following table
showing the results of the examination of the lung in 1,205 fatal
cases which occurred in the General Hospital at Fort Pitt, may
be adduced in proof.   It has been framed in part from the necro-
logical register which is kept in that hospital, and in part from
my own notes, the latter from 1834 to 1839, both years included,
—a period when I was in medical charge of that establishment,
including the lunatic asylum of the army then at Fort Clarence.

Phthisis pulmonalis, recognised as such during life, and confirmed
   by autopsy 415
Chronic catarrh and hæmoptysis with tubercles and cavities 68
Other diseases, with cavities and tubercles 131
Other diseases, with tubercles 119
Other diseases, with cavities 11
Other diseases, without tubercles or cavities........................... 461
                                                             1205

Thus showing that no less than 61·7 per cent. of the total fatal cases were affected with tubercles; and, as during the period included, all the invalids of the army abroad as well as at home were sent to Fort Pitt with the exception of certain regiments—viz., the Horse and Foot Guards and the Royal Artillery, this vast per centage may be considered as applicable to the troops in general, especially as it is now well established that the Foot Guards, as shown in a preceding table, suffer more when stationed at home from pulmonary consumption than any other corps in the service.

This great prevalency of tubercle, this great mortality from tubercular disease, shows most clearly its importance; and what adds much to the interest of the subject is the presumption that the causes of the malady are for the most part preventible, being of a nature admitting of correction by attention to hygiene, especially in the army, recruited as it is by men who at the time of enlistment, after a strict examination, are inferred to be of perfectly sound constitutions.

Considering that the disease has been investigated in a very able manner by some of the most distinguished pathologists of recent times, the attempt to elucidate it further may appear uncalled for and a labor of supererogation. Two motives chiefly induce me to enter upon the subject—one, the extremely Protean character of the malady—the other, the opportunity afforded in military hospitals of obtaining more exact information relative to the rise and progress of the disease than is commonly procurable in civil hospitals, or in civil practice: I might add to these two motives a third—viz., the reflection of the vast importance of the subject, as already alluded to, in connection with military service,—an importance that cannot be too strongly impressed on the mind of the army surgeon, whether regimental or staff—both of whom should ever keep in mind that tubercular mischief is probably lying latent whenever there is any indication of the function of the lungs not being well performed, and this irrespective of age, but most so in the recruit and the young soldier.

The total number of fatal cases of tubercular disease of which I have notes, including those in which the lesion existed either latent or concealed by other morbid action, amount to 310, which may be classed as follows :—

1.	Latent tubercles, without any apparent disease		8
2.	Latent, connected with insanity		6
3.	Latent, connected with other diseases		10
4.	Acute phthisis		22
5.	Chronic phthisis		13
6.	Ordinary phthisis		185
7.	Associated with pneumathorax		26
8.	,,	,, empyema	21
9.	,,	,, fibrinous concretions in the heart and great vessels	24
10.	,,	,, peritonitis	1

316

This arrangement I propose nearly to follow, beginning with latent tubercles.

1. ON LATENT TUBERCULAR DISEASE.—The term latent is employed in this section as implying the existence of tubercle not suspected during life, its presence in the lungs not having been indicated by any symptoms attracting attention, or apparently interfering with the general health of the individual.

The examples I have to give have been all deaths from accidents, or lives cut short independent of any manifest disease.

Cases 1 and 2.—G. Cuthbert, ætat 26, and W. Hamilton, ætat 25, both of 65th Foot; both killed by a fall.—These men, on the night of 1st January, 1824, when under the influence of drink, intent on going into the town of Edinburgh from the Castle where they were quartered, that they might enjoy the festivities of the evening of the New Year, not being able to pass the sentinel at the draw-bridge, scaled the wall, and, in attempting to descend the side of the rock, fell, and were found stark dead the following morning. Their bodies lay at the foot of a perpendicular precipice, from which they must have fallen, of at least 100 feet, on the top of which are the remains of Wallace's Tower. Hamilton's body was on soft ground; Cuthbert's a few feet apart on a pathway. The injuries sustained were many and formidable, and some of them not a little remarkable; these I shall describe under a different section.

Both men were tailors by trade; both bore a good character; and both at the time were considered in perfect health. Cuthbert had not been in hospital since the preceding September, and then only for a few days, and for a slight ailment; Hamilton not since the preceding March, and then only for three days, on account of "slight pneumonia." Since that time it is said that he had cough now and then, of which "he thought nothing."

The bodies were examined about 34 hours after death. Both were muscular and fat; the limbs rigid; the pupils dilated.

1st. Of Cuthbert's.—In the superior lobe of the left lung there was a cluster of tubercles of about the size of a chestnut. Most of them were small and firm, not exceeding a grape-seed in size; one or two were larger, about the size of large peas; these had undergone softening, and presented a soft, curd-like appearance. In other parts of this lung, and in the right, there was a faint appearance of tubercles; in the latter, a small calcareous concretion was imbedded. Both lungs partially adhered. In no other organ were there any indications of organic disease.

2nd. Of Hamilton's.—The left lung adhered very generally and closely; the right partially. Both abounded in small tubercles, most of them granular and firm; a few in the superior part of each lung were softening, and in the same situation there were two or three minute vomicæ. In the plexus choroides there were a few " ovoid opaque tubercles, hardly as large as grape-stones." No other traces of organic disease were detected.

Case 3.—J. Todoraki, ætat. 38.—Died in Zante in 1824, from a wound of the larynx, self-inflicted, between the upper margin of the thyroid cartilage and the os hyoides, separating the epiglottis from its attachment to the glottis, and lacerating the back parts of the pharynx. He died on the fifth day from the infliction of the wound. The history of this man was briefly the following :—By birth he was a Mainote, and might have been of Spartan descent. He was well made, had dark black hair, and grey eyes. During the last seven or eight years he had been attached to the Police-office in Zante; previously he had served as a serjeant in the Greek Light Infantry. He had had no sickness that was known of, and had not been troubled with cough. On the 31st October he was placed in confinement, on suspicion of theft, the commission of which he strenuously denied. The same evening he cut his throat with a blunt knife. His death was chiefly owing to the inflammation, etc., of the wounded parts, in conjunction with a very debilitated state, resulting from loss of blood.

Autopsy 12 hours after death.—The body was muscular, but without any superfluous fat; the parts about the wound were in a state tending to sphacelus; the bronchia were very red, and contained a puruloid fluid. The right lung was much diseased; it abounded in small tubercles, many of which exhibited puruloid softening; they were least numerous in its upper portion. This lung was very red and heavy; it weighed about two pounds, contained a good deal of blood, and was in some measure hepatized. The left lung was much less diseased, and contained comparatively few tubercles; they were similar to those described, and were seated chiefly in the inferior lobe. The other viscera bore no marks of organic disease; but the position of many of them was peculiar, and may be deserving of mention, as showing in a striking manner the effect of tight girding for the sake of a fine waist—the pride of the people to whom this man belonged. The heart lay nearly over the spine, projecting more towards the right than the left side; the right carotid was nearly in a straight line with the innominata; a large portion of the transverse colon, as well as the whole of the omentum, was pressed up and hid under the diaphragm; a large portion of the small intestines was hid in the cavity of the pelvis; the stomach was small and contracted, especially its pyloric portion.

Case 4.—C. M'Kenna, ætat. 24; admitted into regimental hospital, Malta, 8th May; died 19th May.—This man was described as of drunken habits, but in good health previous to a fall from a height of between twenty and thirty feet when drunk. It occurred in the evening of the 8th May. The fall did not render him insensible. Seen about fifteen minutes after by the surgeon, he was conscious, able to walk, his pulse natural, and no function apparently disturbed. On examination the left temple was found to be bruised and slightly cut; there was some ecchymosis round the left eye and over the skin of the right leg, which was also bruised and slightly cut. His breathing was unaffected. No suspicion even was entertained of fracture, or, indeed, of any hurt of the thorax; nor were there any indications discoverable of fracture of the cranium. Until the 15th the wounds appeared to be doing well. On that day some erythema was noticed about the hurt of leg, with some œdema of foot. On the 16th red lines were seen extending from the leg to the thigh; his pulse slow. On the following day delirium was reported, with a tendency to coma. On the 18th there was much incoherency; pulse, skin, respiration natural; occasional subsultus; the wounds of a more healthy appearance. Towards the evening he became comatose, and so remained till he expired on the following day. The treatment at first was merely such as the visible hurts seemed to require. Between the morning of the 17th and the evening of the 18th he was twice blooded, first ad deliquium; 16 oz. were abstracted each time; the blood was neither buffed nor cupped.

Autopsy 16 hours after death. The body well formed and muscular; some discoloration of skin of left side over the false ribs; the principal lesions discovered, the effects of the fall, were a comminuted fracture of the orbitar process of the sphenoidal bone and a simple fracture of the upper part of the sternum, the latter extending from close to the articulation of the left clavicle to the insertion of the third rib. A small portion of the anterior lobe of the cerebrum, about the size of a shilling, corresponding to the fracture, was in a pultaceous state to the depth of two or three lines; there was some ecchymosis in the anterior mediastinum and between the fibres of the pectoral muscle, and also a little purulent fluid in the cellular tissue over the fractured part of sternum; the skin above bore no marks of injury; some ecchymosis too was found under the scalp over the parietal and temporal bone, but no appearance of fracture externally. There was considerable œdema, of the left leg, and a small abscess under the skin near the ankle, with some ecchymosis under the integuments and between the muscles of the calf; the bone was not injured. The lungs were free from adhesions, except between the middle and inferior lobe of the right lung; both lungs contained much blood, chiefly in their inferior portion;—for several days he had been lying on his back; the inferior lobe of left lung contained many tubercles undergoing softening, of about the size of a pea, or a little larger; in some of them there was a little puruloid fluid; a few tubercles of the same kind were found in other parts of this lung and also in the right lung; the bronchia were much redder than natural, especially the larger branches contiguous to the gorged lung. The cavities of the heart and the great vessels were much distended with coagulated blood and fibrinous concretions, especially the venous trunks; the large intestines were much distended with air; there was no softening of the stomach; putrefaction had made no sensible progress. The aorta and cardiac valves in contact with blood were only just perceptibly stained red.

Case 5.—J. Harrison, ætat. 34; 94th Regiment; admitted into regimental hospital, Malta, 20th May; died 22nd May.—This man, previously in the enjoyment of good health, on the evening of the 19th May fell on the stone flags from the terrace-roof of his barrack, a height of about 18 feet. When brought to the hospital on the following morning the only hurt discoverable was that of the head,—a small wound of the scalp penetrating to the occipital bone, but without any fracture of the cranium. He complained chiefly of excessive pain between the shoulders and right breast, preventing his moving or taking a deep inspiration; his pulse was 74; skin moist. Blood was twice abstracted, affording a little relief, but that only temporary. His breathing became more and more oppressed till he died. He was conscious to the last moment. There was no paralysis.

Autopsy 21 hours after death. Body stout. The spinous process and the left transverse process of the 6th dorsal vertebra were found fractured, as was also the body of this vertebra, the latter transversely. The only other lesions that could be attributed to the accident were some coagulated blood effused in the posterior mediastinum and the compression of the right lung owing to air accumulated in the pleura. How the air gained admission was not discovered; the lung was blown into and forcibly distended without the escape of air. There was no emphysema. The left lung partially adhering contained many clusters of grey granular tubercles; they were confined to the superior lobe. The viscera generally were sound.

Death in this instance it may be inferred, judging from the symptoms, was mainly owing to the accumulated air in the pleura, which during life unfortunately escaped detection. That the air gradually collected was clearly indicated by the gradual increase of difficulty of breathing. Could it have been secreted? It is more probable that there was a very minute rupture of the lung.

Case 6.—David Marshall, ætat. 37; S. and M.; killed by the blow of a stone.— This man when in perfect health was struck in the forehead by a large stone projected from a mine about 200 yards distant; his death was instantaneous. The accident occurred at Vido, one of the Ionian Islands, at 6 p.m. on the 14th July, 1826.

Autopsy 16 hours after. Body fat and very muscular. The frontal bone and parts of the parietal bones were found broken in, the integuments perforated and the anterior portion of the cerebrum smashed. One of the internal carotids, just at its entrance into the cranium, was torn. There was a good deal of blood at the base of the brain and effused into the lateral sinuses; there was also some extravasated blood in the substance of each corpus striatum. The lungs were almost free from adhesions; the surface of both was darkly mottled and thickly studded with small granular bodies little larger than a mustard seed, of a white or grey color, chiefly seated in the pleura pulmonalis. A few minute accretions, black and solid, were found in the substance of each lung. The bronchia generally were of a pretty dark red, and contained a little frothy mucus. The bronchial glands were considerably enlarged; the heart was empty and contracted. The thoracic duct contained a small quantity of chyle, of the appearance of ass's milk. The stomach exhibited the hour-glass contraction in a slight degree; in its pyloric portion there was a mass of undigested food, nearly spherical, of about the size of a small orange; a much larger quantity of the same kind of food was found in its upper compartment; it contained no liquid, was nearly colorless and was not softened. The duodenum was empty; there was air under its epithelium here and there, as if artificially injected, also in its cellular structure. There was no offensive smell indicating even incipient putrefaction. There was a good deal of half-digested food in the lower part of the ileum; in its upper portion and in the jejunum there was air. There was very little fecal matter in the larger intestines. The greater part of the colon was perfectly empty, of about the size of the little finger, soft, moist and white. The gall-bladder contained about four drachms of bile. The abdominal viscera generally were of healthy appearance.

These few cases which I have given, though of unequal interest and weight, the last indeed questionable, I trust are sufficient to prove the proposition that tubercles, the germs of pulmonary consumption, may exist and even make some progress without perceptibly affecting the health of the individual. In the two following sections and in the after pages, further proofs innumerable will be found of the latency of tubercles.

In brute animals, it is well known that tubercles are not of uncommon occurrence in the lungs without apparently impairing the general health, judging of that by the condition and degree of fatness of the animals. This is remarkably the case in the instance of sheep: a large proportion of those slaughtered for the market, I have been assured, are so affected, little less than one-third; and this in a hilly district, considered peculiarly fitted for them, and they of a breed hardy and suitable to the climate.*

If then it be a fact that tubercles in their early stage, and it may be even when they are a little advanced, are not incompatible with apparently good health, what a warning ought it to be to all medical officers employed in examining men for the public service, and even for life-insurance companies! Mere form is deceptive;—tubercles may exist in the lungs of persons with chests of ample capacity. Respiratory sounds are hardly to be trusted, or respiratory power. I am disposed to think that the heart's impulse is the indication most likely to be useful, and that if that impulse is at all diffused, however healthy the individual examined may appear there is ground for suspicion of latent tubercle.

2. ON TUBERCULAR DISEASE, RENDERED LATENT OR MORE OR LESS OBSCURED BY INSANITY.—The degree of latency of phthisis in connection with insanity is best shown by necroscopical results. Of 141 fatal cases which occurred in the lunatic asylum at Fort Clarence from its opening in 1819 to 1834, the following is an abstract of the state of the lungs:—

29 Were cases of manifest phthisis, the organic lesions and symptoms according.

28 Were of latent phthisis, the organic lesions in the lungs, tubercles and excavations, having existed without the pro-

* I have examined the tubercle of such common occurrence in the lungs of the sheep, and have found it very similar to that of the human lungs, consisting chiefly, as seen under the microscope, when washed, of granular matter, and containing besides the granules a little oleine and stearine. In the lungs of the lamb tubercles are very rare; they are also rare in those of the ox. According to an intelligent butcher, abundant fat is quite compatible with the presence of tubercles in the sheep in their early stage, and if there be any difference in the quality of the meat owing to their presence, it is the increase of tenderness.

duction of symptoms,—the fatal disease, *quoad* the ordinary symptoms, latent throughout.

9 Were cases partially latent, that is, the lesions were not indicated by symptoms, till greatly advanced and within a very short period, a week or a fortnight of death.

11 Were cases in which granular tubercles were detected in both lungs, but so little advanced that independent of insanity, they were not likely to have been productive of symptoms.

23 Were of other diseases of the lungs and pleura, such as pneumonia, empyema, etc., without any tubercles.

20 Were cases in which the lungs were found free from disease of any kind, apparently sound.

16 The residue of the whole 141, were cases in the autopsy of which the lungs were not examined, only the brain.

That so large a proportion of the fatal cases in this asylum should have been complicated with disease of the lungs, and most of all with tubercular disease, is hardly surprising, taking into account two things—one, the prevalency, as already shown, of tubercles in the lungs of men belonging to the ranks of the army; the other, the peculiar structure of the building at Fort Clarence. Originally designed to be what its name implies, a fortification, and for which it might have been well adapted with bomb-proof roofs and casemates, its underground passages and cells, it was totally unfit for the purpose, the reception of the insane, to which it was applied; indeed in its want of light, in its deficient ventilation, its low temperature and the difficulty of warming its subterraneous apartments, it was better calculated to engender disease than to preserve health or promote recovery.*

* Fort Clarence was one of the line of works constructed during the war at a vast expense, under the dread of a French invasion. Its detailed history would be instructive, especially as showing the wretched and costly effect of a misplaced and false economy in converting it into a lunatic asylum. Its selection was founded on the principle of saving the expenditure that would have been needed to build a proper asylum: even in the vain attempt to warm its subterraneous rooms and passages thousands of pounds were wasted. After repeated reports of medical officers on its unfitness it was closed in 1844, and its inmates were transferred to Shorncliffe; afterwards to Yarmouth, and eventually—viz., in 1854, the establishment was broken up; the officers were removed to Cotton Hill Institution, Staffordshire; the privates to Bow Asylum, Middlesex. The mortality in the asylum, in connection with its principal cause, tubercular disease of the lungs, in the three different classes of patients—viz., officers, privates and women, is strikingly corroborative, keeping in mind their different accommodation. Of the officers,—they residing in a house of ordinary construction—the mortality from 1819 to 1834 was at the rate of 19 per cent.; of the women, the wives of soldiers nearly similarly quartered, it was 18 per cent., whilst of the privates quartered in the casemates it was 39 per cent.!

In describing the following cases, illustrative of the latency of tubercular disease under the influence of insanity, I shall abridge little else than their histories; the morbid appearances will be detailed as they were originally noted down by myself at the time of the *post mortem* inspection.

Case 1.—Of latent phthisis, with tubercles and cavities in the lungs, and ulcers in the cœcum.—J. Robinson, ætat. 29; admitted into the asylum, 11th December, 1835; died 26th August, 1837.—This man, when he enlisted in 1824, was considered a good recruit. In a short time he became eccentric, but he performed his duties correctly till 1832; then he became inconsiderate and slovenly. In 1835, when he was admitted into regimental hospital, he was incoherent in conversation, and occasionally violent, his bodily health continuing good. When transferred to Fort Clarence in December of that year he was somewhat incoherent, but his manners were natural and orderly. Towards the end of December he showed a proneness to pilfering, and also to the tearing of his clothes; his general health continued good. He improved so much mentally that in April he passed three boards and was discharged to barracks under probation. There he had an epileptic fit, and immediately relapsed into his former incoherent state of mind, without appreciable disturbance of bodily health. In April, 1837 he began to lose flesh; his countenance became haggard, his gait weak and tottering; his pulse was feeble; bowels regular; appetite always good; he had no cough. During the last month his feet and ankles became œdematous. On the 25th August he appeared to be much as usual; had taken his food well, and his exercise in the airing-ground. On the morning of the following day his appearance was as usual; he had dressed himself after rising; whilst folding up his bed, he fell down and almost immediately expired. His face was pale at the time, and he was supposed to be in a fainting fit.

Autopsy 30 hours after death. Cadaver but little emaciated; nails not curved; chest capacious; some hair on it. The inner table of cranium was strongly marked with vessels. Pretty much fluid was found under the arachnoid, in the ventricles and at the base of the brain. The pia mater adhered very firmly to the cerebrum, detaching, when removed, portions of the cortical substance. The vessels were large; the substance of the brain firm. Both lungs were partially adhering, chiefly their superior lobes. The left pleura contained 4 oz. of serum; the right 6 oz.; the pericardium 1 oz. In the upper part of the superior lobe of the left lung there was a cavity capable of holding a walnut, and several smaller ones, with very many tubercles, in different stages of progress. A few tubercles, but little advanced, were found in the inferior lobe accompanied by some œdema and consolidation. The greater part of the right lung was covered with a false membrane, as was also the costal pleura. In the upper part of the superior lobe of this lung there was an excavation capable of holding a good-sized orange, also several small vomicæ. In one vomica a tubercular mass was found, loose, and softening externally; there were many tubercles in the middle lobe, and a few in the inferior; in all three lobes there was some congestion of blood and serum. A large bronchial tube, ulcerated, terminated abruptly in the excavation in this lung. There were some large ulcers in the cœcum; the cartilages of the patella were partially softened and partially thickened.

The recovery of reason for a time in this case, the progress of tubercular disease exempt from the ordinary symptoms of phthisis, the ulceration of the cœcum without bowel complaint, are some of its noteworthy circumstances ; another is that the blood was liquid ; in no part was any coagulum found. Was the sudden death owing to spasm of the heart ? In favor of this conjecture it may be mentioned, that no blood was found in its ventricles, though there was some in the auricles and great vessels. Also it may be mentioned that the margin of the mitral valve was slightly thickened, and that there was a thickening of the inner membrane, with a thinning of the inner of the arch of the aorta, with some contraction, from the same cause, of the great vessels rising from it.

Case 2.—Of latent phthisis, with cavities and tubercles in lungs, ulcerated trachea and intestines.—J. Manning, ætat. 24 ; admitted into the asylum 9th December, 1836 ; died 27th May, 1837.—This man was an habitual drunkard ; his character very bad. It is stated that he had several attacks of delirium tremens when in Corfu ; and that in the latter part of that year the action of his heart (previously subject to palpitation) had become irregular and tumultuous, suggesting organic disease. In 1836 he was sent home laboring under mental malady, the first symptoms of which appeared in March of that year, and it is noted, with a total subsidence of the cardiac disturbance. He had first melancholia, which lapsed into amentia. When admitted into Fort Clarence, there was a total loss of reason ; his bodily health was apparently good ; the heart's action natural. About a week after admission he had an epileptic fit ; it did not recur. It was ascertained that a sister of his had been epileptic and insane. In the middle of April he began to deteriorate in appearance and to lose flesh, becoming wrinkled and haggard, with a feeble pulse. His appetite throughout was exceedingly voracious and depraved ; if allowed, he would have devoured his own fæcal matter. In the morning of the 27th May, he appeared no worse than usual ; he took his breakfast and dinner in his ordinary manner. At 2 p.m. his breathing became oppressed and laborious ; his pulse rapid and very feeble ; he died at 11 p.m.

Autopsy 41 hours after death. Body much emaciated ; feet œdematous ; nails not curved. The inner table of the cranium was strongly furrowed ; the arachnoid partially opaque ; the pia mater adhering firmly to the cortical substance, and its cellular tissue was slightly infiltrated with fluid. The glandulæ Pacchioni were unusually large. The lateral ventricles, though unusually capacious, contained but little fluid. The under surface of the fornix was soft and adhering to the velum interpositum. The pericardium contained 3 oz. of serum ; the left pleura 5 oz. of turbid serum ; some lymph was deposited on its costal side. A cavity of moderate size was found in the superior lobe of the left lung, with two or three smaller ones. There were in both its lobes several tubercular masses. Portions of this lung were consolidated. The condition of the right lung was very similar to that of the left, there being a large excavation in its upper lobe and smaller cavities in it and in the middle lobe ; the walls of the excavation were almost gangrenous. Numerous small ulcers were found in the trachea, and a deep ulcer just below the right chorda vocalis. The heart was small but not apparently diseased. There were numerous ulcers in the jejunum, ileum and cœcum, a few in the transverse colon and a small abscess at the verge of the anus, with some hæmorrhoidal tumors ; in one of these was a thick reddish matter, such as might result from the softening of a blood-clot.

It is worthy of remark that during the whole period that this man was under observation in the asylum, where he was daily seen by a very attentive medical officer, there were no symptoms of any of the many lesions above described,—there was no cough, no diarrhœa. Another noteworthy circumstance is the change which was observed in the heart's action on the invasion of insanity, passing then from a diseased to an apparently healthy state and so continuing.

Case 3.—Of latent phthisis, with tubercles and cavities in the lungs and ulcers in the duodenum and other intestines.—George Buxton, ætat. 37; admitted into the asylum, 13th Nov. 1831; died 11th April, 1837.—This man was admitted into the asylum on his return from India, where he had been ten years, and during the two last laboring under insanity. No other information accompanied him. When admitted he was outrageously violent; shortly he became stupid and taciturn. His appearance indicated a constitution much impaired by disease; he was sullen and emaciated. Up to the second year from his admission, no change worthy of remark was observed in the state of his mind. From that time he lapsed into amentia. His bodily health improved. At times he was comparatively rational, for about a week at a time; then relapsed into fatuity; and these two states alternated with tolerable regularity. During the last two years his eyes were frequently inflamed. On the morning of the 11th April, besides his usual stupid appearance nothing observable was the matter with him; he took his breakfast as well as usual and was present at parade; at dinner he sat down but ate nothing; very shortly after his head was observed to droop, then, almost immediately, he fell down, and in two or three minutes expired. It was reported that when this took place his face became of a purplish hue. He had not been subject to fits. During the whole time that he had been in the asylum there were no symptoms of pulmonary or other organic disease.

Autopsy 96 hours after death. Body sub-emaciated; nails large and curved; limbs flexible as in life; those of a body kept the same time rigid. The inner surface of the calvaria was strongly furrowed in the course of the arteries; the bone was thin. The falciform process of the dura mater was reticulated in parts as if from absorption, and was weak and easily torn. There was little fluid in the ventricles; pretty much at the base of the brain and in the spinal canal. The brain generally was of very healthy appearance. The pericardium contained 3 oz. of serum. The right cavities of the heart were very much distended with coagulated blood, *not broken up*, and there was coagulated blood in the pulmonary artery, but none in the left auricle, and yet the foramen ovale was partially open; it admitted in an oblique direction the end of the little finger. The left ventricle and the aorta contained pretty much blood, also coagulated. The right lung, free from adhesions, did not collapse; it weighed 2¼ lbs. It abounded in small cavities and tubercles clustered together in different stages of progress and not confined to any one part. The left lung was universally and closely adhering. A bony mass was found in a kind of false cellular membrane between the pulmonary and costal pleura; it was about two inches in length and a quarter of an inch in width. This lung, which weighed 3 lbs., was vastly diseased. In its superior lobe there was a very large excavation, containing a thin reddish sanies, that did not color transmitted light*; the same kind of fluid was found in the bronchia with which the cavity communicated by small ulcerated openings. The excavation was intersected by many columnæ in which were blood-vessels still pervious. Several smaller exca-

* Showing the absence of pus-globules by Dr. Young's optical test.

vations were found in the inferior lobe and some crude tubercles. Very little of the substance of either lung was tolerably sound. The stomach was distended and very thin. In the duodenum, chiefly in its upper and glandular portion, there were numerous small ulcers with ulcerated cavities in its submucous tissue; these contained a purulent fluid (by the optical test.) Numerous ulcers were also detected in the jejunum, ileum and colon; those in the former were comparatively small; those in the colon were large, especially in the cœcum. The mesenteric glands were enlarged and their substance cheese-like.

The fatal termination in this instance was probably owing, as was conjectured at the time, to the bursting of a large vomica, and the discharge of some of its contents into the bronchia,—the very sanies that was found in them. Whether the coagulation of the blood in the heart was concerned in the event is questionable. The circumstance that the coagula found there were not broken up, would denote that the heart's action had ceased before the blood in its cavities had lost its fluidity.

Case 4.—Of latent phthisis, with tubercles in the lungs and cavities, ulcerated intestines and tubercular deposits in testes and vesiculæ seminales.—C. Lewis, ætat. 41 ; admitted into the asylum, 12th March, 1828; died 26th August, 1838.—This man in 1826, refusing to do his duty was punished; soon after his insanity became manifest. On his admission into the asylum he had a lofty manner, considered himself a person of rank, and conversed accordingly. He was quiet and easily managed. His mental malady remained the same throughout. His health was commonly good, until within the last few months, when his breathing appeared to have become affected. On the 10th August, that is sixteen days before his death, he was feverish, his breathing hurried, with wheezing and sonorous râles. The left lower limb became swollen, from the ankle to the groin. The swelling increased until the 18th; from that time it gradually subsided. The pulmonary symptoms, those mentioned, became more and more urgent till he died.

Autopsy 5 hours after death. Body sub-emaciated; nails not curved; the left lower extremity only just perceptibly larger than the left. The pia mater was very thin, as if atrophied. A large glandula Pacchioni projected through the dura mater on the left side of the longitudinal sinus. Very little fluid was found in the ventricles. The brain was of natural appearance and consistence. The pericardium contained 4 oz. of serum; of sp. gr. 1,010 ; there was a good deal of crassamentum, with some cruor* and fibrinous concretion in the right cavities of the heart; less in the left. Both lungs, for most part, were firmly adhering. The superior lobe of the right was greatly condensed; portions of it sunk in water; it abounded in tubercles in different stages, and contained many small vomicæ. Its middle lobe was similarly diseased, but in a less degree. The inferior contained many crude granular tubercles. The left lung throughout was condensed, and abounded in tubercles in process of softening. Many small vomicæ were found in its superior lobe. The lower third of the pleura on this side was covered with a thick shaggy false membrane, and contained several ounces of purulent fluid. On the under surface of the epiglottis there were

* On the following morning this cruor was found coagulated; the coagulum very soft; and the fluid from the pericardium had become slightly turbid, as if from the separation of a little lymph or fibrin.

many small superficial ulcers and also in the larynx and trachea. A few ulcers were detected in the lower part of the ileum, many in the cœcum, and two or three of a large size in the colon. The left testicle was much enlarged; a curd-like matter was deposited in its substance. The tumica vaginalis contained a considerable quantity of the like matter and some whey-like fluid, of which latter there was a discharge by an ulcerated opening. The prostrate, the vesiculæ seminales and the left vas deferens within the pelvis were all much enlarged, as was also the right vas deferens, close to the vesicula; they all contained tubercular, cheese-like matter. The left femoral vein and its branches were completely obstructed by fibrinous concretions and coagulated blood. The concretion extended to the common iliac vein to where it passes under the artery. It was of different hues, and in two or three places contained reddish softened matter. There was very little serum in the cellular tissue of the limb.

This is in many respects a striking example of its kind. There was no bowel complaint; no cough; no difficulty in making water; no complaint made of pain either in the swollen testicle or the swollen limb. From a note of my own, I find that on examining him on the 17th January, that is seven months before his death, when he appeared to be in good health, his temperature under his tongue was 101°; and that on a second examination which I made, this so late as the 4th August, when he was walking about and on ordinary diet, not in the infirmary and consequently not supposed to be ill by the attending medical officer, his temperature was 104°, with a quick pulse and hot skin. Such were the first indications discovered of his fatal disease; they led to the examination of the chest and the detection by the stethoscope of the malady.

Case 5.—Of latent phthisis, with tubercles and cavities in the lungs and partial softening of brain.—J. M'Dermot, ætat. 29; 85th Regiment; admitted into regimental hospital, Malta, 28th September, 1828; died 10th October.—This man was taken into hospital chiefly on account of a very constipated state of bowels. At the same time he complained of slight pain of chest, with cough. It is stated that there was no pyrexia. During the first three days, using aperient medicine, he seemed to be doing well. In the evening of the 1st October indications first appeared of cerebral disease;—there was aberration of mind with increased action of the temporal arteries and a quickened pulse, followed on the 3rd by some difficulty of articulation. From this time to that of his death, no material alteration of symptoms took place. The mental aberration continued; it was more like that of mania than of delirium; the eyes were wild; the countenance haggard; the arms and hands were almost constantly in motion, feeling the bed-clothes and grasping at imaginary objects, as it were, in the air; his hands he often put to his nose and head. His pulse was always much accelerated; the temperature of the skin moderate; the tongue pretty clean; little thirst; some appetite even to the last. He always described himself as well and said he had no pain. Latterly he passed his stools in bed. The treatment was active: leeches, blisters, mercury; the latter used till the gums were slightly affected.

Autopsy 22 hours after death. Body emaciated; penis turgid. The dura mater was of a light pink hue. The pia mater was redder than usual, especially in the fissura Sylvii and its neighbourhood; there it was firmly adhering, a little thickened and studded with minute, almost miliary tubercles, firm and of a white opacity. The lateral ventricles were much distended with a colorless fluid; and there was a good deal of like fluid in the third ventricle and at the base of the brain; the septum lucidum and the walls of the lateral ventricles, and especially the optic thalami and the whole of the inferior cornua (both very large) were extremely soft. There was a softening too in a marked manner of the corpora striata, and in a less degree of the cerebrum generally and of the cerebellum. The pericardium contained about 3 oz. of serum. Its inner surface was in one spot rough, curiously spotted with an apparent deposition of coagulable lymph. Contiguous to this spot, between its serous and outer coat, a thickening, cartilage-like, was found including and compressing the right phrenic nerve. Both lungs abounded in grey tubercles, some of which were undergoing puruloid softening. In the back part of the superior lobe of the right lung there was an excavation, nearly empty, capable of holding a walnut. The bronchia and trachea contained much bloody mucus; the former was very red; the latter less so. The bronchial glands were much enlarged. There were some small superficial ulcers in the ileum, in its lower portion, and there the glandulæ were a little enlarged.

In this instance have we not an example of cerebral disease coming into activity arresting the symptoms, not the progress, of pulmonary disease, and creating as it were the feeling of health? In connection with this feeling, the state of the tongue, the little thirst, the persistence of appetite, the moderate temperature of skin are noteworthy circumstances. The turgidity of the penis after death is not an uncommon occurrence in cases of tubercular disease of the membranes of the brain, and is often preceded in articulo mortis by convulsive seminal emissions.

Case 6.—Of latent phthisis, with tubercles in the lungs and cavities apparently in process of healing.—Captain P., Roy. A., ætat. about 41; was found dead in his room, suspended by his neck, at Malta, early in the morning of 1st April, 1831.— This officer, in the summer of 1829, at the recommendation of a medical board, left Malta, where he was stationed with his company, on sick leave, on account of troublesome pectoral symptoms. He soon improved at home, and was reported to be in good health. In the beginning of 1830, when returning at the expiration of his leave, he became insane at Florence. At Leghorn he was placed under restraint and medical treatment. On arrival at Malta, about a month before his death, he was very low and dejected; he talked rationally on all subjects but one; he fancied that he was accused of an unnatural crime, and that he heard voices always charging him with it. The pulse was quick and feeble; the bowels constipated; his bodily strength much reduced; he had no cough; no indications of disease of the lungs.

Autopsy at 3 p.m.—The body not quite cold, was but little emaciated; the muscles were flabby; a strong mark of the cord was visible just above the arytenoid cartilage; the vessels in the neck below were turgid; the face was pale. Some rough bony points were found in the dura mater on each side of the falciform process. The brain was of normal consistence. There was little blood in its vessels; a moderate quantity of fluid in the ventricles. The right lung slightly adhering, contained very many clusters of grey granular tubercles; they were most abundant in its superior lobe. The upper part of the left lung was very firmly adhering. Its appearance was uncommon; it was of a leaden hue, very hard and much puckered; cut into, its pleural covering was found to be much thickened; cartilaginous lines penetrated into the sub-stance of the lung to two or three small vomicæ, which were empty. One or two large bronchial tubes terminated abrubtly in the diseased mass, which was about the size of an orange. In the same lobe there were a few granular tubercles, and tubercles of the same kind were disseminated through the inferior lobe. The bronchia were very red, and there was much froth in the trachea and larynx. The intestines as to position had a very confused appearance. The transverse colon descended obliquely from the right hypochondrium, where it was attached to the gall-bladder, nearly to the brim of the pelvis; the duodenum also closely attached to the gall-bladder, descended a little below the umbilicus, covering the kidney, then crossed over; a portion of the upper part of the jejunum was found above the small arch of the stomach; a large portion of the ileum was in the cavity of the pelvis. The intestines generally were of dark hue and their vessels gorged with blood. The stomach contained some half-digested food; its mucous coat was not distinctly softened; its pylorus was so large as to admit three fingers. There were hardened fæces in the cœcum and pultaceous fæcal matter in the colon. The spleen was large; and as it were double. The blood wherever found was liquid.

Have we not in this instance the very rare example of a cavity or cavities in the lung in process of healing, and well advanced to that end, as shown by the puckering, contraction, and cartilage-like hardening of the part, where there is reason to believe that active disease previously existed? Such was the impression made on me at the time, keeping in mind the former pulmonary attack and the recovery of health from change of climate, before the invasion of the mental malady.

Case 7.—Of latent phthisis, with granular tubercles in lungs; the os femoris frac-tured, unaccompanied by pain.—M. Murphy, ætat. 30; 88th Regiment; admitted into regimental hospital, Corfu, 17th Feb., 1827; killed by a fall, May 21st.—This man's intellect became impaired when stationed at Fanno. On his return to head-quarters, Corfu, he was taken into hospital. Idiotic at the time, it is stated that he gradually became worse. He was always quiet. The bodily functions were well per-formed; he complained of nothing and he did not become emaciated. On the night of the 12th May he escaped out of hospital and threw himself from a height of be-tween 50 and 60 feet. In his fall, it was inferred, that he first struck a projecting part of the cliff, perhaps 20 feet from the top, where his cap remained, and that from thence he fell perpendicularly to the ground, probably alighting on his feet. A sen-tinel saw him just in the act, and asked him what he was doing there; he replied, "I am going to heaven," and having said so, he threw himself over. He was taken up speechless; his left thigh fractured. No other material hurt could be detected. On the following day he was able to speak. He appeared to suffer no pain from the fractured bone. The limb, it is said, could not be kept in position; "he tossed it about as if nothing ailed it." Till the day he expired he had some appetite; there was little or no pyrexia. His death took place suddenly and unexpectedly; a few hours before, he experienced a severe rigor.

Autopsy 18 hours after death. Body not emaciated; left thigh swollen, discolored and shortened; the sole of the left foot a little bruised. Much fluid in the cellular tissue of the pia mater, especially between the convolutions of the cerebrum and in the ventricles and at the base of the brain. The vessels in the corpora striata were of an unusually large size. The left lung was generally adhering. Numerous granular tubercles were found in its superior lobe; and in the same, one of the size of a large pea, which was opaque and softening. This lobe was much gorged with blood and serum. Some blood was effused under the integuments of the abdomen, especially in the iliac regions and in the cellular tissue within the pelvis; also under the peritoneal coat of the gall-bladder and of the transverse colon. A slight rupture was detected in the inferior concave surface of the liver. The fracture of the thigh was oblique, below the capsule; the trochanter major was also fractured.

This case is given not so much on account of the tubercular disease of the lung as on account of the absence of pain in the fractured limb and the little disturbance of the ordinary functions from lesions so soon to have a fatal issue.

These cases may suffice for the purpose of showing how very serious tubercular disease of the lungs may be masked, its ordinary symptoms suppressed by insanity in its various forms.

Examples of the like overpowering influence are not uncommon in the instance of other diseases. I shall here notice one only, and that on account of its marked peculiarity and its striking character, somewhat analogous to the case last given. It was in a young woman of color whom I saw in Barbadoes, an inmate of the lunatic asylum of that island; besides being insane, she was at the time laboring under elephantiasis. The lower limb affected was at least thrice its natural size, and its weight must have been great. She had a passion for dancing and for almost constantly indulging in it, which she did with a mad vehemence and in an intensely enjoyable manner. The diseased leg was moved with the same alacrity as the sound one, not the slightest difference was to be perceived in the action of the two.

That insanity should have such an overpowering effect, however mysterious it may be, is yet, when strictly considered, hardly surprising, recollecting how mental emotions are known to overcome bodily pain; and how when under the influence of such emotions, impressions made on the organs of the senses, are often not perceived.

The practical conclusion from such cases as these I have related is so obvious that it need hardly be insisted on—viz., that in all instances of insanity, it is not sufficient to see the patients and to question them as to their state of health: it is necessary to examine them carefully, employing all available means to detect lurking mischief, using for the purpose the thermometer, employing percussion and auscultation, etc.

I would add, that when after some experience I had become impressed by the importance of latent organic disease, especially of the lungs, in persons mentally affected, I did not fail to offer suggestions in accordance, to the medical officers (often changed) appointed to the immediate charge of the army lunatic asylum, and I would fain think not without some benefit.

It would be interesting to have investigated why in a certain number of cases of insanity such an influence as that we have been considering is exercised, and in a certain number of other cases either not at all, or only in a slight degree. The subject being one on which I have no information, not even a conjecture to offer, I can only recommend it to the attention of the psychologist, with opportunities to engage in the inquiry.

3. ON TUBERCULAR DISEASE, RENDERED LATENT BY THE CO-EXISTENCE OF OTHER ORGANIC LESIONS.—This is a subject which it is easy to illustrate by examples. I shall adduce only a few : the experienced medical officer will have no difficulty in supplying more, especially the seniors, who in the earlier period of their career had not the same helps in investigating pulmonary disease which are now in common use, and with so much advantage in the way of arriving at a correct diagnosis.

In each of the following cases the name of the disease under which the patient was admitted will be given, to show, as much as can be done by one word, the main impression on the mind of the medical officer by whom it was treated, of its nature.

The obscuring of one train of morbid actions by another train, in other instances besides those of tuberculosis, is not a little remarkable, and yet has not perhaps had all the attention that its importance deserves. The over-sights, the mistakes made in the diagnosis of disease, by men of the first rank in the profession, honestly described, would be an instructive contribution to medical literature ; and might serve the useful purpose of checking the dogmatism of some practitioners, and the hasty decision and energetic practice of others.*

---

* I am tempted to give an anecdote or two of this kind, and exemplifying at the same time that *tactus eruditus* resulting from long-continued and careful observation. A person supposed to be laboring under confirmed and chronic ascites, and treated accordingly by many practitioners, getting no relief, went to Edinburgh to have the advice of the then most distinguished physician of that city. After a careful inquiry and examination the decision before arrived at by his country brethren was confirmed, and a plan of treatment very little different from that before employed was prescribed.

Case 1.—Of latent tubercles and vomicæ in lungs and other parts, treated as rheumatism.—Wm. Garton, ætat 24; R. F.; admitted into Regimental Hospital, Malta, 21st September, 1831; died 9th October.—A young man of full habit, half-a-year at the station; on admission, was supposed to be laboring under rheumatism. He complained chiefly of pain in the back of the neck, and of stiffness of the part. It is stated that there were no constitutional symptoms. Until the 27th he continued to improve; then the back part of the head became the seat of pain, with a pulse rather quicker than natural; leeches were applied. Again he seemed to improve until 4th October, when he was found breathing laboriously, but without pain; the pulse was 100 and full; the tongue foul; much thirst; V. S. to 20 ounces, which produced syncope; a blister to the chest; an anodyne at night. On the 5th there was some amendment. On the 6th there was a degree of torpor, yet he was sensible; he made no complaint of pain. He gradually became worse, without any marked change of symptoms until the night of the 9th, when he expired. A few hours before the event a tumor appeared at the elbow; it was about the size of a pigeon's egg; opened, about a spoonful of pus was discharged.

Autopsy 15 hours after death.—Body nowise emaciated. With the exception of more fluid than usual in the ventricles and at the base of the brain, nothing abnormal was found in that organ. The pericardium contained 4oz. of serum; the left pleura about 5oz. of bloody fluid; its lower portion was stained of a deep red; some coagula of blood there adhered to it, with coagulable lymph. The left lung had scattered

As the patient was quitting the room, the idea occurred to the physician: Might not the abdominal distension, with fluctuation, arise from an accumulation of urine in the bladder, and this even though that fluid was described as being voided naturally, both as to frequency and quantity? The patient was called back, a catheter was used, a great quantity of urine was drawn off—and there was an end of the ascites. This was told me by the late Dr. Abercrombie, the physician in question, when speaking of the tendency often seen in persons advanced in life to unsuspected accumulation of urine in the bladder.

When a student in Edinburgh, I witnessed a somewhat similar though not so striking an instance of a mistake and its correction. The physician's clerk, according to the usage established in the Royal Infirmary, reads the case as taken down by him of any new patient. After hearing the account of the symptoms, which was well drawn up, the physician, after some questioning, dictated a prescription in conformity with the presumed nature of the malady derived from the detail; just on leaving the bed-side, he—it was the late Dr. Hamilton, the last of the old school of doctors who wore the cocked hat and ruffled sleeve—turned round in his quick manner, and put one or two more questions, the answers to which showed that the malady was totally different from the one inferred, in brief that it was diabetes, and that a very different description of it was needed, which it had the next day, in the clerk's journal, and an opposite treatment from that first determined on.

Another anecdote I will venture to give—this not illustrative of the *tactus eruditus*. A lady who had been some years married, fancied she was labouring under hepatic disease, connected with a tumor of the liver. She consulted many physicians and surgeons eminent in their profession, who arrived at the same conclusion regarding her ailment. The last she consulted, and not the least eminent of the number, confirmed the opinion as to the tumor, but hesitated in recommending an operation, on account of risk. A few weeks after, sudden relief was happily obtained by the birth of a child—a daughter—now the joy of her parents, who are still alive.

This mistake recalls to mind the late Dr. Currie, of Guy's, who considered the liver as the *fons et origo* of a large proportion of the maladies to which man is subject, and who believed that he himself was an illustrative example, fancying that he could place his finger over the very spot where his liver was diseased. On a *post mortem* examination being made, almost every organ but the one accused was found to be more or less diseased.

through its substance small vomicæ, or abscesses distended with pus, with some of a larger size, which were irregularly cellular; its upper lobe contained many minute, firm, grey tubercles. The right lung was very generally adhering; several small vomicæ or abscesses were found in its inferior lobe, but no tubercles; the inferior portion of its middle lobe was injected with blood, as in pulmonary apoplexy; the bronchia and trachea were unduly red. An abscess about the size of a hazel-nut was detected in the anterior mediastinum, just over the pericardium; and another of the same kind in the cellular tissue, just over the second floating rib. The spleen rather large, was of a somewhat pultaceous consistence. In the kidneys, and also in the prostrate gland, abscesses were found similar to those in the lungs. Those in the prostrate had discharged their contents by three small ulcerated openings into the urethra, close to the caput galianaginis.

This case is noteworthy for the amount of organic lesions, and the absence of symptoms, such as might have been expected from them. There was no pain of chest, no cough; latterly no difficulty in breathing. The day he died the respiratory sound was distinct generally over the front of the thorax, and the chest sounded well. There was no suspicion of any disease of the kidneys, or of the prostrate. Even so late as the day before his death, the assistant-surgeon in charge thought he might be "malingering." Whether the vomicæ or abscesses in the lungs and in the other parts were of tubercular origin or not—whether slowly formed or rapidly—is questionable.

Case 2.—Of latent tubercles and cavities in the lungs, with ulcers in larynx and intestines; returned Cynanche Tonsillaris.—S. Burrows, ætat. 17; 49th Regiment; admitted into General Hospital, 24th March; died 31st March.—This youth was a laborer by occupation, of three months' service only, and had never before been in hospital. On admission he complained of a severe cold, with swelling of face and legs, and soreness of throat; both tonsils were enlarged. In a few days he spoke of himself as very much better; he continued, however, hoarse, which, he said, was usual with him. On the 28th he suddenly became affected with great difficulty of breathing, with acute pain in the region of the heart, extending backwards to the left side; his face was livid; on his chest there were patches of red discoloration. After V.S. his pulse, before hard, became soft. A like paroxysm occurred the same evening; again on the 29th, and again on the 30th. He continued very uneasy until the evening of the 30th, when he said he felt better; during the night he got up and went as far as the fire-place; according to the report of the orderly, he then appeared to know what he was doing. He was put to bed, and expired a few hours after. From the beginning a mucous râle was audible generally over the chest, particularly its left side; and that side, towards its inferior part, sounded dull on percussion. Except after venesection, the pulse was never below 120. The expectoration, after the first day, was abundant; it was tenacious, with frothy mucus. The treatment besides V.S. was cupping, with tartarized antimony, etc.

Autopsy 8 hours after death.—Body very fat. The dura mater adhered to the calvaria, and the pia mater with unusual firmness to the surface of the brain, when detached bringing with it small portions of cortical substance. This, the cortical portion, was rather soft, and was in patches injected with blood. The cerebral substance generally was very firm. The vertebral arteries and the basilar were smaller than usual. The left pleura contained two pints of serum, with some pus, the globules of which varied in diameter from $\frac{1}{2000}$ to $\frac{1}{7000}$ of an inch; lymph was deposited on this membrane, and mostly on its diaphragmatic portion, partly in patches, and partly in granules resembling tubercles. The lung on the same side occupied little space, it was so compressed; at its apex it adhered firmly; there, there was a cavity capable of holding a large filbert; it contained some small calcareous concretions, and communicated by an ulcerated opening with a large bronchial tube; adjoining it there were many tubercles, two or three of which were softening; and numerous granular tubercles were scattered through the substance of the lobe; the inferior lobe contained many granular tubercles, some of them clustered, some of them softening, and also a cavity capable of holding a hazel-nut; this was in its upper part; the inferior margin was so condensed by pressure as to sink in water; it was otherwise sound, judging from its resistance. In the right lung, in its superior lobe, there was a cavity equal to about a walnut, and contiguous a smaller one holding some calcareous matter; there were also in this lobe many tubercles, some of them softening; the inferior lobe contained many granular tubercles undergoing change, and a tubercular mass about the size of a boy's playing marble, in which was a deposition of calcareous matter; each of the three lobes was partially œdematous, and the inferior was also in part hepatized; the superior lobe of the left lung was in part similarly affected. There was œdema of the glottis and of the epiglottis, and a coating of lymph on both, and also on the lining membrane of the pharynx contiguous. A small ulcer was detected just below one of the sacculi laryngis, and an abrasion of the vocal chord. The inferior trachea was redder than natural, and slightly œdematous; some fluid exuded from it under pressure. The pericardium contained 2oz. of serum. In the right auricle there was much coagulated blood, and firm fibrinous concretion. The valves of the pulmonary artery were unusually thin, and had in them a deposit granular and firm, very like granular tubercles, and a similar deposit was seen on one of the aortic valves. Small ulcers were found in the ascending, transverse, and descending colon. The cavity of the pelvis contained four ounces of serous fluid.

The apparent inconsistencies in this case are not a little remarkable—the variety of the organic lesions, many of them, doubtless, of long standing; the abundance of fat; the absence of symptoms until the invasion of the acute attack, and the rapidity of its progress and fatal termination. He was considered dull of intellect: might not this dulness—the state of brain connected with it—have been concerned in some degree in rendering latent the chronic lesions?

Case 3.—Of tubercles and cavities in the lungs and in other organs, with disease of bone and partial softening of brain, returned "Necrosis."—Charles Solly, ætat. 33; 41st Regiment; admitted into general hospital, 22nd May, 1839; died 12th June.—This man was received into hospital on his return from India, where he had served 14 years and in good health until 1836, when he had an attack of "brain-fever," followed by tumors in different parts of the head. After having been 8 months there in hospital, he experienced dysentery of six weeks' duration, which was followed by anasarca and ascites. He was thrice tapped; 40 lbs. of fluid were drawn off. His liver, then, it was stated, "felt like a foreign body." The dropsical symptoms gradually subsided. On admission into the general hospital he was very feeble and greatly emaciated. He had some cough; but the pectoral symptoms were so slight as not to attract attention, which was chiefly directed to the state of the head. There was an ulcer over both the frontal bone and the saggital suture, discharging purulent matter; the bone forming the latter was exposed and black. He had occasional diarrhœa; gradually becoming weaker, delirium preceded death. The treatment was merely palliative.

Autopsy 17 hours after death. Body extremely emaciated. A considerable portion of the frontal bone, both externally and internally was rough and thickened, as were also the parietal bones at the vertex; there they were destitute of periostum and probably dead. Lymph was deposited on the dura mater under the diseased portions, and under the os frontis the membrane was rough, blood-shot, and slightly excavated, as if ulcerated. A tumor about the size of half a French bean was attached to the dura mater under the parietal bone, close to the temporal bone. The pia mater was infiltrated with fluid, and was extremely thin and tender, as if atrophied. The cortical substance was pale; the fornix was very soft, as was also the septum lucidum. There was an opening in the middle of the latter large enough to admit the little finger; it gave the idea of being produced by absorption. There was a good deal of fluid in the ventricles and at the base of the brain. The substance of the brain generally was soft. The pericardium contained 3 oz. of bright yellow serum, of sp. grav. 1016. There was a little cruor in the right cavities of the heart; no clot or fibrin. In the superior lobe of the left lung, which was pretty generally adhering, there were several cavities containing sloughs of a peculiar tubercular matter. The same lobe was much indurated, and besides the cavities, it contained tubercular masses of various sizes, softening more or less; they were suggestive of medullary tumor. In some of them there was an obscure appearance of vessels. The inferior lobe was in part œdematous. The superior lobe of the right lung contained many clusters of granular tubercles of the ordinary kind. In its middle lobe, towards its inner margin, there was a tubercular mass, about the size of a walnut, softening internally and having a cavity. The part not softened was like medullary tumor, but no vessels were seen in it. The liver weighed 5 lbs. Its color was that of unbleached wax. Two small tubercles, about the size of peas, were found in its right lobe. The gall-bladder contained no bile, but some thick viscid mucus, and many small black biliary calculi. The cystic duct was obstructed by two concretions of the same kind. The spleen was large and firm. The kidneys were large and pale; in their substance were a few small vesicles; and in that of the left a tubercular mass of about the size of a walnut, resembling that in the lungs and undergoing softening. There were no ulcers in the intestines. There were 4 oz. of bright clear yellow urine in the bladder. It was of sp. gr. 1006, and was not coagulated by nitric acid.

Have we not in this instance a striking example of severe pulmonary disease, tubercles of two kinds, almost latent? Though he had a slight cough, he made no complaint of difficulty of breathing, nor was there any apparent. Nor were there any indications whilst last in hospital of any of the other lesions discovered *post mortem*. Was the mean cause of this negation the severe cranial disease and the diseased state of the brain?

Case 4.—Of a large excavation in lung and small cavities and tubercles with ulceration of pharynx, glottis and intestines, and disease of ganglia of the sympathetic nerve, returned "Catarrhus acutus."—J. Lovatt, ætat. 30; 60th Regiment; admitted into regimental hospital, Malta, 29th Nov., 1834; died 13th December.—This man shortly before admission was considered in good health; and was of "a middling full habit of body." For a considerable time he had not been in hospital. His regiment had recently arrived; during the voyage he had been active at his duty, as he had also been since landing. He stated that he had been ill two days before reporting himself sick. What he complained most of, was cough, which was severe, but without pain of chest. The tonsils and fauces were much inflamed, and there was superficial ulceration about the uvula, with some pain in swallowing. The pulse was quick, the skin hot, the tongue foul; thirst; the bowels were regular. Tartar emetic solution was given for some days with an alum gargle. The cough continuing with much mucous secretion from the fauces, and the ulceration not improving, nitrate of silver was applied; a blister externally and the steam of hot water frequently inhaled, the antimonial medicine being continued with the addition of nitre and tincture of digitalis. Under this treatment, it is stated, that the cough was relieved and also the irritation about the fauces. But the pulse continued rapid, and the ulceration never put on a healing appearance or anywise improved. About the 14th day from his admission, his respiration became much oppressed and he rapidly sank.

Autopsy 17 hours after death. Body emaciated. Brain not examined. The left pleura contained 8 oz. of serum. The left lung, at its superior portion was firmly adhering. This portion contained a large excavation lined with false membrane; so large was it, that it occupied a considerable part of the lobe. Some smaller vomicæ were found in the same lobe. The inferior lobe contained numerous granular tubercles, some of which were softening; a large portion of this lobe was crepitous. The right lung also adhered at its upper extremity. In its superior lobe there were several small cavities, much induration and many tubercles, more or less softening. Similar tubercles were found in the middle lobe, accompanied by a few small vomicæ holding a puruloid fluid or a reddish sanies. The inferior lobe abounded in granular tubercles, little advanced. The pharynx, velum pendulum palati, epiglottis, rima glottidis, were ulcerated, and that very generally. The uvula was small, hard and granular, "apparently secreting pus." The amygdalæ were destroyed; in their place were cavities lined with a false membrane. The margin of the epiglottis was wasted by ulceration, as were also in part the chordæ vocales. The lower portion of the trachea and the bronchia were very red. The bronchial and the lymphatic glands of the neck were much enlarged. The second and third ganglion of the sympathetic nerve were both enlarged; the latter on each side was much diseased, pale, of granular feel, and very hard, as if it contained tubercles. The nervus vagus was apparently sound. The mesenteric glands were considerably enlarged. Many of the lacteals were varicose and obstructed by an opaque white curd-like matter. Several ulcers were found in the jejunum, some even in the duodenum, and very many in the ileum, deep, excavated and bloody, with the usual increased vascularity of the peritoneal coat corresponding. The valvula coli was in great part destroyed by ulceration. There were large ulcers in the cœcum. The appendicula vermiformis, of about thrice its natural size, was ulcerated internally. Portions of the sigmoid flexure were unusually thin, as if atrophied. The stomach, especially its pylorus, was thicker than natural, and generally softer.

It is worthy of remark that through the whole of the progress of this case—so rapid in its fatal progress after admission into hospital—there had been no suspicion of the existence of the lesions found in the lungs or in the bowels. The breathing was not complained of; there had been no diarrhœa, rather constipation. His death was unexpected by the surgeon, an old and attentive medical officer. Yet the man himself, it was afterwards reported, had a presentiment of his fate, he having been heard to say on admission that he should never leave the hospital alive. The probability is that he had long been ailing, though not complaining, and that he had been doing duty when unfit for it, the disease escaping detection, there being no manifest symptoms. What was the effect of the diseased state of the ganglia of the sympathetic nerves?

Case 5.—Of cavities and tubercles in lungs, with partial softening of brain, and ulceration of intestines; treated as pneumonia.—T. Kennedy, ætat. 27; 7th Regiment of Foot; admitted into Regimental Hospital, Malta, 23rd September, 1830; died 8th November.—This man was of intemperate habits. In July he had been under treatment in hospital for a short time with catarrhal symptoms. When last admitted, it was in consequence of the officer of his company noticing his difficulty of breathing when in the ranks. His breathing was found to be quicker than natural; his pulse 100; the skin unduly hot. He reluctantly acknowledged that he had occasionally cough, with pain in his left side. V.S., tartar emetic, and saline medicines were used, with a blister to the chest. He seemed pretty well till the night of the 1st Oct., when he was reported by the orderly—he denying it—that his cough had recurred with difficulty of breathing. At this time he could make a full inspiration with ease when requested; his appetite was good; bowels regular; pulse between 90 and 100. On the 24th of the same month he felt weak, after coughing up much muco-purulent fluid, which he wished to conceal. His features now became collapsed, his feet and legs œdematous; yet his appetite and spirits continued good. On the 27th there was an appearance of ascites, with general anasarca. On the 2nd November diarrhœa supervened, with hectic fever and night sweats; the dropsical symptoms now subsiding. From this time he rapidly declined. Though losing strength and flesh, there was no impairment of his appetite, and his spirits continued excellent. Three days before his death he was at times delirious; he had no cough or diarrhœa, and there were no remains of anasarca. His death at last was sudden.

Autopsy 5 hours after death.—Body much emaciated. The mammillæ were unusually developed, so as to be very like virgin mammæ, and this not from fat, but from hypertrophy of their glandular and vascular structure. A good deal of fluid was found between the membranes, in the ventricles, and at the base of the brain. The substance of the brain generally was soft, especially the optic thalami, the fornix, and the pineal gland. The pericardium was adhering to the heart; the adhesions were soft and easily broken. There was a good deal of blood and fibrinous concretions in the right cavities. One of these concretions suggested the idea of its having been formed during life; it was situated in the ventricle, had a smooth surface, was adhering and blood-shot superficially, as if becoming vascular. A good deal of the right lung was pervious to air; it contained, however, many tubercles, most in its superior lobe. The left lung, generally and very firmly adhering, was very heavy, abounded in tubercles, and contained several large excavations; these, communicating with each other, and with ulcerated bronchia, were lined with false membrane, and were traversed by vessels either carrying blood, or, if empty, pervious; they had an external lining of coagulable lymph. Much purulent fluid was found in the bronchia; so much as to completely obstruct them. The bronchial glands were enlarged. There was no ulceration of the larynx or trachea. The stomach showed the hour-glass contraction, but without softening or any appearance of disease in its rugæ. The liver was healthy; the spleen large, but of natural firmness. A few ulcers were found in the jejunum, and very many in the ileum; some with red and elevated edges; others apparently cicatrising. There was an unusual turn of the colon in the pelvis, and a pouch projecting from the lower portion of the ileum. The colon was much diseased, ulcerated in spots, and covered very widely with a wart-like growth, from coagulable lymph probably effused, as, when scraped off, the mucous coat was found smooth beneath. There was a little serous fluid in the cavity of the abdomen; and some blood, effused and coagulated, under the investing membrane of the right kidney. The mesenteric glands were much enlarged.

In this case is there not reason to infer that the elements of advanced phthisis existed whilst the man was at his duty, at which he would have remained had he been allowed to follow his will? His breathing probably was so tolerable from so much of one lung being pervious; and he had so little cough, and so rarely, from the larynx not being morbidly implicated. His sudden death, it can hardly be doubted, was owing to the bursting of a vomica.

Case 6.—Of excavations and tubercles in lungs, with hypertrophy of heart, and diseased aorta; returned asthma.—B. John, ætat 41; 7th Regiment of Foot; admitted into Regimental Hospital, Corfu, November 26, 1827; died 27th November·—This man, an habitual drunkard, when admitted into hospital in the evening of the 26th, was in a state of intoxication, without having, it was reported, any particular ailment. The following morning he was found laboring under great dyspnœa. His pulse was quick and feeble; his face of a livid hue; his extremities cold; a mucous râle. V.S., 30oz. of blood were abstracted, but with difficulty, even when the circulation was excited by a stimulating draught. His breathing was for the instant relieved. He was put into a warm bath, and a blister was applied to the chest. He rapidly sank, without pain, expiring at 5 p.m.

Autopsy 15 hours after death.—Body not emaciated. The arachnoid was in places opaque. The vessels and sinuses of the brain were gorged with black blood. A great deal of fluid was found between the membranes, in the ventricles, and at the base of the brain. The plexus choroides were studded with minute vesicles. The glandulæ Pacchioni were unusually large. With the exception of the corpora striata, which were rather soft, the substance of the brain generally was firm. The pericardium contained 2oz. of serum. The heart was unusually large. The right ventricle and auricle were distended with blood and fibrinous concretions; the latter firmly adhering, and extending into the vessels. The ascending aorta was enlarged, as was also its arch, showing a tendency to aneurism. The inner coat was irregularly thickened, and, where most diseased, its connexion with the middle coat, correspondingly altered, was feeble; it was very easily detached. Both lungs adhered very firmly, and the right pleura was much thickened. The superior lobe of the right lung contained a large excavation, lined with a false membrane, through which the ends of blood vessels projected like bits of vermicelli. A large bronchial tube and some smaller ones, and also a large vein, were traced terminating in the cavity, ulcerated at their entrance. Whether the vein was obstructed by a coagulum, or pervious, was not demonstrated. Several small vomicæ were found in the same lobe. In the middle lobe there was a melanotic mass about the size of a walnut, and numerous tubercles in different stages of progress; portions of it also were hepatized. The left lung was in great part pervious to air; it contained, however, many tubercles, but no large vomicæ. The bronchia and the lower portion of the trachea were of a deep red. The stomach was very capacious, but not apparently diseased. The duodenum and jejunum contained much chyme. Some small ulcers were detected in the ileum and cœcum. The liver was bulky, of nutmeg-like section; of sp. gr. 1044.

This case is noteworthy in many particulars : his never having been in hospital for any pulmonary complaint, such a complaint having never even been suspected ; the variety and severity of organic lesions, without corresponding symptoms ; the absence of emaciation ; his tolerable health ; his intemperate life ; his sudden death. Was the death owing to a sudden invasion of bronchitis, and to mucus poured into the bronchia, preventing the due aeration of the blood ? The dark blood, the state of the bronchia and larynx, the chyme in the small intestines, seem favorable to the conjecture. Might not his free manner of living have protracted life ? and might not the large blood-letting have hastened death ?

Some other cases were selected with the intention of introducing them in this section,—cases showing how other diseases, especially lesions of the large intestines and of the liver, such as the ulceration of dysentery and hepatic abscess, have a controlling power and masking influence over tubercular disease as regards symptoms, but I withdraw them, fearing to overload my pages with examples. In the preceding chapters on dysentery and diseases of the liver, corroborative instances will be found. That serious lesions of other parts should have such an effect as that just alluded to is in accordance with the like controlling influence witnessed in cases of insanity.

Tubercles themselves in their progress seem to create a state of mind in some respects similar to that accompanying mental disease, with however notable differences,—a state commonly though not invariably marked by a peculiar activity of the mental faculties and of procreative power, by a peculiar cheerfulness and hopefulness and indifference to or absence of painful sensations. Provided the stomach and digestive organs be sound and there be no ulceration of the larynx, pulmonary consumption I am disposed to believe may arrive at a very advanced stage without any distressing symptoms, or indeed without any marked ones. Is it that the less aeration of the blood, supposing that less carbonic acid is separated from the blood in respiration, has a soothing effect, a partial anesthesia, or an exhilarating effect, somewhat similar to that of nitrous oxide ?*   In favor of this conjecture I may mention that whenever I have tried the blood of a person who had died of phthisis, or the serum, such as that collected in the pericardium, it was always found surcharged with carbonic acid. The trial was made by agitating the blood or serum with air in a two-mouthed pneumatic bottle, both mouths closed by stop-cocks, one provided with a bent tube.   Cases bearing out the remark just made are probably familiar to most medical men of any extended experience.   One remarkable instance of the kind I may mention : it occurred in Corfu ; a young officer of the Royal Fusiliers was the subject of it.   When in health he was of retired habits and taciturn : his lungs becoming diseased, he became cheerful, social and talkative.   On embarking to proceed home on sick leave, at the recommendation of a medical board, his remark was, in slang phrase, that " he had done the doctors" ; he should go home and get some shooting and rejoin his regiment in the cool season.   At this time there were large tubercular excavations in his lungs, detected by auscul-tation.   On the passage in a sailing packet—it was before the time that steam was applied to navigation in the Mediterranean —he dined every day at table, every day but the last ; on that day, about dinner-time, he said he did not feel so well as usual, or words to that effect, and requested that something should be brought to him in his cabin : it is stated, that he partook of what was brought to him and not sparingly, and was found dead a few hours after.

As bearing on the same argument, that of organic disease of the lungs not expressed by symptoms, at least by symptoms of a kind to excite attention, I shall give a case which came under my notice in Malta in 1833, in which till the last brief fatal attack in January of that year, the symptoms of phthisis were in abeyance.

Captain T., ætat. 42, eight years before had suffered from dysen-

---

* It may be mentioned as somewhat in confirmation of the above that those persons who have been resuscitated after submersion in water, have described their feelings, so long as they were conscious, to have been of an agreeable kind.

tery in Ceylon, and after his return and for several years he labored under disease of the larynx, for which, in London, nitrate of silver by means of a probang was applied with much advantage. Then, more than a year from his fatal attack, he was assured that his lungs were sound.   After arrival in Malta, for about twelve months, his health improved ; he had little to complain of, except dyspnœa on exertion ; he had no cough ; no pain ; no material debility ; his limbs were pretty muscular.   He was married and the father of five healthy children, the youngest about a year and a-half old.   On going his rounds on the night of the 5th January, as acting field officer, he was exposed to a heavy shower and wetted to the skin.   Two or three days after, he felt a little unwell ; he complained chiefly of his bowels, having some diarrhœa.   A day or two later a vomica was reported to have burst in his lungs.   Blood-letting to the extent of 30 oz. was employed with antimonial medicine.   On the 17th the dyspnœa was such that he was obliged to sit up in bed ; the expectoration was copious and glairy, streaked with a black fetid sordes, as if from gangrene ; the pulse 100, of moderate strength ; the cough severe and distressing with pain of the left side.   The fetid expectoration continued with increasing debility until he expired on the 20th.

The body which was slender, but not emaciated, was examined 13 hours after death.   The lungs did not collapse.   The left slightly adhering was very heavy, much infiltrated with serum and in part hepatized ; it contained several small vomicæ and some diffused deposition, like the matter of tubercle.   The right lung was very generally and firmly adhering ; its inferior lobe was hepatized ; part of it was of the consistence of firm liver and of the color nearly of unbleached wax, and, what was remarkable, it was penetrated and traversed by ligamentous-like bands, which, it was conjectured, might have been once blood-vessels, and the spot the seat of a former excavation.   The middle lobe contained a kind of honey-comb excavation ; its cavities were lined with false membrane and had become gangrenous.   The superior lobe contained two or three small vomicæ ; it was in part œdematous and in many places of considerable density from the deposition of matter like that of the grey tubercle.   The trachea was unusually large ; redder than natural, but not ulcerated.   Each bronchus was large ; the right after entering the lung gave off only one branch, and that large, as if dilated; below the dilated part it was pressed on by an enlarged bronchial gland of about the size of an almond in its shell. The epiglottis bore marks of old disease; it was only about half its usual size; was thickened towards its base; much puckered (evidently the effect of healing of former ulceration) and it did not cover completely the glottis. The inner surface of the larynx showed a bluish discoloration in patches, probably the seats of old ulcers. The heart was large; the right cavities contained fibrinous concretions; in the left ventricle there was black blood coagulated and *broken up*. The liver was unusually large, especially its left lobe, which was generally adhering to the diaphragm; its substance was of a pale greyish yellow color. The stomach was small; it was so adhering to the liver as to have its movements impeded. The spleen about twice its natural size was attached to the diaphragm by adhesions. The alimentary canal throughout was free from ulceration.

This case hardly needs any comment, its history and the state of the organs after death so well according. Presuming, if we may so do, that it affords an example of a tubercular excavation in the lung closed by a healing process, that result seems to be rendered more probable by the state of the epiglottis, respecting which, as to the healing of its ulcerated surface, there can hardly be a doubt.

Though the filling up and cicatrization of a tubercular cavity is certainly a rare occurrence, yet cases more or less similar to the preceding as regards a lull of symptoms, a suspension of active disease, and more—a gaining of strength and flesh, denoting to the unprofessional observer, recovery, are far from uncommon. An instance of the kind which made a strong impression on my mind I shall briefly describe, though an apology, at least to the experienced medical reader, may almost be needed for introducing it. The case was that of a young officer sent to the Ionian Islands from the depôt of his regiment at home with the hope that he might benefit from the climate of Greece. On arrival at Corfu, he was so feeble, that he required to be helped up stairs. In a few weeks he was so much improved under a mild tonic plan of treatment that he was able to ride many miles, and in a few more to take some regimental duty. Finding that he had a large excavation in one lung, and knowing that he was the only son of wealthy parents, anxious for his return, I thought it a duty to make him acquainted with the state of his chest and to advise him to quit the service, for which he was so unfit, encouraging him with the idea that with care he might have tolerable health and live some years; advice he declined following, preferring, he said, the stirring life with his regiment, however short that might be, to a dull one, though prolonged, at home. He lived two years. On a *post mortem* examination being made, I was informed that an additional large cavity was found in his lungs, with many tubercles.

Reflecting on the wide spread of tubercular disease in countries advanced in civilization, especially in Europe, it may be a subject for speculation how far even the intellect of a people is influenced thereby, and a question, whether, if man were exempt from tuberculosis, science, literature, the fine arts would have had so many devoted and successful followers. How many a man of genius has been the victim, as it is commonly said, of this cruel malady! Who does not remember a distinguished friend, ill to be spared, cut off by it?

4.—On Tubercular Consumption, not Latent.—I had thought of classifying the cases of this disease of which I have notes, but after the study of them, this appeared hardly practicable except in a very rough way, such as into acute, ordinary and chronic, as before done, there being such a gradation amongst them, so little that is truly distinctive, so much that is exceptional interfering with precise limitation as to render great exactness hardly practicable.

Aiming at brevity, I shall first give as much as possible in a numerical form such particulars extracted from the several cases as admit of being so expressed; next I shall insert a certain number of cases selected for their peculiarities, restricting myself to the two extremes, the acute and the chronic,—these on the whole being most instructive—and I shall conclude with some general remarks.

254 cases have been chosen for this purpose, exclusive of a considerable number of instances of tuberculosis, which I have thought it fit to put aside on account of latency in connection with insanity, or of complication with some interfering formidable organic lesion.

Of these 254 cases 112 have had the character of the acute

form rather than of the chronic; the remaining 147 rather that of the chronic than of the acute.

The average age of the former, the acute, has been 25 years 3 months; the oldest 42, the youngest 18 years.

The average duration of the disease has been 5 months; the longest 13 months, the shortest 1 month.

The average period of service has been 6 years; the longest 20 years, the shortest 3 months.

Of the chronic cases the average age has been 30 years; the oldest 55, the youngest 19 years.

The average duration of the disease has been two years 1 month; the longest 6 years, the shortest 1 year.

The average period of service has been 13 years 7 months; the longest 29 years, the shortest 1 year.

These estimates, of course, as to accuracy are of unequal value. Regarding age they may be held to be a near approach to the truth, as on enlisting the age of the recruit is tolerably ascertained. The same remark applies to the length of service. That which is least certain is the period of the duration of the disease, and this for the obvious reason that the reckoning was made from the time that the patient has come under treatment in hospital, when, in many instances, it can hardly be doubted, that the malady was well advanced. In making the estimate of this element, it is right to remark that a certain number of cases have been thrown out,—cases in which, either for want of documentary evidence, or other obscuring cause, the time of the apparent beginning of the illness could not be fixed. In the instances of acute phthisis one only has been excluded as uncertain; in those of chronic phthisis no less than 55.

I shall now proceed to the more important lesions, beginning with those of tubercles.

1.—These in different stages of progress, but without cavities or vomicæ, have been found in both lungs in 6 cases of acute phthisis. In 1 instance only have they been met with confined to a single lung. In this solitary case, there was an absence of them in the left, which was tolerably sound; the right was very much diseased; it abounded in tubercles.

2.—Tubercles, with vomicæ, cavities or excavations, have been found in both lungs in 80 cases; in the left lung in 14 cases, the right having tubercles only; in the right in 8, tubercles alone existing in the left.   Besides these lesions the lungs, in the majority of the cases, were more or less otherwise diseased, either partially solidified, the result of inflammation, or partially infiltrated with serosity.   In many of the cases also there was an undue quantity of fluid in the pericardium, and even more strongly marked effusion into one or both pleuræ, denoting in- flammation of those membranes.

3.—In other organs tubercles have been found in the following number of instances ; in the pia mater 1 ; the dura mater 1; the liver 1; the kidneys 3; the spleen 4; the peritoneum 2; the omentum 1; bone 1.   In all these instances the quantity of tubercular matter detected was small ; in that of bone—the head of the fibula—it was associated with caries and an abscess.

The most important lesion is ulcer, commonly connected with or originating from tubercle, if that may be considered, as I believe it generally may, its germ.

1.—Of the aspera arteria.   In 15 cases the larynx was found to be more or less ulcerated; the trachea in 8; the larynx and trachea in 13.   The epiglottis, the chordæ vocales, the sacculi laryngis, the base of the arytenoid cartilages were the parts of the larynx most subject to ulceration.   The cartilages were often laid bare.   Often the voice was not perceptibly affected.   Only in one instance was it impaired without ulceration or visible injury of the vocal organs.

2.—Of the primæ viæ.   In 2 cases superficial ulceration was detected in the œsophagus.   The stomach in every case was found free from ulceration.   Ulcers were found in the duodenum in 3 instances ; in the jejunum in 17 ; in the ileum in 63; in the large intestines in 72.   When occurring in the duodenum and in the jejunum they were rarely absent in the ileum and the large intestines.   In the jejunum in 5 instances they were associated with varicose lacteals distended with opaque white curd-like matter.   In the ileum, its lower portion was oftenest their seat. In the large intestines, the cœcum was oftenest ulcerated, next in frequency the ascending and transverse colon, the appendicula vermiformis next, the rectum least of all.   Though diarrhœa was a frequent result, it was far from a constant one.   In many, very many instances of severe ulceration of the intestines, both small and large, the bowels were little disturbed, sometimes even there was a constipated state of them.

There were other lesions occasionally presenting which may be deserving of notice. In 7 cases the brain, chiefly the central parts of the cerebrum, the corpora striata, the walls of the ventricles, the fornix, the septum lucidum, were found more or less unduly soft, occasionally pultaceous. In 3 cases the liver was voluminous in excess, weighing 6, 5½, 6½ lbs. A portion of one dried on paper yielded an oil-stain. In 8 cases a thrombus was detected, consisting of coagulated blood and fibrin; the latter undergoing softening. It occurred in the longitudinal sinus in 2 cases; in the right ventricle in one; in the femoral vein in 2; in the femoral and iliac vein in 1; in the jugular vein in 1; in the large branches of the pulmonary veins in 1. The coagulum in the veins of the lower extremities was in each instance associated with a swelling of the limb. In most instances the quantity of blood in the cadaver was small. In none was it found liquid, *i.e.*, destitute of fibrin: even if in part liquid and in part coagulated, the liquid part coagulated on exposure to the air. In some cases the coagulum in the left ventricle was found broken up, indicating, as already remarked, the coagulation of the blood in the part, before a total extinction of life, before the ventricle had altogether ceased to act. In some instances the blood taken from the heart mixed with quicklime or kali purum afforded an ammoniacal odor; in one or two the result of the admixture was negative. Almost invariably there was great emaciation; there was hardly a vestige of adipose matter remaining. In many cases the nails were hooked; more or less incurved. In many there was much hair on the chest, but more frequently an absence of it. In a few instances that the lens of the eye was examined, it was found soft.

I shall now give the results of the examination of the chronic cases, observing nearly the same order:—

1.—Tubercles have been found in both lungs without cavities in 4 cases.

2.—Tubercles with cavities in both lungs in 113 cases.

3.—Tubercles and cavities in the left lung, tubercles without cavities in the right in 19 cases.

4.—Tubercles and cavities in the right, tubercles without cavities in the left in 12 cases.

5.—A cavity in one lung, without tubercles in either in 1 case.

6.—Tubercles and vomicæ in one lung, the other lung sound, but compressed by fluid in the pleura.

As in the acute cases, there were other and serious lesions of the lungs in the great majority of instances, such as hepatization, or œdema, or emphysema, one or other and sometimes all three ; and often also lesions of the pleura and pericardium, marked by effusion of serum with, or without lymph, or pus, the latter rarest.

The other organs in which tubercles were detected were the following ; in the pia mater in 1 case; in the liver in 3 ; in the spleen in 2 ; in the kidneys in 3 ; in the testicle in 1 ; in the prostrate in 3* ; in the peritoneum, including the omentum and mesentery, in 6 ; in bone, including one case of morbus coxarius, in 3, all accompanied by caries.

Ulceration was met with in the following organs, sometimes in company with tubercles, and probably in most of them having their origin in these accretions.

1.—Of the aspera arteria. In the larynx ulcers were detected in 53 cases; in the trachea in 28. The sites of the ulceration were very much the same as those specified in the acute. In both the acute and chronic cases ulcers were of frequent occurrence in the bronchi and bronchia. I need hardly observe, that where large cavities or excavations existed, these opened into air-passages through ulcerated bronchial tubes.

2.—Of the primæ viæ. In the œsophagus ulcers were found in 7 cases ; in the stomach in 1 ; in the duodenum in 5 ; in the jejunum in 29 ; in the ileum in 80 ; in the large intestines in 100. The remarks made under this head in the acute form are applicable also to the chronic. In 6 instances the lacteals rising from the small intestines were varicose, and, as before, were associated with ulceration of the villous coat, and their contents were of the same kind—a white opaque curd-like matter. In 2 cases fistulæ were discovered in the perinæum, associated with ulceration of the rectum.

The other morbid appearances were chiefly the following :— The liver was found unduly voluminous in 3 cases. One liver weighed 7¼ lbs. ; it was of the color of unbleached wax ; a portion of it dried on paper yielded an oil-stain. Another, of the same color as the preceding, weighed 5 lbs. ; it was very friable. The third, exhibiting the nutmeg-like section, weighed 5 lbs,

---

* These were cavities inferred to have had their origin in tubercles.

In all three cases, there was great emaciation. Judging from the stain on the scalpel, and the feel—very imperfect criterions it must be confessed—this organ was rarely impregnated with oily matter. The brain, in 13 cases, was found more or less softened, and chiefly in those central parts of the cerebrum before described. In a few instances the pia mater unduly adhered to the surface of the cerebrum, detaching, when forcibly separated, portions of the cortical substance. The stomach in 4 cases only was found unusually soft. The spleen in 1 instance was very voluminous, it weighed 17 oz.: the individual had, with phthisis, suffered from ague in Canada. The kidneys were often in a state approaching to that of Bright's disease, but rarely well-marked. In 3 cases small calculi were found in them; one was of oxalate of lime; the composition of the others, if ascertained, was not noted down. Gall-stones in 3 cases were detected in the gall-bladder; one was of cholesterine; the other of the black kind; the quality of the third is not specified. Softening of the cartilages of the joints, with loss of substance, was found in many cases. Caries of bone was detected in 4 cases. A thrombus occurred in 6 cases; in the right ventricle in 2; in the left auricle in 1; in the pudic veins in 1; in the longitudinal sinus in 1; and in the femoral and iliac vein and vena cava in 1. The condition of the coagulated mass in each instance was similar to that already described, and the fibrin centrically was undergoing the softening process. In the majority of the chronic cases, also in the majority of the acute, the thoracic and abdominal lymphatic glands, especially the bronchial and mesenteric, were found more or less enlarged. They often contained distinct tubercular matter; and not unfrequently cavities and matter undergoing softening. In the groin and axilla, on the contrary, the glands there situated, were rarely seen diseased.

This statement of lesions shows how great are the complications of tuberculosis. How far they all truly belong to the disease, or are in part only accidental or coincident, I do not think it necessary here to offer an opinion. I have stated them irrespective of any hypothetical view, with the belief, that even what may appear least important may afford some aid in coming to a right conclusion respecting the nature of this destructive malady.

I need hardly add, that in the *post mortem* examinations from which the preceding results have been obtained, there may have been oversights, and many. All I can pledge myself for is that the lesions noted were actually observed, and never imagined. As medical science advances and the observing power is sharpened by science, under favorable circumstances of time and place, no doubt much will be discovered by the scalpel in the hands of the zealous inquirer, especially when aided by the microscope and assisted by chemistry.

1. *Of Acute Phthisis.*—The term acute I apply to those cases, such as the following are examples of, which have run their course with a certain degree of rapidity, terminating in death in a space of time varying from about three or four months to a year, and commonly accompanied with more or less pyrexia and a rapid wasting, denoting a certain intensity of morbid action and that mostly continued.

Case 1.—Of acute phthisis, of about three months' duration.—Wm. Henderson, ætat. 18; 50th Foot; admitted 9th March, 1840; died, 11th April.—This young man, a mason by trade, on admission had served only two months. On the 25th February he was taken into the Detachment Hospital at Chatham, on account of acute catarrh; on the 4th March he was discharged convalescent. When admitted into General Hospital on the 9th, the symptoms were cough with expectoration of thick matter; pain in left side of chest; pulse 100; tongue loaded; much debility. The preceding night he had experienced a rigor. On the 11th there were indications of some improvement; the respiration was free; the expectoration muco-purulent. On the 20th there was an exacerbation; mucous and sibilous râles were heard all over the chest without the aid of the stethoscope; there were night sweats; no pain of chest. On the 24th he was still worse; there was urgent dyspnœa; he spoke only in a whisper. From this time the disease rapidly advanced; there were profuse night sweats; great emaciation, with increasing and great debility; pectoriloquy was distinct in right subclavian region, with gargouillement. He died "exhausted." The treatment was palliative.

Autopsy 11 hours after death. Greatly emaciated; nails not curved; mammillæ large. The pia mater, very red and very tender, and easily torn, contained some bloody serum in its tissue, as did also the lateral ventricles. The cortical portion of the cerebrum was rather soft. The left lung abounded in tubercles; parts of it were œdematous, parts hepatized. Towards its apex there was a mass of tubercles, about the size of a walnut, in which was a small cavity, freely communicating with a large bronchial tube, ulcerated almost throughout. The superior lobe of right lung, which firmly adhered, contained a cavity capable of holding a large orange, and which freely communicated with the bronchia. Several small vomicæ were found in the same lobe, and numerous softening tubercles; tubercles, too, abounded in the middle and inferior lobe. The substance of this lung was generally more or less œdematous and hepatized. The under surface of the epiglottis was severely ulcerated. A large cavity existed at the base of the right arytenoid cartilage; the cartilage was laid bare and loose. A smaller cavity was found at the base of the left, in which the cartilage was only partially denuded. Ulcers occurred in the sacculi, and the chordæ vocales were partially ulcerated. The trachea was extensively ulcerated; two of its cartilaginous rings were partially destroyed. The bronchial glands were enlarged; one contained some calcareous matter. A few ulcers were found in the lower part of the ileum, and also in the cœcum. The liver weighed 4¼lbs.

This is a striking example of acute phthisis. It can hardly be doubted that when first admitted into hospital, and treated for acute catarrh, he was laboring under the disease in an advanced state. And, is it not almost as certain, that at the time of his enlistment, when apparently in good health, his lungs were tuberculated?*

Case 2.—Of acute phthisis, of rather less than three months, complicated, with serous effusion into both pleuræ.—P. Lalor, ætat 18; 54th Foot; admitted 13th June, 1839; died 15th June.—A laborer by occupation; of five months' service. It is stated that he experienced a "febrile" attack, attended with pain of side, two months ago when at Canterbury; and that, when on his march from that town to Chatham on the 17th May, there was a recurrence of the pain; he was supposed to "have taken cold." When transferred from the Detachment Hospital to the General Hospital, his state was hopeless. There was great dyspnœa; the pulse 138; he expectorated a thick, yellow, viscid mucus. The left side of chest was without respiratory murmur, and sounded dull on percussion; the heart was felt beating more on the right side than usual. The right side sounded well. Lately he had no pain of chest. During the short time preceding his death, the treatment was merely palliative.

Autopsy 37 hours after death. Much emaciated. No well marked lesion of brain. 70oz. of serum were found in the left pleura; 27oz. in the right; 3½ in the pericar· dium; from each it was similar in appearance, straw-colored, and clear. A good deal of lymph was deposited in both pleuræ, especially in the left. The left lung, owing to compression, was almost destitute of air. In its superior lobe there were many granular tubercles, with one small cavity, containing puruloid matter. The inferior lobe abounded in tubercles, and contained a cavity capable of holding a small orange; within it were loose masses of tubercular matter, and a puruloid fluid; its walls were without a false membrane, rough and shreddy. The puruloid fluid under the microscope exhibited a few blood corpuscles, somewhat altered, many pus globules and minute granules. The right lung was generally crepitous. Several crude granular tubercles were scattered through it. The bronchial and cervical glands were much enlarged, and contained cheese-like tubercular matter. There was a good deal of blood in the right cavities of the heart. The stomach was distended with air. There was no apparent lesion of the primæ viæ. The vesiculæ seminales were distended with a cream-like fluid abounding in spermatozoa, in granules, and pus-like globules. The serum from each pleura was of sp. gr. 1019; a little lymph separated from each after exposure to the air and rest. The serum from the pericardium was of sp. gr. 1014; a minute portion of lymph separated also from it. The lymph was in a fine granular state, and was not dissolved by acetic acid [dilute?] The puruloid fluid from the vomicæ was of sp. gr. 1038. Some urine taken from the bladder was

---

* For the information of readers not acquainted with army usages, it may be right to mention that a recruit before being finally approved, is subjected ordinarily to two strict examinations as to the state of his health—one by a staff medical officer at the recruiting station; another on his joining the corps for which he is enlisted, by a medical officer of the Regiment.

of sp. gr. 1016; it reddened litmus, and was rendered slightly turbid by nitric acid. Under the microscope it exhibited many granules, pus-like globules, and very many extremely minute spermatozoa, in length about $\frac{1}{4000}$ of an inch; some of these were seen to move rapidly with a vibratory, some with an undulating motion. I now infer, from no mention of the contrary, that the larger spermatozoa from the vesiculæ were motionless.

In this instance we have another striking example of acute phthisis running its fatal course rapidly, but differing from the former in being accompanied by a double pleurisy.

The cavity, the vomica in the left lung, with its contents, disintegrated tubercle and puruloid fluid, is a good instance of its kind. Had life been prolonged, no doubt it would by the ulcerative process have opened into the bronchia, and in due time become lined with a false membrane.

Case 3.—Of acute phthisis, with a vast excavation in lung, of about four months.— A. Simpson, ætat. 20; 17th Foot; admitted 30th May, 1839; died 31st August.— A stocking-weaver; 7 months' service. He was admitted into the detachment hospital on the 24th April, laboring, it is stated, under acute catarrh, attended with profuse night sweats, and was then emaciated. When transferred to general hospital, he was very feeble, his respiration difficult; had a dry cough; much torpor of system, and disinclination to speak; his face was generally flushed and he perspired much. His chest sounded dull; there was bronchophony under each clavicle. On the 5th June pectoriloquy was perceived between the 4th and 5th rib of the left side. Towards the end of July hectic fever set in and pectoriloquy was reported as heard at the upper part of each lung. About six weeks before death the left leg and thigh began to swell, without any acute pain. The treatment was palliative.

Autopsy 9 hours after death. Body much emaciated; the left lower extremity greatly enlarged with œdema. In the longitudinal sinus a fibrinous mass was found situated in its posterior part, adhering to one side, and partially obstructing the flow of blood; it extended into the sinus beneath. It was not distinctly softened. The appearance of the brain generally was normal. The pericardium contained 4 oz. of serum. The left lung was closely and firmly adhering. There was an enormous cavity in it, situated anteriorly and extending through the lung from its superior to its inferior apex, giving the idea of a wasted organ, yet, when carefully dissected out, it was found to weigh 4 lbs. 12 oz. Posteriorly it was much consolidated and contained numerous tubercles and many small cavities. Two or three small cavities were found in the right lung, with numerous tubercles and some partial hepatization, as if from effused blood. Some tubercular matter was detected in the spleen and in each kidney, and many ulcers in the ileum and colon. The left femoral and iliac vein were obstructed by fibrinous concretion and clot.

The vast excavation in the left lung—I never saw a larger— with so much loss of substance and yet increase of weight, is very noteworthy; as was also the rapidity of the disorganizing process. Another noteworthy circumstance in the history of the case was the dull torpid state of the patient, a symptom so unusual in the advanced stage of phthisis. Was it connected with a partial obstruction of blood in its course through the vessels of the brain, owing to the concretion in the longitudinal sinus?

Case 4.—Of acute phthisis, of rapid progress, with rupture of rectus muscle.—J. Milthorpe, ætat. 24; 6th Foot; admitted 25th Nov., 1835; died 22nd Jan., 1836.— A tanner by occupation, of one year's service. Before admission here, he was twice during the period under treatment in the detachment hospital on account of pulmonary ailment; the last time about a month. He is now much emaciated and very weak; has pain of chest, cough and dyspnœa; his sputa are of a greenish color. There is a strong bronchial respiration under the right clavicle, and pectoriloquy in the axilla, with incipient gargouillement. Little change was observable till the 3rd December; then the pain of chest was much more severe, with increased debility. About this time hectic symptoms appeared; his sleep was disturbed; his countenance anxious. On the 11th he was attacked with diarrhœa, accompanied by much irritability of stomach, continuing till the 16th. Little alteration occurred in the leading symptoms till the 8th January, when the cough became more severe and the expectoration sanguineo-purulent. Without abatement, but aggravation, of suffering, daily becoming more feeble, he died on the 13th. The treatment was merely palliative.

Autopsy 13 hours after death. Much emaciated; chest narrow; nails hooked. Both lungs were generally very firmly adhering. Both were much consolidated and abounded in tubercles, especially the right, in which, in its upper lobe, were several small excavations. The principal bronchial branches were much dilated. Coagulated blood was found in the sheath of the left rectus abdominis muscle; and this muscle was lacerated transversely; the extremities of the torn fibres were rounded and contracted. The omentum majus was much thickened by opaque matter deposited in it, and abounded in granular tubercles: it adhered to the liver, stomach, parietal peritoneum and to the intestines. Tubercles also abounded in the mesentery and the peritoneal coat of the intestines. A few tubercles were detected in the liver. Many of the adhesions were red and distinctly vascular. A considerable portion of the small intestines lay in the cavity of the pelvis, matted together by adhesions. Several large ulcers were found in the mucous coat of the ileum, and one in the colon. The stomach was rather small. The liver was of nutmeg-like section.

The complications of organic disease in this case with the rupture of the rectus muscle, are its most noteworthy circumstances. It was conjectured at the autopsy that this latter remarkable lesion might have taken place during a paroxysm of dyspnœa, to which the patient from time to time was subject.

Case 5.—Of acute phthisis, of short duration, with ulcerated larynx and intestines. M. O'Halloran, ætat. 22; 95th Regiment; admitted into regimental hospital, Malta, 27th April, 1828; died 9th June.—This man came into hospital from the government yacht, in which he had served six months as a mariner, and where, during the last three months, he stated he had been ailing, having had cough, with uneasiness of chest and night sweats; adding, that during the last thirty-three days, whilst at sea, he had felt every way worse. The case was immediately reported one of confirmed phthisis, far advanced. Towards its termination he became deaf; his feet swollen; his voice lost, but he had no pain in the trachea, or of intestines, and he had no diarrhœa. The treatment was merely palliative.

Autopsy 7 hours after death. Greatly emaciated; œdema of lower extremities. The cerebral substance generally softer than natural. Pretty much serosity in the

ventricles, and at the base of the brain. 2oz. of serum in the pericardium. Its surface exhibited a delicately reticulated structure, and a peculiar roughness, from what
seemed to be a deposition of coagulable lymph. This was exterior. The anterior
mediastinum was redder than natural, and somewhat œdematous. On the left side,
close to it, a large vesicle was found full of air (1½ cubic inch*). The air was completely confined; pressure did not expel it. On examination the vesicle was found to
be situated between the parenchyma of the lung and its pleura, and to be lined on
each side by a false membrane. The left lung was excessively diseased; there was a
large excavation in its superior lobe, communicating with the bronchia; and throughout it abounded, the inferior lobe as well as the superior, in curd-like tubercles, and
was more or less hepatized. The right lung also was very much diseased; was in
part hepatized, and abounded in the same kind of tubercles; the vomicæ it contained
were few, and these small. Both the larynx and the large bronchial tubes were extensively ulcerated. The bronchial glands were greatly enlarged; curd-like tubercles
were scattered through them. The posterior mediastinum was œdematous. The
thoracic duct was empty and collapsed. The omentum was spotted with minute
white tubercles, more distinct to the feel than the sight, without the slightest mark
of inflammation of the membrane; and the peritoneum generally was similarly
affected. The mesenteric glands were considerably enlarged. Several ulcers were
found in the jejunum, very many in the ileum, and a few in the cœcum. The glandulæ generally had the appearance of being distended with tubercular matter. The
spleen was rather large and firm. The stomach was moderately corrugated. The
liver was apparently sound; the gall-bladder distended.

What seems most noteworthy in this case was the latency of
the majority of the many organic lesions by which it was complicated. The œdema of the lower extremities and the œdema
of the mediastina were probably owing to pressure on the great
veins by the enlarged lymphatic glands. The air-vesicle had its
origin, it is presumed, in a rupture of air-cells, and a forced
separation of pulmonary pleura, followed by an effusion of
lymph, constituting a closed sac.

Case 6.—Of acute phthisis, of rapid progress, with a tuberculated state of most of
the abdominal viscera.—J. Charlton, ætat. 22; 4th Dragoon Guards; admitted
January 8, 1840; died 7th March.—This man's service was of seven months.
During the last three he was under treatment in hospital at Coventry, on account, as
stated, of catarrh; not improving, he was sent here. He had, besides cough with
copious expectoration, dyspnœa, with inability to lie on his left side, and night sweats
—in brief, symptoms of advanced phthisis. His pulse at the time was 84, and small.
It is reported on the 31st January that he felt better than for a long time. On the
14th February his cough was slight; the expectoration copious; no night sweats; he
was subject to nausea. On the 19th of the same month his sputa were tinged with
blood; his appetite now was "ravenous." On the 24th he experienced some soreness
of throat, and there was an apthous state of tongue. On the 1st March his pulse had
become very quick—it was 124—and he began to be delirious, mostly at night. On
the 6th he spoke of himself as quite well. He died the following day without suffering. The treatment was palliative and mainly anodyne.

* It consisted of 2 carbonic acid gas, 4 oxygen, and 94 azote.

Autopsy 52 hours after death. Sub-emaciated; chest large and well formed. The brain natural; the fornix rather soft. The heart was large. The right auricular ventricular passage was very large, admitting readily five fingers; the left was small: it admitted only three. The lungs were very heavy. The right lung was very generally adhering, through the medium of granular tubercular matter. Both lungs abounded in clustered tubercles; the right was considerably hepatized and partially œdematous; the left was œdematous, and partially hepatized. In the superior lobe of each there was a small cavity, and tubercles softening. There was a superficial ulcer at the base of each arytenoid cartilage. The bronchial glands were much enlarged, and contained tubercular matter. 8oz. of brownish serum were found in the cavity of the abdomen. The liver was adhering to the diaphragm. There was a deposit of tubercular matter very generally on the peritoneal lining of the abdomen and its viscera, on the omentum and mesentery, the tubercles varying in size from a pea to a mustard-seed. Tubercles of the former size were scattered through the substance of the liver, in which also were many cavities full of a greenish yellow bilious fluid; the largest were capable of holding a filbert. The gall-bladder contained some thick viscid bile, of natural color. Its inner coat was studded with innumerable particles, in color and appearance like cholesterine. The spleen was unusually large; it abounded in tubercles like those in the liver, and both internally and externally. Tubercles were found on the surface of one kidney and in the substance of the other. The mesenteric and lumbar glands were enlarged, and contained tubercular matter. A small ulcer was detected in the lower portion of the ileum.

This case is notable as an exquisite example of tuberculosis, of rapid progress, with little suffering. There was no diarrhœa, no alteration of voice; and when the disease was most advanced there was, as is mentioned, a feeling as it were of health; a happy delirium, or a state approaching that. Was the " ravenous" appetite owing to a sound and active state of stomach? Was the absence of malaise connected with excess of carbonic acid in the blood and the lungs, in conjunction, it may be, with a peculiar state of brain? The heart, I find it stated, was distended with coagulated blood, without any fibrinous concretion.

Case 7.—Of acute phthisis of rapid progress, very complicated.—A. Allan, ætat. 20; 71st Foot; admitted 8th December, 1838; died 3rd January, 1839.—A black-smith by trade; of ten months' service; the last seven in Canada, from whence he is just returned. Shortly after enlisting he had small-pox which was followed by pneumonia; and since that attack he has been subject to chest-ailment. On admission here after landing, he had troublesome cough with copious expectoration; his voice was hoarse; the bowels confined; tongue clean; pulse 100; the respiration was rather loud under both clavicles; the chest, it is stated, sounded well. On the 12th December the sputa were tinged with blood; pulse 120. No change is noticed until the 20th, when febrile symptoms occurred with increased hoarseness. Taking calomel in small doses with opium and tartar emetic, his cough became less troublesome, the dyspnœa less; the pulse was never less than 100. Till the 2nd January there was no material change; then he experienced a sudden attack of severe dyspnœa; he was found sitting erect in bed; his breathing loud, sibilant, with great muscular exertion; the larynx and trachea in each act of respiration moving quickly up and down;

the countenance livid; pulse 126; voice almost gone; the epiglottis, under the finger, felt erect and swollen. V.S.; leeches; a blister, followed by relief. On the following day he was able to lie down in bed; the breathing was still loud and sibilant, with increased muscular exertion. The right side of chest now sounded clear; the left rather dull; the pulse 112, small; at 11 p.m. he expired.

Autopsy 14 hours after death. Not emaciated; chest well formed and capacious. Some fluid under the arachnoid; pretty much in the ventricles; a good deal at the base of the brain. 6 oz. of serosity in the pericardium; 2 oz. in the right pleura; 6 oz.* in the left; the same quantity in the cavity of the pelvis. The right lung weighed 3 lbs.; the left 2½ lbs. In the superior lobe of the right lung there were many tubercles softening and two small cavities, each capable of holding a hazel nut; also some œdema and hepatization. The middle lobe containing a few granular tubercles, was generally hepatized; the inferior was similar. In the superior lobe of the left lung there were two small cavities a little larger than the before-mentioned, and several smaller in the inferior; both contained tubercles in a softening state and both were partially hepatized. The bronchia, trachea and larynx were red. The latter was somewhat swollen. The under surface of the epiglottis and its margin were ulcerated; its cartilage partially laid bare. There were ulcers also in the sacculi laryngis and the chordæ vocales were partially denuded. The thyroid gland was large; the bronchial glands enlarged. The heart was rather large; its ventricles were somewhat dilated. Coagulated blood,† without any fibrinous concretion, was found in all its cavities, and likewise in the aorta. There were several ulcers in the ileum, and many deep and pretty large ulcers in the cœcum and colon. The spleen was large and soft; the liver, weighing 4 lbs., soft and friable.

This case is noteworthy not so much for its rapidity of progress, as for its many complications, the severity of the organic lesions—none of them indicated by pain—and for the little emaciation. The fatal result seems to have been owing more to the induration and œdema of the lungs interfering with the aeration of the blood than to tubercular disease, or even to the ulceration of the larynx and trachea. The sudden paroxysm of dyspnœa threatening suffocation, it can hardly be doubted, was caused by œdema of the glottis and epiglottis; it was on this idea that active treatment was then employed. In this instance a striking example is afforded of the little relation between the tubercular diathesis and mere form of chest and general form of body. This man's body might have served for a model, it was so symmetrical, the chest so well made and capacious, the limbs of finest proportion, the hands and feet small, the latter well arched; the second toe, as in the Greek statues, of greater length than the

* That of the pericardium was of sp. gr. 1012; that of each pleura 1016; that of the pelvis 1014. After 20 hours each became slightly turbid from the appearance of a little fibrin in granules, and each on agitation gave off a little air.

† The blood corpuscles were found bordered with air-bubbles; under the microscope, in serum many of them floated erect.

great toe, so seldom seen in the Northern races, and, indicative of strength, the legs and thighs unusually hairy.

Case 8.—Of acute phthisis of rapid progress, with many complications and distended vesiculæ seminales.—H. Winter, ætat. 20; 7th Foot; admitted 12th April, 1838; died 5th May.—A butcher by trade; of eight months' service. It is stated that he "caught cold" in December, but was not taken into hospital until the 20th March. When transferred to general hospital, he had constant cough, with copious expectoration and pain of chest. According to the abstract of his case, pectoriloquy was perceptible in the right subclavian region. On the 13th April, mention is made of his expectoration, which was then copious and muco-purulent, being tinged with blood. On the 25th, it is briefly stated that he was worse, and that he "raved and moaned constantly in his sleep," and had night sweats, and that his bowels were purged. The purging was reported to have ceased on the following day, and that he felt rather better, but the next day worse; "raving constantly" at night and perspiring much. Thus he rapidly declined, the pectoral symptoms continuing until he expired. The treatment was merely palliative; blisters, warm plasters, cough mixture, anodynes.

Autopsy 22 hours after death. Sub-emaciated; neck rather thick; penis turgid. The calvaria in parts was very thin. There was a good deal of fluid in the cellular tissue of the pia mater and in the ventricles and at the base of the brain. The pineal gland, large and adhering posteriorly, contained two or three small cavities; they were well displayed, opened under water. The brain was firm; its section showed many bloody points. The left vertebral artery was the size of the basilar; the right very small. The pericardium contained 2 oz. of purulent serum; the right pleura 8 oz.; the left 3 oz.; all of the same kind. In the right pleura a good deal of lymph was deposited. The right cavities of the heart were distended with fibrinous concretion and blood. In the superior lobe of the right lung there were many clusters of firm tubercles; near its apex there was a mass of about the size of a hazel-nut, consisting of albuminous matter softening and penetrating the pleura, giving the idea that it might have been the exciting cause of the inflammation of that membrane. The larger portion of the inferior lobe was hepatized; it was grey, and contained a reddish purulent sanies. In the superior lobe of the right lung there were many clustered tubercles and two or three small cavities communicating with the bronchia, the largest capable of holding a filbert. The inferior lobe was tolerably free from disease. The bronchial glands were much enlarged. They contained a curd-like matter, and cavities were found in them, in which was a thick matter found to be purulent by the optical test; the including substance, that surrounding the cavities, was unusually vascular. A similarly enlarged and diseased gland, about the size of a large walnut, was found close to the duodenum attached to the pancreas. It contained curd-like matter and a thick puruloid fluid. There were no ulcers in the intestines, and no distinct lesion of any of the abdominal viscera. In the right patella there was a softening spot and a fibrous state of the cartilage. The vesiculæ seminales were large and distended with a greyish fluid, in which were some spermatozoa. There was a good deal of fat in the posterior mediastinum and under the integument.

The tubercular state of the lungs in this instance probably preceded their inflammation and that of the pleura and pericardium, denoted by the fluid contained in them, and very likely existed even at the time of enlistment. The condition of the brain has been described with some minuteness, on account of the unusual delirium experienced. As nothing is known of the function of the pineal gland in health, it is useless to conjecture what is its influence if anywise diseased. In a large number of cases of phthisis it is found somewhat altered, and very often adhering posteriorly. Irregularity too of the cerebral arteries, as regards size, is of common occurrence in this disease. I have before alluded to the state of the penis in the moribund of phthisis. The turgescence of the organ after death from this disease is not unfrequent, and with very few exceptions, whenever I have examined microscopically the fluid of the vesiculæ seminales I have detected in it spermatozoa.* This, and a probable corresponding state of the ovaries, may be one of the circumstances conducive to the amiable and loving feeling which so often distinguishes the consumptive, as well as their procreative power, even when the disease is advanced.

Case 9.—Of acute phthisis, of rapid progress, complicated, with partial disease of brain, and other lesions.—Wm. Tear, ætat. 27; 30th Foot; admitted 7th September, 1837; died 15th November.—A laborer; of 11 years 8 months' service; was reported to have been stout and athletic, and always in good health until last winter, when he had an attack of influenza, and was in hospital a month. After his discharge it is stated that he continued well until about three weeks ago. Then his pectoral complaint began with cough, soon followed by expectoration, dyspnœa, and night sweats, debility and emaciation supervening. There is now pectoriloquy in both subclavicular regions; the chest sounds dull; the symptoms are the ordinary ones, taken altogether, of advanced phthisis. His pulse on the 2nd November was 115. There was extensive gargouillement in left anterior superior region. On the 14th there was delirium at night; other symptoms not urgent; delirium preceded death on the following day. The treatment was purely palliative.

Autopsy 32 hours after death. Much emaciated; nails not curved. The calvaria was deeply grooved. In the frontal bone, on the left side, a small cavity was found, from which a spiculum of bone projected; and corresponding to it there was a perforation in the dura mater. The arachnoid was partially opaque, and the pia mater granular; the latter was most conspicuous where it dipped between the convolutions of the right hemisphere under the parietal bone; there the granular state was owing to the presence of small firm tubercles. All the cavities of the heart were distended with coagulated blood and fibrinous concretions. The lungs were generally and very firmly adhering. They weighed 6½ lbs. They were vastly diseased. A large excavation existed in the upper portion of each superior lobe, with several smaller ones, and both lungs abounded in tubercles in different stages, and were partially hepatized. The under surface of the epiglottis was granular and slightly ulcerated. In the right side of the larynx there was a pretty large ulcer, by which the greater part of the arytenoid cartilage was laid bare. The bronchia were thickened. The bronchial glands were greatly enlarged and softened. The left pneumo-gastric nerve, where pressed on by one of these enlarged glands, was distinctly atrophied. Many ulcers,

* See my Researches Phy. and Anat., vol. i., p. 337, for examples.

with minute tubercles, were found in the lower ileum, and numerous and large granulating ulcers in the cœcum and ascending colon; there were a few also in other parts
of the colon and rectum; the appendicula was severely ulcerated. Nothing remarkable was observed in the other viscera.

This case is noteworthy for the rapidity of its progress and for
the mildness of its symptoms; also for the little apparent relation
between them and the lesions. The granulating, healing state of
the ulcers in the large intestines is another noteworthy circumstance. Shortly after admission he had diarrhœa, which soon
ceased. Only a day or two before death he believed he was
almost convalescent, and was anxious to be discharged from hospital.

2. *Of Chronic Phthisis.*—The term chronic, as in its ordinary acceptation, is used here in opposition to the acute and as
applicable to such cases as the following, which are unusually
prolonged, and in which there is little intensity of morbid action,
little pyrexia, no rapid wasting, little suffering, and which are
equally opposed to the more numerous cases of ordinary phthisis,
these commonly advanced by fits and starts, characterized by
alternating periods of activity and arrest of morbid action; in
the one stage threatening often speedy dissolution—in the other,
exciting hope, almost always delusive, of recovery.

Case 1.—Of chronic phthisis, of uncertain duration, much complicated.—A.
M'Nultie, ætat. 26; 75th Regiment; admitted 13th October, 1837; died 17th Jan.,
1838.—A weaver by trade; of eight years' service; the last seven at the Cape of
Good Hope, from whence he is recently returned. There, it is stated, he had an
attack of pulmonary disease, followed by scurvy; and later by "derangement of
heart." On admission into general hospital, the heart's action was stronger than
natural; he experienced some dyspnœa with cough and the expectoration of tough,
viscid mucus. He improved until the 1st December, when, in a fit of coughing, he
expectorated four ounces of fluid blood. V.S. was then employed with other palliative
means. The expectoration continued bloody for some time. After a cessation it recurred with some severity on the 12th January. On the 14th, the report described
him as very weak, with much dyspnœa. Wine and tonics were now administered.
On the 16th, the day before he expired, it is stated that he had great thirst and occasionally vomited, and that all expectoration had ceased. It is mentioned that he
desired cold drinks.

Autopsy 24 hours after death. Sub-emaciated; nails curved; left upper extremity
flexible; right partially rigid; lower extremities rigid. No hair on the chest; pretty
much fluid in the lateral ventricles; a good deal at the base of the brain. The ventricles very large, as if they had once contained more fluid. 1 oz. of serum in the
pericardium. The heart large; its right cavities contained a good deal of dark blood;
its left very little. The right cavities were disproportionally large and were slightly
hypertrophied. The auricular-ventricular passage was unusually dilated. The
margin of one of the tricuspid valves was thickened and indurated. Granular

tubercles, that is, minute, white firm bodies, were found in the true right auricle situated under its investing membrane. The pulmonary artery was large. The left auricle and ventricle were normal. The right lung was very generally and closely adhering. In the upper part of its superior lobe there was a cavity of moderate size, with several small vomicæ. It and the other lobes abounded in tubercles in different stages of progress, and here and there this lung was hepatized. In the upper portion of the inferior lobe of the left lung there was a cavity capable of holding a walnut; the upper part of the superior lobe was œdematous; in both lobes there were tubercles and a few vomicæ. The bronchial tubes were of a dark red. An elliptical ulcer, about the size of a finger nail (the little finger) was situated in the lower part of the trachea. The lower portion of the œsophagus had partially lost its epithelium, as if from abrasion. There was a general softening of the mucous coat of the stomach; it was pale and almost of pultaceous consistence. The lower part of the ileum was red, and its mucous and sub-mucous coats were slightly œdematous. In the cœcum there were large ulcers in process of healing, and ulcers nearly cicatrised in the ascending colon. The liver exhibited the nutmeg-like section. It weighed 3½ lbs. The spleen was covered with a thin false membrane. Its substance was firm. The vesiculæ seminales, rather large, were moderately distended with a light brownish fluid, abounding in globules and containing a few spermatozoa. The blood from the right side of the heart agitated with common air in the pneumatic bottle, gave off pretty much air.

This case may be viewed as a fair example of chronic phthisis of uncertain duration. On arrival from the Cape, the health of the man was reported tolerable, and that it so continued up to December. His disease was returned " catarrhus;" pectoriloquy, it is said, was never perceived. The state of the right side of heart is deserving of note in relation to the former cardiac derangement. Apart from the thickening of one of the tricuspid valves—a rather rare occurrence—a distension of the right cavities and an enlargement of the pulmonary artery, are, I believe, rather common than rare in connexion with tuberculated lungs; as might perhaps be expected *a priori*. It is worthy of remark that during the whole time he was in hospital, notwithstanding the ulcerated state of the large intestines, the bowels were commonly rather constipated than relaxed; they were never a subject of complaint. Another noteworthy circumstance is the state of the stomach, as found after death, keeping in mind the irritable condition of it and the excessive thirst during the last days of life. The condition of the limbs as regards *rigor mortis* in this case has been mentioned. The mention of it in the foregoing has been omitted, though commonly noted down at the time of the autopsy, and so omitted from the irregularity of its occurrence; in this respect having some accord with the coagulation of the blood, though I cannot say that they are co-ordinate. A similar remark as to omission applies to the absence or presence of hair on the chest, and to the teeth, whether sound or decayed, and in a less degree to the nails, whether curved or not. These, though helping diagnostic indications, are far from infallible; in a large number of cases, especially of chronic phthisis, the nails are found hooked, the teeth good, the chest without hair; but now and then each of these conditions may be found absent, and most frequently in instances of the acute disease.

Case 2.—Of chronic phthisis of long duration, complicated with hydrothorax, etc.— E. Sarsfield, ætat. 66; extra patient; admitted 28th August, 1840; died Sept. 21.— This man was invalided in 1832, after 21 years' service, being "infirm and worn out." Till within a few months, he had been employed in washing for the general hospital. For several years he had been subject to cough; and for a considerable time before admission he had been laboring under dyspnœa. When admitted, he was feeble and emaciated; his cough very troublesome with copious expectoration; his pulse small and feeble; his bowels usually regular. Examined with the stethoscope, there were clear indications of chronic pulmonary consumption, such as pectoriloquy, etc. On the 4th September, it is stated, that low delirium set in with great debility, from which he never rallied.

Autopsy 27 hours after death. Much emaciated; nails curved. A good deal of fluid in the tissue of the pia mater and in the lateral ventricles. The substance of the brain was of natural firmness. The right pleura contained 2½ pints of serum. The right lung, adhering superiorly, was much compressed. A large cavity was found in its superior lobe freely communicating with the bronchia, and two small vomicæ, also many clustered tubercles. These were grey and granular and occurred also in the middle and inferior lobe and in both lobes of the left lung. In the apex of the latter there was a cavity capable of holding an orange. In both lungs there was a considerable portion of their structure pervious to air. The under surface of the epiglottis was studded with small ulcers; one penetrated to the cartilage which was fissured. There were also some small ulcers in the trachea. The aorta was large, especially its ascending portion, as if dilated. Many ulcers were detected in the ileum, and a few in the jejunum and colon; some in the latter were healing. The surface of the liver was rough and granular; its section nutmeg-like; its substance rather soft and friable.

Have we not in this instance a good example of chronic phthisis, very slowly advancing and eventually becoming fatal from complication with hydrothorax? During life there were no known indications of ulcers either in the aspera arteria or in the intestines; and yet it may be inferred that they were of long standing.

Case 3.—Of chronic phthisis of very slow progress, with tuberculated testis and ulcerated intestines.—H. Nevan, ætat. 30; died 16th January, 1837.—This man, a discharged soldier, was employed as an orderly at Fort Clarence. He had been invalided about three years ago on account of pulmonary disease. He had served in India, where he had lost the sight of one eye. During the time, fifteen months, that he had been at Fort Clarence, he had been subject to cough, with mucous expectoration, and had experienced several attacks of hæmoptysis, the last, two months ago.

A month before his death his chest was examined and a tubercular excavation was found to be indicated under the left clavicle. He was kept on as long as possible as a matter of charity. During the last fortnight he was more feeble than usual, yet he did his duty. In the afternoon of the 15th January he was attacked with extreme difficulty of breathing, short and convulsive; his cough was urgent, expectoration difficult; there was irritability of stomach; the face was pallid; the pulse rapid and feeble; was unable to rest in the recumbent posture. He said, that he had had diarrhœa two days previously. The urgency of the symptoms continued unabated, unrelieved by the palliative means employed. He expired at 9 o'clock the following evening.

Autopsy three days after death. Little emaciated; limbs pretty muscular; chest flat and irregularly depressed, especially on left side; cornea of blind eye opaque and sunken. A good deal of blood in the vessels of the brain. The ventricles merely moist with fluid. The substance of the brain of natural firmness. The left optic, never communicating with the blind eye, distinctly smaller than the right. The upper part of the superior lobe of the right lung was firmly adhering. It contained a cavity capable of holding an orange, full of a reddish fluid. This lung generally abounded in crude granular tubercles; with few exceptions its parenchyma was pale and crepitating. The left lung adhered very generally and firmly. When dissected out, it was found smaller and more condensed than usual, containing little air. There was a large empty excavation in its superior portion, lined with a false membrane, and one smaller contiguous. Throughout it abounded in crude tubercles. The bronchia in it were smaller than natural, as if shrunk from disease. There was no well-marked disease of the larynx or trachea. In the cœcum there were many ulcers and marks of old ulceration. The right testis, larger than natural, was closely adhering to the tunica vaginalis; that is to say, the sac was obliterated. There was an abundant deposit of tubercular matter along the whole course of the epidydimis, and small tubercles were found dispersed through the substance of the testicle. The left testis appeared to be sound; the sides of the tunica vaginalis were only partially adhering.

The autopsy in this instance illustrates but little the immediate cause of death or the nature of the last attack. The condition of the left lung is very characteristic of chronic tubercular disease in its passive state; the organ shrunk and consolidated, an excavation empty, lined with a false membrane, indolent granular tubercles, not softening. Had the cavity in the right lung followed the same course, been rid of its contents and become lined with a false membrane, it is easy to conceive that with care life might have been protracted many years. It was remarked that during the first twelve months when this man was at the asylum performing the easy duties of orderly he improved in appearance.

Case 4.—Of chronic phthisis of long duration, without excavation in lungs,—tubercles in excess, with hæmoptysis.—W. Wood, ætat. 38; 53rd Foot; admitted June 22nd, 1837; died June 27th. A married man, of 19 years' service, the last 7 in the Mediterranean, from whence he is just returned. During the last two years he labored under difficulty of breathing with frequent and sometimes violent hæmoptysis. During the last fortnight he has felt worse. Now, June 22nd, he has severe dyspnœa; cough with thick yellow expectoration, respiration 30 in the minute, pulse full and accelerated, sunken countenance, great debility; his bowels are reported regular; he rests always on his left side. Bronchophony is perceived under both clavicles; the lower portions of chest sound dull; there a moist crepitus is heard; on inspiration some pain is felt in the left side. No material change was perceptible, under palliative treatment, during the short time he was in hospital preceding the fatal issue.

Autopsy 16 hours after death. Sub-emaciated; nails curved. The left lung was generally and pretty firmly adhering; the right not at all. Each lung was unusually voluminous and heavy, each weighed 3¼ lbs., both abounded excessively in tubercles, which in some places were coalescing; there were no cavities in the right lung; in the left, in its superior lobe, there were two small cavities full of thick pus. Though the tubercles generally were little advanced, yet they were so numerous, as to leave very little of the structure of either organ in a state to perform its functions. The bronchia were red. The pericardium was generally adhering; the adhesions were easily broken by the pressure of the fingers, leaving a false membrane covering the heart: this false membrane was studded with hemispherical white masses, of about the size of a split pea and smaller, of almost cartilaginous hardness. The heart was rather large, its right cavities larger than usual. Many considerable ulcers were found in the jejunum and ileum. The other abdominal viscera were tolerably natural. The right testicle was very small and flabby and pale; its tubular secreting structure seemed obliterated. Each tunica vaginalis was closed by adhesion.

Many of the lesions in this case are noteworthy, and some of them in connexion with the symptoms; of the former, especially the state of the pericardium; of the latter the vast amount of tubercles in the lungs, with little emaciation; no excavations, and yet frequent hæmoptysis; ulceration of the small intestines without known functional derangement. This man is designated a " married man." I believe that more married men suffer from consumption in the army than unmarried; which, if a confirmed fact, may perhaps be attributable to two causes chiefly—one, that the tubercular diathesis is commonly associated with warm affections tempting to marriage; the other, that the married soldier has hitherto labored under disadvantages, circumstances unfavorable to vigorous health, especially as regards quarters and diet.

Case 5.—Of chronic phthisis of some years' duration, ending in fatal erysipelas.— D. Sinclair, ætat. 55; an extra patient; admitted 12th March, 1822; died 28th April.—An invalided piper of a Highland Regiment. According to his statement, the cough to which he is subject began six years ago, and every winter since it has become more severe. He is now much debilitated and emaciated, his appetite impaired, but without thirst. He has a frequent troublesome cough, with copious expectoration; his respiration is short and difficult, with shooting pains across the chest; he can lie on either side, but with most ease on the left. His bowels are constipated; he has no night-sweats. Using mild tonics with extract of conium, no change took place in his symptoms until the 17th April, when he was attacked with erysipelas of the face, attended with little pyrexia, but great debility. On the 22nd the inflammation was reported to be subsiding, desquamation taking place; yet though the pectoral complaint was not urgent, he did not improve. Shortly before death his appetite entirely failed, his tongue became parched, his pulse very rapid and feeble and his sensations and intellect obtuse.

Autopsy 28 hours after death. Exceedingly emaciated. The pericardium contained only about a drachm of serum. The right auricular-ventricular passage was unusually large, admitting with ease the four fingers. The walls of the right ventricle were very thin. All the valves of the heart were a little thickened. The superior lobe of the left lung, its upper portion, was adhering. It contained a small excavation and numerous granular tubercles, grey and hard, grouped in masses; very few of them softening. Similar tubercles and as numerous were found in the inferior lobe. This lobe was in part œdematous and gorged with blood; yet portions of it were crepitous. The right lung very similarly diseased, was generally adhering. Its superior lobe was so firmly attached and by a substance of cartilaginous hardness (the thickened pleura?) that the scalpel was required to separate it. In this lobe a cavity capable of holding a small orange was found, which was bounded on one side by the indurated and thickened pleura, rather more than a quarter of an inch thick. This lobe contained also many tubercles, as did also the middle and inferior; all of them granular and indolent. A few ulcerated spots, like abrasions, were detected in the trachea. It and the bronchia were red and wet with a puriform fluid. The bronchial and œsophagial glands were much enlarged without softening, as were also many of the mesenteric. Some of the latter were of cartilaginous hardness and appearance. The stomach and duodenum were much contracted. The liver was small; its weight 2 lbs. 3 oz. The cœcum was much ulcerated. The thoracic duct contained a transparent fluid; its upper portion, to the extent of about two inches, was considerably enlarged; where the enlargement terminated superiorly, there was a contraction; a probe could not be passed; it barely admitted the wire of a catheter. Some of the larger arteries were partially ossified.

This case is a striking example of chronic tubercular phthisis advancing slowly with age and winter weather, and rapidly, and may it not be said, prematurely, brought to a fatal end by the supervention of erysipelas.

Case 6.—Of chronic phthisis, without any distressing symptoms.—P. O'Brien, ætat. 32; 7th R.F.; admitted into regimental hospital, Malta, 1st May, 1833; died 18th August.—This man, of intemperate habits, experienced in the Ionian Islands in 1825 and 1826 remittent fever, followed by ague; in 1831, acute catarrh; and again in the following year. In Malta in the early spring of 1833 he had a severe attack of "pneumonia." When last admitted—viz., on the 1st May, his symptoms were the following: acute pain in the right breast, affecting his breathing: a short, dry cough; a full and quick pulse; a dry skin, but not hot. V.S. to the amount of 30 oz. was employed, and calomel with James' powder prescribed; the blood was not buffed. On the following day he was free from pain, and on the 5th he was reported convalescent. On the 9th he was suddenly seized with diarrhœa. Using calomel, opium and ipecacuanha, this ailment gradually diminished. On the 20th he was again reported convalescent, with a good appetite. On the 28th he declared himself quite well and strong, and appeared free of pulmonic symptoms. A slight diarrhœa followed, but was of short duration, taking chalk and opium. Yet, notwithstanding his own good account of himself and the abscence of cough, he was evidently wasting and losing strength. The stethoscope now used, indicated latent disease of the chest. He was put on a milk-diet, and tartar emetic was applied to the chest. During June no decided change was observable; he continued to speak of himself as quite well. In the beginning of July there was a perceptible increase of emaciation and debility, with a slight tickling cough and some puriform expectoration. Now pectoriloquy was audible under the right clavicle. Wasting with increased debility continued, accompanied by œdema of extremities, diarrhœa at times, profuse cold clammy sweats and evening paroxysms of fever. During the latter period of his disease, he never complained of anything; his constant reply was that he was well. His appetite continued good, as it was throughout his illness; he coughed but little; his breathing too was generally easy, and he commonly slept well. Such was his sleep the night before he died. When he awoke in the morning he was unusually cheerful, took some food, and two hours after expired, "not as if from suffocation, but from extreme exhaustion."

Autopsy 25 hours after death. Much emaciated; nails not curved. The left pleura contained 3 oz. of serum. Numerous tubercles were dispersed through the substance of the left lung, especially of its superior lobe; they were granular and clustered; none were softening; there was no vomica. The lung generally was crepitous. The right lung was much more diseased; it was generally adhering. In its superior lobe there were several small excavations; one, capable of holding a large walnut, was bounded laterally by the costal pleura, the pulmonary pleura being, as well as could be ascertained, destroyed. In the middle lobe there were two small vomicæ and several clusters of granular tubercles. There was sanguineous congestion in the inferior lobe with a few tubercles, but no vomicæ. There was no marked disease in the larynx or trachea. The bronchial glands were much enlarged; so too were the mesenteric. There were many small ulcers in the inferior part of the ileum and a few pale ulcers in the colon. The spleen was rather large. The liver was examined for oil: the result was negative.

The feeling of health in this case, when so near death, is one of its most noteworthy features. Another is the fatal result with comparatively only a moderate degree of organic pulmonary lesion. Is the *vis vitæ*, the power of enduring such lesions, a variable quantity—if the expression may be used—in different individuals? Many familiar facts seem to imply as much.

Case 7.—Of chronic phthisis of slow progress, with enfeebled state of mind.— Sergeant R. Campbell, ætat. 27; 42nd Regiment; admitted into regimental hospital, Malta, 7th February, 1833; died 20th April. This man, of a delicate form and constitution, in 1831 had an attack of "pneumonia," cough persisting. He was under treatment for hæmoptysis in November of the following year. When last admitted he was laboring under decided symptoms of phthisis,—cough with muco-purulent expectoration; night-sweats; wasting; debility; pulse 120 and small; œdema of feet and ankles. During the preceding month, it is reported, that his mind was occasionally affected; "mental weakness" was the term used by the surgeon, and there was a recurrence of the same at times through the after progress of his illness. The symptoms mentioned above continued with little variation. Between the 3rd and 6th April he was troubled with a slight diarrhœa, which subsided under the use of compound chalk powder with opium. The debility and emaciation increasing, on the 18th April, in the evening, he experienced a sudden attack of syncope. On the following day he was in a state of great exhaustion; he became delirious towards night, and expired at 3 a.m.

Autopsy 9 hours after death. Much emaciated; extremities slightly œdematous;

pretty much dark-colored hair on chest; chest well-formed. Pretty much fluid between the membranes in the ventricles and at the base of the brain. The surface of brain rather soft; internally of moderate firmness. One vertebral artery was more than double the size of the other. The left lung was not adhering and did not collapse; parts of it were œdematous. Crude tubercles, consisting of curd-like matter, were scattered through it in little clusters. There was no cavity or vomica in it. The right pleura contained 3 pints of turbid serum holding in suspension puruloid matter and flaky lymph. A thick layer of coagulated lymph covered the pleura. This lung was attached by a strong membranous band. Its superior lobe abounded in a remarkable manner with softening tubercles and minute vomicæ, full of pus-like matter. The middle and inferior lobes also contained many tubercles, but these were less advanced. These lobes were much compressed by the effused fluid The pericardium contained 3 oz. of transparent serum. The heart was rather larger than usual. There was pretty much blood in both ventricles. The blood in the left ventricle was coagulated and broken up as if the heart had acted after its coagulation had taken place. There were a few ulcers in the lower ileum. The mesenteric as well as the bronchial glands were much enlarged. Many of the lacteals were varicose and of an opaque white. The viscera not mentioned were apparently free from disease.

One of the most marked peculiarities of this case was the little painful or uneasy suffering experienced during its course; in this respect resembling the preceding. It was specially stated by the surgeon that there was "a total absence of pain and of dyspnœa" throughout. Was this owing to a state of brain similar to that of the insane, in whom when laboring under phthisis, the same peculiarity is so often witnessed. His "occasional mental weakness" seems favorable to the idea. This, the case of a sergeant, gives the opportunity of expressing the opinion, which I am disposed to believe founded on fact, that non-commissioned officers in the army, especially the higher grade of sergeants, are more subject to pulmonary consumption than privates. Examining the cases in my possession, I find that the former are in the proportion of 8 per cent., and the great majority of them sergeants; and this probably is below the true ratio, as no special attention was given in designating the rank. If confirmed, an explanation will not be difficult, keeping in mind that the tubercular diathesis and acuteness and activity of intellect are so frequently associated.

Case 8.—Of chronic phthisis complicated with fistulæ in ano and perinæo, etc.— S. Bull, ætat. 25; 42nd Regiment, admitted into regimental hospital, Malta, 20th February, 1833; died 15th July.—This man joined the service-companies of his regiment in Malta in March, 1832, and was then laboring under anal and perinæal fistulæ, the former of two years' duration, the latter of a few weeks. His general health seemed to be good. Placed under treatment, he was discharged, as it was believed, cured in July. In the following month he was re-admitted, the fistulæ as bad as before. In November he was again discharged to duty. When again re-admitted—viz., on 20th February, 1833, owing to a recurrence of his local malady, his health was still reported good. Various modes of treatment were employed, but with little good effect. Early in May his health began to suffer; he had cough, pain in the right hypochondrium, increased by pressure, anorexia, with frequent vomiting of a bilious fluid. These symptoms continued, occasionally mitigated, it was supposed, by the treatment employed. Towards the end of May diarrhœa set in with hectic fever. His stools were commonly white from deficiency of bile, and unhealthy. He rapidly emaciated and lost strength. During the last week of his life he had three or four attacks of syncope daily. Throughout, the symptoms of pulmonary disease were obscure. The treatment was chiefly palliative. At the beginning, an alterative course of mercury was tried on the supposition of hepatic derangement.

Autopsy 18 hours after death. Much emaciated. The left lung when brought into view appeared healthy; it was collapsed, adhering only at the summit, where there was a small excavation immediately beneath the pleural lining. In the same lobe were many clustered tubercles undergoing puruloid softening. A similar small cluster and in the same state, and a minute excavation were found in the middle lobe. Apart from these lesions the structure of the two lobes was pretty natural. The right lung was very generally adhering. In the upper part of its superior lobe there was a pretty large excavation, some small vomicæ and very many granular tubercles softening. The middle lobe contained many tubercles in the same state; a few also, but not softening, were found in the inferior. The gall-bladder was distended with thick viscid bile. The liver was of a light wax-color. A portion of it dried yielded much oil (elain) which remained liquid on cooling. The stomach was distended with air and fluid; a thick mucus adhered to its villous coat. The lower part of the ileum was very red, but not ulcerated. The colon throughout was very much diseased. Ulcers with sloughing were found in the cœcum, and in the colon to the extremity of its sigmoid flexure; granulations were interspersed, denoting a healing process in progress. The rectum was unusually red and of a flabby consistence. At the verge of the anus there was a large hæmorrhoidal tumor, which was found to consist of varicose veins. In the same situation there were several small sinuses, some opening through the skin, one through and into the rectum. Two fistulæ were detected in the perinæum; these communicated with the urethra by ulcerated openings close to the caput galinaginis. The mouths of the ducts of the prostrate were large and ulcerated. The bladder was sound.

It is remarkable in this case how little demonstrative, as regards symptoms, were the very extensive tubercular disease in one lung, and the very ulcerated state of the large intestines. There is a prevailing opinion, I believe, that phthisis and *fistula in ano* are often associated. My experience does not accord with this notion; even including fistula in perinæo, I find it to occur only in the ratio of about 1 per cent. in the cases I have collected.

The remarks I have to offer shall be brief. And first on the etiology of tuberculosis. It seems to be tolerably ascertained and now generally admitted, 1st, That inflammation is not essential to the production of tubercle; and, 2ndly, That tubercle may be formed and to a certain extent make progress by accretion without any obvious derangement of health, or well marked

14

change in the condition of the tissue in which it has originated.
The facts stated in the 1st section, that on latent tubercle, and
the instances adduced in the 4th of the existence of tubercle in
men of various ages and of various length of service, seem to
afford sufficient evidence in proof; the former in a manner demonstrative, the latter at least presumptive.

That a peculiar diathesis belongs to the phthisical, either
hereditary, or formed *de novo*—the latter in a large number of
instances, seems hardly questionable.   Whilst it may not be an
easy matter to define this diathesis in at all a satisfactory manner,
there appears to be little difficulty in pointing out many of the
circumstances which favor its production.   In the instance of the
British soldier they may be classed under three heads chiefly,
occupation, including habits; diet; and quarters; and, perhaps a
fourth, dress.

Excepting when engaged in active war, the life of a soldier is
monotonous, his duties tedious and depressing mentally.   There
is little to enliven him but the music of the regimental band.
His *ennui* is not often relieved except by dissipation and low
sensuality,* often in their effects undermining his constitution.
In consequence of this *ennui*, this *tœdium vitæ*, when in garrison,
especially at such stations as Gibraltar and Malta, desertion at
the one is nowise uncommon, nor suicide at the other, where
desertion is hardly practicable.†

His diet, his ration, generally, is not what it ought to be,
either as regards variety, or nourishing power, or even quantity.‡

* A faint idea of the dissipation, at least in the Foot Guards, serving at home, and
chiefly in the metropolis, may be formed from the fact, as shown in the statistical
reports of the army, that of the total sickness of these regiments from 1837 to 1847,
as much as 25 per cent. was from venereal disease.

† Even amongst the troops serving at home, self-destruction is in a comparatively
large proportion; according to the same reports, during the decennial period mentioned in the preceding note, in the cavalry it was to the extent of $5\frac{8}{10}$ in every 10,000
of the strength annually, while in the infantry it amounted only to $2\frac{9}{10}$ in the
same number.

‡ "The ration of the British soldier consists at home of 1lb. of bread and $\frac{3}{4}$lb. of
meat, at which rate it was fixed so far back as 1813, and has never since varied, except
that by a Warrant, dated February, 1833, an additional $\frac{1}{4}$lb. of bread was given to
troops encamped in England." "Abroad the ration consists of 1lb. of bread, or $\frac{3}{4}$lb.
of biscuit and 1lb. of meat, either fresh or salt, the additional $\frac{1}{4}$lb. being given to
compensate for the inferior quality of foreign compared with English meat."—Report
of the Commissioners, etc., p. xxi.   "When a soldier enters the service he has the
prospect of dining on boiled meat [beef] every day for 21 years, if he is enabled to
serve so long."—page xxvii.   4d. a-day is paid by the soldier for his ration of bread
and meat, and 4d. a-day for improving the Commissariat ration, for vegetables, &c.,

The meat is too often that of ill-fed animals, supplied at a low contract price, and on foreign stations, with the exception, it may be, of one or two, deficient in fat. Salted meat has been frequently issued in place of fresh meat, and with the worst effect within the tropics. The proportion of vegetables used has almost invariably been small. Butter and oleaginous matter, milk and cheese have never formed a part of his ration.* Till within a few years the soldier has had only two meals a day, breakfast at half-past seven, dinner at half-past twelve, leaving a fasting interval of nineteen hours.

If his solid food has been supplied on no scientific consideration of what is requisite to constitute a wholesome, invigorating diet, no better attention has been given to his drink. For most part he has been left to provide himself. Rarely has any wine been allowed or beer, and only occasionally a portion of rum. Bread mostly has been the chief article of his breakfast, dry bread with tea or coffee according to the individual's means and taste. Not supplied with any wholesome beverage, and with so long an interval between meals till recently that a supper has been provided, is it surprising that he should have become intemperate and have been tempted too often to drink to excess with little or no regard to the quality of his liquor, whether new and unwholesome rum, such as he carouses with in the West Indies, or the drugged porter, or British spirits, at home.

As to quarters, the soldiers' barracks hitherto have been constructed with little or no regard to sanitary requirements. Their ventilation has been neglected and often their drainage. They have been too commonly crowded; their dormitory and day-room the same; the space—the breathing space—of air, too limited as to cubical capacity; and all the circumstances conjoined the least favorable that can well be imagined to health.† No barrack

and for providing an evening meal; the remaining 5d. of his pay he has clear, unless under stoppages for under-clothing, etc.

* In Ceylon and India, more oily matter enters into the diet of the soldier, from the use of curries, and there phthisis is less prevalent than in most other stations; and may it not be in part owing to this peculiarity of diet?

† "The dormitories or barrack-rooms are very confined, the minimum cubic space allowed to each soldier by regulation being only 450 feet, and a reference to the returns numbered xxxv. and xxxvi. in the appendix, will show that in a majority of cases even this minimum is not attained, and that in a number of barracks there is a deficiency of one-third and in some instances of more than one-half of the space allotted by regulation."—Report, etc., p. xvii.

The following is from the same report:—"The soldier sleeps in a fetid and that I have inspected has been provided with a water-closet, or with decent privies to which access could conveniently be had under cover ;* no barrack-room has even been furnished with chamber-pots ; baths and washing-rooms have been almost equally ignored.†

In the dress of the soldier, till very recently, effect on the eye seems more to have been regarded than either comfort to the wearer, or his health. The tight buttoned-up coatee so long in use when on parade and duty, and especially on march, was better contrived to interfere with healthy respiration than to allow the lungs their free action. This portion of the dress was open to other objections ; nor were other articles, such as the stock, the cap, etc., of a kind to be exempt.‡

Now, if tuberculosis, if pulmonary consumption, be an asthenic disease, as, I believe, is now generally admitted, whatever cause tends to impede the due aeration of the blood, either directly, as by compression of the chest, or indirectly, as by stinting the supply of air, or by circumstances vitiating its quality ;—whatever tends to weaken the bodily frame, as by not affording a sufficiency of wholesome food, and in that wholesome

unwholesome atmosphere, the habitual breathing of which, though producing for the most part no direct immediate effects, probably lays the seeds of that pulmonary disease which is so fatal to the British army."

In reply to a question put by the commissioners, a non-commissioned officer said— "I have [in visiting the barrack-rooms before the windows were opened in the morning] often retired to the passage and called to the orderly man to open the windows. The air was offensive both from the men's breath and from the urine-tubs in the room; and of course some soldiers do not keep their feet very clean, especially in the summer-time."—P. xvii.

* The privy of the oldest barrack in Barbadoes, "the stone barrack," was 179 yards distant from it. This was reported on time after time by the Inspector-General of Hospitals, but in vain.

† "We recommend (say the Commissioners) that every barrack should contain ablution-rooms and baths, laundry and drying-room and workshops; and also that suitable provision be made for non-commissioned officers' and married soldiers' quarters." "That day-rooms be constructed for the use of the men in some of the principal barracks at home, and, if found advantageous, that they be extended to all barracks."—P. xxxii.

‡ "Of late years [since the Russian war] great improvement has been made in the clothing of troops. The form of the tunic now adopted affords protection to the hips and belly of the wearer, which the coatee did not. The material is stated to be better than that formerly in use, and the fashion of tight clothing is for the present at least discarded." "The stiff stock is condemned by almost every one who has given his opinion upon it." "The great coat worn in the British army is of very bad material, of little use against cold, whilst it readily imbibes and retains wet."—P. xxviii.

On enlistment now (1861) the soldier gets 1*l.* and a free kit, which includes all his clothing, upper and under, the latter 3 cotton shirts, 3 pair of socks; afterwards to be provided at his own expense.

variety required; whatever further has a tendency to depress the spirits and create mental weariness,—cannot but be operative in predisposing to and favoring the growth of tubercle. But, in the instance of the soldier, we see that all these causes have more or less acted together. Can we then be surprised that pulmonary consumption should have been so prevalent and fatal as it has hitherto proved in the British army.

With these few remarks I shall dismiss the etiology of Phthisis. The medical officer and the medical inquirer will find on consulting the best authorities that I have been guilty of no exaggeration in what I have stated. In the voluminous Blue Book, the " Report of the Commissioners appointed to inquire into the regulations affecting the sanitary condition of the Army," published in 1858, and in "The Evidence and Appendix" attached, they will find very instructive particulars and details bearing on all the matters at which I have glanced. It is some satisfaction to think that the causes assigned are, as before observed, of a remediable nature, and that the correction of them, judiciously carried out, will at the same time equally conduce to the efficiency of the army, and, by a saving of life, to a saving of expenditure.

The great experiment made in the Crimea in the late Russian war, led to the appointment of the Commission just referred to, some of its results were so terrific. These results, so well recorded, it is to be hoped will never be forgotten. There it was demonstrated, as had been so often demonstrated before, though never in a more striking manner, that hardy and enduring as the animal man is, disease and death to a frightful extent must ensue, if the soldier is overworked, ill fed, ill sheltered, ill clad, in the manner the army was during the greater portion of the time that it was actually employed before Sebastopol ; and *vice versâ* what excellent health the same army, *i.e.* its residue, enjoyed when properly cared for, as it was towards the end of the campaign, when, owing to the feeling excited at home in the public mind, the Government was compelled to take measures requisite to correct the pre-existing evils.

It may perhaps be asked how, with such accumulated experience as is now possessed, how in such an advanced state of science as the present, there should have been so great a neglect shown in relation to the health-concerns of the troops, and this up almost to the present time ? There are other things as strange which we witness, about which a like question might be asked. How is it that clairvoyance, table-turning, spirit-rapping, and the like delusions have in these enlightened times had their benighted believers ? Is it not because a portion of society, and that we fear not an inconsiderable one, is wanting in the elements of sound knowledge ? So, as regards the ruling authorities, have not they too been wanting in that knowledge of hygiene, without which army administration, so far as the health and efficiency of the soldier is concerned, can never be well conducted. Hitherto a Board of general officers has regulated the clothing of the army; the Commissariat has had the supplying it with provisions; the Royal Engineers have been the architects of hospital and barrack buildings. And in each of these important matters the medical officer has had no influential voice. Knowledge is said to be power, and so it is when used; and ignorance is power, and a terrible one in an obstructive way, as the history of army administration has so well displayed. Let us hope that the future will make up for the past, and that in the new era that is opening, if a medical officer is to be attached, as has been recommended* to every army taking the field, as a sanitary officer at the head of the Sanitary Police of the force, it will be in a really responsible capacity and with as much authority as the good of the service will permit.

I have hitherto offered no opinion concerning the nature of tubercle and its development, a subject so obscure that I might well pass it by, and yet so interesting and important that it can hardly fail of having the attention of every inquiring mind. I need not particularise here the many views which at different times and by different pathologists have been taken of it. That tubercle is not a vascular body seems to be well determined. That it is not an organized body, a living entity, any more than a urinary calculus or a biliary can be considered organised and possessed of life, seems also to be admitted as well ascertained. Chemically viewed, it appears to differ but little from coagulable lymph,—an albuminous matter with a little oily or fatty matter constituting its principal ingredients ;—its increase—growth it cannot be said to have, having no reproductive cells—being either owing to accretion from without, the addition of tubercular gra-

* Op. cit. p. xxi.

nules, these an exudation from probably unhealthy blood; or, from epithelial cells from within, these abortive. In favor of the former idea it may be urged that the changes to which tubercle is liable are much the same as those to which coagulable lymph and fibrin are subject, especially that of softening, so well exemplified in that kind of lymph which is yielded by unhealthy blood, separated during life, and often found forming concretions in the ventricles of the heart and great vessels, therein not only softening, but passing also into a semifluid pultaceous state. Even healthy fibrin, I have found, may by the absorption of oxygen, and the removal of a portion of its carbon, become liquid.* Another circumstance which may be mentioned as favorable to it is, that tubercle is found chiefly to occur in those tissues to which it is most allied in composition,—the white serous and cellular tissues and the parenchyma of organs, such as the lungs, liver, spleen, kidneys, lymphatic glands and bones, of which the latter tissue forms a part; but rarely if ever in those tissues, the composition of which is different, such as muscle, and brain and nerve-substance.

Whether tubercle when formed be removable or not is a problem hardly yet solved. I am inclined to agree with those pathologists who reply to the question in the affirmative; and who consequently do not consider phthisis pulmonalis an incurable disease, or in more correct words, a disease absolutely fatal. That tubercles soften and are eliminated is well known; and if few, and the formation of fresh ones be prevented, the disease is arrested. And there are many cases recorded in which this happy event seems to have been realised.

---

* I find that fibrin, obtained from healthy blood, after having been well washed, undergoes even in vacuo (that made by a good air-pump) the softening process, evolving much carbonic acid and ammonia. After about a month (the pump worked daily to remove the carbonic acid generated) at a temperature of about 55°, it was converted into a turbid fluid with a sediment. This fluid under the microscope, viewed with a one-eighth of an inch object glass, was found to abound in minute granules just distinctly visible. The fluid itself, judging from its coagulation by heat and by the mineral acids, had the qualities of pretty strong serum. It was rendered transparent by acetic acid and by aqua ammoniæ and potassæ, which dissolved the granular matter. The coagulum by heat was also dissolved by the acetic acid and the alkalies, and likewise by the strong mineral acids in excess aided by heat. This serous fluid had a very offensive, sickening odor (like that of the putrid sanies so common in tubercular excavations) which it lost in great measure by exposure to the air. I have given these details of the experiments, not being aware that the conversion which it shows of fibrin in part into serum and granular matter has ever before been noticed. The fibrin used was from the blood of a fattened pig.

On the general treatment of the disease I shall offer but few remarks. On the ground that phthisis is an asthenic malady, it seems now to be generally admitted that the tonic, the invigorating method, comprised in whatever conduces to the general health, is the practice that affords the best chance of affording relief; and the only chance, if that be possible, of effecting a cure : of course the complications to which the complaint is so especially subject, its epiphenomena, will demand special attention, and must be dealt with according to their nature, keeping in mind the character of the main underlying infirmity, and that no more reducing means should ever be used than are absolutely necessary, if necessary at all.

By change of climate, it is to be feared, little good can be effected, even in the earliest stage of the malady,—the possible remedial stage,—unless, indeed, it could be clearly shown that there is any one station tolerably exempt from the disease, and which can afford examples, like some stations in the United States of America, of cases of decided consumption having there recovered.*

At present, do not motives of humanity and regard for army efficiency alike dictate the propriety of invaliding as soon as possible every soldier laboring under the malady, when well ascertained, sending him to his home, and not detaining him month after month to die in hospital, as has been too much the practice hitherto.

The great aim of the medical officer should be in the first instance, by the most careful examination of recruits not to admit into the service those predisposed to the disease, if that be practicable ; at all events to reject every recruit in whom the function of respiration is anywise defective, leading to suspicion

* Some interesting cases of the kind will be found in the valuable medical statistics of the United States army. The stations most remarkable for exemption from phthisis are those inland and elevated, where the air is usually very dry. There is much in these statistics, and the reports which form a part of them, made by the medical officers of the United States army, deserving of the attention, indeed of the careful study of the medical officers of the British army, and the authorities at the War Office might profit by their perusal. On opening the work, in search of some other information, I find the following, reminding me of a great want, that of gardens being attached to barracks, especially in our foreign stations, so often recommended by medical officers, but in vain. "The troops in various portions of New Mexico have been afflicted with scurvy ; the result of the usual causes of that disease—the use of salt meats and absence of all vegetables. With the cultivation of company and post gardens, the disease has almost entirely disappeared."—P. 429.

of the existence of tubercles. Another great aim should be to prevent in the sound and enlisted soldier the production of tubercle,—and with this intent seeing to everything that can be done to preserve in health and vigor the men entrusted to his care,—enforcing all sanitary rules that can be enforced, and suggesting to the commanding officer all such measures as can be carried into effect which promise on the principles of hygiene to prevent disease. It is an almost God-like office, his; and with the increased power the medical officer is now likely to have, and the increased means at his disposal, he will have much to answer for, if he fail in his duty.

CHAPTER VI.

ON PNEUMATHORAX.

Remarks on it, viewed as an Epiphenomenon of Tubercle.--Detailed cases of.—Observations regarding its Semeiology, Pathology and Treatment.

ALTHOUGH pneumathorax has not a place in the list of army diseases, that which is, I should rather say, was authorised for medical returns, yet on account of its interesting nature and not unfrequent occurrence, it may be deserving of being considered apart from phthisis, with which it is so commonly connected.

The cases of which I have notes and which I propose to describe, 26 in number, with one exception, were all of the kind just mentioned, being associated with tubercles in the lungs, and owing their origin to a perforation into the pleura, either by an excavation communicating with a bronchial tube, or by a bronchial tube itself ruptured opening into that membrane.   Apart from this epiphenomenon, if I may so designate pneumathorax, all the cases, with the exception of one, were varieties of phthisis, and might be given as examples of the kind in their different stages of progress.

Of the whole number, 15 were of the right side ; 10 of the left ; 1 of both sides.

Of the whole, 6 were recognised during life ; the remainder not before the *post mortem* examination.

Of the former, 4 were operated on by paracentesis with immediate, but only temporary relief.

The air contained in the pleura was examined in 7 cases.   It was found to consist of azote and carbonic acid in variable proportions, or of these gases with a variable admixture of oxygen.

In every instance but one the collection of air was accompanied with that of serum, or of a purulent or puruloid fluid.

When in the following cases the treatment is not specified, it is to be understood to have been merely palliative ; when the hospital is not named, that it was, as already mentioned, the

General Hospital at Fort Pitt; and further, it may be as well to premise, that when paracentesis was performed the author took upon himself the responsibility of operating.

It was my intention at first to have given a selection from these cases; but, on re-examining them, and finding in each some peculiarity, it seemed best to include the whole. Many of them are less satisfactory than could be wished, owing to the imperfect manner in which they are detailed, that, too often, arising from the defective manner in which, during life, the patients were examined, in consequence either of the medical officer under whose immediate care they—the earlier cases—were, not being familiar with the use of the stethoscope, or, if familiar, omitting the use of it, and of appropriate means of detection. These cases, I would fain hope, will not be held to be valueless: serving as warnings, they are well adapted to expose the danger of routine practice, to which there is so great a tendency in those of our profession who do not take an interest in medicine as a science, and have not constantly in mind the necessity of that wholesome doubt leading to inquiry.

Case 1.—Of pneumathorax, without inflammation of pleura, preceded by diabetes. —T. Holmes, ætat. 33; 60th Rifles; admitted 22nd July, 1840; died 2nd August.— This man was sent home from his regiment, to be invalided on account of diabetes. On admission the symptoms of advanced phthisis were distinct, but not urgent. From the abstract of his case it would appear that he had been ailing for a year and a-half, and that during the whole time there had been an undue secretion of urine and that sweet. On the 30th July 7 pints were voided in the 24 hours: it was of sp. gr. 1036; evaporated it yielded a dark brown extract, rich in urea, but without saccharine matter. On the same day he complained of pain in the right axilla. His death was sudden and unexpected.

Autopsy 5 hours after death. Greatly emaciated. The right side of chest sounded tympanitic. When perforated much air rushed out. The quantity was estimated at 8 pints, so much water being required to fill the void space in the pleura. The pleura contained no liquid and "bore no marks of recent inflammation." Air forced into the lungs by a bellows, found vent through two or three oblique openings in the pleura communicating with a cavern of honeycomb form in the lower part of the middle lobe. The inferior portion of the superior lobe and the whole of the middle and inferior were hepatized and contained tubercles in different stages of progress, also several cavities. The left lung was very similarly diseased. There was a small ulcer at the base of each arytenoid cartilage. The liver contained a globular cyst, about the size of a billiard ball, full of what appeared to be dead hydatids in course of change, greyish membranes matted together. The capsules of the kidneys were unusually tender; their cortical substance very red.

Pneumathorax in this instance was not suspected during life; it probably took place only a very brief time before death, and may have been the immediate cause of death. It is remarkable that whilst the patient was laboring under diabetes the disease of the lungs was latent. In the abstract of his case, it was stated that " he had not been troubled with any pectoral complaint." On admission into the general hospital it was detected only by means of auscultation. It is curious to observe how towards the termination of life, the urine whilst retaining a high specific gravity had lost its saccharine quality. It reminds me of a case of diabetes in the Royal Infirmary of Edinburgh, which I watched when a student, remarkable for retaining a high specific gravity with an alternation of quality; at one period of the 24 hours there being abundance of sugar in it without urea; at another period, the opposite, much urea and no saccharine matter.

Case 2.—Of pneumathorax, from minute perforations in the pulmonary pleura, rapidly fatal.—F. Diamond, ætat. 23; 83rd Regiment; admitted 11th August, 1838; died 24th September.—This man's illness commenced in May last in Canada, with pain of chest, soon followed by symptoms of phthisis. On admission, immediately after his return, there was obscure pectoriloquy in the right lung and other indications confirming the diagnosis. He improved till within five days of his death, so as to be considered almost convalescent. The unfavorable change was marked by hoarseness and difficulty of swallowing. The evening before he died he was suddenly seized with extreme dyspnœa and difficult expectoration, increasing till he expired.

Autopsy 21 hours after death. Moderately emaciated. The right side of chest sounding tympanitic, denoting the presence of air, the abdomen was first examined. The liver was found partially displaced towards the left side, the diaphragm on the right having been pressed down nearly to the margin of the false ribs. Some of the air in the right pleura was collected in a gum elastic bottle. This was effected by laying bare the pleura, at an intercostal space, and immediately breaking through the membrane and turning the stop-cock the instant the bottle was distended. 12 measures of the air thus obtained were reduced by solution of potash to 11; by phosphorus to 9·5. The minute quantity of oxygen thus indicated may have been contained in the apparatus used. On opening into the chest, the right lung was found very much compressed and covered with a false membrane, except towards its apex, where its surface was puckered. On blowing air into the lung under water, small bubbles passed out at this part, as if through pores in the pleural lining. In the substance of the lung within, there were several minute cavities communicating with bronchial tubes, two of them contiguous to the pleura. This lobe abounded in tubercles: the middle lobe contained a few; the inferior still fewer and more granular, and though compressed was tolerably sound. The pleura contained two or three ounces of serous fluid; its cavity was lined with a coating of lymph, which over the diaphragm was very thick, and there had a kind of cellular structure. The left lung, generally adhering, was even more diseased than the right, abounding in tubercles with cavities and in part œdematous. The epiglottis was abrupt, as if its apex had been cut off; its margin was rough; it did not entirely cover the glottis; a portion of it probably had been destroyed by old ulceration. There were a few small ulcers in the large intestines.

In this instance as in the preceding, pneumathorax was not

suspected during life. Had it been recognised by the medical officer in charge, and an operation performed, the fatal effect might have been warded off, at least for a time. It was conjectured at the autopsy that the sudden hoarseness and difficulty of swallowing might have been owing to the pressure of air superiorly in the pleura. Another conjecture was, that the air had escaped into the pleura by a larger perforation than was detected, afterwards concealed and closed by lymph thrown out.

Case 3.—Of pneumathorax complicated with empyema.—R. Roberts, ætat. 28 ; 1st F.; admitted into regimental hospital, Barbadoes, 22nd June, 1845; died 24th October.—This man, of 11 years' service, was supposed on admission to be laboring under catarrh of a mild character, and until 1st July he seemed, it was said, to be doing well. On that day he had a sudden fit of coughing and expectorated about 3 ounces of blood. From that time, though expectorating frequently small quantities of blood, he appeared to improve slightly. On the 15th August his disease was returned phthisis, the symptoms of which were then pretty well marked. The expectoration streaked with blood had become purulent. He had occasionally diarrhœa. On the 23rd September the respiration at the upper part of the right lung was reported to be cavernous. Some pain complained of in the larynx was relieved by a blister. On the 30th his feet and ankles became œdematous. From this time he gradually sank.

Autopsy 7 hours after death. Hands and lower extremities œdematous. Right side of chest distended and tympanitic; also the abdomen. The liver was found displaced; its inferior margin was below the umbilicus. The diaphragm on the right side tense and tympanitic, was convex inferiorly, and protruding about two inches below the false ribs. On the left side it was normal. On puncturing the diaphragm on the right side, air rushed out with much force ; some of it collected extinguished a light. A purulent fluid followed the discharge of the air; it was of a greenish hue ; its quantity, measuring what was contained in the pleura, was altogether 112 fluid ounces. The right lung, owing to compression, occupied but a small space; it was covered with flaky lymph, of which there was a good deal mixed with serum. In the superior lobe a depression was detected, on its outer surface, about the size of the nail of the little finger, in which was a small opening in the pleural covering, communicating with a tubercular excavation by a narrow fistulous passage about an inch distant. The excavation was capable of holding a filbert. This, the right lung, abounded in tubercles and in small vomicæ and cavities. The left lung was pretty healthy ; it contained only a few granular tubercles. There were many small ulcers in the larynx and trachea, and in the small intestines. The mesenteric glands were much enlarged.

As was remarked in the preceding case, so it might have been said in this, that had the pneumathorax been timely ascertained, and an operation performed, life might have been protracted.

In the autopsy, the calvaria had been removed before the distended abdomen and thorax were opened : it was curious and instructive to see how, owing to the pressure, the cerebral vessels had become injected and distended, and how the blood poured out when they were divided ; and how, on the contrary, when the pressure was taken off by opening those cavities, the blood ceased to flow, and the brain became pale. The liquid blood coagulated on exposure to the air.

Case 4.—Of pneumathorax, rapidly fatal.—O. M'Greary, ætat. 41; 28th Foot; admitted 21st October, 1838; died October 22.—This man, of 17 years' service in India, immediately on his return was taken into hospital, on account of chronic pulmonary disease. The symptoms were not reported as anywise characteristic or urgent. After being under observation eight days he was discharged to barracks· When re-admitted on the 21st October he was laboring under great dyspnœa; had a dull pain in the right side of chest, a feeble pulse, cold perspiration; in brief, was nearly moribund. Stimulants, etc., were used without any good effect. He expired the following morning.

Autopsy 31 hours after death. Sub-emaciated. The right side of chest sounded tympanitic. The liver and the diaphragm on the right side were found much pressed down. On puncturing the latter air escaped. The right lung was much compressed· The pleura contained no fluid and was without a false membrane. Both lungs abounded in tubercles and cavities. In the right lung, in the inferior portion of its upper lobe, there was a small excavation, communicating with the pleura by an opening large enough to admit a goose-quill; the opening into the bronchia was not detected. A portion of the inferior lobe of this lung was pervious to air. The lower edge of the right sacculus laryngis was ulcerated. In the ascending and transverse colon there were many large ulcers; most of them were covered with granulations in process of healing.

The rupture into the sac of the pleura probably occurred only a few hours before his last admission. In the morning of the very day he was brought to hospital, he had been out walking, and on the preceding day he had been down in town buying plain clothes, being about to be discharged the service. That death was owing to the escape of air into the pleura, oppressing the heart and compressing the small portion of lung previously pervious, is hardly open to question. In this, as in the preceding cases, the pneumathorax escaped detection during life, owing to want of proper examination. It may be mentioned that 5 hours *post mortem*, the carotid artery and jugular vein were examined. No air was found in either. Some blood that flowed from the latter, mixed with kali purum, afforded a slight trace of ammonia by the muriatic acid test. It may also be mentioned that some liquid cruor from the right cavities of the heart coagulated after being taken out and exposed to the air, 31 hours at least *post mortem*. In the same cavities there were some fibrinous concretions.

Case 5.—Of pneumathorax, complicated with various lesions, rapidly proving fatal. —W. Phillips, ætat. 24; R.B.; admitted into regimental hospital, Malta, 17th March, 1831; died 25th March.—This man, of drunken habits, between September and

December last, was twice in hospital on account of venereal ulcers and a bubo. When admitted on the 17th March he was laboring under severe symptoms of "pneumonia." On the 19th, after copious blood-letting and the use of tartar emetic in nauseating doses, it is stated that he felt better; pulse 108, no pain; respiration easy; the blood last drawn (24 oz.) not buffed. On the 20th the report was again favorable, also on the 21st. On the 22nd a mucous râle was perceived over the whole chest; there was much dyspnœa, some cough, no pain, slight epistaxis. He gradually became worse, dyspnœa increasing, which, in his last hours, was accompanied by low delirium.

Autopsy 22 hours after death. Not emaciated. The left side of the chest was larger than the right, and tympanitic. The body placed in a bath, the chest was punctured under water; a large quantity of air rushed out; a portion collected was found to consist of 13 carbonic acid, 7 oxygen, 80 azote. The water that entered to supply the place of the air measured 6½ pints. As it was clear when taken out, it may be inferred that there was no pus in the pleura. It was thrown away before its examination was made, as intended, for serum. The lung on this side was free from adhesion, and there was no lymph on the pleura. In the superior lobe and in its inferior surface, about 2 inches from the mediastinum, a small circular opening was found in the pleural covering (its margin red and vascular) which communicated with an irregular excavation and that with a bronchial tube, as was proved by inflating the lung, when air passed freely out. Scattered through this lung there were many granular tubercles, and like tubercles were found on the pleura. Its inferior lobe was emphysematous; the cells very large and distended with air. The middle lobe was in part œdematous and in part hepatized. The superior lobe, besides the cavity already mentioned, contained many sinuses, which were red and lined with a delicate false membrane. The right lung free from adhesions, was, with the exception of the sinuous cavities, much in the same state as the left. Its upper surface was tolerably crepitous and altogether it was less engorged than the left. The mediastinum on the left side was œdematous and the seat of a sinus about 3 inches in depth, from which issued a reddish turbid fluid. There were about 2 pints of serum in the cavity of the abdomen. A sinus was detected in the prostrate, almost encircling it; it was lined with a delicate false membrane and opened into the urethra, close to the caput galinaginis. There was no stricture of the urethra. The penis was distended; just before expiring, he exclaimed "I am suffocated." The mesenteric and lumbar glands were enlarged, as were also the glands in the groin, where during life there were two or three small sinuses.

The ulcerated cavities in the lungs in this case were peculiar. Were they connected with a venereal taint? A similar sinus in the prostrate *perhaps* favorable to this idea. As on the 22nd, two days before death, it is pretty certain that there were no indications of pneumathorax, may it not be inferred that the rupture of the pleura took place subsequently; also that the fatal event was mainly owing to the pressure from accumulated air? Another query was made at the time of the autopsy—viz., whether the ulceration in the mediastinum, close to the œsophagus and par vagum might not in the first instance have been productive of the dyspnœa?

Case 6.—Of pneumathorax temporarily relieved by operation.—M. Partridge, ætat. 28 ; 65th F. : admitted 7th October, 1835; died 23rd October.—This man was received into hospital, to be under observation on his return from the West Indies, where he had suffered from ague and from repeated ulceration of the right leg. His health was reported good. On the 13th October he first complained of cough, which was chiefly troublesome at night, without pain of chest. His aspect was unhealthy. Using a " cough mixture," the cough was relieved until the 20th, when it became more severe, with a sharp pain of right side of chest, much heat of skin, thirst, pulse 120. V.S. to 16 oz.; tartar-emetic mixture. On the 21st there was less pain of chest, but more heat of skin and increased thirst; pulse 120, and small. The right side of chest was now found to be more prominent than the left ; the left on percussion duller than natural.; the right very resonant; no metallic tinkling. At 7.30 p.m., he was very much worse; there was severe pain of chest, which had been preceded by a sensation, as if something had given way suddenly within, followed by great difficulty of breathing. The respirations were 48 in the minute, hurried and laborious ; pulse 130, small and feeble; skin cool, moist from perspiration ; counten- ance pale, livid, very anxious ; a dragging pain in the right hypochondrium; pro- minence of right side more apparent; a metallic tinkling perceptible from the mamilla to within an inch of the right clavicle ; the respiratory murmur very indistinct and distant. On the 22nd the symptoms all were rather aggravated. At noon, after a consultation, paracentesis was performed between the sixth and seventh rib. On withdrawing the stilette much air escaped, with sudden and great relief. It being found by a probe that the lung was collapsed, the canula was left in, covered exter- nally with oiled silk and confined by a bandage. At the evening visit he expressed himself as easy; his respiration was easier. He passed a tolerable night. At 9 a.m. the following day he expired suddenly.

Autopsy 28 hours after death. Sub-emaciated. Opening first into the cavity of the abdomen, the liver was found protruding a little on the right side; the diaphragm there convex, and more transparent than natural, as if there were air in the pleura. Next, opening into the chest, the heart was found pressed a little to the left. Its right cavities contained a good deal of crassamentum and fibrinous concretion; its left ventricle some *broken up clot.* The left lung contained many tubercles, most of them granular. They were most numerous in its superior lobe, in which also there was a small vomica. The right pleura contained 8 oz. of viscid serum, in which were some flakes of coagulable lymph. The lung on this side was so compressed as to be reduced to about one-third its natural volume. Eight pints of water were required to fill the vacant space. The pleura was covered with a layer of soft lymph. The lung was free from adhesions, except its superior lobe, which was attached to the side by a short, thick, very vascular band of almost cartilaginous hardness. On forcing air by a common bellows into the trachea, the superior lobe did not expand ; the middle lobe expanded partially ; the inferior generally ; air passed out through an ulcerated opening in the under portion of the middle lobe. In the superior lobe there were excavations, each capable of holding a walnut, freely communicating with the bronchia ; also one or two vomicæ, and a large number of tubercles but little advanced. In the middle lobe there were a few tubercles and a single cavity which communicated with the sac of the pleura. The cavity was small, capable of holding a hazel nut; the perforation was large enough to admit a goose-quill ; a small bronchial tube terminated in the cavity, and was slightly projecting. The inferic lobe was free from tubercles. There was no marked lesion of any of the abdomina viscera.

This case is noteworthy from the disease of the lungs having been so long latent, showing, as so many other cases show, that if any considerable portion of these organs be tolerably sound, the health may be apparently good. May it not be inferred that in this instance the perforation of the pleura gave rise to the pleurisy as well as to the pneumathorax ?

Another comment made at the time was that the fine bronchial tube opening into the cavity, and slightly projecting, might have acted the part of a valve, allowing the air to be pumped in and preventing its return.

Judging from the *broken up clot* in the ventricle, the heart was the *ultimum morens*.

Case 7.—Of pneumathorax, complicated with empyema.—J. Hogan, ætat. 38 ; R.B. ; admitted 7th January, 1837 ; died February 6th.—For four years this man had been troubled with chronic cough, not however incapacitating him for duty. Three months ago it became more severe. He was first taken into regimental hospital, from whence, not improving, he was transferred to the general hospital. He had then a troublesome cough with some dyspnœa occurring in paroxysms, relieved by the expectoration of muco-purulent matter. His appetite was good ; his bowels regular ; his chest sounded well ; mucous râles were perceived on each side. He continued much the same, his cough easier, until the evening of the 27th January, then he suddenly experienced an unusual sensation in the right side, attended by a great increase of dyspnœa. The ear applied to the chest (the patient in the sitting posture) no respiratory murmur was audible over the whole of the right side. On percussion, the upper portion sounded tympanitic ; the lower, below the 6th rib, sounded dull. In the recumbent posture, the whole of the anterior part sounded tympanitic ; the lateral parts dull. On gentle succussion a fluid was heard moving in air in the right pleura. No marked lesion was detected in the left lung. The heart's impulse was heard in its normal situation. The symptoms not being urgent, the bandaging of the thorax was recommended in consultation, and in case of urgency of dyspnœa the operation of paracentesis. His feet and legs became œdematous, his urine scanty ; hectic symptoms followed with increasing dyspnœa, but, till a few hours before death, not to such an extent as to be very distressing. Coma preceded the fatal event.

Autopsy 26 hours after death. Much emaciated. The liver was found displaced towards the left side and pressed considerably down. The diaphragm on the right side was convex. There were some soft adhesions between its surface and that of the liver, and some flakes of lymph in the right hypochondrium, with about 3 oz. of serous fluid. The body placed in a bath and the pleura punctured under water, much air was discharged ; 38 oz. measures were collected ; some escaped. The air was found to consist of 33·3 carbonic acid, 4·2 oxygen, 62·5 azote. Taken out of the bath and the thorax opened, 6½ pints of purulent fluid with flakes of lymph were found in the right pleura. The first pint taken out was of sp. gr. 1,015 ; the second of sp. gr. 1,020 ; the third 1,022 ; the fourth 1,030. The pleura was covered with a layer of lymph. The lung was compressed towards the spine. It was attached to the costal pleura superiorly by thick and firm bands ; one of them was of the thickness nearly of the little finger, and within, when divided, three blood-vessels were distinct. On inflating the lungs under water, no perforation was detected. Inflated, after having been carefully dissected out, air passed freely through a small opening in the pleura pulmonalis of the inferior surface of the upper lobe of right lung, close to the thick

15

band. The opening communicated with a superficial cavity capable of holding a walnut, in which a large bronchial tube terminated. Within it there was some thick matter and also a small slough, which lay loose over the perforation, and which in the supine posture, might have prevented the escape of air in the experiment of inflation. This lung, besides the cavity, contained only a few firm, grey tubercles. It partially expanded on forcible inflation. In the superior lobe of the left lung there was a minute cavity capable of holding a hemp-seed; apart from this, and with the exception of many crude miliary tubercles in both lobes, this lung was pretty natural. The pericardium was closely adhering to the heart. No other well marked lesion was detected.

The bandaging of the chest was recommended in this case, and not immediate paracentesis, on the idea that the lungs were more seriously diseased than they were found to be. It was a mistake. Had the operation been performed, life might have been considerably protracted.

Case 8.—Of pneumathorax, operated on with temporary relief.—J. Murphy, ætat. 19; 57th Foot; admitted 9th February, 1837; died 17th May.—This man, whilst at his depôt, shortly after enlistment, 13 months ago, suffered from fever, pneumonia and pleurisy. When transferred to general hospital, his symptoms were cough, dyspnœa, general debility. There was no pain of chest; little expectoration. His chest sounded dull on the right, clear on the left side. There was little change until the 17th March, when he complained of pain in the left side, which inspiration increased. Some relief followed V.S. and the use of diaphoretics. On the 6th April, there was a recurrence of the pain, which was relieved by the same means. On the 27th April, in the evening, the dyspnœa suddenly increased, with acute pain of side. On the 29th, when I first saw him, he was apparently moribund. The dyspnœa was excessive; perspiration profuse. The left side of chest was distended and tympanitic; there was a total absence there of the respiratory sound. A grooved needle was passed into the pleura between the 5th and 6th rib. Some air escaped, followed by a little relief. Two hours after, the difficulty of breathing having increased, a small trocar was introduced. Much air escaped, and the ease afforded was great. The canula, which had been allowed to remain in, covered with lint saturated with oil, was withdrawn on the 30th, a cotton thread having been previously introduced through it. There was a considerable "thin discharge from the chest." On the 1st May, the left side became emphysematous, the emphysema extending towards the neck and groin, with some soreness of throat. The skin was now hot and dry, the pulse rapid and small; the breathing easier. At 3 p.m., the emphysema having increased, it had reached the face and the right side of chest, a trocar was again introduced. About 5 oz. of serum escaped and some air. The canula was left in covered with oiled lint. From this time there was a copious discharge of thin sero-purulent fluid, occasionally as much as 16 oz. in the 24 hours; latterly it was greenish. On the night of the 4th May, during a fit of coughing, the canula was ejected; it was not replaced; the opening was merely covered with oiled silk. The discharge continued. By the 10th the emphysema had almost entirely disappeared. He gradually sank.

Autopsy 50 hours after death. Much emaciated. The left lung was found collapsed. The left pleura contained 8 oz. of purulent fluid and was covered with a dense layer of lymph. An opening into the sac was detected capable of admitting a goose-quill, situated in the inferior lobe and communicating with a small cavity. There were a few excavations in this lung and numerous crude tubercles. The right lung, firmly adhering, contained some small cavities and many tubercles. There were some small ulcers in the lower portion of the ileum.

Of this case I saw less than I could wish ; and was unavoidably absent when the *post mortem* examination was made. The cotton thread, it may be remarked, was introduced to prevent the closure of the artificial orifice, and to allow of the escape of air and fluid, the emphysema which occurred not being anticipated.

Case 9.—Of pneumathorax, with pleuritic effusion, rapidly fatal.—J. Tinan, ætat. 32; 1st Foot; admitted into Fort Clarence, 7th June, 1825 ; died 14th October.— This man was received into the asylum on his return from the West Indies, where his mind had become deranged in 1833, when convalescent from yellow fever. On admission he was sullen, often using foul and abusive language. His health seemed good. After a short time he became less morose ; his conduct more orderly; his conversation tolerably rational. Up to the 8th October he appeared to be in excellent health. Then he looked unwell, yet no symptom of disease, it is stated, could be detected; his pulse was natural ; his breathing free ; there was no cough, and he declared he was quite well. Thus he continued until the evening of the 10th, when his respiration had suddenly become laborious and wheezing; his pulse rapid and very small. Next morning his breathing was somewhat easier; in the evening it was more oppressed, with increased feebleness of pulse. On the 12th he seemed rather better; some viscid mucus was expectorated ; his pulse was stronger. On the 13th all the symptoms were worse, yet he continued to say that he had no pain, no uneasiness. He expired during the night, about 79 hours after the first symptoms of disease had been noticed.

Autopsy 33 hours after death. Nowise emaciated. There was more fluid than usual in the brain. The cavities of the heart were distended with coagulated blood. The left pleura contained a good deal of air, which had no offensive smell, and about 8 oz. of serum, with some loose coagulable lymph. The left lung from compression occupied very little space. It contained several tubercles undergoing softening, and a cavity capable of holding a walnut, which communicated both with the bronchia and the pleura. It was superficial and situated in the lower part of the superior lobe. The substance of the lung, apart from its condensation from compression, was pretty natural. The pleura was very little thickened; a little shreddy lymph was deposited on its costal surface. Both the superior and middle lobe of right lung were partially hepatized and contained softening tubercles and some vomicæ full of a thick matter. The inferior lobe was without tubercles and tolerably sound. A few ulcers were found in the ileum and cœcum. There was much blood in the body, abundance of fat, and the muscles were of good color and no way atrophied.

This case deserved a place in a preceding section—that on tubercular disease masked by insanity. How noteworthy is it that so much disease should have existed in the lungs, not only not indicated by any symptom, but, what is more remarkable, by no emaciation—no deficiency of adipose matter ! The pneumathorax, probably of only four days' duration, seems to have been the immediate cause of death.

Case 10.—Of pneumathorax, with pleuritic effusion, rapidly fatal.—J. Crummay, ætat. 27; 5th Foot; admitted into Regimental Hospital, Malta, 20th December,

1834; died 25th December.—This man was relieved off guard and brought to hospital, having when on duty been suddenly attacked with acute pain of chest and difficulty of breathing. His pulse, it is stated, was tranquil; his skin cool; his tongue clean. V.S. to 28oz., followed by a blister to the right side, the seat of the pain, and a saline aperient with tartar emetic. On the 21st he felt easy but weak; the pulse hurried and small; "respiration free." In the evening there was much abdominal tension, and dyspnœa almost to suffocation; the pulse tremulous. On the 22nd, after an alvine evacuation, there was temporary relief, soon succeeded by great difficulty of breathing. On the following days till he expired, there were lulls and exacerbations, with a rapid increase of weakness and feeling of exhaustion.

Autopsy 13 hours after death. Sub-emaciated. The right side of chest was larger than the left, and tympanitic, as was also the abdomen. On opening into the abdominal cavity, the liver was found displaced; the greater part of it was on the left side of the spine. The diaphragm on the right side was convex, and it pressed on the liver. Punctured under water, a vast quantity of air rushed out. Some of it collected was found to consist of 16 carbonic acid and 84 azote, without any oxygen. The lymphatic vessels, before joining the thoracic duct were large, distended with a transparent colorless fluid. The right pleura, covered with a false membrane, contained 17oz. of serous fluid, with some loose flakes of lymph. The right lung was small, and compressed close to the spine; its lobes were adhering one to the other, and its superior lobe at its apex to the costal pleura. In this lobe there was a small cavity, which communicated with the sac of the pleura by an ulcerated opening large enough to admit a crow-quill; and with the bronchia by a large branch that terminated in it abruptly. This lung contained many tubercles; they abounded most under its pleural lining, where they were most advanced. Its parenchyma was pale, and so condensed from compression that it sank in water. The left lung contained many grey granular tubercles, and one small vomica, full of a thick puruloid fluid; it was generally crepitous.

This patient was described as delicate, and subject to "pulmonary ailment," yet not to the extent to incapacitate him for duty. Had not the small vomica in the right lung penetrated into the pleura, he probably might have continued many a month or even year in tolerable health. It was matter of regret that the pneumathorax was not discovered during life. Had the operation of paracentesis been performed early, considering how much of each lung was in a tolerably healthy state, the result might have been favorable.

Case 11.—Of pneumathorax, operated on with temporary relief.—S. Black, ætat. 27; 3rd Light Dragoons; admitted 23rd July, 1837; died August 15th.—This man was a volunteer to the 3rd Light Dragoons under orders for India. He marched from London to Canterbury, and from thence to Sittingbourn, shortly before admission into the general hospital, where he was brought to be under observation, having been considered by the examining Staff Surgeon unfit for foreign service, it having been ascertained that he had been subject to chronic cough for twelve months past, and some little difficulty of breathing, but not hindering him from doing his duty. Previously in his ordinary health, early in the morning of the 31st July he awoke with a feeling of suffocation, as if about to die; his breathing was spasmodic and most difficult. The orderly officer immediately abstracted a few ounces of blood, which was followed by slight relief. At 9 A.M. he was again in a most distressing state, suffocation threatening; he was propped up in bed; his breathing rapid, short, and difficult; pulse very quick and small; some pyrexia; pain a little to the right of the scrobiculus cordis, increased when he attempted a full inspiration. The lower part of the thorax was somewhat tympanitic, and without distinct respiratory murmur. This side was rather more ample than the left. The heart's action was felt towards the left clavicle. In consultation it was thought advisable to perform the operation of paracentesis. An incision of about two inches was made through the integuments, between the sixth and seventh rib, about half way between the sternum and spine, and through the muscles, with the intention to lay bare the pleura, on the supposition that it would be pressed out. It not being seen, a small trocar was carefully introduced, its point directed upwards. The stilette withdrawn, a little air came out. A long probe introduced, was not stopped till nearly its whole length had entered, showing that the lung had collapsed. Presently, a fit of coughing occurring, a large quantity of air was expelled, also a small quantity of serum. Considerable relief followed. Now, using the probe, its entrance into the pleura was prevented, as if the lung had become re-distended. The canula was left in, covered with oiled lint. On account of the pyrexia, in the evening he was blooded to the extent of 16oz. He passed a tolerable night. On the following day he was lying comparatively low, and his breathing was tolerably easy. A good deal of serum had been discharged. The next day the report was similar. The pulse had greatly abated in quickness. There was much fluid and air discharged, and some air gained admission. The fluid was at first serous; it afterwards became puruloid. On the 5th August night sweats were reported, and some delirium at night. There was little alteration until the 14th, when he was attacked with diarrhœa. He sank with little uneasiness of any kind. After the operation he never required to have his head much raised. His voice though feeble was distinct. The general treatment throughout was directed merely to the relief of the more distressing symptoms.

Autopsy 7 hours after death. Sub-emaciated. The liver was found in its natural situation. There were several large ulcers in the cœcum and transverse colon. The right pleura contained about a pint of puruloid fluid. It extended nearly two inches above the clavicle. The lung on this side was collapsed and contracted towards the spine, to which it adhered. In its superior lobe, its upper part, that in the axillary region, there was a small excavation, capable of holding a cherry. There was an ulcerated opening from it into the sac of the pleura, large enough to receive a goose-quill, and it communicated with the bronchia by a large branch, ulcerated, *projecting within it*, so as to act the part of a valve. The same lobe contained several minute vomicæ, and numerous tubercles softening. In the middle and inferior lobe there were many grey granular tubercles. The left lung was generally and firmly adhering. In its superior lobe there was a considerable excavation, full of a reddish sanies. It contained also two or three small cavities, and numerous tubercles in different stages of progress. The inferior lobe abounded also in tubercles of the same kind. The bronchia and trachea were very red. There was an extensive and deep ulcerated cavity under each chorda vocalis.

This case, like the preceding, is noteworthy, and even more so, for the latency of tubercular disease, and for the direful effects of air accumulating in the pleura. The operation may be considered so far successful that it afforded relief of suffering, some prolongation of life, and, may it not be added, an easy death.

Case 12.—Of pneumathorax, with empyema, etc., rapidly fatal.—F. Aspinall, ætat. 27; 7th F.; admitted into regimental hospital, Malta, 17th January, 1834; died 25th January.—This man, of known intemperate habits, had experienced during the eight years of his service, chiefly in the Mediterranean, attacks of various disease. The last for which he had been under treatment was a slight pain of side with cough. When relieved, he was discharged at his own request and was employed as an orderly. It is stated that no organic disease of the lungs could be discovered either by percussion or auscultation. Only two days later—viz., on the 17th January, he was re-admitted with "fully developed symptoms of tubercular disease of the lungs" and of effusion into the cavity of the chest. His breathing was short, his cough troublesome, expectoration purulent; pulse 110; brown fur on tongue; bowels constipated. Pectoriloquy was perceived on the right side; metallic tinkling on the left. He rapidly sank; expiring on the 25th.

Autopsy 9 hours after death. Both sides of chest were sonorous on percussion : the left was the largest. The stomach unusually large, distended with air and liquid, reached the right iliac region; its pylorus was turned over the cœcum. The diaphragm on the left side was pressed downwards and was tympanitic. Punctured, some air escaped. It had a strong smell of sulphuretted hydrogen. A small portion collected by applying to the opening a vial filled with water, was found to consist chiefly of carbonic acid and azote. The left pleura contained 3 pints of turbid serum mixed with pus; it was lined with a thick layer of granular lymph. The left lung, with the exception of a small portion of its inferior lobe, was collapsed. In its superior lobe there was a small cavity, in which a large bronchial tube terminated, an ulcerated opening, of a size to admit a goose-quill, effecting a communication between it and the sac of the pleura. The same lobe contained many firm grey tubercles scattered through its substance, and a few minute cavities. The inferior lobe was tolerably sound and in part crepitous; it floated in water. The bronchia of this side were very small; and the pulmonary veins, where they entered the heart, unusually small. The right lung filled the cavity of the chest, and was unusually distended with air. Its bronchia were very large, as were also its pulmonary veins; the former were obstructed by pus, as if death had been owing to suffocation, which indeed the symptoms indicated. Its superior lobe contained numerous small vomicæ; the middle lobe many minute grey tubercles; the inferior a small number of the same kind. The trachea was red and its surface granular and slightly ulcerated. A small ulcer was detected close to the chordæ vocales. The valve of the colon was slightly ulcerated, and there was a large ulcer in the cœcum.

In this case, judging from the little accord between the symptoms and the chronic organic disease, it is difficult to avoid the conclusion that the stethoscopic examination referred to was hastily made. The tolerance of so much organic disease as must have existed at the time is remarkable, even allowing for the aversion which soldiers, especially drunkards, have to be in hospital.

Case 13.—Of pneumathorax, preceded by diabetes.—T. Durant, ætat. 18; 41st F.; admitted 22nd December, 1835; died 18th March, 1836.—This man, shortly after enlistment, seven months ago, had an attack of fever followed by emaciation. His ailment was called atrophy. When transferred from the detachment hospital to the general hospital, he was found to labor under diabetes, with great emaciation and general debility. His skin was rough and dry; his appetite inordinate. The only pectoral symptom noticed was a slight tickling cough. Up to the 25th January the quantity of urine voided in the 24 hours varied from 3 to 8 pints. It was found to contain saccharine matter. On the day last mentioned, it is stated that he had " a catarrhal attack," and that he expectorated a large quantity of frothy mucus. A sibilant râle was perceived on the right side, with pectoriloquy. On the 15th February there was some œdema of the right side of face, and of the feet and ankles; and increased expectoration, said to be purulent. His urine now was about 5 pints. Little change occurred until the 21st February, when a sudden pain was experienced in the left hypochondrium. A cavernous râle with gurgling, was perceived in the right subclavian region. Hectic now set in with night sweats; his pulse was 124; his cough short with purulent expectoration. Leeches were applied to the pained part; some relief followed. On the 14th March, the symptoms much the same ; the quantity of urine voided was about 3 pints; it now abounded in urea, without sugar. Though his appetite continued good, and it continued good to the last, the debility increased. He was delirious a few nights before his death. Opium was the principal medicine used; it was given with sulphate of quinine and dilute sulphuric acid. He took at one time two grains thrice a day ; with the increase of the pectoral symptoms it was diminished.

Autopsy 28 hours after death. The diaphragm on the left side was found convex inferiorly. It sounded tympanitic. Punctured, much air escaped from the pleura. The stomach was small; its mucous coat corrugated; its appearance healthy. The investing membrane of each kidney was removed with undue facility. There was no ulceration of the intestines, or any well marked disease of any other of the abdominal viscera. The left pleura contained about 3 pints of milky serum, in which were numerous small, soft, globular masses of lymph. The sides of the sac were lined with a similar substance. The lung on this side was much condensed and its volume reduced. In the lower part of its superior lobe there was a small cavity capable of holding a hazel-nut. It communicated with the pleura by an ulcerated opening and by a narrow sinus with a large bronchial tube. Nearer the apex there was a very large excavation traversed by bands containing blood-vessels. The inferior lobe contained many crude tubercles and some which were softening, and two or three small cavities. In the superior lobe of the right lung there was also a very large cavity and many tubercles. The middle and inferior contained a few small vomicæ. The bronchial glands were much enlarged. The larynx, just below the chordæ vocales, was slightly ulcerated. The heart was small, as if atrophied. It was lying on the right side of the spine.

In this instance complicity of organic lesions is very note-worthy, and also the masking effect in relation to symptoms. Whilst diabetes lasted the pectoral symptoms were as much latent as is occasionally witnessed in cases of advanced phthisis, complicated with insanity. To what extent, it may be asked, were the active functional state of the stomach, the healthy condition of the intestines and the peculiar state of the kidneys (if in diabetes these organs are affected) concerned in the prevention of the distressing symptoms which usually occur on the invasion of pneumathorax ? Many other queries might be proposed, as to the influence of the large excavations in the lungs, the great emaciation, the anæmia, etc.

Case 14.—Of pneumathorax in an advanced stage of phthisis.—J. Lane, ætat. 25; 59th Foot; admitted 24th January, 1837; died 18th June.—This man was taken into hospital on his return from Gibraltar, sent home on account of " pulmonary ailment,'' which began in April, 1836. On admission, he had cough, with difficulty of breathing, and his expectoration was streaked with blood. No morbid sound, it is stated, was perceived in the chest, excepting unusual loudness of the heart's action. In April he experienced a severe pain in his ear, with a purulent discharge, which yielded to a blister. Then night-sweats began, and "bronchial respiration and moist râles" were perceived in the right side. The expectoration was viscid, and still streaked with blood, and occasionally it contained tubercular matter. The symptoms gradually became more decided; gargouillement was heard, followed by pectoriloquy and cavernous respiration in the right lung; the left at the same time giving indications of extensive disease. No mention is made of any acute pain or distressing dyspnœa preceding the fatal termination.

Autopsy 39 hours after death. Exceedingly emaciated. The right side of the chest was larger than the left, more distended, and was tympanitic even over the region of the liver. When the abdomen was opened, the diaphragm on the right side was found convex and very tympanitic; extending downwards beyond the false ribs it was so low as to come in contact with the upper end of the kidney. The greater portion of the right lobe of the liver was on the left side. The stomach was pressed close to the spleen and to the diaphragm. A trocar to which a flaccid bladder was attached, was passed through the distended diaphragm. On withdrawing the stilette within the bladder, air rushed from the pleura and filled the bladder. Its neck was secured by a ligature. 23 measures of this air by lime water were reduced to 20; no further reduction was effected by phosphorus. It extinguished a light. In the right pleura the lung was found collapsed, pressed close to the spine, and almost free from adhesions. The pleura showed no marks of inflammation; it contained 4oz. of serum, but no lymph or pus. In the lung, in its superior lobe, towards the axilla, there was an opening through the pleura pulmonalis capable of admitting the little finger, communicating with a superficial excavation nearly full of thick pus: it was capable of holding a small walnut: irregular sinuses proceeded from it into the substance of the lung. The communication with the bronchia was not detected. This lung abounded in small vomicæ, and in tubercles in different stages of progress. The left lung was similarly diseased. In some places, superficially, it was emphysematous. There was a good deal of thick pus in the bronchia. There were some ulcers in the ileum and cœcum; and some tubercular matter in a fine granular form on the epidydimis of testicle. The right cavities of the heart were distended with crassamentum and fibrinous concretions; the left with coagulated blood alone; no fibrin had separated.

In this case it is probable that the pneumathorax escaped detection during life from unwillingness on the part of the medical officer to subject the patient in the advanced stage of phthisis to a careful examination of the chest. It may also be conjectured that it took place shortly before death. The state of the pleura, free from inflammation, seems in favor of this idea. And, moreover this absence of inflammation, and the presumed time of the perforation of the pleura, may account for there being no acute suffering.

Case 15.—Of pneumathorax, with empyema; operated on with temporary relief.— J. Weston, ætat. 25; 73rd Foot; admitted into regimental hospital, Malta, 24th January, 1822; died 13th February.—This man, it was stated, had an attack of pneumonia in the preceding September, for which he was under treatment in hospital till the 23rd October, when he was sent to an out station for change of air. At this time he was described as delicate, emaciated, and troubled with cough. The cough continuing, and the emaciation increasing, he was re-admitted on the 24th January. He gradually became worse; and, in addition to the other symptoms, he suffered from diarrhœa. On the 11th February the chest on the right side was found protuberant, and sounded tympanitic, without any respiratory murmur; the lips were livid; the respiration hurried and difficult; the pulse very rapid; there was much anxiety. He said he sometimes heard a noise in his chest like that produced by water shaken in a bottle not full. The operation of paracentesis was performed between the 7th and 8th rib. Some air rushed out, followed by about two pints of pus. Immediate relief was obtained. The canula was left in corked. No more fluid passing by it, it was withdrawn the following day. Very little suffering of any kind was experienced during the remaining two days of his life.

Autopsy 10 hours after death. Greatly emaciated. The right side of the chest was protuberant and tympanitic. The liver was a little lower in the abdomen than natural. Some air escaped on opening into the right pleura. The pleura contained about two pints of purulent fluid, with which were mixed flakes of lymph; it was lined with the same. The lung on this side was much compressed. Ulcerated sinuses, two or three in number, were detected, communicating between the sac of the pleura and the bronchia; there was no intermediate excavation. In the superior lobe a tubercular excavation was found, of moderate size, empty and collapsed, lined with a false membrane, and communicating with a large bronchial tube. This lung contained very many grey granular tubercles. So dense was its parenchyma rendered by compression that it sank in water. It was quite free from hepatization. The left lung was of natural appearance externally. It contained one minute abscess, of about the size of a pea, full of a pus-like matter. It abounded in tubercles, all of the granular kind. It bore no marks of inflammation, and was crepitous. The heart was large. Its cavities were distended with coagulated blood. The coagulum was slightly *broken up* in the right ventricle; and in a more marked manner in the left. There were some small ulcers in the lower part of the ileum, and many large ones in the cœcum and colon. Most of them were healing; one was quite healed, and had left a depression, as if there had been no restoration of the mucous coat, the cicatrix being in the cellular; it was covered with a thin epithelium.

The situation of the perforation in this case is noteworthy. Is it not probable that the early attack designated pneumonia was pleuritic, and that the empyema disclosed at the autopsy preceded the pneumathorax? The chief intent of the operation was to give relief, and afford a chance of recovery: when performed, the suffering was great, and death imminent.

Case 16.—Of pneumathorax, with pleuritic effusion.—J. Gilligan, ætat. 29; 73rd Regiment; admitted into regimental hospital, Malta, 10th June, 1833; died 16th August.—This man on admission was under medical treatment for pneumonia. Symptoms of phthisis supervened—viz. : cough with fetid expectoration, dyspnœa, night sweats, a very rapid pulse, much emaciation; there was also œdema of the lower extremities. Examined carefully about a fortnight before his death, a large tubercular excavation was indicated in the superior part of the left lung, with pneumathorax in the right pleura and empyema. The right side was enlarged and tympanitic; and on shaking the trunk a sound was heard as of fluid in air. Though there was considerable difficulty in breathing, it was not of a distressing kind. His death was sudden.

Autopsy 9 hours after death. Very much emaciated. On opening into the abdomen, the diaphragm on the right side was found protruding and tympanitic. Punctured, there was a great rush of air from the pleura. Besides air, the right pleura contained 58 oz. of turbid serum. The whole of its surface was covered with lymph. The lung was much compressed. A small excavation was found in its superior lobe, with an ulcerated opening into the pleura, capable of admitting a goose-quill. In the same lobe there were several cavities of the like kind, and many tubercles. The tubercles were about the size of peas, and of a curd-like consistence. In the middle and inferior lobe there were many similar. In the superior lobe of the left lung there was a very large excavation, and several small cavities and softening tubercles. There were small cavities and tubercles also in the inferior lobe. This lung weighed 2 lbs. Only a small portion, and that in its inferior lobe, was crepitous. The heart was large. It was so displaced as to be almost in contact with the ribs. There were several small pale ulcers in the ileum.

The operation of paracentesis was not thought advisable in this instance, after the detection of the pneumathorax, in consideration of, not so much the advanced stage of the disease, as the circumstance of the dyspnœa not being distressing, and the additional one of there not being the faintest hope of any lasting benefit from it.

Case 17.—Of pneumathorax, suddenly proving fatal.—J. Boyd, ætat. 27; 11th Foot; admitted Nov. 23rd, 1840; died 17th January. This man was taken into hospital on his return from Canada, where two years ago he had an attack of hæmoptysis with pain of chest. Previously his health had been good. From that time he had always been ailing. On admission he had pectoral symptoms, but not so severe as to confine him to bed. They were chiefly cough, with muco-purulent expectoration, dyspnœa, hoarseness, with much uneasiness in the laryngeal region. Only the day before his death he was walking about and anxious to go to his home in Ireland. His death was sudden.

Autopsy 12 hours after. Greatly emaciated. The left side of chest sounded tympanitic. On opening the abdomen, the diaphragm on the left side was found much pressed down, the left lobe of the liver "doubled up," and the stomach displaced almost to the right side of the spine. On puncturing the left pleura a good deal of air escaped. The heart was much displaced towards the right side. The pleura contained 8½ pints of sero-purulent fluid. Its surface was lined with opaque, rough lymph. The lung was greatly compressed. In its superior lobe there were two cavities; one near its apex of moderate size; the other near its centre. This communicated with the sac of the pleura by two small valvular openings. In the same lobe and also in the inferior there were a few small cavities and many crude tubercles. In the right lung there were similar cavities and tubercles. They were mostly confined to the superior lobe. The middle lobe was hepatized, as was also the inferior partially. The trachea was much ulcerated; one of the arytenoid cartilages was laid bare by ulceration, and a small ulcer was found in the under surface of the epiglottis. There were many ulcers in the ileum, cœcum, ascending and transverse colon.

In this case, the stethoscope, it would appear, not having been used, the pneumathorax was not discovered during life. His dyspnœa, though latterly severe, was no more in degree, according to the medical officer in charge, than might be referred to a greatly disorganized state of the lungs.

Case 18.—Of pneumathorax, with empyema.—G. Hicks, ætat. 39; 90th F.; admitted 9th July, 1837; died 26th September.—This man, of 20 years' service, when employed with a recruiting party in London experienced an attack of pulmonary disease, from which, it is stated, he had suffered eight months previously. On admission he was emaciated, had cough, with muco-purulent expectoration, dyspnœa, and pain of chest extending to the shoulders. There was little change reported until the 31st July, when he had an attack resembling ague, which, he said, he had been subject to in the Ionian Islands; it yielded in a few days, taking sulphate of quinine. Again, there was little change noticed until 3rd September, when a hollow sound on percussion was heard in right side of chest. From this date all the symptoms became worse; there were hectic flushes, night sweats and other indications of advanced phthisis. Diarrhœa set in on the 22nd. He gradually sank. No mention is made of any severe suffering.

Autopsy 36 hours after death. Much emaciated. The right side of the chest was tympanitic and more prominent than the left. On opening into the cavity of the abdomen the diaphragm on the right side was found pressed down to the margin of the false ribs, and was tympanitic. When punctured some air escaped. On opening into the chest, the right lung was seen occupying the upper portion of the pleural cavity. A quantity of turbid serum filled the inferior space, and air the superior. The fluid amounted to 3 pints; pus was mixed with it. The lung was firmly adhering and required to be dissected out. There was a large excavation in its superior lobe; one also of considerable size in its inferior, and many small vomicæ in both, with masses of tubercles in different stages of progress. The larger cavity freely communicated with the bronchia; the lower, both with the bronchia and the sac of the pleura. From the situation of the perforation, the air must have passed in, it may be inferred, under the fluid, a circumstance which might have prevented any great influx of air; and the condition of the lung altogether might have conduced to the same, for hardly any of it was pervious to air; where there were no tubercles, there was œdema or hepatization, or a condensation of substance from pressure. The left lung was very much less diseased. There was a small vomica in the superior lobe and clusters of tubercles in it and in the inferior. A small ulcer was detected in the left bronchus and another in the upper part of the œsophagus. A small fibrinous concretion was found in the right ventricle; it was adhering and undergoing *softening*. The ascending portion of the aorta was enlarged and slightly sacculated; the inner coat of the arch and of the thoracic portion was irregularly thickened and partially ossified. The mouths of the great vessels rising from the former were a little contracted; those of many of the intercostals were more so, and some were entirely closed. The liver weighed 4¾ lbs.; its section was nutmeg-like; a portion dried on paper left an oil-stain. The lower part of the ileum was much ulcerated and there were a few ulcers in the cœcum.

In this case the pneumathorax was not discovered during life. "The hollow sound on percussion observed in the right side of chest," should, it might be supposed, have led to its detection; but, unfortunately the staff surgeon in charge of the medical division at this time was little familiar with the signs of thoracic disease, those afforded by auscultation and percussion.

Case 19.—Of pneumathorax, with gangrene of lung, etc.—J. Chisholm, ætat. 30 ; 60th R. ; admitted 22nd June, 1837; died 17th July.—This man was received into hospital on his return from the Mediterranean, from whence he was sent home on account of pulmonary disease, said to have been of four months' duration. On the voyage he had several attacks of hæmoptysis. On admission his cough was distressing, with muco-purulent expectoration, urgent dyspnœa, pain in chest, pectoriloquy in right lung. On the 4th July pectoriloquy was reported in the left lung, its superior lobe, and night sweats. On the 12th diarrhœa set in, after which he rapidly sank.

Autopsy 36 hours after death. Greatly emaciated. The right side of the chest over the inferior lobe of lung sounded tympanitic. On opening into the abdomen, the liver was found in its usual position. On opening into the chest the inferior lobe of the right lung was found compressed by air and an offensive fluid, about 5½ oz. In the superior lobe there was an enormous excavation, occupying the greater part of it and extending into the middle lobe. In the inferior part of the latter there was a cavity which communicated with the sac of the pleura; the opening was circular, about the size of a split pea and not valvular. The walls of both cavities were nearly in a gangrenous state. The inferior lobe, as well as the other lobes, abounded in tubercles. In the superior lobe of the left lung there was a cavity capable of holding an orange; it freely communicated with the bronchia. In the same lobe, and also in the inferior, tubercles abounded in different stages of progress. The base of one of the arytenoid cartilages was partially laid bare by ulceration, and there was a small ulcer in the right chorda vocalis. There were some deep ulcers in the cœcum, and in the ascending and transverse colon. The cartilages of the patellæ were in part sodden and soft, and there was a partial thinning of the cartilage of the head of the humerus.

In this instance the absence of anything like a valve in the cavity communicating with the pleura, may well account for the small quantity of air collected in its sac.

Case 20.—Of pneumathorax, with hydrothorax, etc.—J. M'Loughlin, ætat. 36 ; 6th F. ; admitted 2nd April, 1840; died 15th April.—This man had served many years in India from whence he had been twice sent home on account of "chronic hepatitis." On his last return in June, 1838, he came to Fort Pitt as an invalid. After being a week under observation in hospital, he was discharged "fit for general service, having recovered his health." Subsequently he was employed on the recruiting service, until December, 1839, when he was again taken ill. On re-admission into general hospital, he had a troublesome cough, laborious breathing, œdema of feet, pulse 126 ; relaxed bowels; night sweats; curd-like pellets in his expectoration; pectoriloquy at the superior parts of both lungs. On the 12th December he com- plained of severe and general pain of chest; pulse 130. On the 15th the pain was somewhat less; the tongue dry; sordes on teeth. He died "exhausted;" he was sensible to the last.

Autopsy 19 hours after death. Much emaciated. The diaphragm on the left side was found protruding into the abdominal cavity, and was tympanitic. On puncturing an intercostal space on this side, much air rushed out. The pleura contained 40 oz. of serum with some loose flakes of lymph; there was no deposition of lymph on its surface; the lung was much compressed. When water was poured into the pleura and the lung blown into, using a bellows, there was an escape of air from the inferior lobe, through an aperture of a sinus—a narrow ulcerated cavity—extending beneath pulmonary pleura. A large excavation was found in the superior lobe, and in it and in the inferior were many vomicæ and softening tubercles. The right pleura contained 12 oz. of serum, somewhat turbid from shreddy lymph suspended in it. In the superior lobe of the right lung there was a large cavity and many vomicæ and softening tubercles. Vomicæ and tubercles occurred also in the middle lobe, and many clustered tubercles in the inferior. There was a small ulcer at the base of the right arytenoid cartilage. There were many ulcers in the ileum and large intestines. 14 oz. of serum were contained in the cavity of the abdomen. The liver weighed 4 lbs.; its section was nutmeg-like.

In this case pneumathorax was not detected during life; it probably took place shortly before death, about the 12th. Considering the state of the lungs and of the liver, as ascertained after death, is it not probable that the former were more the seat of the disease than the latter when in India?

Case 21.—Of pneumathorax, with advanced phthisis.—J. Beauland, ætat. 25; 51st F.; admitted 1st June, 1837; died 14th July.—This man, of two years' service, about 7 months ago became unfit for duty from pain of chest, with cough. When transferred to general hospital, he had in addition dyspnœa with copious fetid expectoration. There was little change until the 17th June, when he began to improve. Four days before his chest had been examined; the right lung appeared to be normal; in the superior lobe of the left lung, the respiratory murmur was hardly audible. It is stated that he went on improving; the cough having ceased, his expectoration greatly diminished, and that he was gradually gaining strength and flesh. On the 12th, at the morning visit, there was no unusual symptom. At the evening visit a great change was found to have taken place. He had severe pain in the left hypochondrium, extending upwards and downwards; a troublesome cough, profuse expectoration; urgent thirst; pulse 115, not full; flushed face. A very strong cavernous râle was perceived over an extensive surface in the left lateral and mammary regions, with a clear sound on percussion in the same regions; "the right lung normal." The next morning the symptoms were less severe. During the day the patient was reported to be in "a promising condition." Towards midnight his breathing became laborious, his cough urgent, until about 5 a.m., when he said he was better. At 8 a.m. he expired, dying rather suddenly.

Autopsy 28 hours after death. Sub-emaciated. The left side of chest, its lower portion, tympanitic. Opening into the abdomen, the diaphragm was seen nearly in its usual position. The sternum removed, the left lung, with the exception of its inferior one third, was found adhering. The pleura contained some air and about 5 oz. of purulent fluid. The lung was compressed upwards and towards the mediastinum. In its superior lobe there was a cavity of irregular form, with several sinuses, freely communicating with the bronchia. A perforation was detected in its lower part into the pleura, large enough to admit the end of the little finger. In the same lobe higher, there was a very large excavation. The lung as a whole was an extraordinary mass of disease; scarcely any part of it was without cavities and vomicæ. The substance of the right lung was tolerably natural and crepitous. In its superior lobe there were only a few small vomicæ, and in its middle and inferior only a few clustered tubercles. The bronchia and the lower part of the trachea were full of a glairy mucus. There was an ulcerated cavity in the left chorda vocalis. The upper portion of the trachea was granular. There were a few ulcers in the ileum; and some large ones in the cœcum and in the ascending and transverse colon.

The little apparent connection as regards severity between the organic lesions and the symptoms is very noteworthy; and especially the improvement for a while and its interruption, so soon ending in death. Was that sudden interruption owing to the perforation of the pleura?

Case 22.—Of pneumathorax, with complicated organic lesions.—J. Keeffe, ætat. 33; 46th F.; admitted 2nd March, 1839; died 27th March.—This man's illness began at Gibraltar in August last, and has continued ever since. On admission, shortly after landing, he was found to be laboring under well marked symptoms of advanced phthisis. Pectoriloquy was shortly detected in the right lung. During the last fortnight of his life he was subject to night sweats and diarrhœa. Shortly before death his intellect, it is stated, had become confused.

Autopsy 11 hours after death. Greatly emaciated. The right side of chest sounded tympanitic. The right pleura contained some air and about 6 oz. of serum, compressing moderately the lung. In the anterior surface of the superior lobe of the right lung two ulcerated openings were found, from $\frac{1}{10}$th to $\frac{2}{10}$ths of an inch in diameter, each leading to a small cavity in the parenchyma, through which, it was inferred, the air had found a passage into the pleura. Higher in the same lobe there was a large cavity and many softening tubercles; tubercles abounded also in the middle and inferior lobe. The left lung was generally crepitous; it contained many tubercles and two small cavities. In the right ventricle there was some cruor and several small rounded fibrinous masses, externally pretty firm, softening within and containing a reddish puruloid fluid. The aorta was enlarged; its inner coat thickened throughout; the mouths of the intercostal arteries were contracted; the cœliac at its origin was so even in a higher degree. The spleen was about twice its natural size. There were several ulcers in the cœcum. In the prostrate there was a small cavity. The cartilage of the left patella towards its inner margin was soft, depressed and shreddy.

The variety of lesions in this case is noteworthy. There is no mention of any acute suffering, nor of severe dyspnœa. The pneumathorax, which was slight, probably occurred only shortly before death; it was not detected during life.

Case 23.—Of pneumathorax, with comparatively little disease of lungs.—F. M'Pharlane, ætat. 26; 79th F.; admitted 5th Nov. 1835; died 31st December.— This man had experienced hæmoptysis in Canada in June, and was sent home for change of climate. On admission he had some dyspnœa with cough and expectoration, and a constant pain of chest. His pulse was 80; appetite good; his chest sounded clear; and, excepting under the right clavicle, the respiratory sound was natural, there "it was crepitating with strong bronchophony." There was little change until the 20th November, when severe pain of right side was experienced, which abated after treatment. On the 9th December there was a recurrence of hæmoptysis in a slight degree. On the 15th of the same month he had severe pain under the right clavicle, said to have been relieved by a blister, his cough and dyspnœa continuing. On the 23rd there was an aggravation of all the symptoms. Again some relief of pain followed the application of a blister. On the 26th the respiration was described as easier. On the following day the dyspnœa suddenly became very urgent, with lividity of face, cold extremities and an almost imperceptible pulse. A little relief was afforded by the use of antispasmodics and warm applications. On the 30th there was a return of all the distressing symptoms, which lasted a few hours ; when these somewhat abated, he became hot and restless. Another exacerbation, and especially of the dyspnœa, preceded his death, on the following day.

Autopsy 28 hours after death. Sub-emaciated. The right side of chest was more prominent than the left. On opening into it, much air escaped. The right lung was collapsed and compressed ; the heart was pressed unusually to the left. The pleura contained about half a pint of serum with flakes of lymph ; its surface had a very thin coating of lymph. A considerable ulcerated opening was detected in the pulmonary pleura ; it communicated with a small cavity—a sinus—situated in the lateral part of the superior lobe, and that by a minute aperture with a cavity in the same lobe, of a size capable of holding a hazel-nut ; a bronchial tube terminated in it. A few crude tubercles were found in this lobe and also in the superior lobe of the left lung. The lungs otherwise were pretty natural. No well marked lesions were found in the other viscera.

It was a matter of regret that the pneumathorax, which, probably, was the immediate cause of death, was not detected during life : it was not even suspected. The weather was cold ; and, in consequence, it was said, the chest latterly was not examined. The operation of paracentesis might have at least afforded relief of suffering, and probably a prolongation of life. The case was a favorable one for its trial, so much of both lungs being pervious to air and in a tolerably healthy state. The intermitting character of the symptoms suggested the idea that the occasional lull, or relief, might have resulted from a partial absorption of the air, thereby diminishing its noxious pressure.

Case 24.—Of pneumathorax, with pleuritic effusion.—J. Duffy, ætat. 40; 74th Regiment; admitted 11th August, 1838 ; died 22nd August.—This man, of 20 years' service, the last five in the West Indies, from whence he is just returned, is stated to have been laboring under pulmonary disease since April, 1837, and sent home invalided in consequence. On admission he was much emaciated; had pain in the left side of chest, with cough and muco-purulent expectoration. There was a small tumor on the sternum, which dilated on inspiration. No marked change was reported to have taken place till within two days of his death, when he had occasional rigors, followed by cold sweats. The death was said to have been sudden and unexpected.

Autopsy 9 hours after death. Sub-emaciated. The left side of chest tympanitic. On opening into the cavity of the abdomen, the diaphragm on the left side was found pressed down, but to no great extent. On exposing the costal pleura on the same side, between the sixth and seventh rib, it was pressed out, and was tympanitic.

Punctured, some air escaped. 57oz. of turbid serum* were contained in the pleura. The lung adhering to the side by several thick long bands, was greatly compressed; it was destitute of air; in its superior lobe there was a collapsed excavation, lined with false membrane; a large bronchial tube terminated in it. Many granular tubercles were scattered through both its lobes. Some of them were softening; these were about the size of cherry stones; two such were situated immediately under the pleura pulmonalis, raising that membrane about a quarter of an inch; air forced into the trachea, escaped close to one of them by an extremely small aperture, so small that it could not be demonstrated by the scalpel and probe: the inference was that the aperture extended from the pleura into a bronchial tube, and that, owing to the covering of lymph, it escaped detection. The right lung partially adhered; it was very voluminous, contained much air, and did not collapse. There were several small vomicæ full of thick matter in its superior lobe, and many tubercles, some of them softening. In the middle and inferior lobe there were many granular tubercles. The small tumor in the sternum was found to be composed of a curd-like matter, differing little from softened tubercle. The cavity of the abdomen contained 30oz. of a straw-colored fluid.† The liver weighed 4lbs.; it contained much blood. There were a few small ulcers in the sigmoid flexure of the colon, and some large ulcers red and congested, in the rectum. He had been subject to tenesmus. There was a softening and partial atrophy of the cartilage of the patellæ.

The record of the symptoms in this case was very brief and imperfect. No examination of the chest was made during life; and consequently none of the principal lesions were detected. It may be inferred that there was little acute suffering arresting attention.

Case 25.—Of pneumathorax (double), with complicated organic lesions.—T. Godfrey, ætat. 26; 24th Foot; admitted into Fort Clarence, 16th July, 1839; died 24th January.—This man, of delicate frame, was twice in hospital in Canada for bowel complaint. Whilst recovering from an attack of this kind in February, 1838, he had an epileptic fit, followed by furious madness, into which, after amendment, he thrice relapsed. He was admitted into the asylum with amentia. Towards the end of August, as his mind improved, pulmonary disease became developed. On the 19th November there were decided symptoms of phthisis: resonance of voice was perceived under both clavicles. On the 6th December pectoriloquy was stated to be distinct on each side: "thick tubercular matter" was then expectorated. On the 19th he was fast sinking; the signs the same, with the addition of hectic. During the last month his death was daily expected; there was little action; a great languor of functions approaching the hybernating state. During the entire period that he was in the asylum, his stomach was very irritable, vomiting the greater part of his food. The bowels were frequently relaxed. A day or two before the fatal event, he experienced "a pleuritic attack" of right side, for which leeches were applied.

Autopsy 27 hours after death. Greatly emaciated. Both sides of chest sounded

* This fluid agitated with common air, gave off pretty much gas. Under the microscope it exhibited many pus-like globules of somewhat irregular form, and many granules.

† Put aside, after two hours, it was found coagulated. The coagulum was pretty firm, semi-transparent, moderately contracted, and surrounded by serum. Under the microscope it exhibited an interlacement of dotted filaments. The serum agitated in the pneumatic bottle gave off pretty much air.

tympanitic. The calvaria was very thin. Much fluid was found in the cellular tissue of the pia mater, in all the ventricles, aud at the base of the brain. The walls of the fourth ventricle were unusually soft. On opening into the abdomen, the diaphragm on each side was found lower than usual and tympanitic. There was air in both pleuræ: most in the left. The left lung was collapsed. It was covered with a delicate false membrane, as was also the costal pleura. In the sac of the pleura there was a little turbid fluid, about an ounce and a half. In the lung, in its superior lobe, there was a large excavation; it communicated freely with the pleura, by an ulcerated opening, not valvular, large enough to admit a goose-quill. There were several smaller cavities in this and in the inferior lobe, and numerous tubercles in different stages of progress. The substance of the lung was more or less indurated. The right pleura contained 7oz. of serous fluid. The lung on this side was partially collapsed; it was free from adhesions; nor was there any false membrane on the pleura. In the superior lobe, at its apex, there was an irregular cavity, capable of holding a large walnut; it communicated with the pleura by two considerable ulcerated openings, not distinctly valvular. All three lobes contained tubercles: those in the superior and middle lobes were undergoing softening; in the inferior they were less advanced. The bronchi, trachea, and larynx were severely ulcerated. One of the cartilaginous rings of the trachea was laid bare. The under surface of the epiglottis and the angle of the vocal chords also were ulcerated. Ulcers were found in the stomach, duodenum, jejunum, ileum, and colon. Many of them were deep and extensive; those of the stomach varied in size from that of a sixpence to that of a split pea. There was a deep ulcer in the upper part of the appendicula vermiformis. The pericardium contained 3oz. of transparent serum. There was coagulated blood with fibrinous concretion in the right cavities of the heart. In the right ventricle, entangled amongst and firmly adhering to the columnæ carneæ, were little masses of fibrin more or less rounded, pretty firm externally, softening within, something like a boiled pea in its rind.

This case is noteworthy both for the great variety of organic lesions, and more especially for the double pneumathorax, and the ulcerated state of the primæ viæ, including the stomach. May it not be inferred that air escaped first into the left pleura, and only shortly before death into the right? The apathetic state of the patient so long before death is remarkable. Was it owing to the great variety of the lesions, and the great debility and wasting—a wasting of the blood as well as of the solid tissues—the effect of long-continued disease?

Case 26.—Pneumathorax, without tuberculated lungs, with abscess in liver penetrating into the lung.—J. Tavron, ætat. 31; 7th R.F.; admitted into regimental hospital, Malta, 15th September, 1831; died 28th January, 1832.—According to the report of the assistant-surgeon, who had charge of the case, this man on admission into hospital was laboring under catarrh. The disease, it is stated, gradually increased, resisting varied treatment, and at last assumed "the character of phthisis." During his illness he had one or two severe attacks of diarrhœa; during the last fortnight his bowels had been regular, and the night sweats, which previously had been great, had ceased. He expectorated at one time a considerable quantity of blood. The expectoration latterly was copious, with an odor said to be like that of "old beer." Till the day of his death his appetite continued good.

Autopsy 4 hours after death. Excessively emaciated. The right side of chest tympanitic. On puncturing the right pleura, a taper held near was extinguished by the air which rushed out. It had a most offensive smell. The plural cavity contained about three pints of brown, turbid, fetid fluid. It was lined with a layer of coagulable lymph. The lung adhered in some places to the costal pleura, and generally *apparently* to the diaphragmatic. The inferior lobe was very much diseased and ulcerated. On careful examination it was found to communicate with the pleura, and through an ulcerated opening in the diaphragm with a large abscess in the superior part of the liver. The superior and middle lobes were condensed, but did not seem materially diseased. No tubercles were found in them, nor in the inferior. A long probe introduced into the trachea passed into the pleura, through an ulcerated opening of a valvular kind in the inferior lobe. The abscess in the liver had a dense, almost cartilaginous-like sac. It contained a curd-like matter, which, it was conjectured, might have owed its origin to an hydatid. The substance of the liver generally was pretty natural. The gall-bladder was distended with greenish bile. The left lung, rather more distended with air than usual, was crepitous throughout. It contained no tubercles or cavities. Comparing its bronchi and those of the right lung, there was a marked difference of size, those of the right were so much smaller and compressed. There were some cicatrices of old ulcers in the cœcum. The appendix vermiformis was obstructed midway; a bristle could not be passed through the stricture. The peritoneal coat thereabout was unusually thick. The spleen was about twice its natural size, and nearly of the firmness of liver.

None of the more important lesions in this case were discovered during life, owing, no doubt, to the omission of a careful scrutinizing examination.

In perusing these cases one cannot but be struck by certain symptoms mostly in common, such as the distressing dyspnœa, the sharp pain—both of sudden occurrence—the greatly accelerated and feeble pulse, the cold sweats—these most strongly marked in the acute cases. All of these symptoms, with certain morbid appearances commonly found on the *post mortem* examination, such as the effusions into the serous cavities and cellular tissue, seem to be referrible to that which gives a name to the disease, itself generally an epiphenomenon—viz.: the escape of air into the pleura, and its accumulation there, making pressure on the lung, diaphragm, heart, great blood vessels, and some of the principal nerves. And this pressure, it is easy to imagine, and the facts seem to bear out the conjecture, cannot but be powerfully operative, conducing to the disturbance of the functions of organs, and the production of other effusions from the oppressed circulation.

Further, in reading these cases we find a marked difference in the nature and quality of the contents of the pleura into which the air has found admission: 1, air alone; 2, air and serum; 3, air and pus; 4, air and offensive pus, more or less putrid. Do not these differences point to differences as to the time of duration of the malady, and the kind of communication established between the lung and the pleura? Does not the presence of air alone in the cavity denote a very recent attack; on the contrary does not the accompaniment of much serum with lymph denote one of longer duration; and longer still, if in place of serum there be pus, and that pus putrid? Inferences, and somewhat of the same kind, seem to be deducible from the nature of the air. It appears to be well established that all the gases concerned in pneumathorax may be absorbed, and some more readily than others, by the membrane with which they are in contact— oxygen and carbonic acid also more readily than azote.* Consequently the more recent the attack, the larger should be the proportion of oxygen; the longer the time from its invasion, the greater should be the proportion of azote. And, may not the power which the membranes have to absorb air help in the more chronic cases to account for the mitigation of symptoms, which even in the worst is occasionally witnessed?

Another circumstance which can hardly fail arresting attention is the variety noticeable in the opening, the perforation, admitting the air into the pleura—in some instances very small; in others large; in some connected with a valvular structure allowing air to pass, but preventing its return; in others without such a structure, and permitting the air not only to enter but also freely to pass out. These differences hardly need comment as to their influence on the amount of distention, and the degree of severity of the symptoms arising from distension.

The vast amount of organic disease, and that various, and of various organs, occurring in so many of the cases, accompanied with comparatively little suffering or complaint of pain, is remarkable, and confirmatory of the opinions before expressed, that complicity of lesions has a masking effect, and that with oppressed respiration there may be accumulation of carbonic acid in the blood, exercising an anodyne, an anesthesic influence on the nervous system.

Relative to the treatment of pneumathorax I shall restrict myself to a very few remarks. I believe it may be laid down

---

* See the Author's Researches, Anat. and Physiol., i. 257, et seq.

as a principle, that each case requires special consideration, and, it may be, peculiar management. When the distension from accumulated air is great, threatening the extinction of life, the propriety of an operation cannot be questioned: the operation is sure to afford immediate relief, with a chance of a considerable prolongation of life. I have put on record in a former work* an instance in which these results were happily obtained ; the patient surviving the operation from the 13th May to the 29th July, and a good part of that time in a state of ease. On the contrary, if the symptoms are not distressing, if there be but little distension, then, I believe, it is better not to interfere, trusting rather to the powers of the system to check by absorption accumulation of the distending air, than to attempt its partial removal—for generally it can only be partial—by an operation. It is right to keep in mind that in operating a danger is always incurred of admitting atmospheric air, and that undiluted, directly into the pleura, with an aggravating effect in the way of exciting inflammatory action in the pleura, and putridity of its contents. And, further, and most of all it should be remembered, that, as to a permanent cure, the vast majority of the cases are hopeless— these being engrafted on tubercular disease, of which the special lesion, the pneumathorax, as already intimated, is merely an accident. And, viewed in this light, the general treatment indicated is the same as that for pulmonary consumption.

In considering the origin of pneumathorax, I have not thought it necessary to discuss the question whether air—*the air*—is not sometimes secreted, as it is presumed to be in the air-bladder of fishes ; nor is it now my intention to enter upon it, the source of the air in all the preceding cases being so obvious ; and it being a rule in science not to seek for another cause when the cause assigned is sufficient to account for the phenomenon.

* Op. cit., i. 249.

CHAPTER VII.

ON EMPYEMA, HYDROTHORAX, PERICARDITIS.

Remarks on their unfrequency.—Connection of Empyema and Hydrothorax with Tubercles.—Peculiarities from complications.—Illustrative cases with comments. – Statistics of Pericarditis —Cases of.—Some general remarks on these several diseases, as to origin, pathology and treatment.

EMPYEMA, judging from my experience, is comparatively of rare occurrence amongst British troops. The same remark applies to hydrothorax and pericarditis. Neither of them has a place in the nomenclature of army diseases ; carditis is indeed to be found in the list, and pericarditis has probably commonly been returned under that designation.

Empyema and hydrothorax, like pneumathorax hardly deserve to be ranked amongst idiopathic diseases, being rather epiphenomena, the results, the consequences of inflammation. Moreover, like pneumathorax, they are almost invariably complicated with other affections, especially with tubercles and thereby rendered often obscure and apt to escape detection. Of the total number of fatal cases of which I have notes—viz., 22, tubercles were detected in 12 ; of the other ten, 2 were the sequelæ of measles ; the remaining 8 followed fevers contracted in a warm climate, and dysentery,—both, especially the latter, notorious for impairing and debilitating the constitution.

Of the whole number, with the exception of the three of hydrothorax, the age of the men was little advanced, the average of the whole being but 22 years ; 9 were of the age of 20 and under ; 4 were from 21 to 26 ; 5 from 29 to 48. This circumstance of age is in accordance with their complications, and both together seem to be strongly confirmatory of a pre-existing low, feeble state of vitality.

Owing to the complications, almost every case exhibited well marked peculiarities. On this account I shall give most of them and with some minuteness of detail. This seems advisable, for the same reason as that before assigned under the head " of " tubercular disease rendered latent by co-existence with other organic disease." The human body out of health may aptly enough be compared to a machine out of order. Now, if we fix our attention on the latter, how very different shall we find the derangement of its action, if instead of one part being injured, many parts are injured; and these in various degrees and diverse manners! If this be true of the machine of human invention, how emphatically is it true of the human machine, so vastly more complex in construction and delicate in structure.

1. OF EMPYEMA.—Of the cases of empyema the following are all I have collected with the exception of four, these the least remarkable.

Case 1.—Of empyema, with tuberculated lungs.—G. Bull, ætat. 30; 60th R., admitted 23rd May, 1836; died June 27.—This man had been under treatment in Malta, from whence he is just returned, for fistula in ano in January last. He is now laboring under dyspnœa with a troublesome cough, difficult expectoration, and pain of chest increased by a full inspiration. The heart is felt beating on the right side of the chest; the left side is enlarged and sounds dull; respiration there is inaudible; he lies always on the left side. The operation of paracentesis was proposed, but was not performed, he objecting; and it was not urged as his general health was tolerable; his appetite pretty good; his strength sufficient to allow of his rising and walking about. Between the 30th May and his death, there were occasional febrile paroxysms, sometimes accompanied with purging. Latterly his dyspnœa and cough were more severe. The night before his death, he experienced a sharp febrile fit, followed by copious sweating. In the morning of the 27th June he was oppressed by orthopnœa; his countenance was livid; his extremities growing cold. The operation was again proposed, as affording the only means of relief; but his consent could not be obtained. He expired at 2 p.m.

Autopsy 48 hours after death. Much emaciated. On opening into the abdomen the diaphragm on the left side was found very convex, pressing down the stomach, pancreas and spleen; a considerable portion of the pancreas lay on the right side. On removing the sternum the heart was seen entirely on the right side. The pericardium contained 2 oz. of serum. In the left pleura there were 8 pints of purulent serum; above, the fluid was nearly transparent; towards the bottom it was opaque, differing little in appearance from pus of an abscess, and was proved to be pus by the optical test. There was much lymph deposited on the pleura, and much also mixed with the fluid contents. The false membrane was in some places soft; in others of almost cartilaginous firmness. The lung adhered closely to the spine, and was much condensed by compression. In its superior lobe, at its apex, there were two small tubercular excavations with ulcerated openings into the sac of the pleura, and a pretty large bronchial tube terminated in each of them. The parenchyma of this lung exhibited no other lesion, for though condensed it did not appear diseased. The superior lobe of right lung was in part œdematous. This lobe and the others contained many granular tubercles. The tissue surrounding each tubercle was pale. A small ulcer was detected just below the left inferior vocal chord. There were adhesions between the colon and liver, and the left lobe of the latter and the diaphragm. There was a small ulcer in the jejunum, many in the lower ileum and one in the cœcum. The mesenteric glands were much enlarged. Some of the lacteals in the mesentery were distended with a whitish matter, as were also the villi of the jejunum, and in consequence were very conspicuous. The thoracic duct was large but empty. The left testicle, somewhat enlarged, contained a tubercle about the size of a small bean, consisting of a cheese-like matter; its two tunics were adhering and some lymph was effused into the cellular tissue of the scrotum.

Is it not probable that pneumathorax in this case preceded the empyema? The openings from the lung into the pleura suggest the query. It is easy to conceive that as the unelastic fluid increased, the elastic might diminish, and by absorption. No doubt, could assent to an operation have been obtained, the life of the patient might have been protracted. During life the disease of the testicle was not known. As no complaint was made by the patient, it may be inferred that the tubercle in its indolent state not having excited inflammation in the part, occasioned no pain.

Case 2.—Of empyema, with tuberculated lung, relieved for a time by an operation. —J. Thornley, ætat. 22; 8th F.; admitted 7th October, 1836; died Jan. 30th, 1837. —Of one year and nine months' service; the last twelve in Jamaica, from whence he is just returned, laboring under pulmonary disease, which began shortly after enlisting, and was attributed to "cold." His symptoms now are hoarseness, cough, muco-purulent expectoration, dyspnœa, pain of left side and in the region of the heart; decubitus always on the left side; a circumscribed flush of cheek; night sweats; the left side of chest more capacious than the right; sounds dull; absence of respiratory murmur except faintly posteriorly close to the spine, and anteriorly a little below the clavicle; the heart's action regular, but its impulse most evident on the right of the ensiform cartilage; the tongue clean; the bowels regular. The right lung seemingly free from disease. On the 16th October the operation of paracentesis was performed; 16oz. of greenish fluid were evacuated; a tent was introduced and a bandage applied to the chest. His breathing, which was before difficult and hurried, was relieved. On the 23rd, the operation was repeated; now, the 6th rib was perforated, about its middle, and a canula introduced and allowed to remain in. 7½ oz. of a similarly colored fluid was discharged. He felt much relieved. It is stated that every day after the last operation, a large quantity of serum escaped by the canula, and this for a considerable time. A month after he was much improved, his breathing very much easier; his appetite increased; also his strength; he was able to walk about the ward. The discharge now averaged little more than an ounce *per diem*. Now, there was a recurrence of the pain of chest, followed in a few days by a rather copious discharge of puruloid fluid mixed with a little air. All the symptoms became worse, the discharge profuse and very fetid, with hectic fever and night sweats. He was conscious to the last. On the 13th December, seven weeks after the perforation of the rib, a small circle of necrosed bone came away.

Autopsy 36 hours after death. Greatly emaciated. Nails much hooked. The left side of chest somewhat smaller than the right, as if from contraction; the former sounded dull; the latter resonant. The left pleura contained 2¼ pints of *puruloid* fluid. The pleura was covered with a thick false membrane, granular and red as if organised, and vascular. The lung was greatly compressed and was bound down firmly close to the spine. Its superior lobe contained many firm, granular tubercles, and one small cavity capable of holding a hazel-nut. The substance of the lung was dark; it contained no air. The right lung was voluminous, but not heavy; it did not collapse. In its superior lobe there were many granular tubercles. Its middle and inferior lobe were somewhat œdematous and of a dark color. The left bronchia were very small and pale. The trachea and larynx were also pale. The right chorda vocalis was bare and partially destroyed by ulceration. The mesenteric glands were much enlarged; some were of the size of walnuts and contained a central cavity in which was a puruloid fluid. There were many small ulcers and granular tubercles in the lower part of the ileum. There was a partial softening of the cartilages of the knee-joints, and a partial loss of substance of the lining cartilage of each acetabulum.

This case at one time, after the second operation, was very promising, and great hope was entertained of a recovery until another attack of inflammation of the pleura occurred. Had there been an absence of turbercles and of that tendency to inflammation, the common accompaniment of tuberculosis, the hope might have been realised. Paracentesis by perforating a rib, it need hardly be remarked, is as old as the time of Hippocrates. Its chief advantage is that the opening obtained by it is so easily closed.

Case 3.—Of empyema, complicated, with tubercles of lungs and gangrene of pleura; paracentesis performed.—W. M'Clintock, ætat. 19; 10th Foot; admitted 15th May, 1823; died 20th July.—This young soldier, it is stated, had an attack of pneumonia in March, which was subdued by V.S. often repeated, etc., leaving him very feeble; and followed by fever of the typhoid type in April. After about three weeks, when seemingly convalescent, œdematous swelling occurred in the feet and ankles. Transferred from regimental hospital, on admission into general hospital his symptoms were chiefly the following: cough, with scanty expectoration; pain of chest; decubitus solely on left side; hot skin; thirst; nightly exacerbations and sweats; pulse 120; bowels loose; moreover he was very pale, feeble, and emaciated; his appetite was good. Carefully examined on the 18th May, the left side of chest was found dull on percussion, and œdematous. On the 20th paracentesis was performed; about 15oz. of pus were drawn off, with some immediate relief. During the following month there was no favorable change, but the contrary; he became more emaciated and debilitated. Daily there was a discharge from the chest, which latterly became very fetid. On the 25th June a small fluctuating red tumor was noticed on the left side, between the fifth and sixth ribs; punctured, about 1lb. of fetid fluid was discharged. On the 20th July it is stated that the discharge by the first opening had continued, and in considerable quantity, and always excessively fetid, excepting last week that it had become less in amount. Bed-sores now occurred in those parts most subject to pressure, and two of the ribs, their convex portions, owing to ulceration of the skin, were laid bare. His appetite to the last continued good; his bowels unaffected. Insensibility, with slow and convulsive breathing, preceded death.

Autopsy 18 hours after death. Excessively emaciated; feet and legs œdematous. The left pleura of a dark color, and in some places almost black, as if gangrenous; was much thickened, and almost of cartilaginous hardness; it contained four pints of fetid purulent fluid. The lung on this side was greatly compressed, and in part hepatized, as indicated by its ready friability under pressure; there were dispersed through it a few minute, grey, translucent tubercles. Similar tubercles were found in the right lung; otherwise it was pretty healthy. Its air-cells were rather large.* The stomach was nearly empty, and was very small and contracted. No disease was detected in any of the abdominal viscera.

This case was of the most unpromising kind at the time of the operation, the powers of the constitution were so reduced. The goodness of the appetite to the last is a noteworthy circumstance in connexion with the very sound state of the stomach and intestines. The quality of the air found in the right lung after death may, perhaps, account for the insensibility that preceded by some hours that event.

Case 4.—Of empyema, with tuberculated lungs, enlarged liver, and ascites.—D. Cavanagh, ætat. 26; 65th Foot; admitted January 26, 1836; died November 23.— This man, of five years' service, had during the last four years three attacks of pulmonary disease. The last occurred in December, 1835, and was of the three the most severe; he was blooded largely, with merely mitigation of symptoms. When admitted into general hospital, transferred from the detachment hospital, his symptoms were the following: obtuse pain in the upper and lateral portion of thorax, most of right side, impeding respiration; pain also in right hypochondrium, extending to the shoulder; inability to lie on his left side without increase of pain and dyspnœa; dry cough; tongue clean; appetite indifferent; pulse firm; bowels regular. His aspect, it is added, was unhealthy. Two days later, rigors were reported. On the 1st Feb. it is stated that no respiratory murmur was audible in the right lung, and that that side measured more by an inch and a half than the left, and was dull on percussion. On the 7th February paracentesis was performed between the fifth and sixth rib, about midway between the sternum and spine, and 10oz. of well-conditioned pus were evacuated. On the 9th the trochar was again introduced, the wound having closed; 17oz. of pus were discharged. On the 13th, 16oz. more came away. On the 14th the respiratory murmur was heard below the right mamilla. Up to the 15th there was improvement, the discharge continuing profuse through a valvular opening. On the 22nd there was a discharge of 2oz. of fetid pus. There was now some hectic, with profuse perspirations and emaciation; his appetite moderate. On the 28th the dyspnœa and cough were reported to be easier; the emaciation continuing; the quantity of purulent discharge variable; the right side contracting. In March and the succeeding months there was occasional griping and looseness of bowels, and occasional pain in epigastrium, followed by tumefaction of abdomen. In the beginning of September there was some tenderness of abdomen on pressure; diarrhœa, with tormina and tenesmus. On the 23rd October it was stated that his expectoration was occasionally mixed with blood, that the swelling of the abdomen had increased, and that there was fluctuation. Paracentesis was now performed; 7 quarts of serum were drawn off; the urine scanty, and of high color. On the 6th November the abdomen was again much distended; the operation was repeated, and again on the 19th, 10¼ and 7½ quarts of serum were drawn off. A discharge of pus from 2 to 4oz. daily continued from the chest until the 20th November, when it had nearly ceased.

* Some air collected from them in the superior lobe was found to consist of 10 carbonic acid, 3 oxygen, 87 azote.

Three days before death he became nearly comatose, and the abdomen at the same time tympanitic. The medicines used were conium, quinine, etc., iodine-ointment, etc. Autopsy 32 hours after death. Greatly emaciated. The abdominal cavity contained 11 pints of clear serum. The liver, of the color of unbleached wax, was very voluminous; it weighed 5lbs., and a portion of it dried yielded pretty much oily exudation. The pancreas, excepting its head, was small; it was very firm. The spleen was large, and of firm consistence. The kidneys natural. The mesenteric glands were enlarged, and softening in their centres. Some ulcers were found in the cœcum. The right pleura contained about a pint of pus, and was much thickened· The lung, partially adhering, was greatly condensed, and was destitute of air. In its superior lobe there was a small excavation, and many tubercles about the size of a pea undergoing softening. The left lung, slightly adhering, was free from tubercles, and without any marked lesion. The right cavity of the chest was smaller than the left, and this distinctly from a shrinking of its parieties and contained parts. Two of the œsophageal glands were enlarged and soft, as if suppurating.

The quantities of purulent and serous fluids discharged in this case were very noteworthy. By three operations, 50 pints of serum were obtained from the abdomen. The quantity of pus from the pleura was about 54 pints, at the rate of about 3oz. daily. Had it not been for the very serious complications, recovery probably would have taken place.

Case 5.—Of empyema, complicated, with diffuse cellular inflammation and abscesses. —Wm. Daly, ætat. 31; 24th Foot; admitted 19th December, 1836; died 18th Jan., 1837.—For eight years this man had suffered from ulceration of the left leg, connected with varicose veins. On the 16th a radical cure was attempted by operation, after Sir B. Brodie's method, followed by pressure. The wounds healed. In about three weeks small abscesses occurred in the situation of the divided veins, accompanied by a feverish state, on account of which he was transferred from the surgical to the medical division. On the 17th December the features were shrunk, the tongue black, with sordes on teeth; there was a catching at imaginary objects; severe pain of shoulders, of elbows, and of wrist-joints. He seemed moribund. Abscesses shortly appeared in the pained parts, and a large one over the sacro-iliac synchondrosis : these were opened. The unfavorable symptoms gradually abated; and he gained some strength, using calomel and opium, sulphate of quinine, wine, etc. In December his ailment had assumed the character of thoracic disease. He had slight cough from the beginning; early in November it was accompanied with some uneasiness of chest, and occasional night sweats, his appetite continuing good. On the 9th December some improvement was reported; his cough was chiefly troublesome at night. On the 15th the left side of thorax had a sunken appearance, and measured was found less than the right—viz., as 15½in. to 17in.; it sounded dull, and was without any respiratory murmur. Emaciation and debility increased, without frequency of pulse, dyspnœa, or febrile exacerbation. In the middle of December an ulcer formed on the back of the sacrum, which spread and discharged much fetid pus. He complained most of pains in his hip and knee-joints, increased by any motion or pressure, but without external redness or swelling. He died, it is stated, " gently, without dyspnœa."

Autopsy 24 hours after death. Much emaciated. The left pleura was lined with a thick false membrane. It contained 2¾ pints of very thick puruloid fluid, in which were suspended flakes of lymph. The lung was compressed close to the spine, and was destitute of air; dissected out (it adhered firmly), it sunk in water; no tubercles were found in it; its structure, apart from condensation from pressure, appeared to be sound. The right lung was more or less œdematous; when incised much serous fluid flowed from it. Its superior lobe contained a few granular tubercles in small clusters. The stomach was small and contracted, but not diseased. A few abrasions were detected in the œsophagus. The gall-bladder was distended with bile of natural appearance. It contained two rather large calculi, and three small ones; the former of the black kind; the latter consisted of cholesterine. Many of the joints were much diseased. Each acetabulum and head of femur was very red, as if gorged with blood, and the former contained some bloody fluid. The round ligaments were red and wasted. The cartilage both of the head of the bone and of the acetabula was in part absorbed, and correspondingly there was a loss of substance of bone. A sinus distended with puruloid matter was found close to the small trochanter. It was about four inches long; it passed under the crural arch, but without communicating with the joint. The synovial fringes of both shoulder-joints were of a deep red, and the cartilages of the heads of the bones and their cavities were in part wasted. A like lesion was detected in the right sterno-clavicular joint. Some lymph was effused into the cellular tissue surrounding the right wrist. The veins of the leg operated upon were generally small; there was no appearance of any obliteration of the divided vessels.

This case is noteworthy for the diffuse cellular inflammation which followed the operation for varix, for the associated low fever, and more especially for the after lesions—*i.e.*, those which afterwards became conspicuous. Is it not remarkable that with such disease of pleura there was so little dyspnœa and pectoral suffering? Was the exemption owing to the very acute and active inflammation in the joints, concentrating as it were sensation; or to the state of the lungs, one simply condensed, the other partially œdematous, the œdema probably occurring only shortly before death?

Case 6.—Of empyema, with gangrene of lung.—J. Pearce, ætat. 48; 7th R.F.; admitted into regimental hospital, Malta, 7th Nov., 1832; died 24th December.— This man, of 28 years' service, was of intemperate habits, especially during the last 12 months, having had with increased pay as assistant armorer more means of drinking. Since then he has suffered from a variety of ailments, such as fever, colic, dysentery, delirium tremens. When last admitted he had pain of side with cough. Under treatment, he appeared to be mending; the cough and pain were relieved; he could lie on either side. On 20th December he had a feverish attack at night with a severe paroxysm of coughing, during which he expectorated "about a quart of puriform fluid mixed with blood." It is stated that he had no pain at the time. On the 22nd another violent fit of coughing came on, when "matter and blood flowed from his mouth [were expectorated?] and continued so to flow until the next day, when he expired."

Autopsy 24 hours after death. Much emaciated. The arachnoid generally was opaque, thicker and stronger than usual. There was a good deal of fluid in the cellular tissue of the pia mater, in the ventricles, and at the base of the brain. The substance of the brain was very firm. The pericardium contained 2oz. of serum, in which were flakes of lymph. In the right pleura there were 2 pints of putrid blood. On removal by dissection, the greater part of the inferior lobe of right lung was found in a state of gangrene; it was black, fetid and easily torn. It exhibited confusedly the appearance of an abscess, or of an excavation, but without tubercles. The middle and superior lobes were gorged with bloody, offensive fluid. The left lung was tolerably sound. The liver was rather large, of the color of unbleached wax. There was pretty much healthy bile in the gall-bladder. The inner coat of the large intestines exhibited some redness and pulpy thickening.

This obscure case was considered one of chronic hepatitis, and was treated as such. No suspicion was entertained, by the medical officer in charge, of pulmonary disease. May not that state of brain produced by habitual intemperance have an influence like that of insanity in masking and rendering latent the lesions of other organs? Is it not probable that the thoracic disease had its origin in the parenchyma of the lung and not in the pleura, and was originally an abscess, beginning with partial engorgement—that engorgement which is so often the consequence of alcoholic poisoning? His last illness was immediately after an excessive drunken debauch.

Case 7.—Of empyema, with softening of brain and incipient gangrene of pleura.— M. Sweeny, ætat. 20; 31st F.; admitted 25th June, 1840; died 26th August.— This man's complaint began two months ago with pain in the left side of chest, for which he was bled and blistered. On admission into general hospital the side complained of was protuberant, dull on percussion, and without respiratory sound; the heart was felt beating under the right mamilla; decubitus on left side; cough, with pretty copious expectoration; dyspnœa; feeble pulse; appetite pretty good. On the 13th July the left side of chest measured 2½ inches more than the right. "An abscess, then pointing under the left mamilla, was opened;" 7oz. of pus were evacuated, with temporary relief; and a good deal afterwards. He continued to improve up to the 4th August, when diarrhœa came on, followed by swelling of the belly and night sweats. On the day of his death he experienced some pain of abdomen, and shortly after, a few hours before the fatal event, there was loss of speech, dilated pupils, and stertorous breathing.

Autopsy 11 hours after death. Much emaciated. The brain generally was soft, the fornix and septum lucidum pultaceous; the pia mater so very thin that it was difficult to detach it except in shreds. The left pleura contained 7 pints of fetid pus; the pleura was almost black from incipient gangrene. The left lung was excessively compressed, and was close to the spine; it was very compact and firm, but no wise hepatized, and was free from tubercles. The right lung was pretty healthy throughout. The bronchia were red, and contained some purulent fluid. The pericardium adhered closely and firmly to the heart, which lay on the right side of the spine. There were 6 pints of serum in the cavity of the abdomen. The omentum adhered to the diaphragm on the left side. The liver was small. The spleen was large, and its capsule thickened.

This was a very favorable case for paracentesis. Why the operation was not performed I am ignorant: I find no reason assigned in the too brief abstract. The condition of the brain is noteworthy, especially contrasted with that described in the preceding case.

Case 8.—Of empyema, with pneumathorax and obstructed femoral vein.—J. Rogers, ætat. 18; 27th Foot; admitted 2nd August, 1838; died January 12th, 1839.—This man had measles in June. Two days after leaving hospital he was re-admitted, laboring under "catarrhus acutus." This was on the 9th July. At the same time, it is stated that he had severe pain in the right side. When transferred to the general hospital on the 2nd August he was greatly emaciated; the scapulæ were projecting; the left side of the chest was ¾ inch larger than the right, and was dull on percussion. He had no longer any pain there, and could lie on either side. During the next six weeks there was little change; occasional night sweats; diarrhœa occasionally. On the 16th September there was a return of pain in the left side, and the protuberance there had increased; the heart's impulse was felt in the right side. On 2nd October mention is made of vomiting at times, as well as of diarrhœa. On the 21st of the same month he had an attack of dyspnœa during the night, with profuse expectoration. On 12th November profuse diarrhœa was reported with night sweats, and two days later the expectoration of fetid matter of a dirty grey color. On the 27th it is stated that "an abscess" had burst exteriorly in the lower part of the left side of chest, and had discharged a large quantity of thin, fetid matter; the pulse was 100. On the 1st January there was a continuance of the fetid discharge, and with it some air. On the 11th January his cough was very troublesome; the discharge dark, fetid, and profuse. His left foot was much swollen; both feet cold. On the 12th his stomach had become very irritable; nothing, it is stated, was retained but wine. The teeth and lips were covered with sordes; in brief, he was moribund; he expired during the night.

Autopsy 33 hours after death. Much emaciated. The calvaria very thin and light. The dura mater apparently wasted, especially its falciform process, which in part was cribriform. The pia mater also very thin and tender. The lower part of the left side of chest was tympanitic. In the pleura of this side there was some very offensive air, and about 22oz. of putrescent dark brown fluid, which, agitated in the pneumatic bottle, gave off much gas. The pleura was lined with a false membrane, so discolored as to be almost black. The lung was attached to the side by a long thick band. It was extremely compressed, and was close to the spine. No tubercles were found in it. In its superior lobe there was a superficial cavity opening into the pleura, and communicating with one or two bronchial tubes. The abdominal viscera appeared to be sound. The left iliac vein was found to contain a fibrinous concretion undergoing softening; in one direction it extended into the beginning of the vena cava; in the other into the femoral vein. In the latter there was a clot, in which was a cavity nearly empty. In one of the larger branches of the same vein there was a fibrinous concretion completely obstructing it; it was firm exteriorly; within it, as it were in a cyst, was a pus-like fluid.* The femoral vein, so far as it was traced, contained coagulated blood, as did also the right iliac vein. The coats of these veins had no appearance of disease.

This case might be called pneumathorax, but empyema seems more applicable to it, on the supposition that disease of the

---

* It did not change the color of turmeric paper, or give off ammonia when mixed with kali purum. Under the microscope it was seen to consist of particles of various sizes: some about equal to pus globules, others, and the majority, much smaller, and of irregular forms.

pleura and effusion into its sac preceded the opening from it into
the lung, permitting the entrance of air.   As regards the operation of paracentesis, the same remark applies as in the former
instance, only with the difference that on admission into general
hospital, the disease was so much more advanced.   In both
cases the absence of ulceration of the intestines, with absence of
tubercles in the lungs is noteworthy.   The fibrinous concretions
preceding death in the veins of the lower extremities are worthy
of remark, as is also the puruloid matter detected in one of them.

Case 9.—Of empyema, with caries of ribs.—W. Hart, ætat. 20; 41st Foot; admitted 17th October, 1839; died May 3rd, 1840.—This man was transferred from the
detachment hospital to the general hospital, after an attack of "pneumonia," which
began early in September, 1839.   On admission, he was very feeble; there was dulness on percussion over the lower third of each lung; a short cough, without expectoration; pulse 84.   On 8th November there was much pain in the left hypochondriac
region, with increase of cough, followed shortly by night sweats and an increase of
dyspnœa, especially when lying on the right side.   On the 7th December the integuments of the left side were found swollen, pitting on pressure; there was an increase
of pain there, and his cough was more severe.   On the 1st January a distinct fluctuation was reported under the left mamilla; a puncture was made the following
day; much pus was discharged, and continued to be discharged daily.   A few days
before the fatal termination, his debility and emaciation rapidly increased; his teeth
became covered with sordes; though unable to expectorate, it is stated that he was
conscious to the last, and that there were no indications of disease of brain.
Autopsy 30 hours after death.   Greatly emaciated.   There was pretty much fluid
in the tissue of the pia mater, in the ventricles, and at the base of the brain.   The
pia mater adhered with unusual firmness to the cerebral surface, portions of which
came away in detaching this membrane.   The fornix and septum lucidum were pultaceous, and the brain altogether was of unusual softness.   The left pleura contained
8oz. of purulent fluid; it was thickened, and its costal surface was partially destroyed;
many of the ribs were carious, and covered with soft lymph.   The left lung adhered
superiorly; it was so compressed as to be destitute of air; its substance was apparently sound.   The right lung was pretty generally adhering, and through the medium
of soft lymph, which was deposited in flakes in considerable quantity; like the left,
it was free from tubercles, and also sound.   The pleura contained 10oz. of serum,
turbid from flakes of lymph suspended in it.   In the abdominal cavity there were
24oz. of turbid serum, in which also some flakes of lymph were suspended.   There
was no well-marked lesion of any of the viscera not mentioned.

This case is closely analogous to the two preceding, and might
call for the same commentary.   In this, as in the last, the
morbid state of the brain, without any symptom indicative of
it, is noteworthy—a state of brain somewhat similar, at least as
regards softness, to that of the infantile brain.

Case 10.—Of empyema, with tuberculated lungs.—J. May, ætat. 24; R.B.;
admitted 2nd September, 1836; died 10th September.—This man is just returned
from the Ionian Islands, where a little more than a year ago his illness commenced,

with cough and dyspnœa, which still trouble him. On examination, the right side of the chest is found to be unduly prominent and to sound dull on percussion; the respiratory murmur also is inaudible, except obscurely in the sub-clavicular region. During the short time he was under observation, little change was noticed with the exception of a certain degree of drowsiness, two or three days before death, which rather increased, but never passed into coma. He died at night suddenly and unexpectedly; not a single day, not even the last, had he been confined to his bed.

Autopsy 36 hours after death. Not much emaciated. Some œdema of extremities. The right side of chest very much larger than the left. On dividing the vessels of the scalp and on opening the sinuses of the dura mater, much blood flowed out which did not coagulate on exposure to the air. In each choroid plexus, there was a bony concretion of about the size of a pea, and there was a similar one in the pineal gland. The abdomen laid open, the diaphragm on the right side was found protruding about 2 inches beyond the false ribs, the right lobe of the liver proportionally displaced; it covered the greater part of the kidney. The stomach was pressed into the left iliac fossa, and a large portion of the intestines into the cavity of the pelvis. The instant that an opening was made into the right pleura, fluid gushed out with much force. 17 pints of serum of a milky hue were collected; its sides were covered with a rough false membrane. The lung was exceedingly compressed; it weighed only 6 oz. It contained several tubercles softening. Its structure generally appeared sound; its bronchia were very small. In the left lung there were also many tubercles and of a larger size, about that of filberts; some were of almost cartilaginous firmness, others of the consistence of soft putty; one had a central cavity communicating with a bronchial tube. About 1½ oz. of serum in the pericardium. The heart was pressed very much to the left side. The suprarenal glands contained tubercular matter like that found in the lungs. No marked lesion was discovered in any of the abdominal viscera.

Had the operation of paracentesis been performed in this case, life probably might have been prolonged. It was proposed, but the patient would not submit to it. The little suffering attending the great distension of the pleura, is very noteworthy. Was it owing to the state of the blood, probably containing carbonic acid in excess: or to the pressure producing sanguineous and especially venous congestion? And might not death have been owing to the same cause? The considerable flow of blood from the brain when its vessels were divided before the great cavities were opened, the forcible gush of fluid from the pleura when that distended membrane was punctured, and the œdematous state of the extremities, are circumstances all seemingly favorable to the conjecture, as is also the drowsiness which occurred and was increasing a few hours before death.

2. OF HYDROTHORAX.—The two following cases of hydrothorax are given chiefly on account of their complications.

Case 1.—Of hydrothorax, with disease of brain and other complications.—A. Cross, ætat. 27; 72nd F.; admitted 5th Feb., 1836, died 6th June.—This man's illness commenced two years ago with epileptic fits at the Cape of Good Hope, from whence he has recently returned. When first admitted, after landing in February, there was a partial paralysis of the left side. For some time previously the epileptic seizures had been of irregular occurrence; his general health pretty good. The day after entering the hospital furious delirium came on, requiring the straight waistcoat, followed by continued violent cerebral symptoms; every third or fourth day a paroxysm occurred marked by tremors, moaning, foaming at the mouth, coma. In the intervals he was almost entirely deprived of motion in the right side. After about a fortnight there was some remission, but of short duration. Early in March the fits were more frequent and more severe. They were preceded by violent pain in the left side of the head and attended with much dyspnœa, leaving him very weak; he was much emaciated. In April he improved, and he continued to improve in May. He was able to walk out; his articulation though imperfect was less indistinct, and he gained flesh. There was a cessation of the fits, and all the functions were well performed. On the 4th June he was discharged, preparatory to his appearing before the invaliding board at Chelsea Hospital. On the following day he was re-admitted, brought in laboring under hemiplegia, with urgent dyspnœa and "oppression of chest." He was quite conscious, but with a tendency to sleep; there was pain of the left side of the head; his pulse was full; the temperature of the body increased; urine was voided naturally; the bowels were costive. A vein was opened; when 4 oz. of blood had been taken, he became faint. At 3 p.m. he was moribund; at 6 p.m. he expired. On first admission the treatment was various; V.S., cupping, setons, etc., but without any apparent immediate good effect.

Autopsy 20 hours after death. Sub-emaciated. The right side of chest sounded dull. The dura mater adhered closely and firmly over a considerable portion of the anterior of the left hemisphere of the cerebrum; when separated the surface of the cerebrum corresponding was seen of a yellow hue and was found to be of a flabby consistence and to contain cavities, in which was a kind of false cellular tissue, infiltrated with serum. Though flabby the diseased part was tougher than natural and was cut with greater difficulty. The pia mater and the arachnoid in the same situation were hid in a layer of lymph two or three lines thick. The ventricles of the brain were considerably distended with fluid and there was a good deal at its base. No other morbid appearance was discovered in the encephalon, with the exception of the pineal gland, which was adhering posteriorly and unusually abounded in gritty matter ;* and the lateral ventricles, which inferiorly were a little softened. The right pleura contained 4 pints of serum. The lung on this side was much compressed; its apex was attached to the costal pleura by a band, about ¼ inch thick, of almost cartilaginous firmness; and it was generally adhering by numerous soft bands and fibres of a red color to the same surface. On its inferior lobe there were two false membranes—one inner, of considerable firmness, the other, on that, and of soft consistence, as if recently formed. This lobe contained many granular tubercles, indeed it abounded in them; most of them were of the size of a small pea and were of soft consistence; its middle and superior lobe were free from tubercles. The left lung, though not adhering, did not collapse; it was very much heavier than natural; a great part of it was hepatised as if from the infiltration of lymph and the coloring matter of blood. In its superior lobe there were some clusters of granular tubercles. There was some œdema of the anterior mediastinum. The pericardium contained 3 oz. of serum. The heart was rather large; there was a good deal of coagulated blood and fibrinous concretion in its cavities. In the cœcum and ascending colon there were several cicatrices of old ulcers, marked by depressions, a dark hue and an irregular granular surface. In the

---

* It was examined and found to consist of phosphate of lime, of a little carbonate of lime, and animal matter; no oxalate of lime could be detected.

ileum, and chiefly in its lower portion, there were numerous ulcerated spots. The other abdominal viscera appeared tolerably sound.

This case is equally noteworthy for the recovery when that was almost despaired of, and for its sudden and fatal termination. In the first instance was not the cerebral disease complicated with pleuritic inflammation and effusion? And was not the death owing to a recurrence of the latter? The symptoms and the lesions seem to indicate as much. Does not the ochry stain of the diseased portion of the brain denote that blood was effused on the part, and was afterwards absorbed, leaving its iron, the coloring matter of the stain. That the active treatment first employed had little or no good effect was inferred from the improvement occurring after its discontinuance, and when little or no medicine was used.

Case 2.—Hydrothorax, with disease of pancreas.—J. Wilmore, 7th R.F.; admitted into regimental hospital, Malta, 27th December, 1830; died 5th Feb., 1831.—This man, of intemperate habits, of robust make, during the last three years had several attacks of disease; "dysentery" in December, 1828; "enteritis" in June, 1830; "pneumonia" in December of the same year. In January, when considered convalescent, he was suddenly seized with dyspnœa and pain of chest, which relieved by treatment, recurred at different times, as it were in an intermitting manner, gradually however increasing, until the fatal termination, and that apparently from suffocation, for unable to lie down from the extreme dyspnœa, he expired in the sitting posture. During his illness V.S. was often repeated. The medicines prescribed were chiefly diuretics with blue pill, hyoscyamus, etc.

Autopsy 23 hours after death. The right side of chest larger than the left, sounded dull; slight puffiness of that side and of the right side of face; slight œdema of the hands and feet. A little fluid in the ventricles and at the base of the brain. On opening into the abdomen, the diaphragm was found pressed down on the right side to the margin of the false ribs, presenting a yielding protuberance, not tympanitic. The liver was beyond its ordinary boundary; the gall-bladder was so low as the umbilicus. The small intestines were situated almost entirely in the cavity of the pelvis, and were collapsed so as to occupy as little space as possible. The larger intestines were in a similar state, excepting that the cœcum was moderately distended with flatus, and contained a small quantity of scybala. On opening the thorax the heart was found unusually to the left, evidently from the effect of pressure. It was small. The right auricle was full of coagulated blood and fibrin, these bearing the form of the cavity when turned out. The small quantity of blood-clot in each of the ventricles was in a *broken state*, as if acted on after coagulation had taken place. Coagulated blood was found in all the large vessels. The pericardium contained 5oz. of yellowish serum. There was some reddish fluid in the posterior mediastinum. The right pleura was greatly distended; it contained 10¾ pints of reddish brown serum, colored by blood, as was shown by subsidence of the coloring matter, the fluid being taken out and left to rest. Both surfaces of the pleura were covered with a thick layer of lymph, which on the costal side was flocculent; over the diaphragm was in minute granular masses. The lung, its substance apparently sound, was so compressed that it occupied little space, was entirely destitute of air, and consequently sank in water.

17

The left pleura contained about a pint of serous fluid. The lung on this side was adherent in many places; its inferior lobe was much condensed; it was generally pretty healthy. No tubercles were found in either lung. In the abdominal cavity there were many adhesions between the liver and colon and mesentery, and between the intestines and peritoneum. The pancreas was small and hard; its cellular coat was unusually dense and strong. Between it and the left lobe of the liver there was a peculiar firm structure, as if formed of condensed cellular tissue. Cut into, it was found to be cavernous; its cavity irregular, somewhat like that of the vesiculæ seminales; one or two of its sinuses penetrated into the substance of the liver; it also communicated with the pancreas by a lateral opening into its duct, which, when laid open, was seen in some places much enlarged, in others contracted, and in one or two apparently obliterated. The cavity contained a little fluid, and some small concretions, the largest nearly the size of a pea.* The liver was of ordinary size and apparently sound. The common duct, where it passed through the coats of the intestine, was so contracted that there was difficulty in introducing a small probe. The mouth of the pancreatic duct was normal.

The intermitting character of the disease in this case is remarkable, as if arising from a struggle between the vital powers and the morbific causes—the one at one time the more effective, the other in their turn acquiring the mastery. Had the hydrothorax been detected during life, probably much relief might have been afforded by an operation, and life might have been prolonged. The tumor between the pancreas and liver, connected with both, and the concretions in it, probably derived from both, are curious and uncommon.

3. OF PERICARDITIS.—Of this disease the four following cases are striking examples.

Presuming that no distinction was intended to be made in the naming of army-diseases between carditis and pericarditis, it would appear from the army statistical returns that inflammation of the heart, or rather, I would say, of its sac, is of very rare and uncertain occurrence. Referring to these returns, we see how for years, at one station, there has not been one instance of it, and yet in other years, and these sometimes consecutive, cases of it have occurred. Thus, in Canada, from 1817 to 1836 inclusive, with an aggregate strength of 64,000 men, of the 11 cases of carditis given, of which 3 proved fatal, not one took place during the first five years of that period—yet three, one in each year, took place in the three following years; other three

---

* Their color was partly white, partly black; they appeared to consist of albumen and of the matter of the black biliary calculus; they burnt with flame, emitting a smell like that of albumen, crackling before taking fire, and leaving very little ash. They were insoluble in alcohol.

occurring in a single year, 1830—this after an interval of five years; and five in the last two years, viz., 1835-1836, in the intermediate years not a single case being recorded. At all the other stations included in the army returns, the like is noticeable, seeming to indicate, though it must be confessed obscurely, that even in the instance of the most sporadic diseases, the causes productive of them, are either only occasionally present, or if present, varying greatly in their intensity of power.

Case 1.—Of pericarditis, with empyema, and a mediastinum-abscess.—M. Skelly, ætat. 30; 7th Regiment; admitted into regimental hospital, Malta, 27th Feb., 1832; died 20th April.—This man, previously in good health, was brought to hospital laboring under pain of left side, with cough, much pyrexia, and some difficulty of breathing. On the following day there was an increase of the pain and dyspnœa; the pulse was 100 and full; the face flushed; great thirst. A vein was opened in both arms; very little blood could be obtained; it was described as "dark and ropy." A blister was applied to the pained part, and calomel and antimony were administered. Slight relief was experienced. On the 29th there was an increase of dyspnœa, with indications, it was stated, of bronchitis. V.S. (24 oz.); the blood buffed. On the 1st March the symptoms were more unfavorable; he was restless during the night, and at times delirious; his pulse 140; pupils dilated; tongue dry; cough troublesome; expectoration difficult; skin hot. V.S. (8 oz.); blister to nape of neck. Calomel, gr. ii., every hour, with a draught every second hour containing 5 grs. of carbonate of ammonia, and 30 minims of T. Scillæ. On the 2nd, the pulse was 126; the breathing "thick and laborious;" the pupils less dilated; cough less severe. 20 leeches; a blister along the course of the spine; the same medicine. On the 3rd the report was more favorable; he could make a full inspiration without coughing; the pulse was 104 and soft; the tongue moist. On the 5th he was free from pain, and considered improving. The calomel was now omitted, and T. Digitalis 8 min. with Liq. Ammon. Acetat. 3 drachms given every third hour. From the 5th to the 13th there was little change; he continued free from pain. On the 13th his breathing became laborious; his pulse full and quick; there was much pyrexia. Leeches were again applied to the chest, and small doses of tartar emetic prescribed with some relief. Again for several days there was little change; his cough occasionally severe. On the 23rd there was much œdema of ankles, also some œdema of face and chest; his breathing was shorter. Digitalis, with subcarbonate of ammonia and stramonium, were now given, with temporary relief, and an increased flow of urine. Thus he continued until the 4th April, when he experienced an attack of diarrhœa, which, it is stated, "was relieved by the usual means." On the 8th, during a violent fit of coughing, he expectorated a considerable quantity of blood. From this time he became anasarcous, and never rallied; "he gradually sank" without any marked change of symptoms, with the exception of a feeling of much drowsiness during the latter hours.

Autopsy 24 hours after death. Considerable general anasarca; lividity of inferior part of left side of chest; the left side sounded obtusely. The brain was rather soft, especially inferiorly; there was pretty much fluid in the lateral ventricles, and at its base. In dissecting off the muscles of the chest, the sinus of an abscess was detected a little below the left mamilla. It passed obliquely, and communicated with a collection of pus in the anterior mediastinum, at the inferior margin of the pericardium. The pericardium was greatly distended; it contained three pints of pus. The heart was pressed a good deal towards the left side, and appeared outside, as it were, the pericardium, from the false membrane which had formed. All its cavities were empty and compressed; the ventricles were very small; the auricles, especially the right, and venæ cavæ unusually large. The left pleura contained 40 oz. of purulent fluid, collected in its inferior portion. The lung on this side was so compressed as to be destitute of air. After having been washed, to remove the little blood that was in it, it was of a grey color and spongy texture, tough and strong, yielding, but not breaking, under powerful pressure—that of the thumb-nail and end of index-finger— and considerable force was required to tear it. Where the pus was collected, there was a false membrane; the upper, and indeed all but the lower, portion of this lung was adhering. The right lung adhered very slightly; it contained a good deal of blood, and was heavier than natural. In its substance, close to its pleural covering, was a closed sac of almost cartilaginous firmness, full of a soft, putty-like matter, which was found to be composed of phosphate of lime, with a little carbonate of lime and animal matter. The abdominal viscera were free from any apparent lesion.

No suspicion of pericarditis was entertained during the life of the patient, although the chest was examined more than once with the stethoscope. It sounded well, it was stated, on the right side, but dull on the left; the respiratory murmur at the same time being distinct in the right lung, indistinct in the left, except in its upper part, where there was a slight râle. Empyema alone was conjectured. Had the diagnosis been perfect, considering the complications, the result probably would have been the same. The anasarca gradually increasing, the feeling of drowsiness felt towards the end of life, the very quick breathing and pulse, etc., the state of the heart in relation to its cavities, and the condition of the adjoining venæ cavæ, accord well with the distended state of the pericardium. Was not the pressure from this distension, gradually increasing, ultimately the cause of death by arresting the heart's action?

Case 2.—Of pericarditis, with hydrothorax and ascites.—J. Duffy, ætat. 19; 27th F.; admitted 12th October, 1837; died 20th January, 1838.—This young man had been in the service only 3 months. He was transferred from the detachment hospital, supposed to be laboring under phthisis. On admission into general hospital, he had cough with dyspnœa; the other symptoms were not minutely detailed, nor were they during the progress of the disease. Up to the 13th November it was stated that he was sometimes better, sometimes worse. Then his cough had become more trouble-some and his pulse irregular. On the 27th December, œdema of the lower extremities was reported. On the 2nd January mention was made of purging, of night sweats, and of great debility; and of some relief from acid drinks and opium. The pulse, it is stated, had become weaker and more intermitting, and the dyspnœa greater. His death was sudden; he talked rationally only five minutes before.

Autopsy 16 hours after death. Limbs œdematous. The pericardium was nearly an inch thick from a deposition of lymph. It contained 20oz. of turbid serum, from which, on rest after removal, flakes of lymph subsided, and some pus globules, proved to be such by the optical test. The right auricle and ventricle contained pretty much blood, with a little clot, but no fibrinous concretion.* All the cavities were small; the right were empty; all the valves were sound. No coagula were found in the veins. The left pleura contained about 4 oz. of reddish serum, with some soft lymph and coagulated blood. The lung on this side, partially adhering, contained many granular tubercles. Its inferior lobe was in part œdematous and in part hepatized. The right pleura contained 18 oz.† of serum. Two coagula of blood were found in its inferior lobe. All the lobes were denser and heavier than natural, as if from a slight effusion of lymph; and granular tubercles were scattered through all of them. In the abdominal cavity there were 32 oz. of a clear yellowish serum. The liver was rather denser than natural; it weighed 3 lbs. In the cœcum there were a few small ulcers. The testes and vesiculæ seminales were small. The left vesicula contained two kinds of matter, one opaque and white, like scrofulous matter; the other of the appearance and consistence of gelatinised starch. In the other vesicula there was a dark greenish, almost black fluid.‡

This case is as noteworthy for its chronic as the preceding was for its acute character; and in point of suffering they present as great a contrast. Comparing the two, their epiphenomena are seen to have a certain resemblance, and yet not without differences. What significance should be attached—if any—to the result of the trial of the blood and other fluids found after death? I hesitate to offer an opinion.

Case 3.—Of pericarditis, with hydrothorax and partially hepatized lung.—C. Sheppard, ætat. 19; 65th Regiment; admitted into detachment hospital, Edinburgh Castle, 16th February, 1824; died 19th February.—This young soldier, in consequence of the illness of the surgeon of his regiment, was transferred from his own hospital to the detachment hospital adjoining, accompanied by the statement, that when he first came under treatment—viz., on the 19th January, his tonsils were enlarged, the fauces inflamed, deglutition difficult, and that there was pyrexia; further, that he had been relieved by V.S. (20 oz.) by a blister to the neck and the use of tartarised antimony. It was added, that on the 4th February he experienced pain at the scrobiculus cordis, accompanied with great dyspnœa, cold extremities, a pulse only just perceptible, and extreme prostration of strength; that the pain was relieved by a blister, and that taking wine and bark, he so far rallied, as to permit of his removal. The case now appeared to be hopeless. The breathing was short and quick, but without pain; indeed he had been altogether free from pain from the beginning except a slight degree complained of in the act of swallowing, and that which he had experienced at the scrobiculis cordis; he had no appetite; his voice was feeble and altered, his bowels relaxed; his debility extreme; yet his intellect was clear. He lingered on till the 19th without any change of symptoms deserving of record.

Autopsy 12 hours after death. Much emaciated; no œdema of extremities. The

* Agitated with common air in the pneumatic bottle there was a slight absorption; and again the following day.

† The fluids from the pericardium, pleura and abdomen, similarly agitated, gave off pretty much gas.

‡ No spermatozoa could be detected in either fluid, or in the little fluid obtained from the testes and vasa deferentia; granules in each were seen, etc.

abdomen tympanitic and somewhat distended. The right side of chest dull on percussion; the left resonant, almost tympanitic. The peritoneum was first carefully
exposed. The intestines were seen through it greatly distended. There was no free
air in its cavity. Opening into the latter, the stomach was found greatly distended
and the diaphragm pressed upwards into the thorax. Now, when the stomach was
drawn down, and percussion repeated on the left side of chest, the sound was very
dull, showing that the contrary sound in the first instance was owing to the inflated
state of the stomach. Independent of distension, neither this organ nor the intestines
showed any marks of disease. There were some scybala present. The other abdominal viscera appeared to be sound. The pericardium was very large. It contained
2½ pints of pus, with which was mixed much loose, soft coagulable lymph, not unlike
curd in appearance. On the whole inner surface of the membrane there was a deposit
of granular lymph, which, over the heart was about two lines in thickness. All the
cavities of the heart were contracted; the left ventricle very closely so; it contained
no blood; the right ventricle and auricle contained very little. In the left auricle
there was a small fibrinous concretion, flat, thin, and of oval outline and of firm consistence; it suggested the idea of having been formed during life. The muscular substance of the heart was paler than usual. The left pleura, covered with a thin layer
of rather soft coagulable lymph, contained a pint and a half of serum, with some loose
lymph. The lobes of the lung were adhering together and to the pericardium and
diaphragm by soft lymph in an unusually large quantity. This lung was much compressed; its inferior lobe was hepatized; it sank in water. The inferior lobe of the
right lung was in the same state, though in a somewhat less degree, and the middle
lobe less still, the superior nearly natural. There was a little puruloid fluid in the
bronchia of left lung; more in those of the right. The posterior mediastinum was
œdematous and contained a good deal of reddish serum. The larynx and trachea were
of a deep red. Contiguous to one of the sacculi laryngis was a small sinus burrowing
under the mucous membrane; its orifices—they were two and small—had a black,
gangrenous appearance. On the other side, close to the rima glottidis, there was a
large burrowing sinus, which in one direction opened into the pharynx, in the other,
just under the epiglottis. In the cellular tissue of the larynx, immediately under its
epithelium, there were three or four little abscesses, about the size of peas and of a
like form, full of "healthy pus." The vessels of the neck were much gorged with
blood. The thyroid gland was unusually red. A small abscess was detected between
the internal jugular vein and the carotid artery; it was situated in the cellular
structure, which was thickened.

This case is noteworthy in many particulars, especially compared with the two preceding. How remarkable that with
such severity of lesions, and these peculiar, there should have
been so little pain, so little distress in breathing, or distressing
feeling of any kind! Was it the complicity of the morbid
actions that conduced to this? or, was it owing to pressure on
the par vagum? The tympanitic state of the stomach and of the
intestines, and the absence of œdema of the extremities, are also
noteworthy. Was the former anywise connected with the presumed pressure on the nerves just named? It came out after
death and after the autopsy that three months before enlistment

he had been wounded in the chest with a pitchfork. Whether that was concerned with the origin of his disease, there is barely occasion for conjecture, all the minute circumstances of the accident being unknown.

Case 4.—Of pericarditis, with hepatization of lung.—W. Phibbs, ætat. 20; 12th Foot; admitted 29th April, 1840 ; died 23rd July —This young man, of 4 months' service, on admission had some soreness of throat and headache, with enlargement of tonsils. Two days after, an eruption like that of scarlatina appeared, with an increase of soreness of throat. On the 7th May the symptoms were subsiding. On the 24th he was reported convalescent. On the 6th June he attempted to poison himself by laudanum (he had been an apothecary before enlisting). An emetic timely given, followed by drinking largely of warm water, arrested the effects. Up to the 7th July it is stated that he continued well. Then, after drinking some cold milk, he had an attack of colic, with sickness of stomach; there was great thirst; the pulse 110. After five or six days there was occasional vomiting, and he refused food; he experienced some pain in the left side of chest, chiefly in the region of the heart, and also slight abdominal pain ; the pulse was small and irregularly intermitting; the bowels relaxed ; there was much debility. The symptoms, according to the brief report of the case, continued much the same to its fatal termination. He was conscious to the last; he expired suddenly, a few minutes after returning to bed from the close-stool by its side. The treatment was " in the first instance antiphlogistic; latterly, nourishment and stimulants."

Autopsy 7 hours after death. Sub-emaciated. The brain appeared to be perfectly sound. The pericardium contained 22 oz. of pus.* Its surface was covered with a thin, rough, false membrane. In all the cavities of the heart there was a little coagulated blood and fibrinous concretion. Both lungs were adhering. The right lung weighed 3 lbs. Its inferior lobe, fully distended, was hepatized throughout. Its color was grey and brownish. In its substance were several small cavities, of irregular form, communicating one with the other. They conveyed the idea, in the absence of tubercles, of being formed by the softening and disintegration of the consolidating matter. The middle lobe was partially hepatized. The superior lobe was very small, as if compressed by the others ; it was pervious to air. There was some frothy fluid in its bronchia. No notice is taken of the state of the left lung, from whence it may be inferred that it was normal. There was a small ulcer at the base of one of the arytenoid cartilages. The pancreas was very hard, and its lobules more closely compacted than usual. There was no distinct lesion of the other abdominal viscera.

This case seems most noteworthy in a negative point of view. Neither the pneumonia nor pericarditis was detected during life. Were the symptoms so obscure and so little urgent, as they appear to have been, owing to the reduction of vital force, the result of the preceding scarlatina? or was there a state of brain, an approach to that of the insane, such as the attempt at suicide would seem to indicate, which had a masking effect? The brain weighed 3 lbs. 2¼ oz.

* It was of sp. gr. 1030. Under the microscope it exhibited, besides the ordinary pus globules, numerous granules.

On the foregoing cases I shall offer but a few additional remarks. Regarding the origin of the disease, reviewing the
several cases of empyema, it was probably no wise identical. In
some, on the *post mortem* examination, a communication, we
have seen, was traced between the sac of the pleura and the
bronchia, suggestive of the idea, as in the instance of pneumathorax, that the inflammation productive of the effusion might
have been occasioned by the presence of air—air which afterwards might have been absorbed. The more common cause,
however, seems to have been idiopathic inflammation of the
membrane itself—a pleurisy often combined with pneumonia.
Whether a softening granular tubercle, formed on the surface of
the pleura, might have excited such an inflammation, is a question more easily started than answered : I mention it, finding
the query appended to one of the cases, and suggested at the
moment of drawing it up.

In noticing the fluid accumulated, mention has been made of
difference of quality—sometimes puriform, oftener puruloid, and,
I may add, occasionally little more than serum : serum rendered
slightly turbid by suspended globules or granules, or by delicate
shreds or particles of lymph. Another circumstance may be
worth recalling and fixing attention : in every instance in which
the effused fluid was tried by agitation with common air, it gave
off some gas. What the gas was, was not determined ; the probability is, that it was chiefly carbonic acid and azote. The
evolution was most strongly marked in those cases in which the
fluid had acquired an offensive smell, approaching more or less
to the putrid. Such an odor results from fermentation, and
that—the putrid, like any other fermentation—it is commonly
understood, cannot be excited without the presence of oxygen.
If this be granted, we can hardly avoid the conclusion that
oxygen may exist free in the fluid in sufficient quantity—a very
small quantity only is required—to give rise to the fermentation ;
and, inasmuch as in some instances no communication could be
discovered between the pleura and the lungs, in other words, no
false passage admitting atmospheric air, the facts seem to accord
with the theory. Instances such as that noticed in Case 15, in
which putrid pus was discharged on opening an abscess, though
rare, are well known—instances these in which we are certain
that there was no direct communication between the cellular

tissue, the seat of the inflammation, and the open air. As in the examples of empyema with putrescence, these discharges seem always to denote a feeble state of the vital powers, and most imminent danger of life; and for this reason, it may be presumed, that if the system is tolerably vigorous, the probability is, that the oxygen introduced into the blood in respiration will be expended in the ordinary way to feed the flame of life, if I may so speak, and will not pass into any of the secretions, in them to have a contrary effect, that of promoting death and decay.

The state of the lungs in most of these cases, so little of them pervious to air, owing to condensation from pressure, often accompanied with hepatization from effusion of blood and lymph, may well excite surprise, as showing how small a degree of respiration, or of aëration of the blood, is sufficient for the continuance of life. They in this respect remind one of the hybernating animals; and in these cases of disease, as in those animals, may not what we know of the one be inferred of the other—viz., that there is a certain accordance, a certain harmony between the action of the lungs and the action of the other viscera—in brief, a feeble action throughout; and further, that there is, as was conjectured in pneumathorax, an over-charge of carbonic acid in the blood; this conducing probably to diminished acuteness of sensation, a condition approaching to that of anesthesia, and, it may be imagined, humanely ordered to insure a more easy death—an euthanasia.

On the treatment of empyema, the few remarks made on that of pneumathorax are, I believe, not inapplicable, especially as regards the operation of paracentesis. The drawing off the accumulated and oppressing fluid is sure to afford temporary relief, and probably, in the majority of cases, only such relief, inasmuch as in so large a proportion, the effusion is associated with tubercles and other chronic lesions. In a certain number of cases, however, the chances of doing well might be greater, especially if performed at an early stage; but in these, if detected, there would generally be, it is to be apprehended, an aversion on the part of the patient to submit to the operation. In the four cases described, in which paracentesis was performed, the treatment was of the simplest kind: no injections were attempted into the pleural sac. This is to be regretted; judging from analogy, it seems probable that some such application might be useful. Wine was employed by the ancient physicians; a solution of iodine, found so serviceable in hydrocele, is more deserving of trial. As coal-tar has been found serviceable in checking putridity, a poultice containing it might be useful applied to the chest, should the discharge from the pleura become offensive; the injection, too, of tar-water, or of a weak solution of creosote, might deserve a trial. Whether, when an operation is indicated, it should be performed between the ribs, or by perforating a rib, as proposed in the Hippocratic writings, is, perhaps, not of much importance: the latter has some advantages, sufficient, I am inclined to think, to justify a further trial of it. To promote as much as possible the chances of recovery, it need hardly be added that all precautions should be observed which conduce to the general health, and more especially to the prevention of pyrexia, foremost amongst which are good air with perfect ventilation,* great cleanliness of bedding and dressing, with a nutritive tonic diet.

---

* These can hardly be secured unless the patient have a room to himself, constructed on approved sanitary principles. In a great military hospital it would be well were there such rooms, and an adequate number, provided. In a crowded ward, or one not even unduly crowded, the operated on, whatever the malady, are placed to disadvantage.

CHAPTER VIII.

ON THE COAGULATION OF BLOOD IN THE VESSELS DURING LIFE AND THE SOFTENING OF ITS FIBRIN.*

Connection with some of the preceding diseases.—Recent knowledge of the phenomena.—Importance of the subject pathologically.—Instances of the diseases with which associated.—Specification of the vessels the seat of the coagulation.—Description of cases.—Remarks on the changes and products.—Their pathology reverted to, as probably explanatory of certain sudden deaths, etc.

I AM induced to treat here of the subject enunciated above, from a certain analogy which the phenomena seem to have to the diseases or epiphenomena which have just passed under review. As in them, the changes in question are commonly associated with a state of debility—a cachectic state—well contrasted with the state mostly observable in cases of aneurism, in which, if there be not an excess of vital force, there is rarely a deficiency ; and in which the coagula formed, instead of showing a tendency to liquefaction, more frequently exhibit the contrary one—that to become more compact and resisting.

Although this kind of coagulation and softening has come under notice only in recent times, for I believe no mention is to be found of the phenomena in any of the older writers, not even in Morgagni or in the morbid anatomy of Dr. Baillie, yet judging from my own experience they are far from unfrequent occurrences ; in proof I may state that in the short space of two years, those of 1837 and 1838, when my attention was specially directed to their detection, I found them in no less than 14 cases. This

* The Thrombosis of Virchow, who too often has had credit for having first observed this change in the fibrin of blood. The observations of Mr. Gulliver "On the Softening of Coagulated Fibrin," published in the Trans. of the Roy. Med. and Chir. Society of London, in 1839, preceded those of the Berlin professor by many years. As long ago as 1829, I had ascertained that fibrin is subject to softening and deliquesence with the production of heat and the evolution of carbonic acid and ammonia. See Res. Anat. and Phy. ii., 343; and as early, I had noticed, the change in question in the cadaver, as is shown by some of the following cases. To Mr. Gulliver, undoubtedly, the merit is due of having first shown clearly that fibrin by softening can acquire a puruloid character ; and can become a pathological element distinct from pus. The whole of this chapter, and indeed the MS. of the entire work, was sent to the printer before I had seen Professor Virchow's work on Cellular Pathology.

was at the General Hospital, Fort Pitt, where during the same time the number of bodies examined was about 174.

Of their importance in a pathological point of view I shall at present say little; probably it has been hardly duly appreciated. Be this as it may, they are surely interesting and deserving of minute and continued inquiry. The investigation may perhaps throw light on the nature of tubercle, and on some other diseases, such as fistula in ano, and peritoneal inflammation arising from perforation of the intestine, diseases commonly connected with a feeble diathesis or with a cachectic state of the system, and, it may also aid in explaining sudden and unexpected deaths.

Of the total number of cases of which I have a record, these 43 in number, softening had taken place in the coagulum in 33 instances; in the other 10 it had not commenced, or at least was not observed. The following table shows the diseases in which it was detected and the number of instances.

Phthisis pulmonalis	24
Hæmoptysis	1
Pleuritis, with gangrene of lung	1
Dysenteria chronica	2
Scorbutus	2
Peritonitis from perforation of intestine	1
Peritonitis, with pleurisy and tubercle	1
Cancer of stomach	1
General dropsy	1
Hæmatemisis	1
Disease of heart	2
Rupture of mesenteric vein	1
Ascites	1
Anasarca	1
Lumbar abscess	1
Malignant tumor	1

The ages of the persons in whom it was found, varied at the time of their decease from 18 to 51 years; the average of the whole was 33.

The next table shows the part in which the coagulation took place, and the number of times in the same place.

Right ventricle of heart	4
Right and left ventricles	1
Left ventricle	3
Right ventricle and aorta	1
Coronary vein	1
Large branches of pulmonary vein	1
Internal jugular vein	1

Longitudinal sinus*	3
Longitudinal sinus and left ventricle	1
Longitudinal sinus and left iliac and femoral vein...................	1
Vena cava	2
Vena cava and iliac veins..	3
Iliac and femoral veins	8
Iliac and pudic veins...	1
Femoral veins	2
Hæmorrhoidal veins	1
Pulmonary artery	1
Pulmonary vein	1
Epididymis...	1
Vena portæ	1
Hepatic veins... ·	1
Sac of aneurism..	1
Muscular substance of heart..	1
Under pleura pulmonalis (?)...	1

The situations in which the coagulation has taken place, as shown by this table, those mostly where there is the greatest tendency to stagnation, may be adduced further in evidence of the phenomenon depending in part on a debilitated state of the system.

Of these cases, five of those which occurred at Fort Pitt, have already been briefly given by Mr. Gulliver in an excellent paper " On the Softening of Coagulated Fibrin," communicated by him to the Royal Medico-Chirurgical Society, and published in their Transactions for 1839. Those I shall introduce shall be given somewhat more in detail, selecting such as appear to be of most interest and most suggestive. I have abridged the account of symptoms in the majority, and I might have abbreviated the description of the morbid appearances with a saving of time and space, but by so doing, I cannot but think, any value which the cases may have would be diminished. In several instances there are omissions, made at the time of the *post mortem* examination, which now I can only regret : those who are engaged in researches of the kind can make ample allowances for them.

Case 1.—Hæmorrhoidal tumor of mesenteric vein; coagula in vena cava inferior and iliac veins.—G. Darlington, ætat. 39; 80th Foot; admitted into regimental hospital, Malta, 15th March, 1828; died 28th March.—This man, previously in good health, was first admitted into hospital on the 27th February with pain of abdomen,

* In one instance the coagulum is described as about the size of an orange pip, having a central cavity, in which was a little pus-like matter. It is mentioned as remarkable that the little mass of fibrin was in the midst of coagulated blood and free, *i.e.*, not attached to the side of the longitudinal sinus. The case was one of phthisis.

between the margin of the false ribs and the umbilicus. He was discharged on the 6th March, and was re-admitted on the 15th with the same ailment. The pain was severe and fixed, not extending to the shoulder or affecting the breathing. He was blooded copiously, and had purgative medicine. The blood was not buffed. On the 17th the abdominal pain had ceased. On the 19th the glands of the groin became swollen. On the 21st the swelling had diminished, the pulse was natural, and he was otherwise well. On the 22nd he complained of pain in the lower part of the chest, extending round to the back. On the 24th there was a swelling in the right hypochondrium, hard, circumscribed, and painful; pulse 80   On the 27th there was a great increase of pain, not relieved by warm fomentations; a blister, and anodyne. It now extended down the side, with loss of power of the extremity of that side, which became much swollen, and with a turgid state of its veins. The limb was of a livid color, and much colder than the left. The pulse was so weak as to be scarcely perceptible; he had no longer any appetite, but much thirst. A warm bath without relief. On the 28th the stomach became irritable, and nothing he took was retained. There was less pain of leg; the lower part was black; both legs cold. He died at 1 p.m. It is remarked that the day he died he could move the limb, though with difficulty, and that he had sensation in it as far as the knee, but that below the knee the skin was senseless. The case was first considered one of hepatic disease, and aperients with mercury were the medicines chiefly prescribed. The alvine evacuations were at times bilious; latterly of a dark color.

Autopsy 21 hours after death. Not at all emaciated. The thoracic viscera presented no appearance of disease. The right cavities of the heart were considerably distended with blood; and in both the auricle and ventricle there were fibrinous concretions firmly adhering, giving the idea of having been formed before death. A tumor, capable of holding about a pint and half of fluid, was found in the abdomen, resting on the duodenum, and covered by the omentum, which in a puckered state adhered to it, and also to the pancreas. It was full of grumous blood, not unlike the matter of black vomit. Whilst under examination it became ruptured, and its contents were poured out. The ruptured part was thin, and almost gangrenous. The thickness of the sac varied from 1 to 3 or 4 lines. When cut it had a grisly feel, almost as if cartilaginous. Its inner surface was smooth, not unlike that of the urinary bladder, with here and there small cavities or sacculi. At one spot, where it was attached to the duodenum, there was an ulcerated space to the extent of a sixpence, almost black, and the mucous coat of the intestine corresponding to it was discolored. On minute examination an opening was found in the sac, where a large mesenteric vein entered it. The vein entered very like the ureter into the bladder very obliquely, and was continued in part some way along the sac, as if half of the vessel had been destroyed, and the other half left. On a portion of the sac interiorly there was a layer of red coagulated blood, pretty firmly adhering. In the vena cava there was a coagulum, extending from its commencement into both iliac veins. That passing into the left was cord-like and tapering; it adhered firmly to the side of the vessel, and appeared to be composed of compact fibrin. Where thickest, it was little thicker than a crow-quill; was irregularly flattened, and did not prevent the return of blood. There was some fluid blood in the veins of this extremity; the limb was not swollen or discolored. On the right side, the coagulum completely filled the iliac vein, adhering to it firmly, and descended into the femoral, gradually becoming softer. All the veins of this limb were distended with black blood, very feebly coagulated. The coats of the iliac vein, through its whole course, were thickened, and its calibre contracted—most at its lower, least at its upper part: that is, most nearest the femoral, least nearest the cava. The upper portion of the coagulum—

that in the cava—was nearly conical; .it completely prevented the return of blood from the right extremity, but allowed it to pass from the left. There was an effusion of lymph along the course of the obstructed vessel. The whole limb was livid, and distended with serum and lymph, but it did not pit on pressure. The right femoral and iliac arteries were empty, and much contracted. The aorta internally was perhaps a little rougher than usual, but not distinctly diseased. A considerable portion of the small intestines were in the cavity of the pelvis; these were of a dark reddish hue. The abdominal viscera generally were free from disease.

This minute description has been given on account of the singularity of the lesion, which I infer—the inference resting on the appearances and symptoms—was a rupture of a mesenteric vein, the formation of a hæmorrhoidal tumor, and an after co-agulation of blood in the vena cava and veins of the extremities, but more especially of the right. I have to regret that no notice was taken at the time of the interior state of the concretion.

Case 2.—Coagula of blood in the venous trunks; sudden death.—J. Foley, ætat. 43; 85th Regiment; admitted into regimental hospital, Malta, 19th March, 1830; died 16th June.—This man, shortly after admission, had the ordinary symptoms of advanced pulmonary consumption. These became mitigated under treatment, and to such an extent that on the 13th May the functions were reported to be healthy, with the exception of his respiration. During the last three weeks of his life he took no medicine, and his bowels, it is stated, were regular. He died suddenly in bed at 4 a.m.

Autopsy 11 hours after death. Greatly emaciated. The lungs were extremely diseased, containing cavities and vomicæ, and abounding in tubercles. There were no ulcers in the trachea or larynx; but there were many and large in the colon, and a few small ones in the lower ileum. The stomach was sound, and contained some chymous fluid. The vena cava superior and the right auricle were much distended with coagulated blood. In the right ventricle there was also some fibrinous concre-tion. The left ventricle contained coagulated blood *broken up* "*in pieces.*" There was also much coagulated blood in the pulmonary veins, and in the left auricle. Some in a soft state was found in the abdominal aorta and the iliac arteries. The inferior cava was exceedingly distended with coagulum. The vena portæ and its branches contained a little—the hepatic veins a good deal; all much of the same character, as if quite recent, and suggestive of the idea that death—the sudden event—was owing to the sudden change in the condition of the blood.

Case 3.—Fibrinous concretion obstructing the left iliac vein, and coagulated blood the femoral, without disease of those vessels.—A. Craig, ætat. 23; R.B.; admitted into regimental hospital, Malta, 26th September, 1830; died 22nd January, 1831.—This man, when laboring under confirmed pulmonary consumption, experienced during the night of the 28th December acute pain extending from the left groin to the foot. The limb became first slightly œdematous, afterwards swollen. The pain for a time increased in the *groin*, so as to be of great intensity, yet, *there* there was no swelling or redness. It gradually subsided, but it never ceased entirely. He had the use of the limb and was able to walk. I could not learn that there had been any numbness or diminution of its temperature; it was always wrapped in flannel. He died as it seemed "from exhaustion."

Autopsy 13 hours after death. Much emaciated. The left lower extremity was swollen and œdematous. Both lungs were extremely diseased and abounded in tubercles and vomicæ. The pericardium contained 6oz. of transparent serum. There was much fibrinous concretion in the right auricle and ventricle. The left ventricle contained some coagulated blood "broken into fragments." There was a fibrinous concretion in the left iliac vein and coagulated blood in the femoral and in its larger branches, gradually decreasing in firmness downwards and ending in the veins of the leg a little above the ankle. The concretion superiorly reached nearly the entrance of the vena cava. Its substance was firm and nearly colorless. There was no appearance of disease of the inner coat to which it adhered firmly. The cellular coat of the vessel was in some places thickened and generally infiltrated with serum, as was the cellular tissue of the limb throughout. Whether the concretion was opened or not is not stated: it probably was not, my attention at that time not having been drawn to the subject of the puruloid softening of fibrin. The aorta and its branches were examined; no lesion was found in them.

Case 4.—Fibrinous concretion in heart and in common iliac vein; in the latter softening and puruloid.—A. Galena, ætat. 46; a native of Malta; admitted into the civil hospital, 10th March, 1832; died 11th May.—This man's disease was called "general dropsy." When much reduced in strength and without any abatement of the dropsical symptoms, diarrhœa supervened, and death speedily followed.

Autopsy 20 hours after death. There was general anasarca of the trunk and extremities. The right lower limb was more swollen than the left. The right pleura contained 2 pints of serum; the left 1½ pint; the cavity of the abdomen 3 pints. The cellular tissue of the intestines was œdematous, and there were patches of lymph on the mucous membrane of the colon and rectum. There was a rounded fibrinous concretion in the right ventricle of the heart. A fibrinous concretion was found in the right common iliac vein, just before its passing under the corresponding artery. It was about the size of a common almond, of a pretty firm consistence and adhering posteriorly to the vein. It contained a puriform fluid like that of an abscess, as if the fibrin had become changed into pus. There was a smaller concretion of the same kind, and containing a similar fluid in the left iliac vein. When detached, the surface of the vein beneath in each instance was seen to be yellowish and rough, and firmer than other portions of the same vessels. The femoral vein also in each limb contained coagulated blood. No abscess could be detected in the adjoining parts, or elsewhere.

Case 5.—Coagula in the left iliac and femoral vein; closure with suppuration of appendix vermiformis.—T. Keir, ætat. 23; 73rd Regiment; admitted into regimental hospital, Malta, 23rd October, 1833; died 3rd May, 1834.—This man, whilst in hospital, in addition to the ordinary symptoms of advanced pulmonary consumption, had great hoarseness of voice. On the 1st May he felt a pain in the left lower extremity, attended with swelling, which continued, but without severity, till he died, three days after.

Autopsy 17 hours after death. Much emaciated. The left lower extremity swollen and œdematous. The right cavities of the heart were distended with coagulated blood, *partly broken up.* The left cavities contained a small quantity of coagulum, which in the ventricle was similarly broken. There was no separation of fibrin from the blood in either cavity. In the left lung there was a vast excavation. The right abounded in tubercles and vomicæ. The epiglottis, trachea, and bronchi were more or less ulcerated. There were small ulcers in the jejunum and colon. The appendicula vermiformis was singularly diseased. Its middle portion was distended with puruloid matter, as it were encysted, being contained in a delicate false membrane closing the passage. The left iliac and femoral vein were distended with coagulated blood, as were also the deep veins of the leg and foot, and the saphena of the thigh. There was no apparent disease of the coats of these vessels.

The closure of the appendicula vermiformis is a noteworthy circumstance; to me it is a solitary instance of the kind.

Case 6.—Fibrin in the thoracic duct, with ulceration and puruloid softening.—M. Deveril, ætat. 42; an armorer; died in Malta, 23rd May, 1833.—This man for many years had been intemperate, and had been subject to asthma. Latterly he became dropsical; he was twice tapped. During the last fortnight of his existence delirium, very like *delirium tremens*, set in. His kidneys became very active; the œdema of limbs and the other dropsical symptoms disappeared, and his breathing, before difficult, became easy.

Autopsy 20 hours after death. Much emaciated. The cerebrum was softer than natural; the septum lucidum pultaceous; there was much fluid in the ventricles. The heart was hypertrophied. There was some œdema of the lungs, and also of the nurilema of the par vagum, especially where it gives off the recurrent. The thoracic duct was enlarged, especially its receptaculum. A thin coagulum of blood adhered to it, and it contained besides a reddish fluid; near its end there was a layer of lymph covering an ulcerated spot, which communicated with a small outer cavity, little larger than a cherry-stone, full of a puruloid fluid similar to that resulting from the softening and liquefaction of fibrin. At the time it was called an abscess, and the fluid, pus. In the pelvis there were about two pints of serum. There were no marked lesions of any of the abdominal viscera.

The state of the thoracic duct in this instance is very remarkable, especially considering its little disposition—even less, I believe, than veins—to take on a diseased action. It may be open to question whether the origin of it was *ab interno* or *externo*, and also what were its morbid influences.

Case 7.—Vena portæ and splenic vein obstructed by coagula; death from hæmatemesis—R. Oliver, ætat. 30; 94th Foot; admitted into regimental hospital, Malta, 10th September, 1833; died 11th October.—This man, of intemperate habits, of a weakly and sallow appearance and dyspeptic, just before admission vomited about a quart of blood, nausea preceding, attended with pain in the region of the spleen. On the 14th and 15th September he vomited about a pint each day. There was no return of the hæmatemesis until the 1st October; but in the interval his health greatly deteriorated, his appearance becoming leucophlegmatic, with general debility, distension of abdomen, œdema of feet and scrotum; his pulse small and quick. On the 1st October he vomited about three pints of blood; on the 8th a pint and half; on the 9th at different times about a quart; on the 10th and 11th a very large quantity. The blood first ejected was liquid; latterly it was partly in clots. His stools were like coffee-grounds. He expired, it was said, "completely exhausted" from the frequently repeated hæmorrhage which continued to occur within a very short time of his death. The treatment was such as is commonly employed to arrest hæmorrhage.

Autopsy 7 hours after death. Anæmic appearance, with a slight degree of general anasarca. The upper portion of both lungs was pale and crepitous; the lower gorged with serum. There was much serum in the bronchia, suggesting suffocation as the immediate cause of death. It was coagulated by nitric acid. The left pleura contained 6 oz., the right 3 oz.; the pericardium 2 oz. of serum. There was no blood in the cavities of the heart; this organ was normal. In the venæ cavæ there was a little blood, and that so dilute as to resemble colored serum. The mesentery was loaded with fat; the cavity of the pelvis was almost filled with fat. The liver was small; it weighed 2 lb. 14 oz. It was of a rough, tuberculated appearance; of moderate firmness; of the color, somewhat lighter, of unbleached wax. A portion of it dried on paper imparted no stain of oil. The stomach was large, and contained a large quantity of bloody fluid, and some clots of blood. It seemed sound in texture. The small intestines were flabby, and contained a reddish fluid. In the large intestines there was a good deal of dark, pitch-like matter. In neither was there any ulceration. A firm coagulum was detected in the vena portæ, which extended into two branches in the liver, and in the opposite direction into the veins terminating in the vena portæ. The obstruction in all appeared to be complete. In the splenic vein, the coagulum reached the spleen. Near that organ the vein was much distended. There the coagulum was softening in its middle, and was partly reddish, partly white. The outer coat of this vessel was ossified to the extent of about half an inch, and about one half of its circumference. Most of its larger branches within the spleen were full of dark, coagulated blood. The spleen was about twice or thrice its natural size; it weighed 2 lbs.; in substance, it was rather pale and soft. The coagulum in the vena portæ and in the hepatic branches, and in the superior mesenteric vein was almost of ligamentous firmness and whiteness, and was strongly adhering. Even in its central substance there was present some bony matter. The veins of the stomach were without coagula. The splenic artery was large, but not ossified. The kidneys were pale and anæmic.

I shall offer here little or no comment on this singular and singularly obscure case ; merely remarking that there was no knowledge of the individual having ever received any injury which could have been concerned in the production of the disease. It should have been stated in the description that the part of the vein that was ossified was its external cellular fibrous coat. Etiologically, whether the ossification preceded the coagulation, or the coagulation of the blood the ossification, I apprehend must be left in doubt.

Case 8.—Softened fibrin in the lung; branch of pulmonary artery ulcerated; death from hæmoptysis.—W. Read, ætat. 26; 89th F.; admitted 25th May, 1835; died 17th September.—This man was sent home invalided from the West Indies on account of chronic catarrh of 3 years' duration. When admitted on landing, he had most of the symptoms of advanced pulmonary consumption. There was a kind of lull of them until six days before his death. At night then he was suddenly seized with what was called "a vomiting of blood," which lasted half an hour. From this time he rapidly declined. Another attack of the same kind, which occurred also during the night, almost immediately proved fatal.

Autopsy 15 hours after death. Sub-emaciated. Chest large and very sonorous on percussion. The lungs, partially adhering, were very voluminous. Of each a large portion was emphysematous. Under the pleura of one there were large vesicles distended with air.* Both lungs had a singularly lobulated structure. In the right lung, in the upper part of its middle lobe, there was a cavity capable of holding an

---

* About 4 cubic inches of air was collected from them, immersed immediately after removal in water. It was found to be azote, not being diminished either by lime water or phosphorus.

orange, full of coagulated blood. A large branch of the pulmonary artery opened into it,* and also a large bronchial tube. In the superior lobe of the same lung there was the appearance of a cicatrix, produced by grizzly bands intersecting a small condensed mass; it contained also many grey miliary tubercles. Tubercles of the same kind were found in the superior lobe of the left lung. In the substance of its inferior lobe there was a collection of soft albuminous matter resembling *softened fibrin*.† Attached to the inferior portion of the same lobe, between it and the diaphragm, probably under the pleura pulmonalis, there was a similar mass and larger, about the size of an orange. There was a good deal of coagulated blood in the bronchia and some in the stomach, probably swallowed. The lining membrane of the organ was stained red. There was no appearance of disease in any of the abdominal viscera. The pericardium contained an ounce of serum. There was much coagulated blood in both auricles and ventricles of the heart. The coagulum in the right was firmer than that in the left, as if longer coagulated. There was also a little fibrin in the right cavities and a little cruor; this set apart after three hours remained liquid; agitated in the pneumatic bottle it gave off a good deal of air.

This case, strictly rather belongs to the preceding than to the present section. It is inserted hypothetically, on account of the masses between the lung and the diaphragm yielding a matter similar to that resulting from the softening of fibrin, and suggestive of the idea in consequence that the masses themselves may have consisted of fibrin, and have undergone a like change.

Case 9.—Fibrinous concretions in the heart with puruloid softening.—J. Christopher, ætat. 35; 68th F. ; admitted 20th September, 1836 ; died 22nd March, 1837.—This man for many months labored under lumbar abscess, without his general health materially suffering. Early in January an unfavorable change took place; the purulent discharge became copious; debility rapidly increased with hectic and a short tickling cough; bed sores formed on the hip, and before death there was anasarca, especially of the lower extremities.

Autopsy 32 hours after death. There was hepatization and tubercular disease of the lungs, with effusion into the pleura. There was also varied abdominal disease; effusion (9 pints of serum) with marks of peritoneal inflammation, and caries and exostis of the lumbar vertebræ, with extensive sinuses, etc. The pericardium adhered to the heart. The cavities of the heart were nearly empty. In the left ventricle, in its inferior part two small masses of fibrin were found adhering to the columnæ carneæ; one was about the size of a large cherry and spherical; it contained a pus-like fluid; the other, rather larger, was of a less regular form, somewhat globular, tapering in one direction, and shreddy. Whether it contained any softened matter was not ascertained. Both were partially tinged by the coloring matter of blood. The spherical one resembled a cyst; its shell—applying the term to the containing

---

* The artery was not in a band traversing the cavity. It had been interrupted and destroyed by the ulcerative process, like a bronchial tube. A large probe passed readily through it, pushing before it a little loose spongy lymph. Probably the hæmorrhage was so rapid that the blood in part flowed over and entered the stomach, from whence it was rejected by vomiting.

† Under the microscope it exhibited very much the same character—viz., globules of different sizes, the largest about the size of pus-globules. With aqua potassæ it became viscid, and gave off no ammoniacal odor.

part—was about a line thick and so strong as to admit of inflation with the blow-pipe after the discharge of its contents. The fluid it contained was about the consistence of the pus of an abscess. It did not distinctly produce colored rings when tried by the optical test.

In the history of this case no symptom is mentioned that could be associated with the small concretions in the heart.

Case 10.—Concrete fibrin, undergoing puruloid softening in the longitudinal sinus and in the left ventricle of the heart.—J. Smith, ætat. 18; 17th Foot; admitted 25th March, 1837; died 28th August.—This man had been ill about two months before his admission into the general hospital. His symptoms were those of a complication of peritonitis and dysentery. He gradually sank. On the 28th August his pulse was hardly perceptible. For several days before the event he was pronounced to be moribund; his extremities cold; facies Hippocratica; slight delirium; no expression of any painful suffering.

Autopsy 7 hours after death. Exceedingly emaciated. In the middle of the longitudinal sinus there was a small mass of pale fibrin softening in the centre; pretty firmly adhering; it did not completely obstruct the passage; an extension of it was found in two venous branches. Both before it and behind there was some coagulated blood. There was a little serosity in the ventricles, and pretty much at the base of the brain. The substance of the brain was pretty natural. In the cavities of the heart there were fibrinous concretions. There was an extension of the mass in the left ventricle into the aorta. The portion in the ventricle contained some softened matter, which, like that in the longitudinal sinus, was not iridescent. In the arch of the aorta two thread-like portions of coagulable lymph were detected, each coiled, and bearing a certain resemblance to a small cylindrical earth-worm. There were a few curd-like tubercles or accretions between the pleura pulmonalis and the diaphragm, where the lungs were adhering; and some interlobular emphysema. There were no tubercles in either lung. There were numerous lesions within the abdomen; tubercles in the omentum, firm and white, less in size than small peas; adhesions of the several viscera and abscesses. One of these, which was between the edge of the liver and the upper part of the duodenum, contained about an ounce of highly iridescent pus; another, more properly a sinus, in the right iliac fossa, extended upwards to the kidney, and downwards to the external inguinal ring. It was beneath the peritoneum, and by a perforation of the intestine communicated with the adhering cœcum; it contained a reddish sanies. There was a perforation also in the ileum which communicated with a small sac, as it were, of false membrane, which had formed between two folds. There were large ulcers in the colon and rectum, and also ulcers in the ileum. Another and more remarkable lesion remains to be noticed, viz., an ulcerated opening between the appendicula vermiformis and the lower portion of the ileum. The two were adhering together and to the brim of the pelvis; and the extremity of the former, it may be inferred, owing to the extension of penetrating ulceration, had sloughed off into the latter.

In this case we have a remarkable example of complicated organic disease slowly making progress, with the display of an effort as it were to repair or correct certain lesions; one is very noteworthy, viz., the last described, the penetration of the ileum, and the reception within it of the extremity of the vermiform appendix, and that laid open by ulceration.

Case 11.—Aneurism of aorta, containing softening fibrin; closure of a branch of the pulmonary artery by coagula.—J. Sherron, ætat. 33; 60th Foot; admitted 25th July, 1837; died 19th August.—This man's illness began suddenly in November last, and was attributed to playing the bugle. Whilst in hospital, after his return from the Mediterranean, the predominant symptoms were—great dyspnœa, cough with copious expectoration, rapid wasting, and constant nausea. Between the 7th and 17th August his appetite became voracious. On the 18th his pulse was almost imperceptible; his voice hardly audible. He expired a few hours after.

Autopsy 26 hours after death. Greatly emaciated. The lungs were much diseased, containing cavities and tubercles. The heart was rather small; its structure natural. An aneurismal tumor was found within the pericardium, just above the semilunar valves, contiguous to and pressing on the pulmonary artery. Its sac was capable of holding a large walnut. It had a rough lining membrane, continuous with that of the aorta. The entrance into it was of a size to admit three fingers. It contained a little loose clot, and a small portion of fibrin. The latter was adhering, and was softening interiorly. The corresponding portion of the pulmonary artery was rough. One of its larger branches—its right—was closed from the pressure of the tumor, its sides adhering as if glued together by lymph; a small force, however, was sufficient to separate them. The same branch beyond, and its ramifications so far as they were followed, were plugged up with coagulated blood and fibrin, adhering to the coats of the vessel, and evidently of some standing, but when cut into, no softening could be detected in their centre. With the exception of the site of the aneurism, the aorta was free from disease.

In this case we have the unusual association of tubercles with aneurism, and of aneurism with softening fibrin.

Case 12.—Fibrinous masses containing puruloid matter in left ventricle of heart.—R. Winkworth, ætat. 58; admitted into Fort Clarence Lunatic Asylum, 19th May, 1819; died 8th February, 1837.—This man was transferred from the Hoxton Asylum to Fort Clarence, when the latter was opened for the reception of army lunatics in 1819. He had been in confinement since 1805, after trial for murder, and acquittal on the plea of mental imbecility. His person was diminutive, voice effeminate; he was beardless, and the organs of generation were imperfectly developed. When first admitted he had mammæ of considerable size, which became atrophied. His mental faculties were feeble; his manners gentle and childish; he was tractable, and made himself useful. His health was good until November, 1836, when he became subject to diarrhœa, and in the following month to cough with mucous expectoration, and hurried breathing. Pectoriloquy was tolerably distinct in the right subclavicular region. He gradually declined in strength, without urgency of cough or diarrhœa. His appetite was good to the last. His pulse was small and quick; during the last ten days it was not perceptible.

Autopsy 52 hours after death. Emaciated. No hair on chin or pubes; legs and feet œdematous. The cranial bones were very thin. There was much fluid under the membranes and in the ventricles of the brain. The corpora quadrigemina were very small, as indeed was the encephalon generally. Its substance was very firm. The posterior moiety of the septum lucidum was deficient. Both lungs abounded in tubercles, and contained many cavities. The larynx was very small. The left cavities of the heart were distended with coagulated blood, the right nearly empty. In the left ventricle, adhering to the columnæ corneæ, there were numerous small white masses, many of them globular. Cut into, they were found to contain a fluid of the appearance of pus —rather thicker than benign pus, and having a red tinge. On glass held before a candle there was no iridescence; the transmitted light was yellowish. It was not materially affected by muriate of ammonia, and had no offensive smell. Externally the little masses were pretty firm. One had the appearance of being vascular, but whether really so was uncertain. The largest was about the size of a hazel-nut; the smallest about that of a pea. Nothing peculiar was observed in the substance of the heart. Mixed with the coagulated blood there was no ordinary fibrinous concretion, and the coagulum was not broken, thereby denoting that it was a *post mortem* formation. The thoracic aorta was very large, the abdominal smaller than natural, especially above the origin of the common iliacs, which were unusually small. The generative organs—penis, testes, vesiculæ seminales, prostrate—were all very diminutive. There was no albuginea; the vasa deferentia were distinct; the epididymis exceeded in volume the testes. There were some masses of fat adhering to the right cord—masses nearly the size of an almond. The intestines were free from ulceration. Their position was abnormal.

In this case we have a good example of congruity of organs in partially arrested development.

Case 13.—Concrete fibrin in internal jugular vein, and in the right iliac and right and left femoral vein, with puruloid softening.—C. Buckley, ætat. 33; 63rd F.; admitted 26th October, 1837; died 2nd November.—This man, of 14 years' service in India, was sent home on account of varicose veins. Brought to hospital immediately on landing, he was found in a feeble state, with cough, pains in the legs, considerable œdema of both lower extremities and some effusion into the abdomen. His pulse was very feeble; the urine not coagulable. Auscultation afforded no morbid indications. Under a course of diuretics and tonics, the dropsical symptoms subsided and his general health improved so much that he was discharged on the 30th September. On the 26th October he was re-admitted, with cough, dyspnœa, pains in the legs and a dropsical state of the feet and ankles. On the 28th the report was favorable; his cough and breathing were relieved, and his pulse, which had been very feeble, was of better strength. On the 1st Nov. a great change for the worse had taken place; the pulse was scarcely perceptible; his extremities cold; in brief, he was moribund, yet his intellect was undisturbed. He expired the following day at 11 a.m.

Autopsy 26 hours after death. The lower extremities œdematous, the right limb more than the left. The pia mater was very thin and was detached with difficulty. Corresponding to the posterior part of the right parietal bone, there was a considerable depression in the substance of the cerebrum, holding about half a drachm of fluid, which was rendered turbid by nitric acid. The pia mater over the depression was thickened, as was also the arachnoid; its boundary substance was unusually firm, and to the depth of two or three lines was of a brownish hue. There was much fluid in the ventricles and in the occipital fossæ. The corpora quadrigemina* were small; the pineal gland very small. The substance of the brain generally was firm. In the neck, in each side, in the situation of the curvical glands, sinuses were found containing pus or a puruloid fluid; they extended upwards to the jaw and downwards to the axillæ. The glands too were diseased, enlarged and many of them were suppurating. There was no appearance in them of tubercular matter, nor was there any redness of skin externally. The sterno-clido-mastoideus muscle immediately over the glands was involved in the suppuration, being wasted, and as it were corroded. A small fibrinous concretion was detected within the right internal jugular vein: it was

---

* The testes and penis were very small, as was also the larynx. There was no hair on the pubes. By his comrades he was considered as averse from the sex.

adhering and softening. The right lung was bulky and heavy; its dependent parts œdematous; portions of it, not exceeding a filbert in size, were hepatized. The left was collapsed and tolerably sound. The heart contained a very little coagulated blood and fibrin, and was nowise peculiar, excepting the fossa ovalis, which was of unusual thinness, with several small openings in it, two large enough to admit a goose-quill. The liver weighed 2¾ lbs., was adherent to the diaphragm and contained imbedded in its substance two small collections of puruloid matter, in volume not larger than a pea. The spleen was firm; its capsule partially thickened. The kidneys were unusually hard, almost of gristly consistence. The rectum was red and flabby. The right iliac and both the femoral veins were filled with coagula, the former to its junction with the vena cava. The coagulum in the right femoral vein was thick crassamentum; in the iliac of the same side it was fibrinous, partially tinged red, of a firmer consistence externally, softening internally. Just at its entrance there was a little reddish sanies, which under the microscope was seen to abound in globules, many of them like pus-globules. In the left femoral vein, a little below Pompart's ligament there was a mass of fibrin, very slightly adhering, which was rounded superiorly, firm externally and resting inferiorly on dark red crassamentum. When punctured, a cream-colored fluid came from it, exceedingly like pus and very like that of the sinuses in the neck. It was somewhat thicker than laudable pus. Under the microscope it was seen to consist of globules, not quite so regular as pus-globules, and of numerous granules. Compared with the matter from the neck there was no well-marked difference. The cavity from which it issued was of considerable size and contained a residue of similar matter colored slightly reddish.

This case has been given pretty much in detail on account of its many peculiarities. The patient was under the care of a very intelligent and attentive medical officer, and during life there was no suspicion of suppuration in the neck, or of coagula having been formed in the veins of the inferior extremities; nor in the abstract of his case, which accompanied him from his regiment, was there any mention of apoplexy or of cerebral disease at any former period. The legs after death were examined for varicose veins; none could be found; the superficial veins were not larger than usual. Not the least noteworthy circumstance in this instance is the similarity of the matter found in the neck, the liver and the veins; and suggestive (may it not be surmised?) etiologically, of a like origin.

Case 14.—Concrete fibrin, with puruloid softening in the ascending vena cava and iliac veins.—P. Long, ætat. 35; 86th Foot; admitted 11th May, 1837; died 7th August.—This man, when taken into hospital, had recently arrived from the West Indies in a very enfeebled state from diarrhœa of four months' duration, and with a constitution impaired by attacks of other disease during a service of 17 years. Under a mild treatment he appeared to be slowly improving until the 21st June, when an œdematous swelling began in the left lower extremity, with considerable hardness and pain along the course of the femoral vein, and especially at the place of junction of the saphena Gentle frictions employed, the pain rapidly ceased, and the swelling gradually. On the 24th July the right leg became œdematous, and a hardness was perceived soon after in the direction of the vein, but attended with little uneasiness, with very little pain. The swelling of the limb was at its maximum about the 28th July; after that it slowly diminished. The bowel complaint continued with little interruption or abatement to the end. He gradually lost strength and appetite, and latterly fell into an extremely languid state, dozing a good deal, which might perhaps have been partly the effect of the opium which he took.

Autopsy 23 hours after death. Extremely emaciated. The left lower extremity pretty much swollen, pitting on pressure; the right hardly perceptibly. The membranes of the brain had an atrophied appearance. The fornix was soft. There was a good deal of fluid in the ventricles. The lungs, with the exception of a bony concretion in each, about the size of a hazel-nut, appeared to be sound. Together they weighed 1 lb. 6 oz. The heart was small, as if atrophied. The liver weighed 2 lbs. 8 oz. There was a small calculus, of the lithic acid kind, in the pelvis of the left kidney. The lower ileum bore marks of old ulceration. The colon throughout was more or less diseased. It exhibited ulceration in its different stages; many ulcers were still open, some were healing by granulation, and some had healed, marked by a bluish discoloration. The vena portæ contained liquid blood; in the other vessels generally, and in the heart, there was very little blood. Its quantity in the body was small, denoting a very anæmic state. In the femoral and iliac veins of each side, extending into the ascending cava as far as the emulgent veins, coagula were found, more or less obstructing these vessels. The right femoral and iliac were more distended than the left. In the right femoral vein the coagulum was of the appearance and consistence of the fresh crassamentum of venous blood. In the left it was much firmer and paler, as if the coloring matter had been in part removed, but not equably. The coagulum in the vena cava was nearly of the same hue. Laid open it was found to be formed of layers of fibrin, within which was a semi-fluid puruloid matter. In the coagulum in the right iliac vein there was a small quantity of the same kind of matter. The left iliac contained a little firm fibrin. The saphena of the same side, which at one time, it may be inferred, held a coagulum, now was empty.

In this case it may be inferred, as in so many others, that a debilitated state of the system conduced to the formation of the fibrinous concretions in the veins; and that these when formed were not without effect in shortening life can hardly be doubted. The anæmic condition of the body, in connexion with these accretions of fibrin, is noteworthy.

Case 15.—Concrete fibrin, with puruloid softening in right ventricle of heart, and in the aorta.—J. Owen, ætat. 39; 56th Foot; admitted 25th June, 1837; died 28th August.—This man had suffered from fever and other complaints in the West Indies. Since 1836 he has had repeated attacks of hæmoptysis. On admission, after his return home, he was in the advanced stage of phthisis. During the last week of his life a troublesome diarrhœa supervened with tenesmus. The emaciation was great, as was also the debility, yet he is reported to have died rather suddenly and unexpectedly.

Autopsy 27 hours after death. Both lungs, very closely and firmly adhering, abounded in tubercles in different stages of progress. In each there was a small excavation, and portions of both were hepatized. Under the pleura pulmonalis of the right lung there was a cartilaginous mass.* The heart was large. All its cavities,

* It was about 3 inches by 1 in extent, and on careful examination was found in parts to be enveloped in a fibrous tissue, portions of which were in bands and like

as well as the principal vessels, were distended with coagulated blood, without cruor. When the clot was turned out of the right ventricle, three masses of lymph of a reddish hue, and containing a semi-fluid matter of the same color, were found in the lower part of its cavity, amongst its reticulated structure. The matter was neither iridescent, tried by the optical test, nor had any unpleasant smell. The largest mass was about the size of a hazel-nut; but less regular in form. Its surface was slightly· softening. The adjoining part, as well as the heart generally, was of ordinary appearance; there was no trace of ulceration. Nothing but clot was found in the left ventricle and in the ascending aorta. In the thoracic portion of the latter, two small masses of lymph were detected, one about the size of a cherry, the other about that of a pea. Both were firmly adhering to the vessel. Where they adhered, there the inner coat of the aorta was thickened and indurated, the middle wasted and thin. Each little mass was firm externally; each contained a semi-fluid matter, of a light brown hue, and not iridescent. There were a few ulcers in the ileum, and many large ones in the colon. The other abdominal viscera were of natural appearance.

Is it not probable that death in this instance was owing to coagulation of blood in the heart?

Case 16.—Obstruction of the left iliac and femoral veins by coagulated blood.—J. Gleson, ætat. 20; 27th F.; admitted 30th May, 1837; died 22nd July.—This man was admitted in the advanced stage of pulmonary consumption. On the 6th of July the left leg and foot became œdematous and rather painful. Amongst his latter symptoms were severe pain at scrobiculis cordis, with a tendency to retching and slight convulsions when making any attempt to drink. On the 17th the œdema of the lower extremity had extended to the thigh. Just before death he had a severe and protracted fit of coughing.

Autopsy 11 hours after death. Greatly emaciated. The left lower extremity œdematous. There was a large cavity in each lung and both abounded in tubercles. The larynx was ulcerated. There were ulcers in the jejunum, ileum and colon. The left iliac and femoral veins were obstructed by coagulum, which in the former was soft of a light reddish hue; in the latter, its upper part, it was partly soft and partly firm, and nearly of the same color; whilst in its lower portion it was of the color of ordinary crassamentum. The coagulum extended superiorly to near where the iliac vein passes under the iliac artery. There, there was a cluster of slightly enlarged and very red lumbar glands, which, it was conjectured, by their pressure in retarding the flow of blood, might have promoted its coagulation. No puruloid matter was found in any portion of the coagulum, nor was there any appearance of the softening which in other instances has been observed associated with the presence of that matter.

In this instance we have an example of coagula in their early stage formed in the veins ; not differing apparently from ordinary crassamentum. Had life been long protracted, in all probability the coagula would have become fibrinous concretions.

Case 17.—Fibrinous concretion and coagula, the former with puruloid softening in the femoral veins.—J. Edwards, ætat. 20; 41st Foot; admitted 30th May, 1837;

tendon. A section brought to view a cavity containing loose, irregularly formed masses of bony matter; bony matter entered also into the substance of the cartilaginous—altogether giving the idea of a nisus formativus, an effort, as it were, to form bone, cartilage, and tendon.

died 5th July.—This man, when transferred from the detachment hospital to the general hospital, had been ill and under treatment there since the 13th April, with symptoms resembling those of pulmonary consumption. Pectoriloquy had been perceived in the right side of chest. Expectoration was at first copious and purulent. On the 27th June the integuments ulcerated over the cartilages of the 7th and 8th ribs and a large discharge of fetid matter took place and continued from a sinus communicating with its source in the chest. No swelling was noticed of the lower extremities until the 4th July, the day preceding death, nor was there any mention made of pain having been complained of in the limbs.

Autopsy 40 hours after death. Much emaciated. The lower extremities œdematous. Portions of the ribs on the right side of the chest below the mamilla, where the sinus was situated, were carious. The fistulous opening communicated with a large cavity in the substance of the lung. It contained about 3 pints of turbid fluid.* Its walls were gangrenous. This lung was pretty generally and closely adhering to the costal pleura; its parenchyma was considerably condensed, owing to the pressure, no doubt, of the fluid contained in the cavity formed in it. No tubercles could be detected in it or in the left lung. The latter was in part emphysematous and partly œdematous. Coagulated blood was found in all the cavities of the heart. The liver weighed 5 lbs. and was pale as if anæmic. The other abdominal viscera were apparently sound. Both femoral veins were completely obstructed by fibrinous concretion and by coagulated blood, the former to the extent of about 2 inches from Poupart's ligament; the latter, beginning where the former stopped, reached nearly to the knee, gradually diminishing in firmness. The large venous branches were also filled with coagulum. The fibrinous concretion was pretty firmly adhering. When taken out, the vessels appeared internally unaltered; externally, however, their cellular fibrous coat was condensed, and each vein adhered with unusual firmness to the adjoining artery. The concretions opened were found softening inward, and to contain a pultaceous matter. Beyond the obstructed veins, the iliacs and vena cava were perfectly pervious, though rather small; they contained a very little blood and a little fibrinous concretion.

This case, irrespective of the veins in the lower extremities, is noteworthy on account of the abscess (a pure phlegmonous abscess?) in the substance of the lung; a lesion, according to my experience, amongst soldiers of rare occurrence. One remarkable example of it I remember to have witnessed in the hospital of the 42nd at Malta, and that was a case which recovered completely after life had been despaired of. The expectoration for a while was most copious and offensive, indicative of gangrene and frequently threatening suffocation.

Case 18.—Fibrinous concretion in heart and in the iliac veins with partial puruloid softening.—J. M'Laughlin, ætat. 38; 89th F.; admitted 25th May, 1838; died 7th November.—This man, of 19 years' service, was taken into hospital in a very debilitated state on his return from the West Indies. His disease shortly exhibited the well marked characteristics of pulmonary consumption, pectoral and abdominal symptoms alternating,—the latter chiefly pain in the region of the stomach, vomiting and diarrhœa. Six days before death the left lower extremity became slightly swollen, and some pain was felt in the course of the femoral vein.

* This fluid taken out and put aside, coagulated: the coagulum was soft.

Autopsy 44 hours after death. Extremely emaciated. The lungs were greatly diseased. A large cavity in one lung communicated freely with the pleura, giving rise to pneumathorax. The right cavities of the heart contained a little coagulated blood and fibrin. In the left ventricle there was a good deal of fibrinous concretion; near its apex a mass of fibrin was found in which was an empty cavity, as if its contents had escaped. In the right iliac vein, where it joins the vena cava, there was a mass of fibrin, firmly adhering, in which was found a pus-like matter that was slightly iridescent. The vessel was not so completely obstructed as to prevent the flow of blood The femoral vein communicating with it was empty. The left iliac and femoral vein and its branches were all distended with blood, strongly adhering, but not of firm consistence. Where the first-named vein passes under the iliac artery, it was closed, its sides in contact and closely adhering together with the exception of two small apertures just large enough to admit a pin's head, through which it may be inferred the blood passed till the coagulum formed below obstructing its flow. The intestines were free from ulceration. A few small ulcers, pale and depressed, were found in the mucous coat of the stomach.

The appearance of the coagula in the veins of the right and left lower extremities would indicate different periods of formation. That the fibrinous concretion was of much longer standing than the soft coagulum, cannot be doubted, but in the history of the patient no clue could be found to the exact time of its production. It may be worthy of remark, that the inner coat of the veins containing the coagulum of blood was strongly stained red, whilst the right cavities of the heart, also containing coagulated blood, were free from stain ; seeming, in the difference, to denote that the former was in a state more advanced to putridity.

Case 19.—Fibrinous concretions in the right and left ventricle of heart, with puruloid softening.—C. Marriott, ætat. 22; 98th Foot; admitted November 8th, 1838; died 9th November.—This man, before his transfer to the general hospital, had been laboring under pulmonary and abdominal disease eight months. On arrival he was moribund, the extremities livid, great dyspnœa, a very feeble pulse. He was conscious at the evening visit, expiring the following morning at 4 a.m.

Autopsy 33 hours after death.* Not emaciated. A small portion of the substance of the cerebrum was detached with the pia mater, and correspondingly to the extent of about half an inch by a quarter, the cineritious matter beneath was blood-shot and pultaceous ; the brain generally firm. The left pleura, on which was deposited much lymph, contained 70 oz. of yellowish serum. The lung was so compressed as to be destitute of air. Scattered through it were many cheese-like tubercles. The right lung contained a few similar tubercles, about the size of cherries, and was much gorged with blood and serum. The heart was large; the great vessels connected

---

* 12 hours after death the right carotid artery and the internal jugular vein were examined. No air was found in either of them. Two or three ounces of blood flowed from the vein. A portion of it, tested by potash, afforded signs of ammonia; the remainder put aside did not coagulate ; the following morning the red corpuscles had subsided, and were covered with clear serum. Now, the portion to which the potash had been added gave off a strong ammoniacal odor, not needing the approach of muriatic acid as at first to detect the volatile alkali.

with it small, especially the aorta. In the right auricle and ventricle there was some loosely coagulated blood, with pretty much cruor, and a mass of lymph. Near the apex of the latter cavity fibrinous concretions and small clots were found which contained a reddish pus-like matter, slightly iridescent. In the left ventricle there was a little soft coagulum, and near its apex and adhering there were two pretty large masses of fibrinous concretion, nearly the size of almonds. One contained a reddish puruloid matter; the other was empty, and evidently *collapsed;* a section of it displayed a cavity large and smooth within. Besides these two there were several smaller masses. There were about 8 oz. of serum in the cavity of the abdomen. It was collected with difficulty, owing to the manner in which the different viscera were adhering together. A good deal of shreddy lymph covered the intestines. The omentum was gathered up and thickened, so as to resemble a pancreas in form. There was a general granular state of the peritoneum, especially of that portion of it reflected over the intestines. The spleen was large and firm; its section showed a hepatized appearance,—a central portion of a light hue, included in an outer of a darker color. The splenic artery contained a firm coagulum, without any distinct softening; it gave the idea of having been formed during life. With the exception of a small ulcer in the cœcum, the mucous membrane of the alimentary canal was free from disease.

In this case probably death was partly owing to the concretions formed in the heart, especially in the left ventricle. The empty collapsed state of one of them is a noteworthy circumstance; its puruloid contents (supposing them similar to those of the concretion not emptied) must have entered the circulation, and may have acted as a poison.

Case 20.--The vena cava ascendens obstructed by fibrin undergoing puruloid softening.—Anne Hartley, ætat. 51; admitted into Fort Clarence, 21st October, 1821; died 13th March, 1839.—This woman, the wife of a private soldier, had suffered in health in India. From the time of her admission into the asylum in 1821, until 1835, she was mostly quiet, tolerably intelligent and obedient; at irregular intervals excited and violent, then her talk was abusive and obscene. In the autumn of the last mentioned year, she was so rational for two months, that measures were taken for her discharge. Her relapse was sudden. During 1836 the paroxysms of excitement were more violent than before, and of longer duration. In 1837 she emaciated, and looked sickly. On the 10th January following she vomited about a pint of blood. On the 21st she was reported convalescent; but she continued to decline, was pale and emaciated, and subject to syncope. On the 4th December of the same year the left lower extremity became swollen, pitting on pressure; the temperature was slightly increased, but without febrile symptoms. The œdema gradually subsided, and on the 21st had entirely disappeared. Her health did not improve; her stomach continued irritable; she had a trifling cough, and expectorated a little mucus; her breathing free; the skin was cool; the pulse feeble, but not frequent; the debility and emaciation still increasing. About a month before death her intellect for a short time was unusually clear. A fortnight later there was a recurrence of excitement, notwithstanding her enfeebled state of body. A few hours before she expired the right lower extremity was observed to be generally swollen from the foot to the groin, and rather hot and red, pitting on pressure.

Autopsy 17 hours after death. Much emaciated. The membranes of the brain had an atrophied appearance. The cerebral substance was generally firmer than common.

The lateral ventricles were much distended with transparent fluid, and there was a good deal at the base of the brain. The lungs were partially œdematous. There was a little coagulated blood in the right cavities of the heart, and in the left ventricle. The stomach, chiefly its middle portion, was greatly diseased. Its whole circumference was the seat of cancerous tumors, in texture resembling medullary tumor; the largest was about the size of a pigeon's egg. Several of them were ulcerated, and covered with a brown slough. The stomach generally was much contracted; its cardiac and pyloric portions were free from disease. The liver, pancreas, spleen, and kidneys were small, but without marked disease, except a portion of the pancreas—its head—which was large and hard in texture, very like that of the tumors described. The lower portion of the inferior vena cava contained a fibrinous concretion, apparently quite closing it. It was about two inches long, and resembled an almond nearly in form. Cut into, it was found to consist of an outer coat, comparatively firm, and of an inner fibrinous mass, formed of successive layers of lymph. At its upper extremity a softening seemed in progress, and there, between the outer coat and the inner mass, a little puruloid fluid of a reddish hue was collected. There was an extension of the concretion into the left iliac vein; where it was under the iliac artery it was compressed, beyond it was protuberant; it was very dense, reminding one of the fibrin of an aneurismal sac. Like that of which it was a continuation, it had a laminated structure. It had no appearance of softening. Where it terminated the lower portion of the iliac vein and the upper portion of the femoral were exceedingly contracted; no blood recently appeared to have passed through them; a probe, however, could be passed, their sides, though in contact, not being agglutinated. The very little fibrin they contained, for they were not quite empty, was chord-like, firm, and hard—where thickest less than whipcord, where finest not thicker than sewing thread. The right iliac and femoral veins contained coagulated blood and fibrinous concretion—the latter softening. Adhering to the lower part of the aorta, just above its bifurcation, were what appeared to be small portions of fibrin, the largest about the size of "the nail of little finger."

This case, apart from the main disease, and the mental state, is noteworthy for the apparent restoration of the left lower extremity to its normal size, notwithstanding the obstruction in the ascending cava and femoral vein.

Case 21.—A fibrinous concretion, including another undergoing softening in the right ventricle of the heart.—J. Fellows, ætat. 26; 8th Foot; admitted 20th May, 1839; died 8th November.—This man, when received into hospital on his arrival from Jamaica, was in the advanced stage of pulmonary consumption, the symptoms of which were severe and well marked. On the 17th October he was reported as very feeble and "sinking;" on the 3rd November as having had a violent attack of hæmoptysis, which did not entirely cease until the 7th, the day before he expired. Some hours before death the dyspnœa was extreme, and he was insensible.

Autopsy 17 hours after death. Greatly emaciated. Both lungs contained tubercles and excavations. The larynx was much ulcerated. There were ulcers in the lower ileum, in the cœcum and ascending colon. There were fibrinous concretions and a little cruor in the right auricle and ventricle; and in the latter there was also a mass of fibrin of singular appearance and structure—if the latter expression may be allowed; it bore a resemblance to a finger in a glove; it consisted of an outer firm case, white and thin, and of an inner of a reddish hue, soft, but not pultaceous. The containing and contained were so slightly cohering, as to be easily separated. The remark made at the time was, "that had life been protracted, the inner portion would probably have become semi-fluid."

The concretion in the heart, so peculiar, is suggestive of its mode of formation—viz., that the included portion and the including were of different ages, and of different qualities in consequence: the outer recent and firm; the inner older and softer.

Case 22.—A fibrinous concretion in longitudinal sinus, with puruloid softening, and a ruptured hæmorrhoidal vein.—R. Evans, ætat 33; 52nd F.; admitted 9th September, 1840; died 14th September.—This man, whilst in the West Indies, had suffered from dyspnœa, with debility. On the homeward voyage he was attacked with scurvy. On admission, just after landing, he was in a very feeble, hopeless state. A low delirium set in a few hours before death.

Autopsy 21 hours after death. Much emaciated. There was a good deal of ecchymosis of the left leg. Over the tibia black coagulated blood was found under the integuments, and also amongst the muscles of the limb and between their fibres. There was a firm fibrinous concretion in the longitudinal sinus, softening internally. The brain was of natural appearance, and there was but little excess of fluid between the membranes and in the ventricles. A considerable portion of the middle and also of the inferior lobe of the right lung was œdematous. In the latter, two large vessels were found full of firm coagulum—formed, it was conjectured at the time, from their appearance, during life, and which might have been the cause of the œdema of the part. The pericardium was generally adhering, but not firmly to the heart. 4½ pints of coagulated blood and serum were found in the cavity of the abdomen. The intestines were blackened externally, stained by dark blood. A clot was detected adhering to one of the hæmorrhoidal veins, at a spot where there was a rupture of the vessel, and from whence it may be inferred the effused blood was poured out. In the upper portion of the jejunum there was a perforation of an unusual kind, so large as to admit the little finger, with smooth edges, as if a piece had been cut out or absorbed, and without any surrounding thickening or marks of inflammation. The liver in parts had a pale anæmic appearance, and in part was rather redder and more congested than usual. In this part some of the veins contained clots of fibrine, portions of which were softening.

This case is very noteworthy for its lesions, illustrative of scurvy. The perforation of the jejunum as if from mere absorption, remarkable, and seemingly indicative of very low vitality.

Case 23.—A fibrinous concretion, with puruloid softening, close to a ruptured valve of the aorta.—H. Sutton, ætat. 18; 17th F.; admitted Jan. 1, 1840; died Jan. 22nd.—This man was admitted with severe hernia humoralis, followed by stricture and irritability of the bladder, the urine depositing a ropy sediment. He had occasionally retention of urine, rigors, headache and shifting pains. He fell into a low state with blunted sensibility, approaching to stupor.

Autopsy 19 hours after death. Sub-emaciated. There was no distinct lesion of the brain. The right lung was slightly œdematous. The heart was large and its cavities distended with coagulated blood and fibrinous concretions. A rupture was detected in the situation of the middle valve of the aorta, which was partially destroyed, ragged lymph adhering to its edges. The cavity at the ruptured spot was capable of holding a hazel-nut. It contained a fibrinous concretion softening. The kidneys were unusually red and vascular; the urinary bladder thickened and the urethra, near its membranous portion, almost closed and greatly indurated.

In this case probably the blood had become materially vitiated, inasmuch as the lesions of the solid structures would hardly account for the fatal event.

These cases, if they do not elucidate the mode of formation of the coagulum, the fibrinous concretion and the puruloid fluid, may at least throw some light on their source, their composition and age, and the changes they are subject to.

That the coagulum (taking a special instance) which first forms in the lower extremity, as indicated commonly by pain and swelling of the limb, is coagulated venous blood, I apprehend does not admit of question ; nor, I think, does it admit of question that the fibrinous concretion, in so many instances associated with the coagulum, is derived from it, in process of time the coloring matter being absorbed, or somehow removed; and further it seems to me, it can hardly be doubted that the fibrin, if not absorbed, as it sometimes appears to be, becomes by an ulterior change softened in part and more or less converted into the puruloid fluid.

The only means we have of judging of the incipient coagulation are by the pain and swelling in the limb. Taking these as a criterion in the several cases, it would appear that the alteration from one state to the other is slow in taking place; that for several days the coagulum retains its color, and differs but little from ordinary crassamentum ; that not till the 12th day or thereabout, the softening of the fibrin begins; and that a longer period is required for the formation of the puruloid fluid. The following cases may be referred to in support of these conclusions : as regards the first, the time the coagulum remains little altered, Nos. 1 and 16 ; as regards the second, more difficult to define, No. 17; and as regards the third, the formation of the puruloid fluid, No. 14. I had expected to have been able to have made more references denoting the probable time of change, but on reperusal of the cases I have failed, finding in how many of them the coagulum was found in the veins after death, undenoted by any marked expression of pain during life.

The qualities of the puruloid fluid—that the most peculiar feature—have been well described by Mr. Gulliver in the paper already referred to. Such observations as I have made on it, accord with his, with the exception that when tested for ammonia, I have found it in the majority of instances, to yield slight traces of this alkali. It may be described briefly, as consisting of corpuscles somewhat less in size than pus-globules and less regular, with which are intermixed granules of various sizes; and as not being rendered viscid either by admixture with aqua ammoniæ or a solution of muriate of ammonia.

From the experiments of Mr. Gulliver it would appear that a fluid or semi-fluid coarsely resembling it, may be obtained by the slow coction of fibrin in a water-bath at blood-heat. This is an interesting fact. In his trials the time was varied from seventeen hours to eighty-four: in that of seventeen hours no change was visible in the fibrin; in the others, the longer the coction, the greater was the softening, the more complete the liquefaction. In all his experiments the fibrin acquired more or less of an offensive smell, and there appears to have been a beginning of putrefaction.

In the softening which takes place in the living body, the fibrin has been free from this odor. Another remarkable circumstance belonging to the latter is that the change is a central one, as if two opposite influences were in action at the same time, the one superficial conducing to the hardening, the other interior, conducing to solution, to liquefaction, suggestive of a *nisus formativus*, directed as it were to the formation of a cyst with fluid contents. These are peculiarities showing a marked difference between the fibrin undergoing change during life, and the same out of the body subjected to coction, or when exposed to the atmosphere or undergoing liquefaction, with much development of heat from the absorption of oxygen and the production of carbonic acid and ammonia.*

An interesting subject for inquiry is the difference manifested in the fibrin in the cases under consideration and in those of aneurism; and, whether depending on peculiarities in the fibrin itself, or on the state of the living organism, in the one— the cases in question most commonly tainted, in the other— those of aneurism—mostly healthy, or on both. That both are concerned, seems to me most likely. I have already adverted to the class of persons, the feeble and cachectic, in whom

* See my Anatom. and Physiol. Res. vol. ii., p. 343.

coagulation and the softening of fibrin are most frequently witnessed. In favor of the idea that some peculiarity, some vitiated state of the blood may also exercise an influence, I may mention that in those cases in which I examined the blood after death, I have found it to contain, as it appeared to me, an undue proportion of the white corpuscles, and also, that in each instance that I tried the blood taken from the cadaver, I have found it, on mixing it with hydrate of lime or potassa, to afford more than the usual traces of the presence of ammonia ; and, I may add, that when the same blood or any fluid effused, was subjected to agitation with common air, there was not an absorption but a disengagement of gas : both results I am disposed to consider as indicative of a morbid condition.

I have ventured to throw out the idea that the occurrence of coagula during life may help to explain sudden deaths : many of the cases in their manner of termination were favorable to the conclusion. Case 2 may be mentioned as a probable example, in which the blood was found coagulated in most of the great vessels ; and in the left ventricle, not only coagulated, but broken up, showing that *there*, at least, the blood had coagulated before the action of the heart had ceased.

Relative to another suggestion which I made in introducing the subject, when speaking of its importance pathologically, that it may possibly throw light on the formation and progress of tubercles, on the formation of fistulæ and some other organic lesions, it would be premature now to dwell at any length. The softening of fibrin as witnessed in these cases and the softening of tubercles, both centrically, and the products of their softening are sufficiently analogous. That a fibrinous concretion softening in a hæmorrhoidal vein may give rise to a fistula in ano by exciting an ulcerative process, can, I think, hardly be doubted. And, may not the same obstruction with softening ending in destructive ulceration in other veins or arteries well account for various internal and fatal hæmorrhages? Case 7 presents a remarkable example of the kind, and the more singular from the state of the vein, in which the coagulum formed was partially ossified.

In all the preceding remarks, diseased action has been supposed to be perpetuated by the fibrin in its course of change: perhaps there are exceptions, and occasionally the fibrin, after consolidation, instead of degenerating into something worse, is without liquefaction, absorbed, as, it may be presumed, happens in cases of recovery from phlegmasia dolens, allowing the blood free course through its wonted channels. The appearances presented in Case 20 are favorable to this conclusion.

CHAPTER IX.

ON PNEUMONIA.

Statistics of.—Influence of climate and of other causes productive of the disease.—Illustrative cases with comments: 1st, of the least complicated; 2ndly, of the complicated, with inflammation of the mediastina and cellular tissue; 3rdly, with hypertrophy of heart, etc.; 4thly, with cerebral disease; 5thly, with peritoneal inflammation; 6thly, with anomalous symptoms; 7thly, with rheumatic inflammation, and deposition of lithic acid; 8thly, with tubercles; 9thly, of chronic pneumonia.—Remarks on the foregoing, as to predisposition, symptoms, duration, treatment, and especially on blood-letting, and on the constitution of man past and present.

THIS disease, as might be expected, considering the conditions of military life, though not one of the most common to which the soldier is exposed on service, is yet not of unfrequent occurrence, nor unproductive of a considerable mortality. This is well shown in the following table, in which the admissions and deaths from the disease are given as they occurred at the several stations named during the periods specified. It is drawn up from the Statistical Reports of the Army, and for 10,000 of aggregate strength. Included in it, for the sake of comparison, are the admissions and deaths from pleurisy, a disease so often connected with pneumonia, but so very different, as the table shows, in the ratio of its fatality.

		PNEUMONIA.		PLEURITIS.	
		Admitted.	Died.	Admitted.	Died.
Great Britain, Dragoon Guards and Dragoons,	From Jan. 1, 1836, to March 31, 1837,	149·2	6·0	14·1	—
Gibraltar, ...	From 1818 to 1836 inclusive	415·4	9·2	4·6	—
Malta, ...	From 1817 to 1836	335·5	10·7	5·1	—
Ionian Islands, ...	,, ,, ...	310·9	11·5	12·2	0·4
Bermudas, ...	,, ,, ...	372·0	10·0	4·3	—
Nova Scotia and New Brunswick,	,, ,, ...	324·0	12·5	15·5	0·4
Canada, ...	,, ,, ...	431·5	15·3	19·0	0·9
West Indies, Windward and Leeward Command, ...	,, ,, ...	224·0	12·9	3·9	0·1
Black Troops, ...	,, ,, ...	442·4	36·4	2·9	0·2
Jamaica, ...	,, ,, ...	135·3	2·9	5·6	—
Ceylon, ...	,, ,, ...	170·9	6·2	—	—
Malays, 1st Ceylon Regiment ...	1818 to 1836	152·2	15·5	—	—
Moelmyne, ...	1827 to 1836	112·9	7·3	—	—
Rangoon, ...	From April 21, 1824, to Sept. 20, 1826	141·0	6·6	—	—
West Coast of Africa, ...	1819 to 1836	81·3	5·4	—	—
Black Troops, ...	,, ,, ...	79·0	10·5	27·7	5·2

		PNEUMONIA.		PLEURITIS.	
		Admitted.	Died.	Admitted.	Died.
St. Helena, ...	1818 to 1837	40·6	5·1	20·3	—
Cape of G. Hope, Cape District,	1818 to 1836	296·2	9·7	—	—
Hottentot Troops,..................	,, ,, ...	234·5	9·6	—	—
Mauritius,..........................	,, ,, ...	226·0	11·1	11·1	1.2

From this table we see that though there is some relation
between the frequency and fatality of pneumonia and the climate,
as to temperature of the different stations, the relation is not a
steady and exact one; indeed, in certain instances, the contrary,
it would appear, is the case. That Canada should stand highest
and Jamaica so much lower in the numerical scale is not surprising; but why there should be so great a difference between
Jamaica and the Windward and Leeward Command as is shown,
they having nearly the same climate, is not a little perplexing.
That the disease should be less frequent and severe in Ceylon,
Moelmyne, and Rangoon than at most other stations, may perhaps be explicable, taking into account that at these stations
dysentery is the prevailing malady, and may, and probably
does, attack those who are enfeebled and predisposed to take on
diseased action, rather than pneumonia. But this remark does
not apply to the Mauritius, where, though dysentery holds rank
amongst the most fatal diseases, there is no unusual exemption
from pneumonia.

This irregularity of occurrence of pneumonia, within certain
limits is not restricted to countries; it is witnessed also as to
seasons, and this in the same countries. The coldest months
may be most productive of the disease, and yet far from being
in the exact ratio of the degree of cold. Of the fatal cases of
which I have notes—cases which occurred at the General Hospital, at Fort Pitt, at Malta and Corfu—the following figures
show the amount for each month at each station:—

	FORT PITT.	MALTA.	CORFU.	TOTAL.
January, ...	4	6	1	11
February, ...	4	3	1	8
March, ...	1	4	2	7
April,....................	1	2	1	4
May, ...	4	1	—	5
June, ...	2	—	1	3
July, ...	4	1	1	6
August	1	—	1	2
September	1	3	—	4
October, ...	—	1	—	1
November, ...	3	—	—	3
December, ...	1	—	1	2

Also, it is worthy of remark, that in the same country, in the same garrison, the frequency of its occurrence and its fatality are not only variable in different years, but also in the same year in different bodies of men; thus in Malta, in the two years mentioned below, the number of cases and the fatality from the disease varied as follows :—

		STRENGTH.	CASES.	DIED.
1830.	Royal Artillery,	155	1	—
	7th Foot,	514	13	1
	73rd ,,	529	10	—
	85th ,,	532	3	—
	Rifles,	542	15	1
1831.	Royal Artillery,	151	3	—
	7th Foot,	491	11	2
	73rd ,,	512	32	1
	85th ,,	500	10	6
	Rifles,	509	14	1

Again, referring to the tabular view first given, we see that colored troops suffer from pneumonia, even when serving in a tropical climate, in either a somewhat higher ratio than white troops, or only in a little lower ratio. The Negro troops in the West Indies are an example of the former; the Malays and the Hottentot troops in Ceylon and the Cape of Good Hope of the latter. At the same time it is worthy of remark, that at each of these stations they suffer most from the disease in the higher and cooler regions, least like their native climate, the very same regions where Europeans enjoy the best health.

The etiology of most diseases is obscure, nor is that of pneumonia an exception. Two causes seem to be in operation at different times: one of a common kind, more or less prevalent in every climate and in every country, productive of the disease in its sporadic form; the other peculiar, an obscure something in the atmosphere, productive of the disease in an epidemic or endemic form, after the manner of influenza. The irregularities of its occurrence, such as those alluded to, and the general statistics of the disease, as shown in the Army Medical Returns, are strongly corroborative of this. In the instance of Ceylon, whilst in five years—viz., from 1821 to 1825 inclusive—the deaths from pneumonia were only 3, in subsequent years—from 1828 to 1832—they amounted to 9.

The pathology of pneumonia will be best illustrated by the fatal cases. Of these cases one of the most remarkable features is their complication, so much so indeed that an instance of the disease unmixed, uncombined with some other lesion, is of rare occurrence.   Of 56 cases of which I have notes, the complications have been the following, viz.: with tubercles, 7; pleurisy, 16;* bronchitis, 12; peritonitis, 3; cellular inflammation, 4; rheumatism, 2; dysentery, 2; disease of liver, 3; of brain, 5; of heart, 2.   And in some of these cases the complication has not been single, but even double or multiple.

Besides the complications, the disease has occasionally shown itself in different forms, these solitary cases, such as the typhoid, bearing a resemblance to typhoid fever; such as the algid, with a resemblance in many of its symptoms to cholera.

As in civil life, so in military, the great majority of the cases have been acute; of the whole number given seven only could with propriety be considered chronic.

In the acute cases, both lungs in the larger number of instances were affected; thus, of the whole number, 41 were examples of double pneumonia; of the 15 remaining, in which one lung only was affected, 10 were of pneumonia of the right side; 5 of the left.   In the chronic cases one lung commonly was sound, at least so far as to be tolerably adequate to the function of respiration.

The subjects of the disease, especially those to whom it proved fatal, have most commonly been men of some years' service, and often of intemperate habits and impaired constitutions.   Of the total of the latter, the following were the ages, viz.: from 17 to 25 years, 11; from 26 to 35 years, 29; from 36 to 47 years, 16. That none should have fallen its victims beyond the age last mentioned may seem singular, but it is easily explained by the fact, that the number of men in the ranks of the army exceeding 47 is exceedingly small, the majority either dying or being invalided as unfit for service before they reach that age: a fact this, I may remark, demonstrative of the great wear and tear of military life, subject as it is in our service to exposure in so many climates, to so many discomforts and often hardships, with hitherto so few precautions taken of a sanitary kind, whether

---

* Pleurisy and pneumonia are so often associated, that it is not surprising that the former in the returns from certain stations—as Ceylon, Moelmyne, Rangoon, the Western Coast of Africa, and the Cape of Good Hope—should be, as we have seen in the preceding table, entirely omitted.

as to quarters, food, or dress. For many years past the army medical officers, as already pointed out, have been reporting on these evils, but their voices have been as of one crying in the wilderness.

That these evils conduce to the production of the disease in question, and to many other diseases, cannot, I think, be doubted. Bad air and defective nourishment, with intemperance, their well known accompaniment, cannot but act as predisposing causes, by lowering the vigor of the system. The ordinary exciting causes are not far to seek; they are closely connected with the predisposing. On a field-day, heated by exercise, in his tight and heavy uniform, especially oppressing the chest, the soldier no sooner had returned to his quarters and was at liberty, than he was prompt to be rid of his encumbrances; he threw off often all but his trousers and shirt, in quest of refreshing coolness, regardless of perspiration suddenly checked. So, too, at night, when overcome by heat in his crowded and close barrack-room, and profusely perspiring, as it may have been, how often was he tempted to rush into the open air, equally careless of consequences.[*]

The comparative frequency of pneumonia in the West Indies, and its severity there in the Windward and Leeward Command, I am inclined to think may in part be explained by taking these circumstances into account. It may be objected to this explanation, that it seems to be refuted by the comparative unfrequency of the disease amongst the troops in Jamaica. The objection does appear strong; the only way I can meet it is, by presuming that, if the causes of the disease there are the same as in the other islands, the predisposition to it, owing to a better diet, may be less. Of the kind of barracks, and their situation there, I cannot speak from my own knowledge, never having been in Jamaica, but I believe, from what I have heard and read of them, that those most used are more roomy and of better construction than the majority of those in the other West Indian

---

[*] In a preceding note some particulars have been given of the dormitories of the troops, and of the imperfect ventilation of barracks: I remember the time when the soldier had not a bed to himself, two or more sleeping together; and in some barracks the beds were arranged in tiers one over the other. Recently I met an old soldier, a sergeant-major of a cavalry regiment, who was invalided in 1835, after 25 years' service, who told me that the first time he had a bed to himself was in 1824, in Piershill Barracks, in the neighbourhood of Edinburgh: they were cavalry barracks, and were of improved construction and recently built.

Islands, and in higher and cooler localities; and, if so, these circumstances may aid in accounting for the apparent anomaly.

The cases which follow have been selected chiefly as examples of the more remarkable, especially as regards their complications. In describing them, the symptoms and the treatment have been given rather more in detail than in any preceding section; the doing so seeming more requisite, especially the latter, the treatment, as bearing on the progress and result of the malady.

1. OF THE LEAST COMPLICATED CASES—In these, nine in number, the pleura and bronchia were more or less involved. So many are given, each case exhibiting some peculiarity.

Case 1.—Of pneumonia, with hepatized lung, treated by large blood-lettings, etc.—W. Abraham, ætat. 24; 88th F.; admitted into regimental hospital, Corfu, 29th March, 1826; died 2nd April.—This man, previously in good health, on admission had severe headache, troublesome dry cough, acute pain of chest, increased by a full inspiration; pulse 100, full and hard. His illness began the day before with lassitude followed by rigors. V.S. (40 oz.) without relief; blood not buffed. V.S. repeated (16 oz.); a blister to chest; a purgative. March 30th—The respiration was easier; pulse 120, hard and strong; great thirst; no headache; bowels freely opened. V.S. (32 oz.), Haust. Sudorificus. 31st—A pretty good night; the respiration easier; the pain less; pulse 100 full; Haustus Catharticus. April 1st—Free from pain; respiration improved; the pyrexia unabated; the pulse very full and hard; cough soft and not troublesome; Haust. Sudor. In the evening there was a recurrence of pain, and very acute. V.S. (48 oz.), a blister to the pained side. 2nd—Relief from pain; a restless night; skin cool and moist; pulse 100, small and compressible; bowels free; vomited several times during the night; tongue loaded; much thirst; Haust. Sudor. 11.30 a.m.—Within the last hour he became delirious; "his countenance has sunk in an extraordinary manner;" pulse weak; before the accession of delirium he vomited a little bilious matter. A blister to the head. During the course of the day he several times vomited a quantity of "greenish-colored bile." His extremities have become cold; pulse feeble and irregular; breathing laborious; deglutition difficult. He expired at 8 p.m.

Autopsy 17 hours after death. Not emaciated. The chest sounded well. Rather more serum than common at the base of the brain. The left lung was, very generally, closely and firmly adhering; its upper surface was crepitous and its appearance natural; its lower and larger portion was hepatised; its pleural covering thickened; its bronchia were dark red and full of frothy mucus. The right lung was partially adhering; its structure was pretty healthy; in its inferior portion there was a good deal of blood. The right cavities of the heart were distended with blood. The stomach, the upper portion of the small intestines, the cœcum and transverse colon, were exceedingly distended with air. There was an unusual redness diffused over the great arch of the stomach. The liver was rather large, but not apparently unhealthy. The gall-bladder was large and distended with bile.

The commentary made by me at the time was, "Perhaps the delirium and death in this case were owing to the abstraction of blood, especially the last, the inflammation not being sufficient to account for the event." Another comment was, "that the flatulent distension of the stomach and intestines might have been partly in fault." A query was added, "Considering the surface-state of the lung, could percussion and auscultation, had they been used, have detected its diseased condition?"

Case 2.—Of pneumonia, with hepatization of lungs, treated by blood-letting, etc.— P. Bracken, ætat. 46; 85th Regiment; admitted into regimental hospital, Malta, 1st March, 1831; died 2nd March.—This man, of very drunken habits, was taken ill a day or two ago, when on guard. He referred the attack to cold. On admission he complained of a dull pain in the inferior portion of the right side of chest. His breathing was quick and difficult. V.S. (18 oz.) A tendency to syncope; the blood was buffed and cupped. A dose of opium in camphor-mixture; relief of pain and a freer respiration, a slower pulse and an increased secretion into the bronchia, but with little power to expectorate. At 3 p.m. there was "general excitement." V.S. was repeated; small and frequent doses of calomel, tartar emetic and opium. In the evening he was easier, but unable to expectorate. March 2nd—A restless night. The bandage slipped from his arm and he lost about 10 oz. of blood. His respiration is now very rapid and feeble. 3 grs. of carbonate of ammonia in camphor julep. There is an enormous increase of bronchial secretion with inability to expectorate. His lips are livid; the pulse exceedingly feeble. He expired at 10 a.m.

Autopsy 25 hours after death. Not emaciated. The pericardium contained 1½ oz. of serum. There was a good deal of coagulated blood and fibrinous concretion in the right cavities of the heart; less in the left. Some soft coagulum was found in the aorta, in the vena azygos, and in the great veins. Both lungs were very generally adhering. The upper surface of each, immediately under the sternum, was of natural appearance and crepitous. The middle and inferior lobe of right lung and the inferior lobe of the left were hepatised; they were of a fawn color and most easily broken. When broken there exuded from them copiously a very thin puruloid fluid. The inferior portions of their upper lobes were hepatized in a less degree. The blood-vessels in the hepatised substance were empty and pale; no coagulable lymph could be detected in their smaller branches. The lower portion of the trachea and the bronchia generally were very red. On the surface of the liver there were a few shreds of lymph. The abdominal viscera appeared to be sound; no lesion could be detected in any of them.

It is noted down that on the day of this man's admission, when the general symptoms indicated much danger, the respiratory sound in both lungs was distinct and indicating *per se* no very serious disease. Men whose constitutions are impaired by drunkenness are notorious for bearing the loss of blood ill. The circumstances of this case, not unlike those of the preceding, might almost allow of a like commentary.

Case 3.—Of pneumonia, with hepatization of lungs and fibrin in bronchia.—Wm. Dixon, ætat. 47; 13th Light Dragoons; admitted May 29th, 1837; died June 2.— This man has recently returned from India with "a broken constitution," so reported by the surgeon of his regiment, after 30 years' service. Whilst there, and during the last three years, he had been under treatment, at different intervals, for dysentery, continued fever, and hepatitis, and lastly for pain of chest. On the homeward voyage his health, it was stated, had become pretty good; it continued so after landing until four days before admission. Then, when perspiring profusely, he took "a cold drink," and caught "a violent cold." When brought into hospital on the 29th May, there were rigors, great dyspnœa, cough, with copious expectoration; much thirst. His chest sounded dull; there were mucous râles in the superior and anterior part of both lungs. Calomel and antimony. 30th.—Feels much better; pulse 98; tongue still white; great thirst. A purgative of calomel and julep. Towards the evening he expectorated much muco-purulent matter, tinged with blood. His pulse was very quick; his face flushed; the skin moist. On the 31st he felt easier; pulse 100 and soft; cough troublesome, with much expectoration; bowels well evacuated. Towards night there was an exacerbation. June 1st—He complains of no pain; pulse very quick and small; expectoration copious. He seems to be fast sinking. He expired early the following morning.

Autopsy 30 hours after death. Cadaver stout and muscular. Brain of natural appearance. The upper surface of the pericardium unusually dry and transparent. The upper surface of the lungs of natural appearance, and abounding in air. Both lungs were adhering inferiorly and laterally, and were separated with difficulty. The right lung weighed 3½lbs.; the left a little less. The greater part of the former, with the exception of its superior lobe (the lower part of that was œdematous, the upper crepitous), was hepatized, and of different hues, varying in tint from dark red to light brown, the latter predominating. It was most easily broken; a purulent fluid (by the optical test) exuded from it. Most of its bronchial tubes, both small and large, were full of fibrin. The blood-vessels were empty. The inferior lobe of the left lung was in the first stage of hepatization; its appearance was very like that of the crassamentum of venous blood. The inferior surface of the superior lobe was œdematous. The bronchia in this lung were free from fibrinous concretion. The lower portion of the trachea was red. The valves of the heart and the lining membrane of the aorta were stained red. The auricles were distended with coagulated blood and lymph. There was some fibrinous concretion in the ventricles and the aorta. There was no well marked lesion of any of the abdominal viscera. The liver weighed 4½lbs.

This case is most noteworthy for the rapidity of its progress, and for the great amount of lymph poured into the lungs and bronchia in so short a time. The red color of the valves of the heart and of the inner coat of the aorta, is called a stain: the term is probably justifiable, considering the season of the year and the many hours between the death and autopsy. Though the deceased was an old soldier of long service, and had been subject to so many diseases, and was designated as of "broken down constitution" before quitting India, yet his general organization was remarkably sound.

Case 4.—Of pneumonia, with hepatization of lungs, preceded by symptoms of cholera.—T. Evans, ætat. 45; 7th Regiment of Foot; admitted into regimental hospital, Malta, 24th October, 1831; died 3rd November.—When brought to hospital on the evening of the 23rd (formally admitted on the following day*), this man was

* For hospital stoppage from his pay.

suffering from vomiting and purging, suggestive of an attack of cholera. Calomel and opium were prescribed and a warm bath; relief followed. At a later hour he was found laboring under difficulty of breathing, with pain of left side; his pulse 100, full and tense; much thirst. V.S. (20 oz.); a blister to the pained part; a purgative. The blood was not buffed. On the following day much relieved; the pulse 76; respiration easy. Saline medicines. From this time until the 30th, his cough alone was troublesome. Pectoral medicines and hydrocyanic acid. On the morning of the 30th he was free from pain; his pulse 72; tongue dry and glazed. In addition to the pectoral medicines, calomel, ipecacuanha, and opium every third hour. From this time there was a rapid aggravation of symptoms, described as "a gradual sinking." He was conscious at the moment of expiring.

Autopsy 21 hours after death. Not emaciated. Rather more fluid than usual between the membranes, in the ventricles, and at the base of the brain. The pineal gland was large; its structure a little altered, and it contained a larger granule than usual.* Both lungs were feebly but pretty generally adhering by soft coagulable lymph. The right lung did not collapse. It was heavy, for most part hepatized, and of a cream color. When incised there exuded from it a puruloid fluid. Its larger blood-vessels were empty and compressed. The left lung was even more generally hepatized; a very small portion of it was crepitous. The bronchia were slightly red. The pericardium contained 3 oz. of serum. The stomach and intestines were much distended with air. The spleen was large, and its capsule partially thickened, and of cartilaginous firmness.

This case is noteworthy for its insidious course and atonic character, lulling suspicion. Till the danger suddenly became imminent, no apprehension was entertained. The stethoscope, I believe, was not used.

Case 5.—Of pneumonia, with enlarged spleen, treated by copious blood-letting.— T. Rowland, ætat. 27; 7th R.F.; admitted into regimental hospital, 18th March, 1833; died 2nd April.—This man had suffered from remittent fever in 1828, and from continued fever in 1830. From that time his health was good until his present illness. When on guard on the 24th March, he experienced an acute pain in the left breast. From thence he was brought to hospital. In addition to the pain and dyspnœa, he was troubled with cough; the skin was hot; pulse 120 and full. V.S. (2 lbs.); some relief. The blood was cupped and buffed. Tartar emetic gr. i. every 3rd hour. In the evening an exacerbation. Again V.S. (24 oz.) March 25th— Still some pain of side. V.S. (24 oz.) 26th—Had a tolerable night; is now free from pain; his breathing more free; the pulse soft and compressible. The blood last drawn natural. A vesicular eruption on lips. 30th—Until yesterday he appeared to be improving. At 10 p.m. he became restless and incoherent. Now no pain nor cough. On the 31st, after a good night, at daybreak had an attack of diarrhœa. His respiration became hurried, with some pain in the left breast, and there was great depression of spirits. His pulse was 80 and soft; tongue clean and moist; skin cool A blister to chest. Tartar emetic, small doses of calomel and opium; blue ointment to be rubbed into the axillæ and thighs. April 1st—Has passed a restless night; constantly changing his position; breathing short, performed in sighs; is without pain; cough and expectoration have ceased; his pulse is quick and small; tongue dry;

* It was examined, and found to consist chiefly of phosphate of lime; and such I have commonly found the little accretion of this part; I have never detected in it oxalate of lime.

dark sordes on teeth; no thirst; eyes sunken. Says he is much better. Expired delirious at 2 a.m.

Autopsy 8 hours after death. Not emaciated. Brain of natural appearance. The lungs did not collapse. The superior lobe of the left lung was hepatised throughout and entirely destitute of air. Its upper part was of dirty white hue; its lower portion reddish. The inferior lobe was red, but crepitous; its bronchia were of the same color; the bronchia of the hepatized lobe were pale. The right lung was tolerably sound; its bronchia were red and clogged with thick mucus. The spleen was enlarged and was about twice its natural size; its substance pultaceous. A portion of its capsule was of an opaque white, of a cartilaginous firmness, and about a quarter of an inch thick. The right lobe of the liver was soft and friable. The other viscera appeared to be sound.

This case comes under the same category nearly as the preceding and is exposed to the same comments, or nearly the same. The diseased state of the spleen is attributable probably to the fevers which he had in former years.

Case 6.—Of pneumonia, with hepatization of lung and incipient inflammation of pleura, treated by blood-letting.—J. Costello, ætat. 29; 85th F.; admitted April 7th, 1822; died 9th April.—This man's illness commenced three days before his admission with rigors followed by heat and profuse sweating. He considered it an attack of ague to which he had been subject. On admission he had pain of right breast with considerable dyspnœa, but little cough; there was considerable pyrexia and an inclination to vomit. V.S. 20 oz., an aperient. On the 8th he experienced some relief. Some blood was taken by cupping. Towards evening the symptoms were all more severe. V.S. was repeated (12 oz.); a blister to chest; calomel and opium. On the 9th he was free from pain; the vomiting continuing; his bowels open; the skin moderately cool. The blood drawn slightly buffed and cupped. The same medicine. 10th—The vomiting has ceased. During the night some delirium; now rational and moribund, lips livid, extremities cold, pulse imperceptible, no pain. He expired in a few minutes.

Autopsy 26 hours after death. Not emaciated, rather an excess of fat. The pia mater was more vascular than usual, and there was more fluid than usual in the ventricles. The right pleura contained a little serum and loose lymph, was very vascular and was covered with a delicate false membrane which was easily peeled off. The lung of the same side was partially adhering; the substance of the adhesion was soft lymph. The lung weighed 2 lbs. 10 oz. The greater part of it was hepatized, and of a pale reddish hue, exuding, when incised, an almost colorless fluid. The left pleura also was very vascular; but there was no lymph effused in it; its portion corresponding to the stomach, its diaphragmatic portion, was most conspicuously red and blood-shot The lung of this side weighed 10 oz., and was of nearly natural appearance. The right lobe of the liver adhered to the diaphragm. The urinary bladder was empty and very much contracted. Parts of its inner coat were very red, "intensely red," as it were from ecchymosis. The other viscera exhibited no marked lesion.

In considering this case, a doubt arose (expressed at the time) whether the abstraction of blood had not been injurious. Was the vomiting, which was a marked symptom, owing to a phlogosis of the stomach (though not detected after death) similar to that of the corresponding pleura? The contracted and partially ecchymosed state of the urinary bladder was most likely the effect of the blister to the chest. After its application, though there was no dysuria complained of, yet the patient was observed to make water often and in small quantity.

Case 7.—Of pneumonia, with hepatization of lung and pleuritic effusion, treated by very copious blood-letting.—H. Crogar, ætat. 42; 13th F.; admitted into regimental hospital, Corfu, August 5, 1826; died 6th August.—This man, an old soldier, had excellent health, and was remarkable for activity. His only bad habit was drinking, which he too often indulged in to excess, and this until about a month ago, when hearing of a brother's death, he "took it to heart" and abstained a good deal from his wonted potations. On the 30th July, after working hard, and when sweating profusely, he drank a large quantity of water. A violent pain in the chest and belly followed, attended with vomiting. Seen a few hours after by a staff medical officer, the pains had abated; he complained most of pain of chest, which was then greatly aggravated by a full inspiration; his pulse was rapid. V.S. (20 oz.); a warm ano-dyne aperient. On the following morning he spoke of himself as very much better; but it being known that he had been delirious during the night, he was sent to hospital, distant at least a mile, to which he walked. His pulse at the time was very rapid, and a full inspiration still occasioned pain. According to the surgeon of his regiment he made little complaint on admission, and he was discharged on the 2nd August. On the 3rd he was very feeble, had been "raving" during the night; his pulse was exceedingly rapid, his breathing quick, with some cough and a deep-seated pain in chest; his manner anxious and restless; he said he felt much better up than when lying down. A blister was applied to the chest and a solution of tartarised antimony and nitre prescribed. Towards night he had nausea and vomiting; said he felt better. On the 4th, after a restless night, he spoke of himself as better; his pulse and respiration were still rapid. The same medicine with diminished tartarised antimony. On the 5th, when visited, he was sitting on a form eating his breakfast; he said his appetite was pretty good. His pulse at the time was 130; his breathing very rapid; pain still deeply seated in chest, and inability to make a full inspiration. He was removed to his hospital, with a note intimating his great danger, and was carried up. At 1 p.m. V.S. (3 lbs.); at 8 p.m. V.S. was repeated (2 lbs.) The blood was much cupped and buffed. He expired at 7 a.m. the following morning.

Autopsy 28 hours after death. Not emaciated; incipient putrefaction; the abdomen tympanitic. A good deal of serum between the membranes of the brain, especially in the tissue of the pia mater, also in the ventricles and at the base of brain. The cerebral substance firm. The left pleura contained 1½ lb. of bloody serum. The lung on this side was unduly red, and its inferior lobe was in the first stage of hepatization. A concretion, of about the size of a filbert, of a pasty consistence, was found in the inferior part of the superior lobe, near its surface, where it adhered to the costal pleura; it was composed chiefly of phosphate of lime. The right lung was extensively adhering by soft lymph; lymph of the same kind was collected in considerable quantity in the inferior part of the pleura. In the same cavity there were about 4 oz. of bloody serum. The lung throughout, with the exception of the superior margin of the inferior lobe was hepatized. The pericardium contained 3 oz. of bloody serum. All the cavities of the heart were distended with air; they contained also a little coagulated blood and fibrinous concretion. The stomach and all the intestines, with the exception of the lower part of the colon and rectum, were distended with air, as were also the omentum and the cellular structure of the gall-bladder. The pancreas and spleen were unusually soft. The liver nearly of ordinary appearance.

This man, having been an officer's servant, was not, when first taken ill, sent forthwith to the hospital of his regiment. The remarks already made respecting the abstraction of blood are specially applicable to this case. The air distending the several organs specified was probably from putrefaction.

Case 8.—Of pneumonia, with hepatized lung, inflamed bronchia, and partial emphysema of integuments of chest, treated by blood-letting.—O. Maguire, ætat. 33; 85th Regiment; admitted into regimental hospital, Malta, 25th March, 1831; died 29th March.—This man, of drunken habits, was admitted off duty, with a slight pain in the right side of chest; his skin was hot and dry; tongue furred; pulse rather quick; the bowels constipated. A purgative of calomel and antimony; four stools. On the following day the symptoms were much the same. V.S. (16 oz.); the blood buffed; some relief. Tartarized antimony. On the 27th his cough was urgent, with slight pain; no expectoration; bowels relaxed. V.S. (14 oz.); faintness, and an outbreak of perspiration. The same medicine. On the 28th, at 1 a.m., there was a sudden change for the worse; he became delirious, and was found out of bed and walking in the ward. His respiration had become hurried, short, and labored; his pulse 130. He died at 5 p.m. The day before, on auscultation, no respiratory sound was heard in the greater part of the right lung; in the left it was distinct, with a slight râle.

Autopsy 11 hours after death. The right pleura was very red and vascular, and contained 6 oz. of serum, in which were flakes of lymph. The right lung, adhering in many places, was in great part hepatized, and was very friable. The left lung was nearly free from adhesions, and, with the exception of its inferior lobe, which contained pretty much blood and serum, was nearly of natural appearance. The anterior mediastinum was red and vascular in a high degree. The aspera arteria, from the glottis to the minute bronchial branches in both lungs, was very red. In the right bronchia there was much mucus. Under the integuments, just below the right mamilla, there was some emphysema. The right cavities of the heart contained much fibrinous concretion, firmly adhering. In the aorta there was liquid blood or cruor. Though a drunkard, the liver was of natural appearance. The spleen was very soft. The stomach was large; its cardiac extremity very soft. There were some cicatrices of ulcers in the large intestines. Many of the abdominal viscera were adhering.

How noteworthy is this case for the rapidity of its progress! On duty, apparently well, on the morning of the 25th—a corpse at 5 p.m. of the 27th! The partial emphysema observed after death, when there were no indications of putrefaction, is remarkable, and as to explanation and significance, how difficult! It would seem to denote a secretion or separation of air from the blood.

Case 9.—Of pneumonia, with hepatization of lungs, pericarditis, and pleuritic effusion; treated by blood-letting.—E. Glynn, ætat. 26; 73rd Foot; admitted into regimental hospital, Malta, 5th May, 1831; died 9th May.—This man, of temperate habits, had been ailing some days before admission. When admitted his symptoms were headache, lumbar pains, pains in the lower extremities, a very hot skin, a loaded tongue, pulse 90. An emetic, with a saline purgative, each of which operated well. On the following day, the 6th May, he was free from headache; the skin dry, the tongue loaded, the pulse quick. Calomel and antimony, after taking which he had several bilious stools, and some moisture of skin. On the 7th, after a restless night, he first complained of pain, and that severe, of the left side of chest; his respiration was hurried; pulse 100; skin hot; much anxiety; his countenance flushed. V.S. (30 oz.); the blood was buffed and cupped. Some immediate relief. A blister to the pained parts. Epsom salts, with tartarized antimony. At noon there was increased heat of skin and dyspnœa. V.S. (32 oz.) The last cup of blood was neither cupped nor buffed; relief; no subsequent pain of chest. On the 8th his respiration was hurried; pulse 120; little cough or expectoration; the expression of countenance anxious; bowels tympanitic. The respiratory sound of the right side was loud and free from râle; so also that of the upper part of the left; but where the pain *had* been felt, there the respiratory murmur was lost, and a tick only occasionally heard. Small doses of calomel and opium, in place of the antimony. 9th—He complains now mostly of weakness; his pulse is small and quick; his breathing very hurried; the cough urgent. He expired at 8 p.m.; his intellect unimpaired to the last.

Autopsy 14 hours after death. Not emaciated. 4 oz. of turbid serum in the pericardium; a little coagulable lymph here and there on the heart. The right auricle and ventricle contained a good deal of coagulated blood and fibrinous concretion, which extended into the pulmonary artery. In the left cavities and in the aorta there was less of both. The vena cava, azygos, enulgent, and other large veins were full of coagulated blood. Both pleuræ were very vascular. The right contained 4 oz. of serum; the left 6 oz. of turbid serum; flakes of lymph were deposited on its surface. The lobes of the right lung were all cohering; their upper surface crepitous; their middle and inferior portion hepatized. The left lung was even more diseased; with the exception of the upper surface of the superior lobe, it was hepatized throughout. Its color was pale red; when incised much fluid flowed from it. The bronchia in this lung and also in the right were very red, as was also the trachea The blood-vessels in the hepatized parts were either empty or contained a reddish fluid. The portions hepatized sank in water. The mucous membrane of the gall-bladder was very red, as if inflamed. There was no bile in the gall-bladder; it contained a small quantity of a whitish semi-fluid substance, but whether mucus or lymph was not ascertained. The spleen was large, and so soft as to be almost pultaceous. The intestines were distended with air.

This case was somewhat anomalous in character. At first it was supposed to be an instance of febrile attack, and it was treated accordingly. In its obscurity it affords much scope for conjecture. Amongst the lesions, apart from the principal one— the very extensive hepatization of the lungs, the state of the blood in the heart and in the great blood-vessels, and the state of the gall-bladder, are noteworthy.

2. OF COMPLICATION WITH INFLAMMATION OF THE MEDIAS-TINA AND THE CELLULAR TISSUE.—These cases, four in number, may be mentioned as chiefly remarkable for their anomalous symptoms : in two, simulating in many respects those of cholera; in one, those of typhus.

Case 10.—Of pneumonia, with symptoms of cholera, partial hepatization of lung, and diffuse cellular inflammation.—B. Jarrett, ætat. 34; 7th Regiment of Foot; admitted into regimental hospital, Malta, 17th September, 1831; died 27th Nov.— This man was taken into hospital on account of a sprained ankle. When recovering from this hurt, he experienced early in the morning of 27th November pain of chest, with headache. When seen at the hour of visit, in addition he had slight difficulty in breathing, a tendency to vomit, and a relaxed state of bowels. His pulse 86; skin of natural temperature; tongue white. Leeches to temples; a blister to the chest; an emetic: after taking it, he threw up much green bilious fluid. He was seen several times during the day, and expressed himself easier until the evening visit, when a great change had taken place. The pulse was scarcely sensible; the extremities were cold; the intellect not impaired; the tongue white and cool; little pain of head At 9 p.m. no pulse could be felt at the wrist, or over the region of the heart; the extremities and tongue were cold; the nails and lips bluish; respiration hurried; the respiratory sound was distinct at the upper part of the chest. Stimulants were given, and a turpentine enema; and hot water was applied to the pit of the stomach and to the extremities, but in vain—the heart could not be excited to act; a vein at the same time was opened, but no blood flowed. He died at 10.30 p.m. It is noted that his countenance was not expressive of cholera.

Autopsy 13 hours after death. Not emaciated; unusually livid, especially the inferior surfaces; the abdomen distended, but not tympanitic. The base of the brain perhaps softer than natural. Very little fluid in its ventricles, or in the spinal canal. Both lungs adhering; both anteriorly crepitous, and of pretty natural appearance; both heavier than natural, especially the right. The inferior part of this lung, close to the spine, was hepatized, was of a brownish hue, and sank in water; the hepatiz- ation diminished gradually towards the anterior surface. The corresponding part of the left lung was less distinctly hepatized; it contained much blood. The bronchia generally were very red, and contained some bloody mucus. The trachea and larynx were of a very dark red, almost livid, as were also the glottis and epiglottis. There was no œdema of these parts; no coagulable lymph effused. The cellular structure round the great vessels in the neck was very much injected with blood; and on the carotid on each side, and in the theca of the par vagum, there were spots of ecchy- mosis. The bronchial glands were large and black; one of them was so soft as to be of almost pultaceous consistence. The small intestines were distended with a yellow, bilious fluid, containing a shreddy matter. The inner coat of the intestines generally was pale and flabby; that of the duodenum was spotted red, owing to a fibrous matter tinged red, probably lymph, scattered over and adhering to it. The spleen was about twice its natural size; it adhered firmly to the liver, and its capsule superiorly was much thickened, and of cartilaginous consistence. In the gall-bladder there was some bile of natural appearance. The other abdominal viscera were apparently sound. Notwithstanding the lividity, there was very little blood in the body gene- rally.

The following queries were appended to the case immediately on recording it:—What was the death owing to? Was it to a sudden invasion of inflammation of the air passages generally, etc., overwhelming the powers of life? Was the apparent in- flammation of the eighth pair of nerves concerned in the event? or the small quantity of blood? or was there a complication of cholera? The clearness of the intellect, the sudden reduction of temperature, the contents of the small intestines, favorable to the last mentioned conjecture.

Case 11.—Of pneumonia, with hepatization of lung and inflammation of mediastinum; treated by blood-letting.—T. Poe, ætat. 25; 28th Foot; admitted into regimental hospital, Corfu, June 20th, 1825; died June 25th.—This man, when acting as cook to his company, was suddenly attacked with pain of chest so severe that he fell down; yet he remained out of hospital six days, suffering all the time from pain in the same part, with cough, and not abstaining from drinking. On admission V.S. (35 oz.); a tepid bath; calomel and antimony. The blood was much buffed and cupped. The following morning, June 21st, he felt easier, but towards evening there was an increase of pain and oppression of breathing, so that "he could hardly breathe or move." V.S. (34 oz.); a blister to the chest; the same medicine. 22nd —Has had some sleep; there is much cough; tongue foul; the expectoration is tinged with blood; he perspires freely. 23rd—No pain now in the right side; complains of pain in the left. His cough is constant; pulse 116, soft; skin moist, bowels open; no sleep; can turn on either side. A tepid bath; calomel and opium with squill. 24th—He slept six hours; pulse 120, and weak; abdomen distended; no stool this morning; other symptoms much the same. A purgative enema; the same medicine. Towards evening he became faint, and his breathing more hurried. After lying on his side several hours during the night, at 7 a.m. of the 25th he suddenly turned on his back and expired.

Autopsy 38 hours after death. Not emaciated. The anterior mediastinum, the outer surface of the pericardium, and both pleuræ, were unusually vascular. Coagulable lymph here and there was deposited on the latter. The lungs did not collapse; they weighed 6 lbs. The left lung was partially adhering by a thin layer of soft coagulable lymph. It had three lobes—a large upper and lower lobe and a small middle lobe—altogether exactly resembling the right. The superior and inferior lobe of each was red and hepatized; portions of them sank in water. The middle lobe of both was only in part crepitous, and tolerably sound. The right lung adhered very generally; the adhesions between it and the diaphragm were short, thick, firm bands, and apparently vascular. The aspera arteria, from the glottis to the bronchia, was inflamed, and in an increased degree towards the latter, judging from the intensity of color. The pericardium contained a small quantity of bloody serum—about two drachms. The right cavities of the heart were distended with coagulated blood and fibrinous concretions. The stomach and intestines were much distended with air. The spleen was small, firm, and pale. No lesion was observable in the other abdominal viscera.

In this case, probably, the disease was fully formed before the admission of the patient into hospital. Acuteness of pain was one of the most marked symptoms; and the great vascularity of the parts where the pain was felt was remarkable, without any serous effusion. May not the latter help to account for the former?

Case 12.—Of pneumonia, with hepatization of lungs and effusion of lymph into the mediastinum and pleuræ.—J. Gregory, ætat. 28; R.B.; admitted into regimental hospital, Malta, 6th January, 1832; died 17th January.—This man had been ailing for two or three days, but he felt no serious indisposition until the morning of the 5th January, when he was on sentinel duty in an exposed situation. Then he experienced

20

pain in great toe and groin, soon succeeded by rigors, vomiting and purging and great weakness. On admission his pulse was exceedingly small and rapid, even beyond counting; his respiration somewhat hurried; there was suffusion of eyes, and the skin of face and trunk had an erythematic blush, and yet the temperature was little above the natural. There was a bluish vesicle on the great toe of the right foot, and a painful swelling at the upper part of the right thigh. V.S. (18 oz.) There was a tendency to syncope during the flow of blood. An emetic the same evening, which had effect on both the stomach and bowels; the ejecta were reported natural. The pulse through the day continued the same, scarcely to be felt; at the evening visit he was found very restless, but when questioned, he said, in a hurried manner, that he was quite well. A warm bath; after it, 10 grs. of calomel, with 1 gr. of opium and a blister to the region of the stomach. On the 7th his pulse was more distinct; his breathing rather hurried; skin of good temperature; tongue much loaded, a dark fur on its middle; much thirst. Says he has no pain. Calomel and opium in small doses every third hour. 8th—Had a pretty good night; pulse 110, of good strength; intellect clear; feels drowsy; urgent thirst; he complains of nothing else; his tongue is red and dry; the bowels open. The calomel and opium omitted. Liquor Ammon. Acetat. frequently. 9th—Delirium during the night; is now collected; pulse 100; skin nearly natural. The same medicine. 10th—He has been delirious since 4 a.m. His tongue at its centre is becoming black; there are apthous spots on its edges; the teeth are covered with sordes; pulse 90. Pulv. Cinchonæ in addition to the saline mixture. During the day there was more or less delirium and occasional hiccough. He lies on his back and sinks towards the bottom of the bed. His pulse is 86; skin cool; one stool. The abdomen is somewhat tympanitic. 11th —No improvement has taken place; the same medicine. 12th—Is very restless; hiccough and delirium during the night. The bark omitted. He is to sip mucilage of gum arabic; small doses of rhubarb and magnesia. 13th—A better night; some improvement of symptoms; pulse 80; skin natural; he asked for something to eat. About 2 p.m. the hiccough and delirium recurred, and continued with occasional inter- missions until the evening of the 16th, when his respiration became labored. He expired at 4 a.m. on the following day. It is noted that through his illness there was no pain of chest, no cough, and till moribund no dyspnœa, and that from the begin- ning he was able to lie on either side.

Autopsy 6 hours after death. Not emaciated. About 2 oz. of serum at the base of the brain. Both lungs were firmly adhering. The right was hepatized and that generally, with the exception of the upper portion of its middle lobe, which was moderately crepitous. The hepatized substance was either of a fawn-color or light red. The bronchia were very red, and contained a red sanies. The blood-vessels in the diseased lobes were empty and collapsed. The left lung was redder than natural, especially partially in patches, where there was an approach to hepatization. Its inferior portion was gorged with blood. A large quantity of lymph was effused into the pleura of this side, and also into the posterior mediastinum and along the course of the great vessels in the neck. The mucous membrane of the œsophagus was very red in several places, and its epithelium there altered, as if acted on by an acrid matter, being rough and easily abraded. The stomach was empty and moderately contracted; its rugæ red. The abdomidal viscera were apparently sound.

How noteworthy is this case for the little connection between the symptoms and the lesions discovered after death! Such negations as those adverted to, are not a little perplexing, and may well check over-confidence in our conjectures concerning the phenomena of disease, the real causes of which are so often only ascertained in part, if at all. The gum arabic was prescribed on the presumption that there might be an abrasion of the epithelium near the cardiac orifice of the stomach, not an unfrequent accompaniment of hiccough.

Case 13.—Of pneumonia, with hepatization of lung and inflammation of mediastinum, pleuræ, etc.—C. Calvert, ætat. 26; R.F.; admitted into regimental hospital, Malta, 11th Jan., 1831; died 16th January.—This man was in good health until attacked by his present illness, which began the day before his admission, with a trembling and weakness of the lower extremities, accompanied by nausea and anorexia. When seen, his pulse was frequent and small; his tongue much loaded; thirst; skin dry and rather hot; bowels tolerably regular. A scruple of ipecacuanha and two grains of tartarized antimony were prescribed, followed by the ejection of some bilious fluid. In the evening he complained of pain in the region of the liver; the stomach was irritable; the pulse very quick and feeble. Blood was taken by cupping; a large blister applied, and 10 grs. of calomel and 1 gr. of opium given. 11th—A bad night; stomach more irritable. When at stool he experienced a convulsive fit of a few seconds' duration. Has a short dry cough; cramps of the abdominal muscles and of the lower extremities; pulse quick and feeble; features shrunk; skin less hot; nothing remains on his stomach. A scruple of calomel with one grain of opium taken was immediately rejected; a bolus of two scruples and one grain of opium was retained, and the stomach after was more quiet. The same bolus was repeated at night. 12th—A better night and he feels better; his gums are tender. Calomel 10 grains, with half a grain of opium. 13th—He slept pretty well; his stomach is tranquil; the cough troubles him at times. His pulse is still quick and feeble; tongue dry at the centre; its edges moist; bowels slow. A purgative enema. After a free evacuation, he slept during the greater part of the day aud appeared decidedly better. So he continued until about 2 p.m. of the 14th, when he awoke with a feeling of oppression of chest and dyspnœa. His pulse was small and rapid; tongue moist and white; skin rather cold; ulceration of gums without ptyalism; a vesicular eruption about the lips; bowels torpid. A blister to the chest; castor oil, which had effect. 15th—Is worse. Has troublesome hiccough, which is alleviated by a strong solution of gum arabic. In the evening there was a sudden change; he experienced a pain shooting through the chest to the spine, and also in the hepatic region; his breathing had become short and hurried; his cough stifling; heat of body much reduced; pulse rapid and fluttering; tongue perfectly dry, eyes sunken and glazed; constant hiccough; great listlessness. Warm flannels were applied; warm negus given. He became colder; the pulse imperceptible. The following morning he expired.

Autopsy 25 hours after death. Not emaciated; much lividity of skin of shoulders and back. Both mediastina were unusually vascular and contained some effused coagulable lymph. There were 4 oz. of turbid serum with a few flakes of lymph in the pericardium. The heart was large. There was much blood in the right auricle. The right ventricle contained a large mass of fibrin, almost without coloring matter, and of a form, as if fashioned by the action of the heart during life. There was a small quantity of similar concretion in the left ventricle. There was cruor without fibrin in the aorta and in the vena azygos, with a little air also in the latter. The left pleura was very vascular, and over the diaphragm there were some spots of ecchymosis. The lung on this side did not collapse; its parenchyma and bronchia were unusually red. The lobes of the right lung were agglutinated by a puruloid coagulable lymph, and were partially adhering superficially. Close to the mediastinum there was a collection of some puruloid fluid between the two surfaces of the pleura. The lung was of a dark red and hepatized, with the exception of a small portion of its superior lobe, which, having a little air in it, did not, like the rest, sink in water. The pharynx was very red, as was also the aspera arteria throughout. The bronchia (intensely red) of the right lung contained a muco-purulent fluid, and there was a similar exudation in the trachea and larynx. The stomach was smaller than usual; its inner membrane was corrugated; it contained only a little brownish fluid; there were some red patches in its mucous membrane. The duodenum presented a similar appearance. The large intestines were partially distended with flatus and partially contracted; their inner membrane was unusually soft and easily separable; in many places it was red and dark red and rough, as if from lymph deposited in a granular form. The cellular coat of the gall-bladder was œdematous. The gall-bladder contained a little thick bile. The liver, spleen, pancreas and kidneys were of natural appearance.

This case like the preceding is open to much comment. When admitted it was designated cholera morbus, and was so returned. Its many peculiarities were probably owing to complications. As the calomel given in such large doses did not arrest the morbid actions, may it not have produced others interfering with recovery? Is it not probable that there was a coagulation of blood in the heart some hours before death, commencing, it may have been, about the time that the sudden change took place, and the impulse of the organ became indistinct?

3. Of Complication, with Disease of Heart.—These cases, two in number, show the aggravating effect of hypertrophy of the heart, well marked by a paroxysmal tendency.

Case 14.—Pneumonia, with hypertrophy of heart and inflammation of mediastina. —G. Finney. ætat. 30; 85th Foot; admitted into regimental hospital, Malta, 16th July, 1831; died 4th October.—On admission this man complained of difficulty of breathing, and of a short dry cough, attributed to "catching cold." His pulse was 100; his skin cool. Small blood-lettings were employed and a strictly antiphlogistic treatment up to the 24th August, when he appeared to be improving. Shortly after symptoms of disease of heart occurred, marked by tumultuous action, and much throbbing of the great vessels, especially of the right carotid; the pulse was rapid, but not irregular. Recourse was had to the local abstraction of blood, and to the use of tartarized antimony in large doses, with hyoscyamus and occasional purgatives. No permanent benefit was experienced. On the 17th September there was an increase of dyspnœa even to orthopnœa, with pain in the region of the heart. The same treatment. The difficulty of breathing continued, and at uncertain periods with paroxysmal violence. Some delirium preceded death.

Autopsy 8 hours after death. Not emaciated. The pericardium contained 4 oz. of serum, and each pleura about the same quantity. The right lung was very heavy; a large portion of it was hepatized, of a red color, and almost impervious to air. The left lung was similarly diseased, but in a less degree. The bronchia and the lower part of the trachea were of a dark red. The heart was about thrice its natural size; its cavities were large; the augmentation of their muscular substance was pretty equal; the valves were sound; nor was there any lesion found in the great vessels; a good deal of coagulable lymph, however, was deposited in the course of the carotids and the jugular veins, just where they make their exit and entrance into the thorax, and most on the right side; and there was a deposition of the like kind in the upper part of the anterior mediastinum. The liver was rather pale; its section nutmeg-like. The spleen was firm when entire; but cut into and pressed there exuded from it a chocolate colored pultaceous matter. Nothing peculiar was observed in any other of the abdominal viscera.

May it not be inferred that the disease of lungs in this case preceded the hypertrophy of the heart, and that the latter gradually aggravated the former; also that the effusion of lymph in the cellular tissue, especially on the right side, had a like effect. Apart from the heart and lungs, the soundness of the organization generally was remarkable; so, too, was the absence of wasting and of œdema.

Case 15.—Of pneumonia, with hepatization of lung, melanotic induration, hypertrophy of heart, and aneurism of aorta.—N. Bennett, ætat. 42; 28th Foot; admitted into regimental hospital, Corfu, 8th April, 1825; died January 1.—This man, of irregular and intemperate habits, before his admission into hospital had been ailing some time with cough and dyspnœa. On admission, he had in addition pain of chest, chiefly in the right side. He gradually became worse till he expired. The most marked symptoms were the pains of chest, a pain in the right hypochondrium, and occasionally at scrobiculus cordis. He had cough, but it was not severe; the dyspnœa was severe in paroxysms, and was increased, as was also the cough, by lying on the left side; he was most uneasy in bed, except his head and shoulders were well raised. His lips were livid; face puffy; some thirst; impaired appetite; an occasionally intermitting pulse; scanty secretion of urine. The treatment was chiefly by aperients, digitalis and other diuretics, leeches and blisters.

Autopsy 16 hours after death. Emaciated. The right pleura contained 5 pints of serum; the left 4 oz. The right lung was attached to the diaphragm and to the costal pleura by some long firm bands, on which were conspicuous minute melanotic tubercles; it was much diseased, including in its parenchyma large masses of melanotic substance, and was also partly hepatized and partly œdematous. The left lung was very much gorged with blood and infiltrated with serum. Very little of either was crepitous. The bronchia were red; the margin of the epiglottis œdematous. The heart was very much enlarged, and contained a great deal of blood. The auricular-ventricular passages were unusually capacious. The left true auricle was much contracted, and full of fibrinous concretion, which was firmly adhering. The aorta was diseased. Just above the origin of the coronary arteries there was an aneurismal sac of considerable size. Its inner membrane was there rough, and elevated into points by atheromatous matter underneath, and the descending aorta exhibited the same kind of roughness. The orifices of the intercostals were diminished and unusually projecting. There were two or three red excrescences, about the size of cherries, and nearly pear-shaped, attached to the mucous coat of the stomach. The abdominal viscera generally were sound; no appearance of disease could be discovered in the liver.

In this case probably the disease of heart and aorta preceded that of the lungs, excepting perhaps the melanotic induration, and was in part the cause of the effusion into the pleuræ and into the air-cells. A suspicion was entertained that the liver was in fault, founded, by the surgeon, on the habits of the man, and the occasional pain (a most uncertain criterion) in the right hypochondrium.

4. COMPLICATION, WITH DISEASE OF BRAIN.—These cases, three in number, are chiefly noteworthy for the manner in which the disease of the lungs was masked. The last of the three is inserted chiefly on account of this masking effect. Considering the morbid appearances in the lungs, the propriety of viewing it as a case of complicated pneumonia is questionable.

Case 16.—Of pneumonia, with hepatization of lung and partial softening, and partial induration of brain.—P. Scanlan, ætat. 35; 60th F , admitted into regimental hospital, Malta, 17th Nov., 1834; died 18th January, 1835.—This man, of 18 years' service, was of intemperate habits, and when drunk violent. On the 26th May, after confinement for five months with hard labor, he was taken into hospital for cough and pain of chest with a faltering in his speech and a paralytic weakness of his right leg. After treatment by purging, cupping and a seton in the neck, he was discharged well on the 18th June. On the 27th of the same month he was re-admitted, the paralytic symptoms having recurred. He had headache, his face was flushed, his intelligence impaired. Some blood was taken from the arm and tartarized antimony was given. Symptoms of mania immediately followed. A seton was inserted as before, and he gradually improved. He was discharged well on the 1st of September Till the 17th November he appeared well and rational. Then derangement of mind recurred, marked as before by a very restless and excited state, sometimes requiring the straight waistcoat, but not yielding as before to medical treatment. On the 11th January he became taciturn; he ate his meals as before. On the 12th his skin was cooler than natural; his pulse slow; he was not able to use his tongue; the hands and wrists were spasmodically contracted. On the 15th the contraction of these parts had increased; his pulse was fluttering. His head was shaved and a blister applied. On the 16th he seemed perfectly sensible, but he could not articulate; when questioned as to pain, he did not point to any part; his pulse was now irregular. He took little nourishment and gradually sunk and expired.

Autopsy 26 hours after death. Much emaciated. The arachnoid in many places opaque. The substance of the brain was of unequal consistence; in some portions more resisting than natural under the knife; in others the contrary. The lateral ventricles were considerably distended by transparent fluid, especially their inferior cornua. The sides of the right inferior cornu towards its apex were adhering; the bounding medullary matter was yellow and soft. A white granular matter was found on the pia mater towards the base of the cerebellum. Some air was detected in the cellular tissue of the posterior mediastinum. The left lung was partially adhering; most of it was hepatized and of a grey color; when incised a thin puruloid fluid exuded from it. The right lung was similarly diseased, but in a less degree; portions of it were emphysematous. The bronchia were very red, and contained a thick frothy mucus. The pericardium contained a small quantity of fluid; it adhered to the diaphragm. There was a large oblique opening in the fossa ovalis, admitting the forefinger. The aorta at its origin was a little dilated, and there was a slight incrustation of bony matter on its inner coat. There was no well-marked disease of any of the abdominal viscera.

It is noteworthy that during this man's last illness there was not even a suspicion of any disease of the lungs, so that the surgeon, a very attentive medical officer, considered the opening of the chest totally unnecessary.

Case 17.—Of pneumonia, with hepatization of lung, pleuritic effusion and partial softening of brain, etc.—J. Watt, ætat. 40; 42nd Regiment; admitted into regimental hospital, Malta, 3rd March, 1834; died 7th March.—This man, of very intemperate habits and of an impaired constitution, had been subject many years to chronic rheumatism. During the last twelve months he had been in a desponding state of mind, threatening to commit suicide. He was reported sick on the 3rd March, after having been during the three days preceding constantly drunk. On admission he had cough and oppressed breathing, with headache and general tremors, especially of hands and tongue. There was a general soreness of surface; the tongue loaded; the pulse 100, and very feeble; his manner confused and stupid. At the time there was no indication by the stethoscope of disease of the lungs; there was no pain of chest. A mild aperient was prescribed and 40 drops of Vinum opii., with a drachm of antimonial wine. 4th—Had a restless night, with some delirium, which has passed off. His breathing is oppressed, his cough frequent, with scanty mucous expectoration; urgent thirst; pulse very quick and weak; much tremor of hands and tongue. Mucous râles are now distinct over the whole of the right side of chest; still no pain. A blister to the chest. Tinct. Camphor. compos. 1 drachm, with the same quantity of Spirit Æther. Nit. twice a day. 5th—Seems somewhat better; had a quiet night; his respiration is more free, the expectoration copious; the bowels open. The same medicine. 6th—Was delirious during the night, and was kept in bed with difficulty; now he is more composed, but his countenance has a wild expression, and the abdomen has become typanitic. About noon there was a recurrence of delirium; his hands and feet became cold; stimulants were administered without effect. He expired delirious at 1 a.m. of the 7th.

Autopsy 9 hours after death. Cadaver unusually fat. The arachnoid was partially opaque; between it and the pia mater there was a good deal of fluid; and there was more than usual in the ventricles and at the base of the brain; a large varicose vein was found in the substance of the cerebellum; the inferior surface of the anterior lobes of the cerebrum was softer than natural. The pericardium contained 2 oz. of serum. There was some coagulated blood and fibrinous concretion in the right cavities of the heart. The right pleura was very red and vascular; it contained a pint of turbid serum. The lung of the same side was partially adhering by soft coagulable lymph. Its superior lobe and a considerable portion of its middle lobe were hepatized, likewise the inferior, but in a less degree. The color of the hepatized substance in the superior lobe was grey; in the middle lobe red; a puruloid fluid came from the former when incised. The left lung was very generally and firmly adhering; its superior lobe was œdematous; the upper portion of the inferior hepatized; the lower portion was tolerably natural. The liver was unusually large, pale and soft; from a portion of it that was dried there was a considerable exudation of oily matter. The mucous coat of the stomach was very soft. The spleen adhered to the stomach and diaphragm; its substance was pultaceous. The omentum, etc., were loaded with fat. The right tibia was much enlarged and irregularly so, from the deposition of bony matter, and also unusually vascular, but without any thickening of the periostum.

Delirium tremens, as partially exemplified in this instance, like insanity, almost constantly tends to render other co-existing disease latent. It is also remarkable how drunkenness conduces to inflammation of the lungs, and of the worst kind. Cases showing this have been given, and I have a large number illustrating the fact: further on, under the head of alcoholic poisoning, more evidence will be adduced in proof.

Case 18.—Of pneumonia, with hepatization of lung, and effusion of lymph on brain, etc.—J. Rotchill, ætat. 24; 28th Foot; admitted 16th May, 1840; died June 7th.—This man, of three months' service only, on admission had a slight cough, without expectoration or pain of chest. He complained chiefly of headache; his tongue was furred; his pulse 76. These symptoms under mild treatment decreased until the 21st May, when his cough became more troublesome; his appetite impaired; the pulse 78; the heart's action diffused. Liq. Ammon. Acetat. was prescribed. The cough soon ceased, delirium occurring at night. On the 28th cerebral symptoms were most prominent; calomel and antimony were given. On the 1st June he was comatose; groaning, but making no reply to any question; he perspired much; his pulse was 84; the urine required to be drawn off. On the 3rd June the conjunctivæ were injected; facies Hippocratica; abdomen tympanitic, painful to the touch; pulse 120; warm fomentations, etc.; after an enema, there were copious offensive evacuations. There was no return of consciousness, it is stated, before death.

Autopsy 38 hours after death.—Not emaciated. The vessels of the pia mater were turgid with blood, and its tissue infiltrated with serosity, with which lymph was mixed; this was conspicuous over the pons Varolii, the optic nerves at their junction, and the crura cerebri. The lateral ventricles were distended with a colorless fluid. The septum lucidum was broken posteriorly, and was throughout very soft, as were also the walls of the ventricles; the fornix was pultaceous. The lungs were gorged with blood. The superior and middle lobe of right lung abounded in granular tubercles. In the former there were two masses of clustered tubercles, about the size of hazel-nuts, and the surrounding parenchyma was hepatized. The bronchia were very red. The lower part of the ileum was rough, from a deposit of lymph in transverse lines, which were bounded by a dark redness of the villous coat. The large intestines exhibited the same appearance, and even more strongly marked.

On admission the case was returned " Catarrhus acutus." That there was bronchial inflammation there can be little doubt; and it was probably combined with inflammation of the parenchyma of the lung, chiefly in its first stage of vascular turgescence. But what is most noteworthy was the cessation of the pectoral symptoms on the occurrence of the cerebral.

5. COMPLICATION, WITH PERITONEAL INFLAMMATION.—These cases, two in number, are remarkable for the variety of tissues involved; for the little distress—in one, from the pulmonary lesions; in the other, from the abdominal.

Cases 19.—Of pneumonia, with hepatization of lung, and peritoneal inflammation, etc.—J. Cage, ætat. 34; 47th Foot; admitted 29th October, 1821; died 3rd Nov.— This man is just returned from India, where he served 15 years, and whilst there suffered from bowel complaint, ague, and rheumatism. His present illness began two days before admission with rigors, followed by heat of skin, headache, and nausea. He now complains of pain of chest, and of a troublesome cough, with some expectoration. His pulse is quick and hard; the tongue foul. An emetic, followed by V.S. (33 oz.), and a large blister to chest; and a draught with hyoscyamus, rhubarb, and antimonial wine. The blood was much buffed and cupped. On the 30th, the cough and pain of chest were less. He complained now more of abdominal tenderness, which was increased by pressure. The pulse was 132, full and sharp; there was much pyrexia; the bowels open. V.S. (20 oz.); a feeling of faintness was experienced from the loss of blood, with vomiting and slight convulsions. The blood again was much buffed and cupped; a portion of it watched was twenty minutes coagulating. No relief of abdominal pain; decubitus on back; knees drawn up; there is great prostration of strength; pulse 130, hard and small. 12 leeches were applied to the abdomen, and after their action a large blister, and castor-oil with vinum opii. On the 31st there was but little abdominal pain, and even less of chest, and no cough; his bowels have been freely opened; there is much thirst; the pulse very rapid; a draught of rhubarb and magnesia, vinum opii and antimonial wine. Nov. 1st—Says he feels better; his tongue is cleaner; he complains most of excessive debility. On the following afternoon there was a fresh and more severe accession of abdominal pain, with much distension, accompanied with great restlessness; the pulse still 130, but small; the extremities rather cold; castor-oil, with a grain and a half of opium. Nov. 3—Relief from the draught; some sleep; tongue pretty clean and moist; pulse 130, very feeble; he says he is much better; the pain and abdominal tension have nearly ceased; his extremities are cold. He desires to have some milk or beer. In the course of the day vomiting occurred, but without a return of pain. At the evening visit he was moribund. He expired at 11 p.m.

Autopsy 26 hours after death. Not emaciated; there was much subcutaneous fat. There was some fluid in the cellular tissue of the pia mater, and more than usual in the ventricles of the brain. The pleuræ were very red and vascular, especially contiguous to the diaphragm; in the right there was rather more than half a pint of reddish puruloid fluid. The inferior lobe of each lung was more or less hepatized. The bronchia were unusually red. The right auricle and ventricle, and the pulmonary artery and its branches, were nearly full of coagulable lymph. The omentum, much thickened and very vascular, adhered to the peritoneum. Scarcely any of the abdominal viscera were free from adhesions, and their peritoneal covering generally bore marks of inflammation. In the abdominal cavity there was about a pint of seropurulent fluid. The cellular membrane surrounding the right kidney was full of pus. There was pus also in the cellular membrane, between the peritoneal lining of the abdomen and the psoas muscles. The fibres of these muscles were exceedingly soft and easily torn. The liver was large, very soft, and easily broken, especially its left lobe: it weighed 5 lbs. The gall-bladder was distended with dilute greenish bile, and the branches of the hepatic duct contained the same kind of bile. The spleen likewise was unusually large and soft. The stomach contained much grass-green fluid; its cardia was unusually red and vascular. Both kidneys were large, and unusually soft and vascular. The intestines, more or less cohering, were covered with coagulable lymph. Their mucous coat bore no decided marks of disease. The scrotum was of a dark color from ecchymosis. Both testes were diseased. The right tunica vaginalis contained some pus, and was covered with a layer of coagulable lymph. The left was very red and vascular. The mesenteric glands were a little enlarged.

How remarkable is this case for its many complications, and for the overpowering influence of the principal disease—the peritoneal inflammation—following, and yet not arresting, the pleuritic and pulmonary! How remarkable, too, the inefficiency of blood-letting, when serious organic disease is once established! How remarkable, further, is the occurrence of so many lesions at the same time, or their co-existence, theoretically considered.

Case 20.—Of pneumonia, with hepatization of lungs and peritoneal inflammation, etc.—J. Hyland, ætat. 32; 60th R.; admitted into regimental hospital, Malta, 16th January, 1835; died 27th January.—This man, of a full habit of body, had frequently been in hospital with cough and rheumatism. His present attack he attributed "to taking cold" a few nights ago, when on guard. He complains now of lumbar pains and of nausea. His tongue is foul, his skin rather hot; thirst; pulse frequent and full; bowels relaxed. An emetic and aperient prescribed, which acted freely. In the evening V.S. (30 oz.) The blood was buffed and cupped. Calomel with antimony and opium. On the following day, no pain of any part. His pulse is frequent, but not so full; skin dry, but cool; solution of tartarized antimony every third hour. 18th—Some cough and oppression of chest; pulse 100, soft; skin cool; bowels rather confined; a purgative enema; small doses of calomel, ipecacuanha and tinct. digitalis. 19th—Much pain of right side of chest, affecting his breathing; it began at 2 a.m; his pulse is full and frequent, his skin hot. V.S. (25 oz.); syncope; the blood much buffed and cupped; a blister to the pained part. 20th—The pain is less; much cough with mucous expectoration; tongue moist; pulse 88, soft; the same medicine. 25th—His breathing is very short; expectoration difficult; pulse small and weak; the digitalis discontinued. 26th—The dyspnœa is increased; is "very low;" skin bedewed with sweat; no stool since yesterday; a small dose of castor oil, followed by an enema, without effect. In the evening, the expression of countenance anxious; the abdomen tense and painful. He expired at 1 a.m. of the 7th.

Autopsy 30 hours after death. Sub-emaciated. In both ventricles of the heart there were fibrinous concretions, rounded and blood-shot, as if formed before death. The left pleura contained 4 oz. of serum. The superior lobe of the left lung was in part hepatized; it felt as if it contained granular tubercles, but none were visible; its inferior lobe was moderately crepitous. A considerable portion of the superior and middle lobe of the right lung was hepatized and of a reddish grey color. The bronchia and lower part of the trachea were red. An œsophagal gland was enlarged to the size of an almond, and was distended with purulent matter. There was a considerable quantity of turbid serum and purulent fluid, with flakes of lymph in the abdominal cavity, especially in both iliac fossæ, in the hypochondria and cavity of the pelvis. The liver was pale and was covered with purulent fluid. Its peritoneal coat was most easily detached; its parenchyma was bloodshot, and so tender as to yield to the gentle pressure of the fingers. A large quantity of purulent fluid was found collected round the spleen, partially confined by "adhesions;" the organ itself was of increased size and very soft; its posterior surface was pultaceous, and bathed in pus and quite disorganized. The other viscera appeared tolerably free from disease.

This case is almost as remarkable for the latency of the peri-

toneal inflammation as the preceding one was for that of the pulmonary ; and likewise for its many and severe complications and
their intractable kind.

6. ABSCESSES IN THE LUNGS.—These cases, two in number,
of this rare disease, are chiefly remarkable for their anomalous
symptoms, to which the complication of cerebral disease may in
part have contributed.

Case 21.—Of pneumonia, with partial hepatization of lungs, and pulmonary
abscesses and partial softening of brain.—D. Bell, 94th F. ; admitted into regimental
hospital, Malta, 6th September, 1834 ; died 14th September.—This man, one of the.
band, his instrument a wind instrument, for some time had been subject to soreness of
throat. When brought to hospital, at 8 a.m. on the 5th September, he was apparently
insensible, and the lower jaw was immoveable as in trismus ; at the same time the skin
was of natural temperature, the countenance of healthy aspect, the eyes clear and
bright, suggesting an attack of mania. The pulse was 100 and rather full. V.S.
(16 oz.); a blister to the nape of neck ; a warm aperient enema. At 3 p.m. he was
convulsed ; for about two hours the convulsions alternated with syncope ; his
extremities were cold ; respiration short and quick, with mucous râle ; pulse 110 ;
twice the bowels were moved. On the 6th he was very lethargic ; skin hot, pulse
120 ; a strong cadaverous smell from the body. At 10 p.m. there was a return of
consciousness of what was passing around and he swallowed some sago with wine.
7th—Is quite sensible, but cannot articulate, the jaw is only partially relaxed ;
" matter" runs from the mouth. 8th—Is able to speak feebly ; pulse 98 ; skin
natural ; bowels open ; tongue furred but moist. He points to the upper part of the
sternum as the seat of uneasiness ; a blister to the part ; Tinct. Digital. with Liq.
Ammoniæ Acetat. 10th—Little change since the 8th, but seems not so well this
morning ; matter is now discharged by coughing. 12th—His debility is increasing ;
about 12 oz. of purulent fluid are expectorated in the 24 hours. He gradually sank
without any change of symptoms.

Autopsy 12 hours after death. Not emaciated. The convolutions of the brain were
rather flattened ; the pia mater and choroid plexus were redder than usual ; the
ventricles contained pretty much serum ; the septum lucidum was softer than natural.
All the cavities of the heart were distended with coagulated blood and fibrinous concretion. The right pleura contained a little serum, and there were some flakes of
lymph on its pulmonary surface. Both lungs were slightly adhering ; neither collapsed ; both contained many small abscesses ; in some of these there was a turbid
fluid ; others were empty, cavities lined with a grey false membrane and surrounded
by " a dense cellular tissue." The inferior portion of both lungs was in part gorged
with blood and more or less hepatized, exhibiting different shades of color. The
bronchia were very red and contained much turbid fluid ; the lower part of the
trachea was of the same color. The epiglottis, especially its under surface, was of a
grey hue and rough, as if from old inflammation ; the sacculi laryngis were of the
same color. No abscess could be detected in the fauces or in the adjoining parts.
The mucous membrane of the stomach and duodenum was softer than natural, and
bloodshot in patches. The gall-bladder contained a little greyish yellow fluid, " more
of the nature of mucus than bile." All the other viscera were apparently sound.

That the purulent discharge in this case came from abscesses
in the lungs seems open to little or no doubt, both these organs

being perfectly free from tubercles. It seems also pretty certain that the pulmonary disease in its early stage was masked by the cerebral, and accordingly as the one abated, the other became more manifest.

Case 22.—Of pneumonia, with abscesses in the lungs and inflammation of pleuræ. J. Kelly, ætat. 47; 36th Foot; admitted 22nd August, 1839; died 23rd August.— This man was brought to hospital immediately after arrival from the West Indies. There, it is stated, he suffered from chronic catarrh, rheumatism, and ague; it is added that he was comparatively strong and healthy during the voyage till within the last few days, when his present illness began. The symptoms on his admission were of the most unpromising kind, and chiefly the following :—Urgent dyspnœa, without cough or expectoration; pulse 100, so weak as to be only just perceptible; dimness of sight; tightness of head; speech indistinct; countenance indicative of distress; much thirst; profuse perspiration; great debility; raves now and then. The chest sounded normal; the respiratory murmur was heard generally without râle. The pulse ceased at wrist some hours before death. Treatment, cupping, etc.

Autopsy 22 hours after death. Of very robust frame, and unusually fat. The vessels of the pia mater were turgid with blood. There was a yellowish brown discoloration of the *surface* of the left hemisphere of the cerebrum, to some extent. The septum lucidum was perforated; the opening, a circular one, was large enough to admit the end of the little finger; shreds crossed it, as if the remains of the entire surface. There was no softening of the septum, nor of any part of the brain. In the lateral ventricles and at the base of the brain there was a good deal of fluid. Both lungs were adhering slightly by soft flaky lymph. Both were unusually red and heavy, and also to a considerable extent œdematous. In the parenchyma of each there were whitish masses about the size of cherries, having a good deal of the character of phlegmon. Of these some were full of a reddish purulent fluid; some of a firmer matter, like the substance of an immature abscess; one or two were empty cavities, their fluid contents probably discharged by the bronchia. The lungs were warm. Tubercles were sought for, but none could be found. The bronchia and lower part of the trachea were red. The right cavities of the heart contained some cruor and fibrinous concretion. All the valves were stained reddish. The liver weighed 5 lbs. The spleen was large and soft. The glands in the left groin were enlarged; there was some ecchymosis, and the left thigh and leg were somewhat swollen. There was no coagulum in the femoral vein. The cartilages of the patellæ and of the bones of the feet were partially rough, and in part absorbed.

The superficial discoloration of the brain in this case would seem to indicate effusion of blood there at some former period. Whether the peculiarity observed in the septum lucidum was congenital or the effect of disease, must, I apprehend, be uncertain. Does not the very corpulent condition of the deceased favor the conclusion that the peculiar lesion of the lungs was of a phlegmonous character, and of rapid formation?

7. COMPLICATION WITH RHEUMATISM.—These cases, two in number, are noteworthy, the first for the manner in which the pulmonary disease was disguised by the cerebral—an additional

complication; the second for the manner in which the rheumatic symptoms were superseded by the pulmonary; and both for the presence of lithic acid in the joints, the accompaniment more commonly of the gouty than of the rheumatic diathesis.

Case 23.—Of pneumonia, with hepatization of lungs, a granular state of kidneys, and partial lithic deposits in joints.—R. M'Illroy, ætat. 36; 50th Foot; admitted 3rd January, 1839; died 6th January.—This man, a pay-sergeant, of 19 years' service, had suffered much from acute rheumatism. Two months ago he had been treated for this disease, and had been under the influence of mercury. Then there were pains in the large and small joints, and the knees and ankles were much swollen. When transferred from the detachment hospital on the 3rd January the case was considered one of rheumatism. On the night of the 5th he experienced an epileptic seizure. On the 6th his intellect was confused; he was continually dozing, breathing heavily. He had no desire for food; the urinary secretion was very scanty. At the evening visit he was much in the same state; his pulse, which on the preceding day had been full, but not quick, had now become small and weak. Apprehending that possibly there might be accumulation of urine in the bladder, the catheter was introduced: no more than two drachms were drawn off. He died at 11 p.m. The treatment was chiefly directed to promote the secretion of urine.

Autopsy 63 hours after death. Nowise emaciated. There was some thickening of the calvaria on each side of the median line. The dura mater in one or two places was unusually thin. The arachnoid was generally opaque and thickened. There was a good deal of serum in the cellular tissue of the pia mater, a little fluid in the ventricles, and pretty much at the base of the brain. The fornix and corpora striata were rather soft. The pericardium contained very little serum, no more than about a drachm. There was coagulated blood in both auricles,* and fibrinous concretion without clot in the ventricles, especially the right. In each pleura there were about 2 oz. of serum. Both lungs were partially adhering. The right weighed 3½ lbs.; the left 2¼. The superior lobe of each was œdematous. The middle lobe of right lung was partially so, and partially hepatized; and the inferior of both was hepatized throughout, and of a light reddish color. The bronchia were red. A concretion about the size of an almond was found in the gall-bladder; it was composed partly of cholesterine, and partly of black matter. The liver weighed 4½ lbs. The spleen was large and "hepatized;" its capsule was partially thickened. The kidneys were indurated and granular; their cortical substance was nearly white. A portion, dried on paper, left an oil stain. There was much turbid serum, with shreds of lymph and white granules, in the left knee joint. On the investing cartilage of the patella, of the head of the tibia, and of the femur, there was an incrustation of an opaque white matter.† In the right knee-joint the appearances were similar, excepting that the synovia was less turbid.‡ The same opaque white deposit was detected on the lining

---

* The small quantity of serum in the pericardium compared with the quantity of blood in the heart, may be adduced in proof of the retentive power of the organ, and that the fluid in question ordinarily is not an exudation, especially taking into account the length of time in this instance between the death and autopsy. A portion of blood from the heart was tested for urea, and with a positive result; a minute quantity, after digestion with alcohol, was detected.

† It was found to contain lithic acid, but whether combined with soda or ammonia was not ascertained.

‡ Some of the turbid fluid from the knee-joint exhibited under the microscope

cartilage of the ankle-joints, on those of the great toes, of the elbows, hip-joints, and the joint of the right wrist. No other joints were examined.

This case is most interesting on account of the deposit on the joints, raising the question whether what was called rheumatism was truly rheumatism or gout. The habits of the individual— a pay-sergeant—during a time of peace, may be considered rather favorable to the conclusion of its being the latter. Yet, had the attacks been those of genuine gout, is it likely that they could have been so mistaken as to be called rheumatic? In my original abstract of the case I find that there is mention made of both the tibiæ being enlarged, a circumstance this pointing rather to rheumatism than gout.

Case 24.—Of pneumonia, with hepatization of lungs and partial lithic-deposit in the joints.—F. Biggen, ætat. 31; 98th F.; admitted 22nd May, 1838; died 26th May.—This man had just returned from the Cape of Good Hope, where he had served 13 years, and in good health, according to his surgeon, until about 4 years ago, when "after taking cold" he had an acute attack of rheumatism, followed by the disease in its chronic form, disqualifying him for military duty. On admission, immediately on his arrival at Fort Pitt, he had pains in the joints of the lower extremities, and also pain of chest with slight cough. The respiration was then dull in the right clavicular region. On the following day there was an increase of the pain of chest and of the cough, with much dyspnœa. There was a crepitating râle perceived over the chest, especially of right side. The skin was hot, thirst urgent, tongue white; pulse 120. V.S. (20 oz.) A purgative. Some relief followed, and he had a good night. On the 24th there was an increase of pain, with a short dry cough and great difficulty of breathing; the crepitating râle stronger. V.S. (12 oz.) A blister to the pained part. He was easier until the evening of the 25th, when the pain, cough and dyspnœa became more severe. His lips were livid; the countenance anxious; the expectoration scanty. Some blood was abstracted by cupping. After a restless night, he expired the following morning. He was sensible to the last.

Autopsy 26 hours after death. Very robust. There was a good deal of coagulated blood, cruor and fibrinous concretion in the cavities of the heart. The lungs did not collapse. The left weighed ⅔ lb.; the right 4 lbs. There was some œdema in the inferior portion of the former, and some frothy fluid in its bronchia. The latter was partially adhering; its superior and middle lobe were hepatized, as was also a portion of the inferior lobe; fawn was the prevailing color; when incised, a turbid fluid, purulent by the optical test, flowed out. The bronchia contained a frothy fluid, and as well as the trachea, were pale; the latter contained fluid of the same kind. The vessels of this lung were full of coagulated blood. The liver weighed, exclusive of ¼ lb. of bile in the gall-bladder, 4¾ lbs.; its peritoneal coat was easily separated; the subjacent surface was unusually vascular. The cartilage of each patella was softened, and in one spot elevated and fibrous. It contained imbedded an opaque whitish matter.* A similar matter was found incrusting the condyles of the former, the cartilages of the

corpuscles of different sizes—some elliptical, some like pus globules—many smaller, and many granules and filaments.

* It was found to consist of lithic acid and animal matter, probably in union with ammonia, as no residue was obtained when subjected to the blow-pipe.

tibiæ of both its extremities, and the first joint of the great toe, and in each instance, in both limbs. The joints of the upper extremities were examined and the sheaths of the tendons of the lower, but the result was negative. The synovial membrane of the joints of the lower extremities was unusually vascular.

This case is suggestive of the same question as the last, and in addition, whether the *dictum* that the lithic diathesis is strictly confined to the arthritic, is founded on a sufficiently extensive induction? The circumstance that the deceased was a private, and must have been actively employed at the Cape, is not favorable to the idea of his becoming the subject of a disease of the extremest rareness in the British army—so rare indeed, that I cannot call to mind a single well-authenticated case of it amongst men of the ranks.

8. COMPLICATION WITH TUBERCLES.—These cases, six in number, might have had a place in a preceding section, that, viz., on the latency of tubercle. Each case had its peculiarities; in three instances there was no appreciable emaciation, in two sub-emaciation only; and in one only much emaciation, that a chronic case. In one, the 26th, there was an appearance in the lung specially noteworthy, from its resemblance to a cicatrix, as if a cavity that had been formed there had been closed up; and in another, case 27, there was an appearance seeming to indicate a like change.

Case 25.—Of pneumonia (so returned) with tuberculated lungs and puruloid effusion into the pericardium and pleuræ.—C. Hughes, ætat. 29 ; 54th F. ; admitted 20th April, 1822; died 23rd April.—This man had recently returned from the Cape of Good Hope, where during the last four years he had been more than once under treatment for severe pain in the right hypochondrium, and for which he had been salivated. After his arrival he was taken into the surgical division of the general hospital on account of scrofulous swelling of the neck with œdema of the lower extremities. About five days ago, after having been discharged relieved, his present illness began. He attributed it to getting wet and cold when on guard. It was ushered in by "cold chills," succeeded by "hot fits," which recurred three days successively, and then he experienced pain in the old situation. Now there is much dyspnœa ; the skin is pungently hot ; the face is flushed, and there is much thirst. V.S. (30 oz.) A purgative. The blood is only slightly buffed. No relief. V.S. (36 oz.) A blister to the pained part. Tinct. of Digital. with solution of tartarized antimony. The blood cupped and buffed. On the following day all the symptoms were more moderate. The antimony was now omitted in consequence of the nausea produced. The pulse being hard and full, and still pain of side, V.S. (8 oz.) was repeated, and calomel and opium were prescribed. During the following night there was some delirium. On the 22nd it was stated that the pain had ceased in the right side, and was experienced in the left. Again V.S. (15 oz.) There was a cessation of pain, but no improvement; he continued restless with delirium, gradually sinking; he expired the following morning at 6 a.m. No mention is made of cough or expectoration.

Autopsy 6 hours after death. Not emaciated. The pericardium externally and also the anterior mediastinum were unusually vascular. The former contained 8 oz. of turbid serum with flakes of lymph, and there was a deposit of the same on its inner surface. The muscular substance of the heart was pale. The left pleura contained about a pint and a half of thin milky serum; the right about 3 pints of similar serum. Both were covered with a deposit of lymph. The costal side of the former was very vascular; the latter was very vascular throughout. The superior lobe of each lung abounded in small firm tubercles, of a grey color; one, larger than the rest, about the size of an orange-pip, was undergoing softening. The inferior lobe of the left lung was red and appeared to be hepatized. The middle and inferior lobe of the right exhibited the same character, but the middle in a less degree than the inferior, which was adhering to the diaphragm. The bronchia were very red, as was also the lower portion of the trachea. The bronchial, œsophageal and mesenteric glands were much enlarged. The latter were softening and contained a curd-like matter. The abdominal viscera generally were tolerably sound, if the liver and speen were not exceptions, which are described as " rather soft and easily broken."

This case is not without instruction on account of the different views taken of it. On admission the disease was named hepatitis on the idea that the liver was the organ affected, founded on pain in the right hypochondrium. Next it was returned pneumonia, the difficulty of breathing probably suggesting that the lungs were the seat of the malady. Now, reviewing the symptoms, imperfectly as they are recorded, may not the correctness of this designation be questioned, inasmuch as there was no cough, no expectoration, and as the demonstrated lesions, those of the pleuræ and pericardium, are adequate to account for the phenomena and the event. If the inferior lobes of the lungs *were* hepatized, and not simply solidified, their hepatization might have been the result of former attacks. The existence of tubercles, denoting a cachectic state of the system, might in part be connected with the failure of the very active treatment.

Case 26.—Of pneumonia, with hepatized lung and tubercles, with a probably filled-up tubercular excavation.—E. Stack, ætat. 30; 39th Foot; admitted 7th Oct., 1837; died 10th October.—This man had recently returned from India, where, it is stated, he had had repeated attacks of pneumonia, bronchitis, and dyspepsia. He was first admitted into the general hospital on account of scurvy, contracted on the homeward voyage. He was discharged on the 23rd September, a month after his arrival. The staff surgeon, under whose charge he had been, then thought he might prove effective. The conclusion, from auscultation, that I came to was different— viz., that he was unfit for further service on account of chronic pulmonary disease. When re-admitted on the 7th October, he stated that he had been unwell for several days, with cough, and difficulty of breathing. V.S. (18 oz.) ; the blood was buffed; a blister to chest; purgative medicine. On the 8th his breathing was reported to be "abdominal;" the countenance was livid, and had an anxious expression; the pulse 120; crepitating râles were heard in the right mammary region, and in the lateral. V.S. (21oz.) ; $\frac{1}{3}$ grain of tartarized antimony every second hour. On the

9th the crepitating râle was more diffused; the expectoration viscid and rusty; pulse 125. Some blood was abstracted by cupping, and the antimony continued. He expired at 8 a.m. of the following morning.

Autopsy 39 hours after death. Not emaciated. The dura and pia mater were very thin. The pineal gland was adhering posteriorly, and it contained no gritty matter. The pericardium contained 2 oz. of serum. The right auricle and ventricle were distended with coagulated blood with a buffy coat. Both lungs were firmly adhering in the axillary region. The superior lobe of the right lung was small and contracted. In its upper portion there were many clusters of granular tubercles, and several small cavities. In one spot there was the appearance of a cicatrix—viz., a cartilage-like induration bisecting a bronchial tube, suggesting the idea of a tuber-cular excavation filled up and contracted after freely communicating with the bronchia. The middle lobe was pale, free from tubercles, and apparently healthy. The inferior lobe, on the contrary, was extremely diseased. It was covered with false membrane of soft lymph, and was hepatized throughout. Detached, it weighed 3 lbs. It was of a brownish hue, and, when incised, there exuded from it some purulent fluid of a rusty color. It contained some granular tubercles, and two masses nearly white of the size of walnuts, "not encysted." In the superior lobe of the left lung, and in its upper portion, there was a cavity capable of holding a small orange, into which a large bronchial tube terminated. The bronchia generally were red. The bronchial glands were enlarged; some of them were softening internally. The liver weighed 3¼ lbs. The spleen was soft. There was the cicatrix of an ulcer in the ileo-cœcal valve.

The noteworthy points of this case hardly need comment. That death was owing to the sudden inflammation of the inferior lobe of the right lung, can, I think, hardly be questioned; or that a large cavity—that in the left lung—pre-existed with tubercles in both lungs, allowing of tolerable health. Further, though not quite so certain, is it not highly probable that an old cavity had closed, and in a manner healed?

Case 27.—Of pneumonia, with partial induration of lungs, accompanied by tubercles and an excavation, as if in process of closing.—J. Crawford, ætat. 28; 87th Foot; admitted 22nd December, 1835; died January 4th, 1836.—This man, of five years' service, had for the last three years been subject to cough, with abundant expectoration; and with difficulty of breathing since November last. On the 19th of that month he was discharged from the general hospital as convalescent from chronic catarrh. Almost immediately after, he was admitted into the detachment hospital with severe dyspnœa; whence, on the 22nd December, he was brought back to the general hospital, laboring under severe pain of chest, increased by inspiration, with cough, copious expectoration, and urgent dyspnœa. He was blooded largely, blistered, and used antimonials. On the following day he was free from pain; the other symptoms much the same; the pulse 90, and soft; the tongue clean; the bowels open. Little change occurred till the 28th, when he complained of pain of bowels, with severe purging, which continued to the 30th, when there was a slight abatement, and of the symptoms generally. On the 31st the purging returned, but he expressed himself on the whole easier; his pulse was full and regular; his skin moist. At the evening visit the dyspnœa had become distressing, and from this time it continued to increase, with abundant rather thick yellow muco-purulent expectoration. Mucous râles were perceived over the whole of the chest; percussion gave pain; the sound was dull. He gradually sank.

Autopsy 42 hours after death. Slightly emaciated. The lungs did not collapse; their upper surface was crepitous; both were heavier than natural. In the upper part of the superior lobe of the right lung there was a tubercular excavation capable of holding a billiard ball. It was lined with a false membrane, and its walls were nearly of cartilaginous firmness. A large bronchial tube opened into it, and the surrounding parenchyma was indurated. In the same lobe there were several clusters of granular tubercles; in the middle lobe there were a few, and also in the superior lobe of the left lung. Both lungs partially adhered to the costal pleura, and the inferior portions of both were gorged with blood. A considerable portion, however, of the parenchyma of each was tolerably sound. There was much coagulated blood in the pulmonary veins. The bronchia were of a dark red, and in them and the larynx there was a good deal of muco-purulent fluid. The cavities of the heart were distended with blood and fibrinous concretions. The liver weighed 2½ lbs. The mucous coat of the stomach was very soft, and was covered with thick mucus. The lower part of the ileum and the large intestines were redder than natural, and moister —somewhat sodden, as it were; and the former was slightly granular.

The cavity in the right lung, which in this instance escaped detection during life, might be considered in progress of closing, and as exhibiting an earlier stage of the healing process than that referred to in the preceding example. The history of the case seems tolerably accordant. The fatal termination was owing, it may be inferred, to partial inflammation of the lungs, and to inflammation of the bronchia. The large abstraction of blood, followed by diarrhœa, probably accelerated the event.

Case 28.—Of pneumonia, with a gangrenous cavity in lung and partial hepatization; treated by very copious blood-letting.—P. Fogarty, ætat. 20; 88th Foot; admitted into regimental hospital, Corfu, 8th June, 1827; died 22nd June.—This man, two days before coming into hospital, had a severe rigor, which lasted about an hour, and was followed by heat of skin and headache, ending in sweating. The next day, he states, he had a similar attack, and at the same time. He now complains of acute pain of right breast, which is increased by coughing. There is flatulent distension of abdomen, and he has vomited much bilious matter. His pulse is 92, and full; heat of skin moderate; tongue white; bowels constipated. V.S. ad deliquium; after two hours a purgative. On the following day there was still some pain; the expectoration was bloody; the skin hot and dry; the vomiting continues; he has had several dark colored stools; his breath is very offensive; there has been no return of rigors. V.S. (38 oz.); the blood is cupped and buffed. V.S. again, after two hours (40. oz.) The blood first collected was cupped and buffed, and only the first. Calomel 15 grs. On the 8th there was cessation of pain and vomiting, and the expectoration was no longer bloody. The thirst is excessive; the urine highly colored; the stools dark and scanty. A cathartic draught. On the 9th it was stated that the bowels had been freely moved, and that the symptoms were less severe. A blister to the chest; tartarized antimony, with compound tincture of camphor. Until the night of the 12th he appeared to be improving; then there was a return of pain in the side, and the cough was more troublesome, with an increase of pyrexia and an irritable stomach; pulse 96. V.S. (32 oz.) On the 15th the symptoms were less severe, but the expectoration and also the stools were very fetid. Between the 15th and 21st he was twice blistered, with temporary relief. There is now an increase of pain, with a hot and dry skin. V.S. (32 oz.) The blood was buffed and cupped. On the 22nd the symptoms were less severe. About 5 p.m. he experienced great dyspnœa; was excessively restless, and said he was dying; his extremities were cold; his intellect unimpaired. In the act of swallowing an anti-spasmodic draught he became slightly convulsed; in a few minutes he expired.

Autopsy 18 hours after death. Sub-emaciated. There was a good deal of fluid at the base of the brain. In the superior lobe of the right lung there was a large cavity; its walls were irregular, sloughing, and almost gangrenous, emitting a putrid smell. A curd-like induration surrounded it, as if produced by a deposition of tubercular matter. The middle lobe was hepatized. The inferior lobe and the whole of the left lung were nearly free from disease. In neither could any distinct tubercles be detected. With the exception of much distension of the stomach and colon from air, nothing unusual was observed in the viscera of the abdomen.

This case was first returned " Febris intermittens;" and in its prodrome affords a striking example of the rigor ushering in inflammation closely resembling that of ague. Whether the cavity formed in the lung was that of an abscess, or the result of the disintegration of tubercular matter, is open to question. Certain it is, that contemporary, or associated with it, there was a partial and severe inflammation of the lung, which the abstraction of blood, so largely practised, did not arrest.

Case 29.—Of pneumonia, with hepatization of lung and inflammation of pericardium, with granular tubercles.—J. Joy, ætat. 18; 69th Foot; admitted 18th February, 1823; died 22nd February.—This young soldier was brought to hospital on the evening of the 17th February, laboring under excessive pain of chest, with much dyspnœa. His pulse was scarcely perceptible; the tongue was white and dry; skin dry. The pain, he says, began a week ago, when on march from the Isle of Wight, after putting on a damp shirt, and that he was previously in good health. Hitherto he has had no medical aid. V.S. (16 oz.) Tartarized antimony, 1 gr.; Ext. Conii, 8 grs.; Hyoscy., 6 grs. On the following morning his appearance was most unfavorable; his lips nearly of the color of venous blood; his cheeks almost of the same hue; little heat of skin; the respiration hurried and labored; no cough; pulse 120, and small; tongue moister; can lie on either side; is now free from pain, and makes no complaint of any kind, and is not in the least aware of his danger. A blister to the chest. The same medicine, with 20 grs. of Digitalis in powder, in divided doses. February 21—During the night he was delirious. His dyspnœa now is rather less. He lies on his back in a careless manner, as if quite at ease. The pupils are rather dilated; the pulse still 120, and feeble; the tongue dry and white. He expired the following evening, and was sensible to the last. Whilst in hospital he coughed very little, and that chiefly at night. He expectorated copiously muco-purulent matter, free from any tinge of blood.

Autopsy 14 hours after death. Stout and muscular. Pretty much bloody serum in the ventricles, and at the base of the brain. The anterior mediastinum was very vascular, as was also the pericardium externally. The latter was adhering on each side to the lung, and when opened was found adhering to the heart at many points by lymph-bands and fibres varying in length from a line to an inch. It contained about 1 oz. of bloody serum, and was covered with a layer of lymph in some places about a quarter of an inch thick. The surface reflected over the heart had a delicate reticulated structure. The heart was large and loaded with fat. Its right auricle and ventricle, and in a less degree the left auricle, and still less the left ventricle, were distended with blood and fibrinous concretion. The valves and the muscular substance of the organ were of natural appearance. The left pleura was unusually red. The right, in addition, exhibited scattered over it dark red and almost black spots, as if from ecchymosis. Its surface was studded also with white tubercles, varying in size from that of mustard-seed to that of duck-shot. Some of them were translucent, some opaque: all were *solid*. Similar tubercles were found on bands of lymph connecting the middle and inferior lobe, and the latter with the diaphragm. On these bands there was the same appearance of ecchymosis. Both lungs were very red, and in part gorged with blood and in part hepatized. When incised, an exudation took place of muco-purulent fluid from the divided bronchial tubes. The right lung contained very many minute white tubercles, similar to those above described. The bronchia were dark red, as was also the lower portion of the trachea. The bronchial glands were much enlarged; the mesenteric less so. The urinary bladder was contracted, and nearly empty. Its lining membrane was incrusted with patches of calculous matter, which, on examination, was found to be lithate of ammonia. The viscera not mentioned had no unusual appearance, with the exception of the pelvis of each kidney, which exhibited spots of ecchymosis, probably the effect of the blister.

The variety of lesions, the rapidity of effect, the comparative ease when there was greatest danger, and this without gangrene, are noteworthy circumstances in this case, as are also the character of the tubercles in so early a stage, and their situation. Another is the robust state of the individual before the fatal attack, if it may be presumed, as I think it may with great probability, that the tubercles were at that time in existence.

Case 30.—Of pneumonia, with partial hepatization of lungs, with tubercles and cavities, and incipient gangrene of œsophagus.—G. Moncreif, ætat. 28; 88th Regiment; admitted into regimental hospital, Corfu, 16th July, 1827; died 9th Sept.— This man, a month before coming into hospital, had been subject to cough, with some difficulty of breathing. On admission he had pain of left breast with pyrexia. After a large blood-letting, and the use of calomel in small doses, he experienced relief The pain twice recurred before the end of the month, and was each time relieved by V.S. The cough and dyspnœa continuing, mercury with squill and digitalis was prescribed and used until gentle ptyalism was produced. The calomel was then omitted. On the 20th August, the cough and dyspnœa becoming more severe, the mercury was resumed. On the 30th dysenteric symptoms occurred; the stools were clay-colored and partly bloody. He was blooded largely and leeched, and had castor-oil and calomel and opium; relief followed. On the 6th September he was distressed by hiccough; the tongue was dry; there was some difficulty in swallowing, and great debility. Dover's powder, æther, and a little wine. On the 7th, 12 leeches to the epigastrium, where pain was felt; some relief. On the 8th the hiccough ceased; the bowels were much disturbed; the stools frequent, clay-colored, and fetid; his skin rather cold; no thirst. All medicine was omitted. Wine, chicken broth. He died on the 7th, and was conscious nearly to the last.

Autopsy 7 hours after death. Much emaciated. There was air under the dura mater, and in the vessels of the pia mater, which were partially injected with blood. There was an unusual quantity of fluid between the arachnoid and the pia mater, and in the ventricles and at the base of the brain—altogether about 4 oz. The superior surface of both lungs had a tolerably healthy appearance; yet the right lung was in great part œdematous. The pleura contained several ounces of reddish serum, and its surface close to the spine was dotted with small white tubercles. The inferior lobe of the left lung was hepatized, and contained, scattered through it in patches, a curd-like tubercular matter, also two vomicæ; these were of an irregular form, and in them, but not filling them, was a similar substance undergoing softening. The superior lobe was similarly diseased, but was without vomicæ. The left pleura was covered with a rough false membrane, which was called " organized," and was spotted with minute tubercles. The left side of the pericardium was similarly diseased. The mitral valves were a little thickened. The lining membrane of the œsophagus was in a state approaching to gangrene; its color was nearly black, and it was most easily detached; this appearance extended from the cardia nearly to the pharynx. The stomach was distended with air and glairy mucus. The duodenum was in part simi-larly distended, so as to look like a second stomach The other intestines were also distended, but chiefly by air. In the large intestines there were patches of bluish discoloration, indicating old ulcers healed. The liver weighed 4 lb. 10 oz.; it was of nutmeg-like section, and rather hard. The gall-bladder contained a very little greenish viscid bile. The spleen was firmer, and of a brighter red than usual. Though the vessels of the kidneys contained much blood, their substance was unusually pale.

In this case may it not be inferred that the tubercles and vomicæ discovered after death preceded the inflammation of the lungs; and that the fatal event was in great part owing to loss of vital force (*that* indicated by incipient gangrene), the joint effect of the varied lesions and the large loss of blood?

9. CHRONIC PNEUMONIA.—These cases, two in number, are well characterized by the state of the lungs, especially the enlargement of the air-cells and the quality of the imprisoned air.

Case 31.—Of chronic pneumonia, with hepatization and induration and emphysema of lungs and thickening of bronchia.—W. Halpin, ætat. 42; 4th D.G.; admitted 4th September, 1837; died 9th Sept.—This man, of 21 years' service, is reported to have had good health until 3 years ago, when he was attacked with pain of chest and cough, for which he was actively treated; relieved, but not cured. According to the statement of the surgeon, he suffered more or less ever after from "chronic asthma and constant dyspnœa." On admission, his dyspnœa was excessive, the cough troublesome, the expectoration scanty and tinged with blood; his breath was peculiarly offensive; the tongue foul; pulse 120 and small; the heart's action indis-tinct; respiration bronchial. During the first two days there was an apparent improvement, especially as to the cough and breathing. On the 7th there was more blood in the sputa; the pulse 132, steady; great thirst; total loss of appetite. On the 8th he felt easier. On the 9th he was unable to rest in the recumbent posture; he was bedewed with a clammy sweat. He died suddenly without a struggle.

Autopsy 18 hours after death. No emaciation, but the contrary, very robust.

Some fluid between the dura mater and the arachnoid; slight œdema of the pia mater; a moderate quantity of fluid in the ventricles; very little at the base of the brain; the cerebral vessels generally loaded; the pericardium contained 1½ oz. of serosity. There was a good deal of coagulated blood and fibrin in the right cavities of the heart. The right auricular-ventricular passage was large. The margin of the tricuspid valve was thickened and almost of cartilaginous firmness. The mouth of the coronary vein was so unusually large as to admit the finger; the pulmonary artery too was very large. There was nothing abnormal in the valves of the left side of the heart. Both lungs were partially adhering. The pleuræ, especially over the diaphragm, were very much thickened. The left lung weighed 4 lbs.; the right 3½ lbs. Both were greatly diseased, showing different stages of hepatization, with œdema intermixed, and emphysema in parts. The emphysema was principally in the lower portion of each lung. Some air was collected from the distended cells; 7 measures of it by lime water were reduced to 5; by phosphorus there was no reduction. This part of the lung examined under water, after the escape of the air, had very much the appearance of the corpus spongiosum urethræ, as if composed of a network of fibres and vessels. Above, bounding the emphysematous part in each, there was a considerable condensation of the parenchyma, with intersecting cartilage-like bands. Macerated for 24 hours and well washed, the blood-vessels of the part were found to be thickened, and likewise the bronchia and the interlobular cellular tissue. The appearance suggested the effect of old inflammation and a condition analogous to the state of the cutis after small-pox, or after corporal punishment. The hepatization was greatest in left lung; the œdema in the right. The color of the former varied, passing from red to brown, and from brownish to grey, œdema more or less intermixed. The bronchia were red and very large. The pulmonary veins were comparatively small; the branches of the pulmonary artery large. Two or three of the bronchial glands were much enlarged, were almost black, and very soft. The liver weighed 5 lbs.; its section was nutmeg-like in a slight degree. Two small cysticerci were found loosely attached to its convex surface. The spleen was adhering to the diaphragm and very soft. The stomach was of unusual volume and unusually heavy. The intestines were sound.

This case is noteworthy for the great amount of organic disease of the lungs and the absence of emaciation; partly, it may be conjectured, owing to the gradual and slow increase of the pulmonary lesions, if the last attack of inflammation be excluded, and a habit of tolerance to some extent acquired; partly, to the sound state of the digestive organs, the stomach seemingly of unusual power; and partly, and perhaps not least, to the absence of cachexia.

Case 32.—Of chronic pneumonia, with hepatization of one lung and emphysema of the other, and an enlarged liver.—J. Thomson, ætat. 33; 6th Foot; admitted June 16th, 1836; died the same day.—This man, of 14 years' service in India, had fever and scurvy at Rangoon, followed by acute rheumatism, with much dyspnœa. On the homeward voyage he rallied from the feeble state in which he embarked; a state so aggravated by diarrhœa that his life was despaired of. He continued to improve and gain strength, till checked by entering a cold climate, when diarrhœa recurred with tormina and tenesmus. On landing, he was taken into hospital on the 23rd May. Then, besides a relaxed state of bowels and rheumatic pains, he had cough and difficulty of breathing. On the 30th he was pronounced convalescent, and on the 7th June he was discharged. Examined a day or two after, he was considered unfit for service on account of serious chronic pulmonary disease. When brought again into hospital he was moribund.

Autopsy 21 hours after death. Sub-emaciated. There was no well-marked lesion of the brain. The pericardium contained 3 oz. of serum. The right auricle was distended with coagulated blood and fibrin. In the right ventricle there was a large fibrinous mass which extended into the pulmonary artery and its branches; when extracted, it exhibited a cast of them, even of the valves. In the left auricle there was a good deal of blood; in the left ventricle only a little fibrinous concretion. The right lung was generally adhering; the left partially; the former weighed 4 lbs.; it was hepatized almost throughout, but in the highest degree in its superior lobe, the color passing from fawn to light red. Under the pleura pulmonalis of the upper lobe there were two cavities, each capable of holding a walnut, full of air, formed, it may be inferred, by the detachment of the membrane forced from the substance of the lung. A bronchial tube terminated in one of them, through which, using the blow-pipe, air passed freely. The left lung was chiefly remarkable for its emphysematous state; some air collected from one of its large vesicles was found to consist of azote, with a little carbonic acid, without any oxygen. Both lungs were free from tubercles. The bronchia of the right lung were very red; of the left less so. The liver was very friable; it weighed 6 lbs. The spleen was firm and rather pale; it weighed 1¾ lb. The large intestines were somewhat thickened and their mucous coat was red and granular. In the epidydimis of each testicle there was a deposit of a putty-like matter.

That life should have terminated so abruptly as it did in this case is not surprising; is it not more so that it was not sooner brought to a close, considering the great amount of chronic pulmonary disease, taking it for granted, as I think we must, that the principal lesions found after death had attained their height, or nearly so, before he was discharged from hospital? Is not this another instance of the comparatively easy tolerance of organic disease from habit gradually acquired?

My further comments on these cases need be but few. The great majority of them are confirmatory of the preceding remark, that an impaired constitution or an unsound state of organization, such as that betokened by tubercle, conduces to the invasion of pneumonia;—a proposition this, I believe, now pretty generally admitted as applicable to the greater number of acute diseases. It might seem to be opposed by the circumstance that in several instances the individuals attacked were rather corpulent than otherwise. But, I need hardly remark that as regards sound and stable health nothing is more deceptive than corpulence,—in itself it may be a disease, and is certainly more frequently associated with a feeble than with a vigorous state of the organism.

Where so great a complication is met with, as witnessed in
many of these cases, it is not surprising that there should be so
great a variety of symptoms, and often much obscurity as to
the character of the disease. Of the influence or effect of the
several kinds I cannot pretend to speak with any precision. The
masking effect of one complication, that of the disease of the
brain, so like the masking effect of insanity, has already been
adverted to : it should never be lost sight of in practice. Rigors,
it would appear, in several cases, neither ushered in the attack, nor
occurred during it. Nor was pain of side always an accompaniment, or pain in making a deep inspiration. The greater variety
of tissues affected, the greater the amount of organic mischief
produced, so much less often was the suffering of the individual; consequently mere pain or distressing feeling cannot
justly be considered a reliable criterion of the degree or amount
of danger. In many of the cases, in their advanced stage,
flatulency of the stomach and intestines with much distension
was remarkable, especially in those in which there was inflammation along the course of the great central vessels and nerves.
Might not the two be associated in the relation of cause and
effect? In one case, that of B. Jarrett, No. 10, there were
symptoms simulating in part those of cholera morbus; in that
instance there was an appearance of inflammation of the pneumo-
gastric nerve; the question just asked might again be proposed.

The rapidity of the disease in running its fatal course is
remarkable, especially reckoning from the time the individuals
attacked came into hospital. The mean time thus calculated
between the admission and death was, in the least complicated
cases only 5 days; in those complicated with tubercles and
disease of the heart, the average was greater, as much as 22
days. In the worst cases, it is difficult to avoid the conclusion that there was a sudden pouring out of lymph into the
parenchyma of the lungs. The buffed and cupped state of the
lungs when abstracted by venesection showed a marked excess
of fibrin in the blood. And, was not the same indicated by the
frequency of the occurrence of fibrinous concretions and crassamentum in the cavities of the heart and in the great vessels?
The peculiar appearance of the concretions in some instances
would indicate that they might have been formed during life;

and the symptoms in dying, and the suddenness of the event in some of the cases, favor the idea.

The color of the hepatization is commonly considered as denoting its age. May not the different hues which the hepatized part presents, depend rather on the nature of the effusion, whether it be of blood alone in the form of crassamentum, or of coagulable lymph, or of a mixture of the two with some other ingredients ?* I am disposed to infer the latter: the shortness of the illness in several of the cases in which the grey hue was predominant; this the last stage of hepatization, as by some authors considered, is hardly, as I think, in accordance with any other conclusions, one excepted, that of tolerance from habit, on the supposition of the lesion being chronic and of gradual increase.

Of the treatment employed, I may remark that it was generally in agreement with the therapeutic doctrines of the time, resting greatly on blood-letting as a means of subduing inflammation; the use of the lancet being regulated very much by the condition of the blood, whether it exhibited or not a buffy coat, excess of fibrin being considered as an indication of sthenic disease, and as such needing a lowering depleting plan of treatment—a doctrine this of very doubtful soundness. The results of the practice are not uninstructive; in the instances recorded, almost invariably, pain was relieved or removed by venesection; but the progress of the disease was not arrested; on the contrary, it may be inferred, was often accelerated, and this by the exhaustion of strength, when venesection was often repeated. Some of the cases strongly displaying the inefficiency of large and repeated blood-lettings were the following :—No. 1, that of W. Abraham, from whom in five days 136 oz. of blood were taken; that of T. Royland, No. 5, from whom in two days the quantity taken was 110 oz.; that of H. Crozar, from whom in seven hours 80 oz. were taken, speedily followed by death. I have said that excess of fibrin, the appearance of the buffy coat on blood abstracted, is no reliable proof of the sthenic condition of the system; more than this, may it not be, should it not be, viewed as the index of a contrary state, the asthenic rather, with which it is so frequently

---

* In the few specimens of hepatized lung, which I have examined chemically, of the grey and fawn-colored kind, I have found a composition not very different from that of tubercle, of which oily or fatty matter formed a part.—See some interesting observations on fatty matter as an element of organic disease, by Mr. Gulliver, in the 26th vol. of the Medico-Chirurgical Transactions.

associated, and not only in the disease under consideration, but in so many more, especially pulmonary consumption, in its advanced stage? This view is now, I believe, the one adopted by many pathologists, and it is supported by numerous facts.

It would be out of place here to enter on the large subject of the treatment of pneumonia. I may briefly remark, that in the slighter cases and in individuals with unimpaired constitutions, it seems now to be admitted, that the tendency of the disease is to spontaneous recovery ; that in the severer cases a mild treatment with good nursing seems to be most efficacious ; whilst, in the most severe, those in which a rapid consolidation of lung takes place, from exudation or effusion of lymph, death in the majority of instances cannot be prevented by any mode of treatment.

Another subject of interest which has lately attracted much attention is that of the constitution of the present generation, whether less sthenic than that of the past ; and if less, consequently less tolerant of the lancet and of severe antiphlogistic treatment. The discussion of the problem at any length would be here misplaced. All I shall venture to remark is, that were I to judge from my own experience, the conclusion I should arrive at would be that the fashion of medical practice, founded we would believe on a sounder pathology, is altered rather than the constitution of man. The average of life now is admitted to be greater than in preceding ages. How remarkable this would be were it associated with a diminished vis vitæ.

CHAPTER X.

ON PERITONITIS.

A disease comparatively rare in the army.—Statistics of.—Most commonly, like pneumathorax, an epiphenomenon, the result of the perforation of some one of the abdominal viscera.—Examples of.—Diathesis.—Illustrative cases, with comments.—Remarks on their pathology, semeiology, and treatment.

ACCORDING to the Army Medical Returns this is a comparatively rare disease: thus, amongst the Dragoon Guards serving at home, and the infantry serving in North America, Gibraltar, Malta, and the Ionian Islands, from 1817 to 1836, with an aggregate strength of 338,440, no more than 76 cases of it appear to have been admitted into hospital, of which 26 were fatal; and, even grouping gastritis and enteritis with it, cognate maladies, and hardly distinguishable except by a *post mortem* examination, the same inference must be made, as, from the returns mentioned, it would appear that the total admissions from the three have been only 30 cases per 10,000 men, and of these 30 treated, no more than 3 had a fatal end. Not questioning this inference, yet I am satisfied, that though comparatively rare, it is, judging from my own experience, somewhat more frequent than those numbers represent, and this owing to the circumstance that a considerable proportion of the fatal cases are not of the idiopathic kind, but the consequence of other diseased action, productive of perforation of one or other of the abdominal viscera, and that perforation in its turn becoming the cause of the peritonitis. Thus, of 39 cases of which I have notes, no less than 30 are of the latter class, and even of the other 9 it is not clear but that some of them too may have owed their origin to the same cause, keeping in mind that a minute rupture easily escapes observation, and is almost sure to escape detection unless carefully sought for. This conclusion would be strengthened by abstracting from these nine cases those accompanied with ulceration of some part of the primæ viæ, leaving only such as are clearly idiopathic, that is, the instances in which the disease began with inflammation of the peritoneum.

I shall first bring under consideration the more complicated cases, those connected with, and, it may be inferred, produced by perforation. This lesion took place in the parts named in the following numbers :—

Stomach	2
Duodenum	2
Jejunum	1
Ileum (its lower portion)	15
Cœcum	1
Appendicula vermiformis	3
Colon	3
Rectum	1
Liver	2

The names of the diseases assigned on admission into hospital were the following :—

Febris remittens	3
„ communis continens	1
Diarrhœa	6
Dysenteria chronica	1
Phthisis pulmonalis	1
Gelatio	1
Rheumatismus chronicus	1
Heptalgia	1
Atrophia	1
Colica	1
Enteritis	7
Peritonitis	3

The average age of those to whom it proved fatal was 29 years; the oldest of the thirty cases was 47; the youngest, 17.

The average time at which death occurred, reckoning from when the perforation was produced, and judging of that event by the sudden invasion of severe pain and other symptoms, was three days,—eliminating those instances in which the invasion was more insidious and not well defined. In a large number of cases the speed of the fatal malady was even greater, rivalling almost the terrible rapidity of progress of cholera ;—thus, in five, death is marked as having occurred in one day; and in two cases in even a shorter time, 12 hours and 17 hours. This great rapidity of progress is very noteworthy, especially contrasting peritonitis with empyema on the one hand and with ascites on the other, suggestive of the more intimate relation with life of the peritoneal membrane than of the plural; and of the more noxious influence of pus* than of serum.

* Not of the *laudable* kind, such as that of the common abscess, free from putrid taint, and containing no air.

As in the diseases hitherto treated of, an impaired constitution has been a predisposing circumstance, so likewise it has proved in this, directing the attention to the morbid actions productive of the rupture or perforation, the immediate cause of the inflammation.

Reflecting on the parts of the primæ viæ in which the perforation occurred, one cannot but be struck by the circumstance of one portion being so much more subject to it than another; the ileum, for instance, than the adjoining cœcum and jejunum; the stomach, the duodenum and rectum, in so much less degree than the ileum. The difference of anatomical structure may help to account in part for the greater proclivity of the one than the other to penetrating ulceration, but not altogether, no more than the difference of structure of the veins and arteries of the right and left side of heart is adequate to account for the contrast between them as regards the taking on of morbid action and the undergoing morbid change. The duodenum is as glandular, even more so than the ileum, yet comparatively how much more exempt from disease. Each portion of the alimentary canal has a function of its own, and it would appear an idiosyncrasy peculiar to it, specially marked by liability to and exemption from certain morbid actions, and not that identity which was presumed in the generalization of Bichat in his doctrine of membranes.

Another subject of interest, and perhaps as obscure and inexplicable, is the habitats of diseases, if I may be allowed the expression,—some countries being distinguished for one kind, some for another. As regards the subject of the present section, it may be mentioned as an example. In Malta and Corfu, perforation of the intestine, especially of the lower portion of the ileum, in the situation of the glandulæ aggregatæ, is far from an unfrequent occurrence: of the total number, no less than 18 took place in those islands during a period of 10 years that I was stationed there; whilst during the three years and a half that I was in the West Indies I witnessed no perforation of the ileum, and only one of any kind, and that in the colon. At Vienna, when visiting the extensive pathological museum attached to the great civil hospital of that city, I did not see a single specimen of the kind, and I was assured by the distinguished Professor who had charge of it, Dr. Carl Rokitansky, that in his vast experience, though he had often witnessed perforation of the stomach, he had never witnessed perforation of any part of the intestinal canal. This information I had from him in 1840. This conclusion, as to the partial localisation of the disease, is confirmed by the data, imperfect as they are, afforded by the army medical returns. Moreover, so far as these returns show, contrary to what *à priori* might be expected, no regular relation, it would appear, exists between the prevalency of peritoneal and dysenteric inflammation, or between the former and elevation of atmospheric temperature, or malaria: then, as regards malaria, whilst out of an aggregate force of 1,843 white troops in Sierra Leone, no less than 739 have died of remittent fever, one only is returned as having died of enteritis, and not one of peritonitis or gastritis—indeed these are not named ; and, as regards dysentery, whilst in Ceylon, with an aggregate strength of 42,978, as many as 993 have died of this disease, chronic and acute, three only have died, according to the return, of peritonitis, seven of gastritis, ten of enteritis.

The following are some of the more remarkable cases of the disease in question of which I have a record. In several of them I have thought it right to notice the observations made in the blood at the *post mortem* examination, partly on account of the indications it may afford, and partly, as in more than one instance the sudden death may have been owing to or connected with its coagulation in the vessels.

Case 1.—Of peritonitis, from perforation of ileum.—J. Davis, ætat. 33 ; 36th Foot ; admitted into regimental hospital, Corfu, July 12th, 1825 ; died July 16th.—This man, a non-commissioned officer, though of intemperate habits, hitherto had good health. When admitted on the 12th July, he came from an outpost, and was laboring under what seemed a slight feverish attack. On the 14th he appeared nearly well ; his pulse slow and soft ; his skin cool. In the evening of the same day there was some febrile excitement, with vertigo and headache. On the 15th there was flatulent distension of abdomen, rapidly followed by symptoms of fatal peritonitis. Much tension and pain of abdomen, nausea and vomiting ; cold extremities ; cold sweat preceded death. He expired at 9 p.m. of the 16th. He was sensible to the last ; and during the last 24 hours was free from pain of head, which previously he had more or less experienced. V.S. and leeches were employed, with little more than momentary relief.

Autopsy 14 hours after death. Very stout and muscular ; the abdomen very tense and tympanitic. On dissecting the muscles from the peritoneum, the latter was found very vascular and distended with air. An opening being made into the cavity of the abdomen, the omentum was seen loaded with fat, very red, and adhering to the cœcum, and there it was thickened and very vascular. Much yellow purulent fluid was found effused, with which were mixed globules of oil ; he had taken castor-oil.

There was a deposit of coagulable lymph on the small intestines, and these were generally adhering. The stomach and large intestines were greatly distended with air, and the small intestines were also distended, but in a less degree. The air beneath the peritoneum, and the oil mixed with the pus, suggested a perforation of the canal. After a careful search a small one was detected in the ileum, within three or four inches of its lower extremity. It was little larger than a large pin's head; fluid passed readily through it; the peritoneal coat surrounding it was dark red, the villous was very little redder than natural, but ulcerated—the ulceration only a little more extensive than the perforation. In the lower portion of the gut there were several small ulcers of the same kind, confined to the mucous coat. The glandulæ aggregatæ were unusually large, as were also the solitary glands in the large intestines. In no other part of the alimentary canal was there any distinct appearance of disease; and the other abdominal viscera were normal, as were also the lungs, excepting that they were generally adhering, and rather gorged with blood.

This case is instructive and doubly noteworthy, as showing how little the health of a robust man may be damaged by a few small ulcers in the ileum, and the imminent danger, the fatal consequence, if the ulcerative process extend beyond the villous coat through the muscular and peritoneal.

Case 2.—Of peritonitis, from perforation of ileum, after convalescence from remittent fever.—T. Allen, ætat. 30; 80th Regiment; admitted into regimental hospital, Malta, 25th July, 1828; died 27th July.—This man, about three weeks before his fatal illness, had an attack of fever, for which blood was abstracted to the amount of 2 lbs. He was discharged after six days. On re-admission on the 25th July, he complained chiefly of weakness and purging; his stools were thin and yellow. On the following day, after an aperient, which removed a great deal of dark fæces, he felt relieved. To-day, the 26th, the pulse is 94; he has some thirst; no fixed pain, but a sense of "stuffing about the chest." A blister was applied to the chest, and some rhubarb and magnesia prescribed, a scruple of each. At the evening visit he complained of "griping;" had had four stools. After having been fomented, a dose of castor-oil; the griping left him. On the 27th, there was much abdominal distension; pulse 120, full and tense; tongue dry and furred; much thirst; no headache. V.S. to 3 lbs; an enema of tepid water; calomel and antimonial powder, 4 grs. of each thrice daily. He bore the V.S. well; only the first cup was buffed. Towards evening the griping pain recurred. 28 leeches were applied to the abdomen, but "they did not draw well." Shortly after he became moribund; his skin cold; breathing quick; pulse rapid and feeble; he complained only of "soreness." He expired at 8 p.m.

Autopsy 14 hours after death. Not emaciated. The chest sounded slightly tympanitic. The abdomen was distended and tympanitic. The lungs were pale, and contained a good deal of air, but little blood. There were some fibrinous concretions and coagulated blood in the right cavities of the heart, and a very little in the left. Some coagulated blood was found also in the aorta, in its arched portion. The vena azygos was distended with liquid blood. The peritoneum was very red and vascular. There was a considerable quantity of puruloid fluid in the cavity of the abdomen, with an admixture of oil. The alimentary canal was generally healthy, with the exception of the lower part of the ileum, to the extent of about two feet. In this portion there were several ulcers, seldom more than $\frac{1}{4}$ inch in diameter; of somewhat irregular form; their edges pale, not elevated, of different depths; in some the muscular coat was laid bare; in one a perforation was detected; it was sufficiently large to admit a common probe. The glandulæ aggregatæ were unusually distinct. The mesenteric glands were red, enlarged, and soft. The spleen was large and soft. The gall-bladder was distended with dilute greenish bile. The liver and other viscera were of normal appearance.

In this case it is noteworthy that there was no vomiting, and that the lungs rather than the stomach appeared to be, if the expression may be used, sympathetically affected. The state of the spleen—so very like that witnessed in the remittent fever of the Mediterranean—was probably the relict of the preceding febrile attack, when also, it is likely, Peyer's glands, the seat of the perforation, first became affected. It may deserve mention, that though only fourteen hours intervened from the death to the autopsy, yet, where the blood lodged in the aorta, there the lining membrane of the artery in contact with the coagulum was stained red: the temperature at the time was not noted down; it was probably above 80°.

Case 3.—Of peritonitis from perforation of ileum, with ulcerated small intestine, preceded by febrile symptoms; a round worm in the cavity of the abdomen.—M. Dean, ætat. 27; R.F.; admitted into regimental hospital, Corfu, 29th August, 1827; died 11th September.—This man on admission had been sent from an outpost, Vido, laboring under febrile symptoms, with headache and tenderness of epigastrium. After V.S. to 20 oz., and the application of 60 leeches to the abdomen, the pain was lessened but not removed. On the 1st August, 25 leeches more having been used, he was relieved of pain, but on the day before he experienced chills succeeded by heat; the bowels were open. Calomel and sulphate of quinine were ordered, 3 grs. of each, every fourth hour. On the 2nd there was "irritability of stomach." On the 3rd, 4th, 5th and 6th, there was no complaint of pain of any part. On the 6th the mouth was affected by the mercury, which was now omitted. The heat was moderate; the skin moist. On the 7th and 8th he continued easy. On the 9th there was no particular pain, but a feeling of general uneasiness; he was evidently emaciating; his countenance was anxious, his voice feeble; the tongue dry and red. Had only one dark stool during the night; a purgative enema, and after its action 2 grs. of extract of opium. The report on the 10th was most unfavorable; during the night he had great uneasiness, particularly about the lower part of the abdomen. Castor oil was prescribed and a warm bath, with temporary relief. As the day declined the pain of abdomen became severe; not the slightest pressure could be borne on the lower part. An enema was ordered and a blister to the hypogastrium. He expired without a struggle at 2 a.m.

Autopsy 8 hours after death. Sub-emaciated. The vessels of the pia mater were much injected. There was a good deal of fluid in the ventricles and at the base of the brain. There was a great deal of fetid serum with some pus and coagulable lymph in the cavity of the abdomen and in that of the pelvis. A living round worm (A. lumbricoides) was found in the right iliac fossa, close to a perforation in the lower portion of the ileum. Portions of the small intestines were agglutinated by lymph; the large intestines were much distended with air; their mucous coat was of a dusky red hue, but not ulcerated. The appendicula vermiformis was slightly ulcerated.

Numerous and large ulcers were found in the lower portion of the ileum; they were of irregular form and deep, most of them having penetrated through the villous coat either to the muscular or peritoneal. In the upper part of the ileum there were a few ulcers of the same kind, and also, but fewer still, in the jejunum. The stomach contained some greenish fluid. Neither the liver nor spleen bore any marks of disease.

In this instance we have a striking example of the inefficacy of blood-letting in subduing an ulcerated state of the small intestines, and also of the inefficacy of mercury. Whether they did not both promote the diseased action is open to question. Brief and scanty as is the history of the case, its insidiousness is well marked. What is most noteworthy is, till the perforation took place, the little relation apparent between the symptoms and the lesions in progress.

Case 4.—Of peritonitis from perforation of ileum, its upper portion, preceded by febrile symptoms.—T. Raennec, ætat. 27; 88th Foot; admitted into regimental hospital, Corfu, 11th Dec., 1827; died 21st Dec.—This man, previously in good health, the night before admission had a rigor with vertigo and lassitude followed by sweating. On the 11th the skin was rather hot, the pulse quick, the tongue white. An emetic, followed by calomel, and that by a purgative. 12th—The medicines operated powerfully. A slight rigor at night; now no perfect apyrexia. V.S. 18 oz. 13th—A chill during the night, now more feverish; tongue dry and harsh; 3 grs. of calomel every second hour. 14th—No chill last night; no pain; skin rather hot; pulse 92; has taken seven doses of calomel; four stools. 15th— The symptoms are nearly the same as yesterday. The calomel to be continued. 16th—Very much purged during the night; his tongue is now moist and clean; feelings easy; the mouth is slightly affected. The calomel to be discontinued. At the evening visit there was much pyrexia; the tongue parched; no pain. A draught with 1 drachm of T. opii. 17th—Had a good night; feels now quite easy; skin and pulse natural; tongue moist; 3 grs. of sulphate of quinine thrice in the day. 18th —No increase of fever last night; no headache or pain anywhere; less thirst; pulse 88; some cough. The quinine as yesterday, and the same quantity of T. opii at night. 19th—Had an exacerbation before taking the anodyne; slept well after and perspired freely. Now the tongue is moist; the skin cool; the pulse 80. The quinine as before, with the addition of 3 grs. of calomel. 20th—Was suddenly seized last evening with pain of abdomen, increased by pressure, and extending to the testes. 36 leeches were applied, and an enema given. The pain continues, with tension of the abdomen. The pulse is 100 and weak; the tongue dry; is much disposed to sleep; the pupils dilated. V.S.; the quantity of blood taken not noted; 12 leeches to head, 36 to abdomen; castor-oil; fomentation. 5 p.m.—Is extremely restless; there is much pain of abdomen and of the body generally; the lips are livid; the pulse very feeble; the intellect clear; only one scanty stool. He wishes for more castor oil, which he vomited; pulse hardly to be counted. He expired at 4 a.m. of the 21st.

Autopsy 31 hours after death. No emaciation; rather excess of fat. The abdomen tympanitic. A general redness of the membranes of the brain. Very little fluid in the ventricles. The thoracic viscera, apart from adhesions of the lungs, seemed sound. The peritoneum was generally inflamed. In the cavity of the abdomen and in that of the pelvis there was much fetid sero-puruloid fluid, with which oil and a little fæcal matter was mixed. The stomach and intestines were distended with fetid air. The intestines were agglutinated together by lymph. In the upper part of the ileum a small perforation was detected, the result of ulceration proceeding from the villous coat. The ulcer was there solitary; no redness, not the slightest, surrounded it. On the peritoneal side, corresponding, there was a deposit of a thin layer of lymph to the extent of about two inches by one, excepting in the situation of the perforation, where, of course, it was deficient. In the lower portion of the ileum, the glandulæ aggregatæ were enlarged, and there were many small ulcers. Two of them were so deep as to have nearly reached the peritoneal coat, on which were patches of lymph. There was a small ulcer on the margin of the valve of the colon. No ulcers were found, or any well marked disease, in the large intestines; they were distended with air. The spleen was large and soft. The liver was adhering to the diaphragm. The stomach was unduly red, but whether from blood-stain, uncertain; the vasa brevia contained blood.

This case was considered on admission as one of remittent fever, and was treated accordingly. It is open to the same comments as the preceding as regards treatment. Though no less than 31 hours intervened in this instance between the death and the autopsy, yet no staining was detected in the vessels containing blood. The temperature of the air at the time was comparatively low, probably not above 50°. The redness of the membranes of the brain was attributed to exudation of blood from the vessels, which, allowing for pressure from abdominal distension, seems not improbable.

Case 5.—Of peritonitis, from penetrating ulcers in the large intestines, of the dysenteric kind.—T. Telford, ætat. 32; 85th Regt.; admitted into regimental hospital, Malta, June 11, 1830; died 17th June.—This man on admission was laboring under diarrhœa; stools numerous and streaked with blood, but without tormina or tenesmus. Sulphat. of magnesia with T. opii. On the 12th it is stated that he had large evacuations of fetid fæces free from blood. Calomel and opium. On the 13th his skin was hot and moist; tongue loaded; no thirst; pulse 90 and feeble. Several stools of a dark color, with grumous blood. A blister to the abdomen; the calomel and opium to be continued. 14th—Very many scanty stools without pain or tenesmus. A suppository of 4 grs. of opium. The same medicine. 15th—Eleven watery bloody stools of rather putrid odor. The same medicine. 16th—Twenty stools of the same character. Pain in the course of the colon; pulse feeble; tongue loaded and dry; skin "temperate;" no tenesmus. The same medicine, with the addition of acetat. of lead, griss and opium gr. i. thrice daily, and friction of the inside of thighs with mercurial ointment. 17th—No mitigation of pain; cold sweats; pulse hardly to be felt; facies Hippocratica. Died at 2 p.m.

Autopsy 21 hours after death. Not emaciated. Abdomen tympanitic. There was no appearance of disease of either brain or lungs. The intestines were found adhering together and to the peritoneum through the medium of coagulable lymph. There was a considerable quantity of puruloid fluid with lymph in the dependent parts. The peritoneum generally was very vascular. The colon was greatly diseased; many deep and extensive ulcers were found in it; one in the transverse portion had penetrated through all the coats; another in the caput cœcum, and a third in the rectum. These perforations were in a manner closed by the folds of intestine in apposition and in the pelvis by lymph effused. On portions of the large intestines, on their mucous coat, there was a warty appearance, as if from lymph deposited; and the same was seen in the lower part of the ileum. The stomach, duodenum and jejunum contained much greenish fluid. The stomach in many places exhibited a delicate arborization of blood-vessels; on gentle pressure, after washing the surface with a sponge, blood was seen to flow from the larger to the smaller branches, and from them to exude in minute drops, illustrating, it was thought at the moment, how hæmatemesis might take place. There was no appearance of softening of the organ. The blood in the vena portæ was liquid. The liver was large. In several places its surface had a fissured appearance, as if from ruptures healed, and beneath each fissure to the depth of two or three lines there was a firm white matter, reminding one of a cicatrix. The spleen was adhering and that generally, and its substance was pultaceous.

This case may be viewed as truly one of dysentery, terminating in peritonitis. And may not this its termination be inferred to have been owing to perforation of the gut, though there was no escape of the contents of the intestine into the abdominal cavity? Yet, though the lesions were dysenteric, the symptoms were not. The state of the liver was noteworthy in its indications. He was a man of intemperate habits, and it was conjectured that from falls during drunkenness, the injuries suspected might have occurred. What was observed too in the stomach may not be unworthy of consideration, both as illustrating, as hinted, hæmatemesis and also black vomit. Had the part been microscopically examined, probably a lesion of the minute vessels would have been found similar to that discovered by Dr. Blair in the same order of vessels in yellow fever—viz., a rupture with a partial loss of substance.

Case 6.—Of peritonitis, from a large penetrating ulcer in the colon, preceded by diarrhœa.—George Hilton, ætat. 37; 71st F.; admitted into regimental hospital, Barbadoes, 12th Sept. 1845; died September 25th.—This man had an attack of diarrhœa early in August; on the 16th of that month he was discharged from hospital, "perfectly cured." When re-admitted on the 12th September, he was laboring under the same complaint; there was a frequent desire to go to stool; the evacuations scanty and mucous. Castor oil. On the 15th there was some tenesmus and tenderness of the abdomen; the pulse quick. On the 17th, in addition to the symptoms already mentioned, there were cramps in the legs. On the 20th he vomited about a quart of greenish fluid. On the 23rd blood was seen to be mixed with the stools, which were very frequent. He vomited much during the night. On the 25th there was pain and tenderness of abdomen; the tongue was dry and hard; the pulse quick and weak; the purging unabated; at 7 p.m. he threw up some blood. He expired at 9 p.m. The treatment from the commencement was merely palliative.

Autopsy 12 hours after death. Not emaciated. Excepting a turgid state of the vessels of the pia mater and an adhesion of the pineal gland posteriorly, nothing abnormal was found in the brain. The inferior lobe of each lung was œdematous. The left pleura contained 6 oz. of bloody serum; the right about 3 oz. The peritoneum was much inflamed. The omentum was thickened at its inferior margin and was there dark and vascular. Much lymph was effused, and the intestines were adhering together. There was a good deal of turbid offensive fluid in the cavity of the pelvis. A large perforation was detected in the transverse colon; it was exposed on removing a portion of small intestine which covered it, using no violence. Besides this penetrating ulcer, there were many more in the colon, and they were large, with more or less œdematous thickening of the cellular coat; some of them were gangrenous. There was no appearance of disease in the small intestines. The large arch of the stomach was unusually vascular.

In this instance no apprehension of danger was felt by the medical officer in charge till within the last twenty-four hours. The case is chiefly remarkable for the severity of the organic lesions, and the comparative mildness of the symptoms. The blood that was vomited shortly before death was probably an exudation from the gorged vessels of the stomach, similar to that which was witnessed in the preceding case at the autopsy. And might not the blood which imparted its color to the serosity in each pleura have been similarly derived?

Case 7.—Of peritonitis, from perforation of jejunum, communicating with an abscess (?) in liver, preceded by dysenteric symptoms.—J. Burns, ætat. 26; R.F.; admitted into regimental hospital, Malta, 27th July, 1833; died 19th August.—This man during the three preceding years had been in hospital for pneumonia, fever and diarrhœa, the one succeeding the other at pretty long intervals. On this, his last admission, he complained of epigastric pain, with thin bloody stools and tenesmus. The pain recurred at times with vomiting. The bowels at first were relieved; latterly they became again more disturbed, and the stools were frequent and offensive. He became daily weaker; the tongue dry and ulcerated; an insatiable thirst, pulse small and rapid; but little pain. In the evening of the 18th he suddenly became "very low," so as to be unable to speak; still without apparent pain. He expired the following morning. The treatment consisted of calomel and opium, blue pill and opium and antiacids.

Autopsy 9 hours after death. Much emaciated. With the exception of slight adhesions of the lungs the contents of the thorax were free from disease. A considerable quantity of brownish fluid was found in the cavity of the abdomen. The peritoneum was generally inflamed, the intestines glued together and the omentum adhering and most of all towards the brim of the pelvis. On minute examination a perforation was discovered in the upper part of the jejunum, communicating with the cavity of an abscess in the liver, situated a little to the left of the lobulus Spigelii and above it. The jejunum was adhering to the liver except at one spot where a rupture had taken place, and through which the contents of the cavity had escaped into the peritoneal sac. The cavity was capable of holding an orange; it was empty; its walls were of a bright yellow. Near it, in the substance of the same lobe, a cyst was found of cartilaginous firmness, containing the thin soft sac of an acephalocyst, granular within and full of a transparent fluid. A portion of the liver dried, imparted an oil-stain to paper. Beyond the jejunum, the small intestines were sound, as was also the stomach. In the large intestines there were several ulcers and marks of old ulceration.

This case is suggestive of many questions, such as the nature of the cavity in the liver, whether that of a true abscess or not; why there was so little pain, and whether owing to two principal lesions, as it were competing; or to the peritoneal inflammation not coming to a height suddenly; or to there having been little flatulent distension?

Case 8.—Of perforation of ileum, with ulceration of gall-bladder and stomach and large intestines, preceded by dysenteric symptoms, without peritonitis.—E. Pritchard, ætat. 29; 89th F.; admitted 21st July, 1821; died 13th September.—This man, whilst in India (from whence he is just returned after a service of 10 years), suffered from pectoral and dysenteric ailments. On admission he was very feeble and emaciated; there was some numbness of the extremities with little pain, and he was still laboring under chronic dysentery, on account of which he had been sent home. His stools were not frequent, but they were white and slimy, with some tormina and tenesmus. During the last two years he had done no duty. Whilst in India he took much mercury, and the numbness of limbs, it is said, followed taking cold when under the influence of mercury. Between the date of his admission and the 4th of September there appeared to be a very slow and gradual amendment. The tongue was clean; there was little thirst; his appetite was pretty good; the bowels were loose but rarely painful; his cough was seldom troublesome, his expectoration free; one night only is said to have sweated; his strength had increased a little. During this time he first took calomel and opium; afterwards rhubarb and opium, with a bitter infusion. On the 4th September the report was as follows:—" Is much the same; bowels loose; but the stools not dysenteric; there is slight pyrexia marked by heat of skin; some œdema of ankles, increasing at night; some cough." On the 8th, cough relieved; six stools, without tormina or tenesmus. On the 10th fifteen liquid stools, without pain; cough rather less; appetite worse. On the 12th—Since yesterday morning has been much worse; nine watery stools, without tormina or tenesmus; the cough is greatly increased; the expectoration, consisting of muco-purulent matter, difficult but pretty copious. He complains of pain of chest and of loins. The pulse is so rapid as hardly to be counted; the tongue red and rather dry; the skin rather hot; much thirst; loss of appetite; features shrunken; great debility. He expired at 7 p.m., when in the act of swallowing a little milk. His death was quite sudden; during the day the symptoms were much the same as during the morning visit.

Autopsy 12 hours after death. Exceedingly emaciated. The left pleura contained a pint of serum; the right about half a pint; and the pericardium about the same quantity. The superior lobe of the right lung was firmly adhering. In it were some crude tubercles and a large excavation. This cavity, capable of holding a large orange, was nearly empty; in it loose was a small triangular concretion, of a greenish yellow color, in a state of incipient putrefaction.* The bronchia and trachea were full of pus, which, it may be inferred, had come from the cavity, and had been suddenly poured out, through a bronchial tube of a considerable size which was found opening into it, and was the cause of the sudden death. Within the cavity of the abdomen there were no marks of peritoneal inflammation. The ileum was found so much distended with air as to resemble the colon. On its peritoneal coat there were numerous small tubercles, some of them softening. In its mucous coat there were many ulcers; some of them were deep, and had reached the muscular coat; some, as

* It resembled a gall-stone, but was differently composed. It consisted chiefly of phosphate of lime, with a covering of lymph.

many as four, had penetrated through that and the peritoneal; they were situated in its inferior portion.*   In the jejunum there were some ulcerated spots.   The caput cœcum was severely ulcerated, and its valve was destroyed.†   There were a few ulcers in the ascending colon.   The liver was larger than usual, but not distinctly diseased.   The gall-bladder adhered firmly to the pyloric portion of the stomach, with which it communicated by two small openings, the result of ulceration; the largest admitted a crow quill.   The stomach was rather contracted, especially towards its pylorus; otherwise it was of natural appearance.   It contained a good deal of apparently healthy chyme, with which some coagulated milk was mixed.   The gall-bladder was much contracted, and its coats thickened.   It contained a large calculus,‡ with barely a trace of bile, indeed there was no space for more, the accretion occupying it entirely, with the exception of its neck.   Where the pressure of the calculus was greatest there the mucous membrane was deficient.   The common duct was pervious.   The mesenteric glands were greatly enlarged; some of them were nearly the size of pigeons' eggs, and were softening.

This case is on many accounts noteworthy : 1. For a vomica without hectic, and for most part with slight cough; 2. For ulceration of the gall-bladder, and a large gall-stone, without pain in that region; 3. For ulceration of stomach, enlarged liver, and enlarged mesenteric glands, with a clean tongue, no nausea, or vomiting, and a tolerable digestion; 4. For an ulcerated cœcum, without latterly dysenteric symptoms; 5. For ulceration and perforation of the ileum, without the escape of its liquid contents, though not prevented by adhesion.

Case 9.—Of peritonitis from perforation of ileum, accompanied with invagination of a portion of the same intestine.—Anna Galena, ætat. 24; a Maltese; unmarried; admitted into the civil hospital, September 5th, 1832; died 7th September.—This young woman had been ill eight days before admission.   Her principal symptoms were excessive pain and distension of abdomen, without vomiting.

Autopsy 17 hours after death.   The abdomen was very much swollen and hard, as if it contained solid matter, owing, as was found, to excessive distension of the jejunum and ileum.   The stomach and liver were pressed up very far into the cavity of the chest.   In the cavity of the abdomen there was about half a pint of bloody serum, with some soft lymph resting on the folds of the intestines, the peritoneal coat of which, especially of the ileum and jejunum, was unusually red and vascular.   A considerable portion of the former—its upper part—was invaginated, and was protruding through a perforation in its lower part, about three inches from its termination.   The portion protruding was everted, and of a livid hue.   There was some dirty greenish

* In the diseased part of the ileum there was a very unusual appearance—a band crossing it from side to side.   It was pretty thick, and covered with mucous membrane, suggesting an abnormal formation, not a morbid lesion.

† Owing probably to the destruction of the valve, there was liquid fæcal matter in the ileum, but none had escaped into the peritoneal sac, owing to the apposition of the parts in which were the perforations—and this without adhesion.

‡ It had much the appearance of a urinary mulberry calculus; it was oval, ·7 inch in length, ·6 inch in width; after exposure to the air for two days it weighed 40 grs.; it consisted of a crust of dark matter, insoluble in alcohol, and of a nucleus of cholesterine.

matter both above and below the invagination. The great distension of the small intestines was between the invagination and the band of the duodenum, where it crosses the spine. The cœcum was moderately distended with air. The large intestines were free from disease. The omentum was adhering to the brim of the pelvis. The stomach contained many round worms.

This case I did not see during the life of the individual. Considering the vast extent of the lesion, is it not surprising that death did not sooner take place, and also that there was no vomiting?

Case 10.—Of peritonitis, from rupture of an hepatic "abscess" (an hydatid?) into the cavity of the abdomen.—A Maltese, ætat. 53; died in the civil hospital, 24th September, 1832.—This man had been ailing several months before his admission into hospital. His disease was designated "Hepitalgia post synochum." Whilst under treatment, a tumor appeared at scrobiculus cordis, with much pain. Three days before death it suddenly subsided, and the pain ceased.

Autopsy 12 hours after death. Greatly emaciated. The thoracic viscera were sound. A large quantity of serum was found in the cavity of the abdomen and in that of the pelvis, with which flakes of lymph were mixed. The liver was adhering to the peritoneal lining of the abdomen, excepting at one spot, just above the lobulus Spigelii, where an abscess had burst into the abdominal cavity. There was very extensive peritoneal inflammation; the intestines were agglutinated together, and the omentum was very red and thickened, and adhering both to the parieties of the abdomen and to the sac of the abscess. The gall-bladder was distended with yellow limpid bile. The common duct and the hepatic duct were obstructed by a dead round worm. There were numerous worms of the same kind in the stomach.

My knowledge of this case was limited like that of the preceding. It can hardly be doubted that the cessation of pain and the subsidence of the tumor were connected with the bursting of what was called an abscess, but, judging from the serum (not pus) effused, was more likely to have been an hydatid.

Case 11.—Of peritoneal inflammation from perforation of ileum, with some ecchymosis on brain.—R. Sandford, ætat. 22; 7th Regiment of Foot; admitted into regimental hospital, Malta, 20th August, 1829; died 21st August.—This man about a week before his fatal illness, had been in hospital for two days, on account of a slight ailment, a looseness of the bowels chiefly, with a little pyrexia. In the morning of the 20th August he was suddenly seized with severe pain at the umbilicus, of irregular occurrence. When seen by the surgeon he was free from pain; the pulse was regular; the abdomen somewhat distended; the bowels confined. Two ounces of castor-oil were given, followed by a saline purgative twice repeated. In the evening there was slight nausea, which he attributed to the medicine not having had effect. There was now great abdominal tension and desire to have an evacuation, but no pain, even on pressure, and the pulse was still regular. A purgative enema was administered without giving relief. The assistant-surgeon was called up in the middle of the night. The distension of abdomen was chiefly complained of. Two drops of croton oil were taken; their effect was slight. In the morning (the exact time is not mentioned) he vomited a large quantity of bilious matter, after which he spoke of himself as well, and conversed freely. At 7 a.m. he was suddenly seized with convulsions, and died.

Autopsy 6 hours after death. Very muscular and fat. Surface of body warm;*
back, arms, and legs livid; abdomen distended. Coagulated blood and fibrinous
concretions were found in the longitudinal and other sinuses. The vessels of the
brain generally, especially the veins, were distended with dark blood. On the right
hemisphere, close to a distended vein in the pia mater, there was a patch of ecchymosis. The pineal gland was of an unusual size, owing to a vesicle containing a
transparent fluid. The substance of the gland was firm, and without gritty matter;
the membrane of the vesicle was strong and fibrous. There was very little fluid in
the ventricles, but pretty much at the base of the brain. The brain was of natural
firmness. The lungs were collapsed, and rather redder than usual, as were also the
bronchia. The pericardium was merely moist with lubricating fluid. The right
cavities of the heart and great vessels were distended with dark coagulated blood and
some fibrinous concretion, as were also the left and the aorta, but in a less degree.
The thoracic duct was empty. The peritoneal lining of the abdomen and the
omentum were very red. Three or four pints of thin puruloid fluid were found in
the abdominal cavity, and in that of the pelvis. The intestines were agglutinated
together by soft lymph, and lymph of the same kind was effused in many places. In
tracing the intestines downwards, no lesion was detected till near the end of the ileum.
This portion of it was in the cavity of the pelvis, and there adhered slightly by coagulable lymph. On drawing it up gently the adhesion yielded, and a perforation was
discovered. It was about half a foot from the valve. There its inner coat was the
seat of a circular ulcer about two lines in diameter, without elevated edges or distinctly inflamed margin. It had penetrated through all the coats by a conical
excavation. On the peritoneal surface there was a minute brownish slough, partially detached. On the villous coat adjoining there were some other ulcerated spots
mostly superficial; a few had penetrated to the muscular coat; they were all of the
same character. The colon was distended with fluid and flatus. The stomach was
capacious, and contained a good deal of greenish fluid. Its mucous coat was soft and
easily abraded. The mesenteric glands were much enlarged. The liver and other
abdominal viscera were apparently sound.

Was death in this case owing to pressure on the brain, from
distended vessels and ecchymosis, or to a coagulation of blood in
the same vessels? The abdominal distension might have conduced to this state of the vessels. Yet there was no vertigo, no
premonitory symptoms of apoplexy. The little painful suffering
experienced is noteworthy, considering the condition of the abdomen and the peritoneal inflammation. Was it owing to some
morbid action at the same time in progress in the brain and in
the stomach, or to excess of carbonic acid in the blood?

Case 12.—Of peritonitis, from perforation of duodenum.—F. Maunara, ætat. 24;
R.M.F.; died August 19th, 1830.—This man, a native Maltese, enlisted in 1824,
and was considered by the surgeon of his corps in good health, and that uninter-

* The calvaria was first removed; the temperature between the hemispheres of the
cerebrum was found to be 96°: immediately after, an opening was made into the abdomen; under the concave surface of the liver the thermometer rose to 101°; two or
three minutes later, an opening was made into the chest; under the heart the thermometer rose to 102°.

ruptedly, and his stout appearance indicated the same. He was remarkable only for an uncommon appetite. On the morning of the day he died he complained of pain in his stomach, and desired to be taken into hospital. He was laid on a ladder for that purpose; but on the way, the pain increasing, he was taken into a house, where in less than an hour he died.

The following day the autopsy was made by the surgeon of the civil hospital. He found the abdomen tympanitic; a large quantity of food, chiefly ripe figs, in its cavity; "the peritoneal coat of the intestines inflamed," and a rupture through which the food had escaped. The stomach and duodenum were preserved, and we examined them together. The ruptured opening was about an inch in diameter, and was situated in the duodenum, a few lines below the pylorus, in its glandular portion. Its margin was quite smooth. It had been attached by adhesion to the surface of the lobulus Spigelii, and from thence, no doubt, it had been separated by the weight and pressure of the figs, etc. A scab—a slough—remained, corresponding in form to the opening, adhering to the liver. Close to the opening, the glandulæ had a diseased appearance, were enlarged, elevated, and of a purple hue. The stomach was of a vast size; it held 13 pints of water, and weighed 15½ oz. It was in a state of general hypertrophy, was every where thickened, but without any appearance of inflammation or of ulceration. It presented no distinct change of form, except at the pylorus, which was so dilated as to be equal in size to the upper part of the duodenum; indeed, where the one ended and the other began, could be determined only by difference of structure. In the external appearance of the organ there was nothing unusual except the large size of its vessels.

This case is very noteworthy, as demonstrative of the little sensibility of the part where the ulceration occurred; also in proof of the little derangement of general health necessarily following such a local disease; and, lastly, as showing how soon life becomes extinct when the contents of the stomach quit their proper place, and pass into the cavity of the abdomen.

Case 13.—Of perforation from ulceration of rectum, without manifest peritonitis; death sudden.—J. Dockrill, ætat. 47; 6th Foot; admitted June 14th, 1839; died the same day.—This man, lately arrived from India, had been sent from his regiment by the military invaliding commission of field officers, and consequently, it may be inferred, not on account of any medical disability. The day before his death he had been drinking to intoxication. In the morning after, he ate his breakfast, it is said, as usual. At half-past eight, he was seized with colic-like pains of abdomen, which were somewhat relieved by pressure. On admission into hospital, the pulse was moderate; the tongue whitish and moist; his bowels had not been regular for some days; he had a scanty stool just before leaving the barrack. The medicine first given was castor-oil with laudanum, which was presently vomited; it was repeated and retained. Next a laxative enema and fomentation were employed, with relief of pain. He slept for three hours. At 7 p.m. there was an aggravation of the symptoms; a great increase of pain; great tenderness on pressure; the pulse now had become extremely weak, and the temperature reduced. He moaned constantly. There had been no alvine evacuation; a turpentine enema was given without any benefit. He expired about 11 p.m., and was sensible to the last.

Autopsy 15 hours after death. Stout, muscular, and fat; abdomen tympanitic; brain normal. In the inferior portion of each lung there was a good deal of frothy bloody fluid. The right cavities of the heart contained much coagulated blood, The inner coat of the ascending aorta was unequally thickened, and its middle coat partially absorbed. On opening into the abdomen, much offensive gas escaped, and fæcal fluid mixed with oil was found in its cavity. All the abdominal viscera presented a pretty natural appearance, with the exception of the lower part of the colon and the rectum, which were ulcerated, the former slightly, the latter severely, and was also perforated. The perforation was through a sinus in the cellular tissue, large enough to admit the forefinger, and nearly its length, which had burst through the peritoneal lining into the cavity of the pelvis. It was black and gangrenous. The ulcerated surface of the rectum was pretty extensive, and of a dark grey color. There were marks also of former ulceration healed, and there was a thickening of the coats and some contraction of the gut, altogether conveying the idea of the effects of chronic dysentery.

This case, like the preceding, is noteworthy for severe local disease, without complaint on the part of the man, and without apparent effect on the general health, no more than that of an ulcer of the same extent of the integuments. It is also noteworthy for the fatal event taking place in so short a time from the rupture, and without the ordinary marks of peritoneal inflammation.

Case 14.—Of peritonitis, with ulceration and perforation of ileum.—D. M'Govern, ætat. 28; 18th Foot; admitted into regimental hospital, Corfu, July 12th, 1825; died July 14th.—This man, employed as an orderly to the commanding officer, had been in delicate health since 1824, when he received a blow in the abdomen. Since, he has had from time to time ailments of different kinds, chiefly cough, pain in the right side, glandular swelling of neck, and looseness of bowels. On admission this last time he had been three days unwell, suffering from vomiting and purging. He has pain in the abdomen, increased by pressure; his pulse is small and quick; the skin cool; the tongue furred; much thirst; stools bilious. 10 grs. of calomel, to be followed by castor-oil and laudanum. At the evening visit he was worse. V.S. to 20 oz.; the blood was buffed. On the following day the abdominal pain, especially in the right iliac region, was much increased. The bilious vomiting continues. The skin is still cool; pulse 102; thirst. 25 leeches to the pained part. Castor-oil and T. opii. At 6 p.m. there was no improvement. Since the morning he had occasional vomiting, but no stool. The abdominal swelling had become more diffused; the pain rather less; pulse 98. 25 leeches more to the abdomen. At 9 p.m. he felt as if "something had burst" in the right iliac region. Is in a cold sweat; his pulse hardly perceptible; the abdominal pain extreme; vomiting frequent. He expired at 1½ a.m.

Autopsy 12 hours after death. Muscular; little if at all emaciated. The right lung was found closely adhering. In its superior lobe there were many small tubercles and minute vomicæ. This lung was denser than natural, and heavy. The left lung was tolerably sound. There was much purulent fluid in the cavity of the abdomen; it was collected chiefly in the hollow of the pelvis, and in the iliac regions. The peritoneum throughout was unduly vascular, as was also the omentum. The latter adhered to the inferior portion of the ileum, and where adhering was thickened. This part of the ileum was greatly diseased; its texture throughout was of various tints, from red to black. In one spot it was ulcerated, and there a perforation was detected, capable of admitting a probe. The inflammation, judging from the discoloration, did not extend quite to the extremity of the ileum, and it gradually diminished towards its upper part. The large intestines did not partake of the disease. The stomach, duodenum, and transverse colon were much distended with air. The mesenteric glands were greatly enlarged. Several of them contained a curd-like fluid. The other abdominal viscera were apparently sound.

In this case it may be inferred that the peritonitis preceded the perforation, at least the sensation, that described as of " something bursting." Yet the inflammation may not have been purely idiopathic : may it not have arisen from the ulcer in the ileum penetrating to the peritoneal coat, and there exciting a diseased action, the beginning of the widely spread peritonitis? The chronic disease of the mesenteric glands and of the omentum, not to mention the state of one of the lungs, might have predisposed thereto.

Case 15.—Of peritonitis from perforation, with ulceration of ileum.—C. O'Keeffe, ætat. 24 ; 18th F ; admitted into regimental hospital, Corfu, 22nd July, 1826 ; died 25th July.—This man on the day of his admission had been suddenly seized with pain in the abdomen, increased by pressure and accompanied with nausea and vomiting; his bowels at the time were relaxed. The progress of the disease was rapid, with increasing severity of symptoms and but little variation of them. At 6 a.m. on the 25th, he walked to the close stool, fainted, and in a few minutes expired. The treatment consisted in the abstraction of blood largely and repeated, and in the use of calomel and opium with castor oil. On the 22nd, 3 lbs. of blood were taken ; on the 23rd, 4 lbs. in the morning, 3 lbs. in the evening. On the 24th 40 leeches were applied. Injections of turpentine were also employed, and fomentations.

Autopsy 4 hours after death. Stout and muscular. The brain was of ordinary appearance ; so were both the lungs ; there was a good deal of blood in their inferior portion. There was also a good deal of coagulated blood with fibrinous concretion in the right cavities of the heart; there was less in the left. The vena cava and aorta contained some. The peritoneum was but slightly red. The omentum was much thickened at its inferior margin and was there adhering. The surface of the intestines was covered with purulent fluid. The small intestines were so distended as to exceed the large in bulk. Many of their convolutions were adhering and their peritoneal coat was unduly vascular. The end of the ileum was attached to the right lumbar region, where the cœcum usually is ; the latter was situated higher. In the former, in its inferior portion, a small perforation was detected, through which some of the contents of the gut had escaped. The penetrating ulcer, internally, was of moderate extent. A little higher another ulcer was found, but this was superficial ; and higher still was the cicatrix of an ulcer, if a deficiency or obliteration of the plicæ of the villous coat allow of the inference. The large intestines were free from disease and moderately contracted.

In this case we have a striking example of the inefficiency of blood-letting in affording relief even from suffering. However, as the inflammation may be inferred to have been caused by a perforation of the intestine, probably no other mode of treatment would have been more successful. It is remarkable how well the large abstractions of blood were borne ; in no instance was there deliquum. Was this owing partly to pressure on the great blood-vessels from abdominal distension? At the autopsy it was conjectured that the sudden death might have been owing to coagulation of blood in the heart after syncope.

Case 16.—Of peritonitis from the bursting of an abscess in the liver.—J. Dalton, ætat. 46 ; 7th R.F. ; admitted into regimental hospital, Malta, 24th March, 1832 ; died 28th March.—This, an old Peninsular man, who for some time past had been ailing, on the 19th January came under treatment for an acute pain of the right side, increased by inspiration; it began suddenly the day before, and was followed by pain in the situation of the ascending colon. His pulse and temperature at the time were little affected. V.S. and leeching were employed. He was pronounced convalescent on the 23rd of the same month, and discharged well on the 11th February. When re-admitted on the 24th March, he complained of a general tenderness; his words were, " tenderness over all of me," with a looseness of bowels. Ease was afforded by a dose of castor oil and opium. During the night he was suddenly seized with lancinating pains extending from the right iliac region to the epigastrium. The tongue was rather dry ; the temperature natural; the pulse regular. Leeches calomel and opium. Ease followed. On the 25th there was a recurrence of the pain, with great severity and increased by pressure. A blister and warm fomentations. In the evening the pain extended from the navel to the throat. There was thirst; the tongue was dry, the bowels loose. Leeches with some relief. Prepared chalk with opium. On the 26th some refreshing sleep during the night. Now has nausea, and has thrown up some bilious fluid. There is an increase of pain, and in the same direction. A warm bath; small doses of Dover's powder. On the 27th he was worse ; there was an increase of nausea ; his knees were drawn up ; his features shrunken, and there was an anxious expression of countenance. Towards evening he became moribund. At 2 p.m. of the following day he expired. He was conscious nearly to the last moment.

Autopsy 20 hours after death. Sub-emaciated. The brain was free from disease. The right lung was very generally adhering, and its inferior part was rather denser and redder than natural. The bronchia in both lungs were smeared with bloody mucus. There was a good deal of coagulated blood without fibrinous concretion in all the cavities of the heart, and also in the pulmonary vessels. In the right iliac region there was a considerable quantity of reddish pus. The omentum and the peritoneal coat of the intestines were very red. The former adhered to the upper margin of the right lobe of the liver, where it was much thickened, close to the opening of an abscess in that lobe, which had burst, its contents escaping into the cavity of the abdomen. The abscess was superficial, capable of holding two or three ounces of fluid; its inner surface flocculent; the aperture was about the size of a sixpence and had a ragged edge. On separating the liver from its attachment, another abscess was discovered, and in its convex part; it was close to the diaphragm, to which the liver there adhered, and in form was hemispherical. It was full of pus. Its sac was like half the sac of an hydatid, smooth inside and cartilage-like. The substance of the liver was generally sound. The gall-bladder and its duct were much distended with thick ropy bile.* The lower part of the ileum was redder than natural, as were also the

* After opening the duodenum so as to expose the mouth of the common duct, pressure was made with the hand on the gall-bladder, but no bile flowed out till much force had been used; yet after it began to flow it continued, though the pressure was removed. The stoppage was ascertained to be owing to the mouth of the duct being obstructed by thick adhering mucus.

large intestines generally. The surface of the latter was dotted with minute red granulations.

It is noteworthy that at no time during life was any suspicion entertained of disease of the liver, and yet it can hardly be doubted that the abscesses in this case were of a chronic kind; and if so, proving—and there are many facts indicating the same— how little an abscess in the parenchyma of this organ affects the general health.

Case 17.—Of peritonitis, from ulceration and perforation of appendicula vermiformis, with disease of brain, etc.—W. Evans, ætat. 44; 68th Foot; admitted 24th January, 1837; died 22nd June.—This man, of 21 years' service, had suffered severely from ague in Canada. After his return towards the end of last year, on his passage from Portsmouth to Chatham in a crowded transport, his feet were frostbitten. On admission the toes of the right foot were black and painful, a redness extended to near the ankle. His appetite was good, his general health little affected. His mind was in a feeble state, and the account he gave of his feelings confused. He refused to have the toes removed by an operation. Toe by toe slowly dropped off, and several of the surfaces, from which phalanges had separated, had granulated, and were covered over. He continued apparently well in health, and seemed proceeding favorably until the night of the 17th June, when he had a rigor followed by headache, "and a disordered stomach." On the 19th it was reported that he had slept ill, that there was irritability of stomach, and that he rejected everything he took. A small V.S. was ordered, and calomel and opium. On the 20th he appeared somewhat better; the pulse was more moderate; the stomach less irritable, and the medicine was retained. On the 21st there was muttering delirium, with floccitation. In the evening his leg was swollen and red; the abdomen tumid and painful on pressure, with distinct fluctuation; pulse 130, small and irregular; his speech was confused and unintelligible. On the 22nd the belly was more tumid, and there was more swelling of the leg, and an increase of redness in the course of the absorbents of the limb. He expired at 9 p.m.

Autopsy 39 hours after death. Not emaciated. There was a good deal of fluid at the base of the brain and in the inferior cornua of the lateral ventricles. In the right corpus striatum, anteriorly and inferiorly, a portion rather larger than a filbert, was found in a disorganized state, yellowish brown, and so soft as to be almost pultaceous.* The surface of the cerebrum generally, and the walls of the ventricles, were less firm than natural. The lungs were tolerably sound, with the exception of the bronchia, which were generally red, as if inflamed. Pus (by the optical test) was found in their minute branches; and a reddish fluid in them generally. Some of the larger were nearly closed by coagulable lymph. The cavities of the heart were distended with blood and fibrinous concretion. On opening into the abdomen pus was found in the cellular tissue under the peritoneum, extending from Poupart's ligament to the hypochondrium on the left side, and some dark serum in the cavity of the pelvis. The vermiform process was perforated and gangrenous. The opening was large, dark, and shreddy. Raised with the forceps a portion remained behind, detached by sloughing; lymph was effused about it, and it was adhering to the mesentery. There was no well marked disease either of the stomach or of the small

* The softened substance under the microscope exhibited globules differing from pus globules: no other particulars are given of them.

or large intestines. The spleen was large, and contained some masses of varied color and firmness; of these one was yellowish brown, in part firm, and in part pultaceous. Contiguous was a sac, capable of holding a small orange, situated between the spleen and pancreas; it was full of a brownish pultaceous matter; more fluid than that in the substance of the spleen. The liver weighed 5 lbs. The testes were hard and somewhat enlarged, and were gorged with blood. One of them contained a spherical mass, of a yellowish hue, destitute of vessels, of about the size of a boy's playing marble. The other contained several smaller ones of the same kind. The large veins of the left leg were distended with coagulated blood of moderate firmness; the veins themselves did not appear to be diseased.

The fatal event in this case, it can hardly be doubted, was owing to the perforation of the appendicula. Some of the other lesions, such as the pultaceous matter in the corpus striatum and in the spleen, were so like fibrinous concretion softened, that I am disposed to hazard the conjecture that such was their nature, and that they had their origin in blood effused. The coagulation of the blood in the veins of the swollen leg, the lymph found coagulated in some of the larger bronchial branches, and the contents of the sac between the spleen and pancreas, so like grumous blood, are circumstances somewhat favorable to this idea.

Case 18.—Of peritonitis, from perforation of ileum and stomach (?) with tubercles. —J. Adam, ætat. 17; 60th Rifles; admitted 17th July, 1836; died 2nd September.— This man, of only eighteen months' service, had done little duty, being weak and ailing. He first came under treatment in regimental hospital in March last, for what was supposed to be disease of the mesentery. When transferred to general hospital in July, he was in a very feeble emaciated state, with much tenderness of abdomen and pain in the region of the liver and spleen. His pulse was 120; he was subject to night sweats, and to palpitation on the slightest exertion; also to dyspnœa, but without cough. On the 26th August the abdomen became tense, and there was an aggravation of pain. From this time he daily became worse, with the addition of "severe hectic attacks in the evening." The day before he died delirium set in. Hydrargyrum cum cretâ was used in the early stage, with iodine externally; leeches, etc., later.

Autopsy 13 hours after death. Exceedingly emaciated. Much fluid was found in the ventricles, and at the base of the brain.* The right lung was generally adhering; the left partially. In the superior lobe of the former there were many clusters of granular tubercles. In its middle lobe there were spots of extravasated blood of a dark hue; and in its inferior, a small cavity, black internally, capable of holding a pea. In the upper part of the superior lobe of the left lung, there was a tubercle about the size of a cherry, undergoing softening. This lung was in part slightly emphysematous, and also in part slightly hepatized and œdematous. The right, with the exception of the emphysema, exhibited the same lesions in a slight degree. The bronchial glands were much enlarged; they contained a curd-like matter.

* The rare occurrence of vessels carrying red blood was seen in the arachnoid, " covering the space between the two prominences of the cerebellum."

Small masses of the same kind were found on the adhesions between the middle and inferior lobe of right lung, and on the diaphragmatic pleura. The mitral valve was a little thickened. It was found very difficult to examine the contents of the abdomen, owing to the very extensive and close adhesions between most of the contained parts—as the omentum to the peritoneum above, the liver to the diaphragm, to the stomach and to part of the colon, and the intestines to one another. In the cavity of the pelvis there were about two pints of fluid, of fæcal appearance and odor. The surface of the omentum and of the intestines, externally, was of a dark grey color spotted with white, from a curd-like matter varying in size and form, deposited on them. The same kind of matter was found in layers between the peritoneum and the muscles of the abdomen, and also on both surfaces of the liver, and on both its lobes. In some places this matter was not merely superficial, but had penetrated, or had been deposited to some depth in the parenchyma. Between the left lobe and the stomach, in the situation where they were adhering together, there was a communication, from a softening of a portion of the intervening matter, accompanied by ulceration, and on the side of the liver with a considerable loss of substance, giving rise to an excavation. The opening into the stomach was large enough to admit the finger. A perforation also was detected of the intestine, the ileum; it appeared to be owing not to an ulceration proceeding from *within*—the mucous intestinal canal being free from disease—but from a tubercle softening in the *outer* coat, and penetrating by ulceration inwards. The spleen was large and firm; it contained a curd-like tubercle; and a similar one was met with in the left kidney. The mucous coat of the large intestines was smeared with a black matter, which was removed by the sponge. The solitary glands were enlarged.

This case is very noteworthy as one of tuberculosis affecting so many organs ; also for its protraction with so much suffering, and this, it may be inferred, even after perforation had taken place, checked, however as to consequences, by the adhesions produced.

These cases sufficiently illustrate some of the preceding remarks, especially as regards the complications of the disease, the variety of organs the seat of the primary lesion, the insiduous nature of that lesion ; and on the occurrence of the perforation, the sudden and unexpected explosion of the worst symptoms, rapidly ending in death.

In the great majority of the cases, it is clear that the perforating ulceration began either in the mucous coat of the hollow viscera or in the parenchyma of the solid ; indeed I cannot point to more than one with any certainty—the case of Adam, No. 18—in which the contrary happened.

That the morbid action ending in perforation, should be insidious so often, and nowise alarming, is not surprising, when we reflect that the ulceration may be limited to a spot only a few lines in diameter, and the rupture, the *causa mali,* be no larger than the eye of a bodkin. The entrance of excrementious matter, such as any portion of the contents of the intestinal canal, or the matter of an abscess, seems invariably to have the immediate effect of exciting peritoneal inflammation. In some instances, as in Cases 5, 6 and 8, it seems probable that such inflammation was started into existence by the ulceration, however limited as to space, reaching the peritoneal coat, effusion being prevented by lymph thrown out and the apposition of an adjoining fold of intestine.

That instances of peritonitis from perforation are so common in Malta and the Ionian Islands, may be owing to the tendency at each station to disease of the glandular structure of the intestines, especially in connection with fever, and more especially that of the remittent kind. We have seen in the fatal cases of fever of these islands that some lesion of the intestines was a common accompaniment, and in its most marked manner in the situation of Peyer's glands, there in the form of granular, elevated elliptical patches, more frequently without, but not rarely with, more or less of ulceration of the villous coat. Now, it is easy to imagine, how after an attack of fever, if the patient be discharged prematurely, before well-established convalescence, the very limited disease of the kind may continue and end in perforation. The little nourishing diet of the private soldier in the Mediterranean, the temptation in his way to intemperance from the cheapness of the country wines, and the habit of making too free a use of fruits often of indifferent quality, are all circumstances favoring the development of the local lesion in question. Not a single death from peritonitis occurred during the same period amongst the officers. In one fatal case of remittent fever in Malta, that of an officer, the glandulæ aggregatæ were found enlarged with slight adjoining ulceration, and one spot was seen where only the transparent peritoneal coat remained, separating the intestinal canal from the abdominal cavity. The coat was firm, indeed unduly hard, giving the idea, that on a former attack—he had had remittent fever in Portugal—the ulcerative process from within, after having destroyed the mucous and muscular coat was arrested at the outer.

That with a certain agreement of symptoms in the fatal cases, there should be considerable variations, is perhaps, no more than might be expected, considering the differences as to the complications and the difference in the seat of the perforation.

Respecting the medical treatment I have but little to state. I have brought forward several cases in which the lancet was freely used, and leeches, but in vain,—merely, perhaps, mitigating the severity of the suffering during the last few hours of life. From such experience as I have had, I am most disposed to the conclusion, that no blood should be abstracted, and that purgatives and even laxatives should be abstained from, and that opium chiefly should be trusted to, as affording the best chance of recovery through an effort of nature—that vis medicatrix, that vis vitæ on which, in disease and health, we are so dependent, and with which, with our disturbing medicine, we are too apt to interfere and check in their sanatory influences.

I have been in doubt whether I should give any of the cases I have of idiopathic peritonitis : after re-perusing them, I find them so little peculiar, comparing them with those resulting from perforation, those least complicated, that I have seen no sufficient reason to add them. Of the nine, two occurred in the Ionian Islands, and were ushered in with symptoms of remittent fever. The remaining seven were in the persons of soldiers in the United Kingdom, invalids sent home from foreign stations, with impaired constitutions and with more or less of chronic organic disease. Blood-letting to a considerable amount, which had a trial in some of these cases, proved as inefficacious as in the others.

CHAPTER XI.

ON CELLULAR INFLAMMATION.

Reasons for using the term.—Statistics of the disease in connection with climate.—The habit of body favorable to its production.—A certain periodicity belonging to it.—Detailed cases with comments, two especially remarkable,—one for a high temperature after death, one for a solution of a large portion of the stomach and diaphragm.—Remarks on its pathology, symptoms and treatment.—Notice of experiments on the effects of pus on animals injected into the pleura.

THE term cellular inflammation is convenient for use on account of its comprehensiveness, being applicable not only to erysipelas phlegmonoides of the older writers, to the diffuse cellular inflammation of some later authors, but also to other of the protean forms of disease which inflammation of the cellular tissue assumes according to the locality, the seat of attack, and the manner in which it may be complicated.

The number of cases which I find in my collection referrible to this head, is comparatively small, only 17 altogether, showing that in its most serious form, that having a fatal issue, this kind of inflammation is comparatively rare amongst our troops. And the same conclusion, I apprehend, must be arrived at from the army statistical reports. Amongst the troops serving at home, including infantry and cavalry, calculating on an aggregate strength of 173,643, it would appear that from 1830 to 1847, both years included, the cases of ordinary erysipelas* admitted for hospital treatment were 665, of which 32 proved fatal; now the aggregate mortality being 2,845, this is in the ratio of little more than 1 per cent. of the total; and, on foreign stations, according to the same documents, it has been even less. Thus, in the Mediterranean, including Gibraltar, Malta and the Ionian Islands, the mortality from it from 1818 to 1836 compared with the aggregate mortality, has been only as 9 to 3,667 ; in the West Indies, includ-

* The term erysipelas as employed in the medical returns of the army, is somewhat vague, being applied not only to erysipelas phlegmonoides, but also to some other varieties or species of Cullen's genus phlogosis.

ing Jamaica, from 1817 to 1836 only as 7 to 13,057, and in North America, including Canada and New Brunswick, where greatest, a little less than in the United Kingdom, being as 1·04 per cent. of the total mortality.

Of the cases which came under my own observation, the majority were idiopathic, three only owing their origin to, or following accidental wounds, viz., one from abrasion of the skin of the palm of the hand from falling on gravel; one from a contusion; the third from phlebotomy.

In the greater number of instances the disease occurred in men of impaired constitutions. In five instances out of the seventeen, tubercles were found in the lungs on the *post mortem* examination, cases these which might have been adduced in treating on the latency of tubercle; and in the other twelve, some lesion was detected indicative of chronic disease. Further, in proof of the influence of an impaired constitution as a predisposing cause, I may mention, that of the whole, thirteen of the cases occurred in invalids, and as such were under treatment in the general hospital, where during the same period, the total number of cases treated of all diseases was 10,256, of which 464 proved fatal.

Like other diseases of an obscure kind—obscure as to their etiology—this disease in its appearance was uncertain and irregular. Its occurrence, it may be inferred, was connected with some peculiar atmospheric condition: thus, whilst for a period of two years between 1821 and 1823, six fatal cases were recorded, about 4·5 of the whole mortality; during a second period—viz., from 1st January, 1835, to the 31st March, 1840, the fatal cases were seven, or only about 2·1 of the total. And, both on foreign and home stations, as regards ordinary erysipelas, the same disparity has been witnessed. According to the army statistical reports, whilst no less than 21 died of the disease in the Foot Guards during 10 years from 1837 to 1847; during the seven preceding years, there was not a single fatal case of it. Another instance may be given: in Canada, whilst from 1837 to 1847 the deaths from it were 21: from 1817 to 1836 they were only 2; the total mortality in the former period having been 1,178; in the latter 982. The inference, too, of an atmospheric condition being concerned in its production seems to be favored by the fact of common erysipelas being of more frequent occurrence in

cold or temperate climates than in warm and intertropical. From
the documents already quoted it appears that in Ceylon, the
Mauritius, the West Indies, including Jamaica and the Mediterranean stations, the mortality from it is only 16 out of a total of
15,371; whilst in Great Britain and North America it is as
much as 101 out of a total of 7,842.

In making a selection of cases for insertion I have been
guided chiefly by the desire to illustrate one of the peculiar
features of the disease, its protean character, simulating so often,
in the symptoms, other diseases, for which it could not fail to
pass unrecognised, were not its true nature discovered by a *post
mortem* examination; and the more to mark this, in giving the
cases, I have retained the name of the complaint first assigned
on the admission of the patients into hospital.

I shall first present two cases in which cellular inflammation
was associated with inflammation of the pleura and peritoneum,
cases which as they might have had a place in two former
sections, may be viewed as connecting those sections with this.
And, need I say that we cannot keep too much in mind, that
such is the tendency of diseases generally—viz., to glide as it
were into one another and become entangled and complicated,
and that they are rarely the entities confined within the restricted
limits assigned them by the systematic nosologist.

Case 1.—Of cellular inflammation, with tubercles and empyema.—S. Coone, ætat.
27; 13th Foot; admitted 10th October, 1822 ; died 2nd December.—"Pneumonia."
—This man's last illness (he had been previously ailing, and was hardly equal to any
duty) commenced in September, with pain in the left side of thorax, attended with
cough and pyrexia, for which he was bled, etc. Shortly after admission into the
general hospital on the 10th October, there was a recurrence of the pain, with great
dyspnœa. On the 24th of the same month there were indications of empyema in the
pained side. A trocar was introduced, but no fluid followed. On the 1st November,
erysipelatous inflammation of the face set in, with augmented pyrexia. Matter
formed beneath each eye in the cellular membrane, without pain, and was discharged by incision. On the 10th November he expectorated a good deal of pus.
There was now a considerable fulness of the left side of the chest, and a sensible
fluctuation. Paracentesis was again performed, and four pints of "laudable pus"
were drawn off. Relief of dyspnœa followed, but no permanent improvement. Up
to the 21st November, from three to six ounces of purulent fluid were discharged daily.
On that day, the opening being much contracted, the trocar was again introduced, but
imprudently *after* a flow of fluid, and in consequence the lung was wounded.*

* This was ascertained at the autopsy. The wound in the lung was found to be
about ½ inch deep; its edges were apparently healing; the surrounding substance
was of a pale red. The operation was performed by myself.

During the next twenty-four hours the discharge was tinged with blood. On the 26th, when the fluid discharged was about 2 oz. daily, his appetite had improved, and was pretty good; there were no night sweats, but a troublesome cough. Two days later he became troubled with diarrhœa; the discharge from the pleura diminished, his appetite failed, and, the purging continuing, he rapidly sank. The treatment for most part, after admission into the general hospital, had been palliative, with nourishing diet.

Autopsy 12 hours after death. Greatly emaciated. An abscess containing 2 oz. of pus was detected in the cellular tissue, between the right carotid and the trachea; and a similar one on the same side, behind the amygdala. There were 16 oz. of seropurulent fluid in the left pleura. This membrane was lined with a thick layer of lymph. The lung on this side was much compressed. It abounded in tubercles of different sizes, and in different stages of progress; the largest were about the size of a hazel-nut. The right lung partially adhered. It, too, abounded in tubercles, and they were similar to those in the left. The spleen was adhering to the diaphragm. The large intestines were somewhat thickened; their mucous coat was rough, and exhibited here and there small ulcers. The lower portion of the ileum also was slightly ulcerated.

The wound of the lung in this instance, it may be worthy of remark, appeared to have had no bad or aggravating effect. It may be mentioned, as serving to prove that the pleura is sensitive, at least in its diseased thickened state, that when a probe, introduced through the canula, was pressed against it, the patient always complained of pain.

Case 2.—Of cellular inflammation, with empyema and peritonitis.—J. M'Kenzie, ætat. 19; 41st Foot; admitted 10th March, 1822; died 30th April.—"Febris com. continens."—This man's illness commenced with rigors and headache at sea, after exposure to wet and cold on the 17th February. He had no medical aid until the 22nd of that month. Then he was in an alarming state; sordes on teeth; great dyspnœa; decubitus on back; knees raised; great pain of abdomen; intolerance of the slightest pressure; pulse 120, small and hard. After V.S., thrice performed on the 23rd, and after being fomented and blistered, there was some alleviation of symptoms; he could change his position, and breathe more freely. On the 3rd March some further improvement was reported; there was a mitigation of the febrile state, and some desire for food. On the 9th there was a recurrence of febrile attack. On the 10th, when transferred to the general hospital, all his symptoms were of the most unpromising kind. There was great debility and emaciation; a dry tongue; abdominal pain on pressure; pulse 116; no appetite; yet he could make a full inspiration with ease. From this date to the 11th April there was increase of abdominal pain, with accession of pain of right side of chest with cough. Boils, too, appeared about the umbilicus, and an oozing of matter took place from the latter. The boils were opened; and, there being a fluctuation of the abdomen, paracentesis was performed; 2⅔ pints of pus were discharged. The feet at this time were œdematous, as were also the left hand and arm. The latter was attributed to a phlegmon in the axilla pressing on the great vessels. It was opened, and 2 oz. of pus were evacuated. A few days later a sinus was detected extending from this abscess half way down the arm. It was laid open, and much purulent fluid was discharged from it. A phlegmon also appeared in the right axilla, and was opened. On the 25th, there being increased swelling of the abdomen, with fluctuation, and likewise clear indications of a collection of fluid in the left pleura, paracentesis was performed; from the former 2½ pints of pus were drawn off; from the latter 4 pints; that from each had the character of ordinary pus, *album, leve, æquale.* He bore the operations well; temporary relief was afforded. On the 28th the operation was repeated on the chest, and 16 oz. of pus were obtained. There was a continued purulent discharge from the abdomen. His intellect continued clear to the last. He died suddenly, just after he had been lifted out of bed at his own request.

Autopsy 9 hours after death. Excessive emaciation; feet œdematous; more or less serous effusion into the cellular membrane between the muscles generally. A good deal of fluid under the pia mater, in the ventricles, and in the spinal canal. Between the abdominal muscles and the peritoneum there was the sac of an abscess, lined with false membrane, and containing about 1½ pint of pus. It was so large that it extended across a little above the umbilicus from one loin to the other, and descended into the pelvis. At the navel there was a small opening, by which it had burst externally. The passage that had been made by the trocar had healed; no trace of it could be detected internally. The liver adhered to the stomach, the peritoneum to the intestines, and the convolutions of the latter loosely to each other, much serous fluid intervening. The stomach and intestines were distended with air and a brown fluid. The lower part of the rectum was red and œdematous. A tubercle, about the size of an almond in its shell, was attached to the mesentery; it consisted of a curd-like matter, and of some gritty matter, chiefly phosphate of lime. An abscess was found between the spleen and the diaphragm; it contained three pints of pus, and its sac was lined with a false membrane. The pancreas was small, and rather hard. The liver appeared sound. The right pleura, covered with coagulable lymph, of considerable thickness, and of a dark red color, contained a pint of purulent fluid. The lung on this side was partially adhering and much condensed, " hepatized and studded with spots of puriform exudation," as shown in its section. The left lung was sound. In each axilla, the cavity of the abscess that had been opened showed no disposition to heal.

The operations performed in this case seemed to be warranted by the circumstances ; but, on after reflection, I was doubtful of their being beneficial, and whether, though affording temporary relief, they did not hasten the fatal event. The immense suppuration in this instance, and its varied seats, were remarkable. The quantity of pus formed and existing about the same time—viz., before an outlet was made—could have been little short of ten pounds. It was also remarkable how little was the feeling of exhaustion, or tendency to faintness: the patient to the last day sat up in bed to have the dressing renewed ; and, excepting his fatal syncope, he never experienced any tendency to faintness. The protraction of the case was remarkable, especially taking into account the peritoneal inflammation.

Case 3.—Of cellular inflammation, with a remarkable communication, owing to solution or absorption of tissue, between the stomach and pleura.—W. Parry, ætat. 20; 1st F.; admitted 6th Feb., 1840; died 11th May. "Subluxatio."—This man was admitted into hospital on account of a slight swelling, with much pain and stiffness of the left ankle-joint from an accident, without any obvious impairment of his general health. On the 8th April a swelling was detected between the tendo Achillis and bone, from a small collection of matter formed there ; 2 oz. were evacuated by an incision. On the 24th April the ankle and dorsum of the foot became red, constitutional symptoms of a typhoid type at the same time occurring; low muttering delirium; subultus tendinum, dilated pupils; dry brown tongue; a full pulse, varying from 130 to 146. These symptoms continued without abatement till he expired. The treatment consisted in the first instance in topical blood-letting, afterwards in the use of alterative doses of calomel, sesquicarbonate of ammonia, etc.

Autopsy 12 hours after death. Sub-emaciated; limbs rigid; left lung œdematous ; cadaver still warm; no signs of putridity. There was a good deal of serum in the tissue of the pia mater and at the base of the brain, but little in the ventricles. Some lymph was effused in the former; and in the pia mater, in the fissures of Sylvius, and at the base of the cerebellum there was a granular deposit like tubercles, with a superficial softening of the cerebral substance of those parts. Granular tubercles were dispersed through all the lobes of the right lung, and a small cavity was found in its superior lobe ; apart from these, the parenchyma had a healthy appearance. In the apex of the left lung there were two or three softening tubercles; in its inferior lobe there was a small cavity; this lobe was partially hepatized. The left pleura contained $5\frac{1}{2}$ oz.* of a reddish brown fluid; the right 3 oz. The upper portion of the great arch of the stomach, between the spleen and its cardiac orifice, contiguous to the diaphragm, was perforated with loss of substance, and to such an extent as to admit the whole hand; moreover, in the diaphragm corresponding, a similar perforation was found, though not quite so large. A few shreddy muscular bands crossed the opening, and the peritoneal lining of the diaphragm was detached round the opening to the extent of about half an inch, as if the fine connecting cellular tissue had been dissolved. It is remarkable that the mucous coat of the stomach generally was not softened, not even close to the perforation; nor did it exhibit any remarkable appearance. There were cavities in the small omentum as if from penetration by solution. There was no appearance of peritoneal inflammation. No fluid was found effused into the cavity of the abdomen inferiorly, only contiguous to the perforation. The inner coat of the duodenum was rather soft; it contained some yellowish chyme, which, put by in a gallipot, after 24 hours had acquired an offensive smell and

---

* It was slightly turbid; had a peculiar cadaverous smell ; reddened litmus paper, but was not perceptibly acid to the taste; it was coagulated like the serum of the blood by nitric acid. Under the microscope, examined about three hours after being taken from the body, it was found to contain blood corpuscles and many globules of different sizes, like oil or fat globules, with some little masses of irregular form. Examined the following day, the blood corpuscles were no longer perceptible, and the globules were less distinct, as if in process of solution.

The inference at the time was that this fluid was in part derived from the stomach, and that inference accords with its reddening litmus paper, and in its resemblance to the little fluid that was found in the cavity of the abdomen. Another inference was that the smaller quantity of fluid of the same appearance found in the right pleura, had passed into it from the left by exudation.

I may mention the result of a trial made to test this conjecture. A stomach, a few hours after the death of the individual from whom it was taken, containing a moderate quantity of fluid which was slightly turbid, reddened strongly litmus paper, and under microscope was found to have suspended in it globular particles and particles of irregular form, was tied at both its extremities and was suspended in a receiver, where it was covered with a plate. After 24 hours, a portion of its contents, about 2 oz., was found collected beneath, having passed through, as through a filter. It retained its acidity, as tested by litmus paper. Yet the inner coat of the stomach was not distinctly softened.

rendered turmeric paper slightly brown. The urinary bladder was much distended. The bursa between the tendo Achillis and the ankle-joint was enlarged ; it contained pus and communicated with the articulation of the astragalus and os calcis ; the car- tilage of these bones was partially destroyed.

The perforated state of the stomach and diaphragm in this instance, so very remarkable in all its circumstances, is, as regards the manner in which it was produced, not a little per- plexing. Was it a *post mortem* occurrence, or did it take place before death ? The latter seems to me the more probable. At present, I am not aware that a lesion of the kind, implicating the diaphragm, has come even within the limits of pathological specu- lation. If the solution was slowly taking place during life, and of the diaphragm as well as of the stomach, it might help to account for some of the anomalous symptoms of the case.

Case 4.—Of cellular inflammation, with an unusual elevation of temperature after death.—J. Brown, ætat. 23 ; 95th Regiment ; admitted into regimental hospital, Malta, 30th July, 1828 ; died 6th August.—" Rheumatismus acutus."—This man on admission had acute pain of the right shoulder, increased by motion and pressure ; there was much pyrexia ; no external swelling. Until the previous night, when the attack began, he had been in good health. 40 leeches to the pained part ; a purgative of calomel and antimony. On the 31st, no relief ; acute pain was also felt in the right hip. The pulse quick and hard ; tongue foul ; much thirst. V.S. 20 oz. Dover's powder 8 grs. every hour *usque ad sudorem.* August 1st—Four powders taken ; profuse sweating produced. The pain of hip is less, that of shoulder unabated. The skin is warm. The blood drawn is slightly buffed. 2nd—A blister was applied last night to the shoulder, without giving relief. The pain of hip is returned, but is less severe. The bowels are costive. A cathartic draught. 3rd—Yesterday the bowels were freely opened. He had some sleep at night after taking 15 grs. of Dover's powder. There is no change of symptoms. 2 grs. of calomel and James' powder, with half a grain of opium every 3rd hour. 4th—Feels much better this morning ; since yester- day afternoon has been almost free from pain. The same medicine. 5th—The pains returned with increased severity in the night and have attacked the left shoulder and hip. Has been much purged. The face is flushed ; the skin very hot, yet moist ; thirst urgent ; tongue loaded ; respiration hurried ; the respiratory sounds natural. Pulvis Cretæ compos. c. opio. in place of the medicine last prescribed. At the evening visit the pulse was still very rapid ; the respiration somewhat hurried. He has taken 15 grs. of the powder twice. Has had three stools. A warm bath, and after it 40 drops of laudanum, with 30 of antimonial wine. 6th—After the draught he slept some hours, and on waking said he was easier. At 3 a.m. he began to talk inco- herently. He complained of pain of abdomen. He continued more or less delirious till 6 a.m., when visited then the skin was pungently hot ; the pulse exceedingly rapid ; the respiration laborious ; the tongue black in the middle ; the abdomen painful when firmly pressed. 36 leeches were applied ; but before they had drawn any considerable quantity of blood he was moribund, and they were removed.

Autopsy 3½ hours after death. Naturally slender, there was no appearance of emaciation. The cadaver was warm ; there was nothing peculiar in its aspect. The pia mater was rather redder than natural. There was very little fluid in the ventricles. The brain was of ordinary firmness. The right cavities of the heart and great vessels were distended with fluid blood, which coagulated on exposure to the air. From one of the mammary veins it sprang out two or three inches, and the jet continued, like the flow of blood from a vein in the common operation of V.S., till stopped by a ligature; and this though the cavity of the abdomen and also of the thorax had previously been laid open. The blood which first flowed from this vessel when divided contained very little coloring matter and fibrin; much less than that which flowed after; yet its fibrin was observed to contract more, much more, in the same time. Besides the liquid blood in the heart, there was with it a little crassamentum and fibrinous concretion. The left cavities contained very little blood, as also the aorta; in the latter it had formed a soft coagulum. The thoracic duct contained a reddish fluid. The lungs, with the exception of being a little redder than natural, seemed healthy. There was some frothy mucus in the bronchia. The gallbladder was unusually red and vascular externally. The bile it contained was dark and very viscid. Portions of the intestines, both small and large, were also redder and more vascular than usual. The lymphatic glands generally were large. The spleen was large, soft, and rather pale. A collection of reddish purulent fluid was detected on each side of the spine of the right scapula. Above the spine, the periostum was detached from the bone to some extent. There was "matter" between the periostum and the bone, and the periostum was covered with coagulable lymph. Below the spine, the abscess was chiefly between the muscles; their fibres were very soft; in some places paler than natural; in some blood-shot. Sinuses in different directions extended amongst the muscular parts to the head of the humerus, where there was an extensive one outside the capsule and towards the axilla. Marks of inflammation—viz., the effusion of serum and of lymph—were very widely spread, even to the neck, the arm, and down the side. In the left shoulder there was slight ecchymosis. In the left hip, close to the head of the femur, over the iliac bone, there was a large abscess full of reddish pus. From it sinuses extended in various directions into the glutei muscles, which had the same appearance as those of the right shoulder. The bone was not denuded. In the right hip there was considerable ecchymosis, but, as in the shoulder of the left side, there was no suppuration. The capsules of the joints interiorly, both of the right shoulder and left hip, were free from inflammation. The temperature of the deep-seated parts was so unusually high, that when the cadaver was first opened, the sensation on touching them was almost "burning," an expression used at the time. A thermometer placed under the left ventricle of the heart rose to 113°; under the liver, to 112°; and then the chest and the abdomen had been opened at least twelve minutes. The air of the room was 86°; this was at 10.30 a.m.: since 7 a.m., the time of the death, the body had been covered only with a single sheet. There were no signs of incipient putrefaction; on the contrary, the redness of the parts designated "unusually red" was of a bright hue; nor did putrefaction take place with unusual rapidity, not indeed so soon as that of the body of a soldier of the same regiment, who had died in the same day of pulmonary apoplexy. It may deserve remark that the three dozen of leeches which had been applied to the abdomen shortly before death, were found all dead the following morning, after having been purged of the little blood which they had abstracted, as if they had been poisoned by the blood.

I have given this case so fully on account of its many peculiarities, and especially the high temperature observed in the deep-seated parts after death. It may be added, and it was specially noted, that at no time during the illness were there any rigors; also, that notwithstanding the extensive disease about the hip, the patient had the power of walking and going to the close-stool. In this instance, as in the last, the question arises—Was the high temperature observed a *post mortem* effect, or the result of diseased action during life? Again I have to express the opinion that the latter seems to me the most probable, and for the simple reason of the absence of any known cause in operation after death adequate to meet the difficulty.*

Case 5.—Of cellular inflammation, with tuberculated lungs.—T. Barrett, ætat. 38; 13th L. D.; admitted 21st June, 1839; died 2nd July.—" Catarrhus chronicus."— This man, recently returned from India, during the 14 years he was there had been often in hospital on account of rheumatism, hepatitis, dysentery and occasional attacks of catarrh. On admission on the 21st June, he was laboring under catarrhal symptoms which began on the 13th On the 25th, when these were rapidly subsiding, symptoms of a different kind set in, such as acute pain of the throat, hoarseness of voice with much pyrexia; the pulse 110; tongue dry and loaded. Towards evening an erysipelatous blush appeared " on the margin of old syphilitic cicatrices on the nose and forehead," which, during the next four days extended over the face and head and from the mouth to the fauces. On the 30th the erysipelatous inflammation began to fade, but with indications of rapid sinking, and with low delirium. The treatment for the catarrh was a palliative "pectoral mixture," for the erysipelas tartar emetic and sulphate of magnesia.

Autopsy 6 hours after death. Not emaciated; limbs muscular. There was much thickening of the integuments of the head from lymph effused, especially *over* the pericranium. The vessels of the brain, both the veins and arteries, were distended

---

* In a former work, in that part which treats of the temperature of the body after death, and in which brief mention is made of this case (Res. Phy. and Anat., i., p. 229), I have assigned the reasons which had induced me to come to the above conclusion. May it not be inferred, I would now add, that the sounder the lungs are during the last stage of life, the better they perform their functions, the better and the more the blood is aerated, the higher will be the temperature at the last moment; and, *cœteris paribus*, the higher it will be found when the *post mortem* examination is made? Does not the case in question favor this, for not only were the lungs free from disease, but the blood also was more than usually florid?

I am aware of the difficulty of the subject, and that other inquirers have drawn an opposite inference—viz., that there is a development of heat actually after death. Dr. Dowler's results are the ones most trusted to by those who take this view. These results, as they are stated, go far to prove that there is an elevation of temperature in certain parts after the extinction of life; but is it clear from them that the increased heat is generated and not simply diffused—*i. e.*, transmitted from the deeply-seated parts to the superficial parts? When the arteries contract, as they do after the heart has ceased to act, the blood is propelled from the arterial into the venous system. This may be one cause of the transfer of heat; and the rigor mortis may be another cause. It may be asked—Why may there not be an elevation of temperature, from changes going on in the blood itself? If there be oxygen in the blood, what is to prevent its acting chemically, and forming carbonic acid as in life, and evolving heat? This is specious, and may be true, but till we have more exact information on the subject, is it not right to suspend our credence? It is well to keep in mind the vast number of *post mortem* examinations that have been made by the ablest pathologists, from the time of Morgagni downwards, and the very few instances in which there have been any indications recorded of *post mortem* elevation of temperature.

with *coagulated* blood. There was pretty much fluid in the tissue of the pia mater; the lateral ventricles contained a small quantity, and there was about an ounce at the base of the brain; it was of the sp. gr. 1,011; on standing it yielded a little coagulable lymph. The substance of the brain was natural. The pericardium contained an ounce of fluid, of sp. gr. 1,027; it jellied on standing; the fibrin collected and thoroughly dried weighed ·6 gr. Some cruor, fibrinous concretions and crassamentum were found in the cavities of the heart. The cruor set aside coagulated. The serum from it was of a dark ale color, and was of the high sp. gr. 1,038. The temperature of the heart was 90°. The left lung adhered superiorly. Towards its apex there was a cavity capable of holding a walnut; within it there were some tubercular masses partially detached; it was lined with a false membrane, and communicated with a bronchial tube; contiguous to it were several clustered granular tubercles and two or three small bony concretions. This part of the lung had a shrunken puckered appearance. The inferior lobe was pretty sound and was free from tubercles. In the superior lobe of the right lung there were a few granular tubercles. There was some redness of the bronchia, and much œdema of the glottis. The epiglottis had the appearance of having lost a portion of its substance from former ulceration. The liver was rather soft; it weighed 4½ lbs. The spleen was large and pultaceous. The stomach was rather soft.

In this case the lesions discovered seem hardly adequate to account for the death. May not the blood coagulated in the vessels of the brain and the high specific gravity of the serum and serosity have been concerned in the event? Apart from the erysipelatous inflammation, the state of the lungs, and especially of the superior lobe of the left, is not without interest in relation to tubercles, and particularly as denoting a healing process in progress, which, if not interrupted, might possibly have got rid of the few tubercles and have been productive of a natural cure.

Case 6.—Of cellular inflammation, without any strongly marked complication, and with seemingly a low state of vitality.—J. Wilson, ætat. 38; 24th F.; admitted 24th September, 1823; died 7th October.—"Erysipelas."—This man has just returned from India invalided, on account of an impaired constitution, after repeated attacks of ague and the use of much mercury. His present illness began on the 21st September, with redness of the left elbow, rigors, heat, etc. On admission the redness with heat and swelling and pain extended from the elbow towards the shoulder and half way down the forearm. There was much pyrexia; the pulse was quick, rather full and resisting; the tongue dry with a brownish crust. V.S. 12 oz., when he fainted. The blood was much cupped and buffed; the fibrin was of a milky whiteness. Pulv. Cinchonæ drachm i.; omni horâ c. oz. i. Mist. seq. Decoct. Cinchon. oz. iv., Liq. Ammon Acetat. oz. ii., Acid. Tart. scruple i., Aq. puræ oz. viii. On the 25th there was erythema and swelling of the left ear. On the 26th the inflammation had extended from the ear to the face and forehead. Whilst at the close-stool he fainted. From the last date to September 30th, there was some improvement; he then felt decidedly better; the pulse was only 74, with apyrexia. The tongue moist and more clean; a better appetite; the swelling of the arm and face subsiding. On the 2nd October a fluctuation was perceived in the forearm; 6 oz. of pus were discharged by an incision. Until the 5th October improvement continued; then there was increased hardness and redness above the elbow, extending nearly to the shoulder.

On the 6th, after a restless night, he was very feeble; the pulse 70, very weak; the tongue dry and brown; frequent vomiting. Towards evening his breathing became hurried; his extremities cold; pulse 60, very feeble and intermitting, in brief he was moribund. The treatment consisted chiefly in the use of bark and its decoction, combined with the acetat of ammonia and aperients as required, with the use of wine in the advanced stage—a treatment which in two other cases of erysipelas that occurred about the same time, with superficial suppuration, appeared to be beneficial, as they recovered.

Autopsy 21 hours after death. Sub-emaciated. There was a deposit of coagulable lymph over the superior portions of both hemispheres, and an unusual fulness of the vessels of the pia mater. The ventricles contained very little fluid. In the left forearm there were several abscesses between the muscles. Under the biceps there was a large one extending from the elbow to the head of the humerus, and communicating with the capsule of the joint, in which was a little pus, and extending also some way under the pectoralis minor. There was no appearance of inflammation of the veins. The left lung was generally and firmly adhering. Both lungs were gorged with blood, and portions of them were hepatized. The bronchia were unusually red, as was also the trachea in part; one portion of it was of a dirty greenish hue, as if from incipient gangrene. There was much blood in the venæ cavæ and the right auricle, and a good deal of fibrinous concretion in the right ventricle. The substance of the heart was rather soft, and was easily broken. The liver was large; its substance soft. There was exceedingly little bile in the gallbladder. The spleen adhered to the false ribs; its substance was firmer than natural, and its external coat thickened The kidneys were large and pale and soft; in the veins of both kidneys a substance was found resembling coagulable lymph, but milk-white (of the same color as the buffy coat already mentioned) and of little consistence. The mucous coat of the stomach and intestines was unduly red, and in places was of a greenish hue, similar to that of the trachea.

In this case we appear to have an example of the failure of the vis vitæ, as denoted by the syncope from the abstraction of a small quantity of blood, by the slowness of the pulse in the last stage, and by the softness of the heart after death.

Case 7.—Of cellular inflammation, very diffused.—Wm. Powell, ætat. 48; 34th Foot; admitted 1st January, 1822; died 11th January.—This man, an old soldier and an invalid, was attacked by his present complaint on the 30th December. It began with rigors, followed the next morning by swelling of the face, with a " burning heat and pain ;" both eyes were nearly closed. He had no headache; the skin was hot; the pulse quick, and rather full. No material change occurred till Jan. 5th, when he complained of pain of throat and difficulty in swallowing. On the 8th the report was, " the swelling of the face has nearly subsided, and desquamation is taking place." There was now considerable swelling of the neck and much pain, the difficulty of swallowing continuing; slight cough; pulse 80 and weak; the skin rather hot; the tongue foul and moist; thirst less urgent; appetite a little better; bowels open. From this date he rapidly sank, with little change of symptoms. The treatment employed was somewhat similar to that used in the preceding case, except that no blood was abstracted, and that antimonials with aperients were given before bark and the compound tincture were administered.

Autopsy 36 hours after death. Sub-emaciated; the neck swollen. A small collection of pus was found in the cellular membrane of the superior palpebra of each eye.

There was a good deal of purulent fluid under the integuments of the head, chiefly on the right side. The cellular membrane in which it was situated was very red, with partial ecchymosis. In some places there was matter beneath the pericranium, and there the bone was bare. The integuments were thickened and puffy. The veins of the brain were turgid, and the pia mater was unusually vascular, with more fluid than usual in its tissue. Several collections of matter were found in the neck. One was immediately between the cutis and the platysma myoides; another between the sterno-thyroid and crico-thyroid muscles; another over the thyroid cartilage, and round the thyroid gland; another, and that an extensive one, in the cellular tissue, between the œsophagus and spine, at least two-thirds the length of the former. Purulent collections were also detected in the anterior and posterior mediastinum, close to the pericardium and the trunks of the great vessels, both veins and arteries. The cellular membrane adjoining, and even the theca of these vessels, appeared very red and inflamed. The inner coat of the same vessels was pale. The outer coat of the pericardium, where in contact with the purulent collection, was very red; its inner coat was slightly red. It contained 1 oz. of "milky serum." The fauces were inflamed. The epiglottis was red, and much swollen; the rima glottidis swollen and contracted. The larynx throughout was marked with red transverse streaks. The bronchia and the substance of both lungs were unduly red, as were also the pleuræ. The inferior lobe of the right lung was of a dark red, and hepatized. The left pleura contained 4 oz. of serum. There was no well marked diseased appearance of any of the abdominal viscera.

That the event was fatal in this case is not surprising, considering how extensive was the inflammation and suppuration, and the situations in which they occurred. It is noteworthy how little pain was experienced, excepting in the neck, and how latent in relation to symptoms was the diseased action in the other parts.

Case 8.—Of cellular inflammation, very diffused.—J. Tait, ætat. 36; 65th Regiment; admitted into regimental hospital, Edinburgh Castle, Jan. 4, 1824; died 8th January.—"Febris communis continens."—This man's illness commenced in the evening of the 2nd January with severe rigors. At the time he had an irritable open bubo in the right groin, after gonorrhœa. He was very stout and plethoric. On admission on the 4th, the principal symptoms were nausea and vomiting; pain along the course of the dorsal spine; slight cough and dyspnœa from pain; no great prostration of strength; the pulse was 96, and soft; a slight increase of temperature; tongue foul; bowels constipated. At the evening visit, after the action of an emetic and purgative, there was less nausea, but an increase of pain. V.S. 24 oz.; deliquium animi. The first portion of blood drawn was buffed and cupped; the second in a less degree. "Pain removed to the right loin." After the V.S., calomel, 3 grs.; pulv. antimon, 2 grs.; ext. opii ½ grain. On the 5th, after a pretty good night, a return of dorsal pain; pulse 98, full. V.S., 36 oz. The blood buffed and cupped, excepting the last portion; the pulse immediately after, 144. On the 6th, after the action of a purgative, acute pain was felt in the right loin, with increase of dyspnœa, and an anxious expression of countenance; pulse 130, very compressible. Nine leeches to the pained part. On the 7th, pain only in the right loin; some delirium; pulse very rapid and small. On the 8th, after a sleepless night, the delirium continued; the pulse was felt with difficulty; respiration rapid; lips livid; said he was free from pain; evidently moribund. An hour and a half before he expired, there was a sudden swelling of the right arm, without redness or pain.

Autopsy 18 hours after death. No emaciation. The vessels of the brain were turgid. In the posterior mediastinum, along its whole course, there was "suppuration," with œdema and effusion of lymph. The quantity of pus found was small, only about two drachms. The cellular structure, the diseased seat, was exceedingly vascular, especially under the œsophagus and round the aorta. The inflammation extended upwards nearly to the pharynx, also along the course of the subclavian artery to the left arm, which was considerably swollen from œdema and the effusion of coagulable lymph. A small collection of pus was found close to the bronchial artery. Round the subclavian and the axillary, the cellular structure was very red and slightly œdematous. In another direction, along the insertion of the diaphragm on the right side, there were marks of the same diseased action—viz., increased vascularity, œdema, and some purulent effusion in the cellular tissue, between the muscle and corresponding peritoneal covering. The pericardium contained only a few drops of fluid. The muscular substance of the heart was very tender and easily broken. There was a good deal of blood in the right auricle; a little in the right ventricle; very little in the cavities of the left side. The lining membrane of each was more or less red, varying in degree according to the quantity of blood contained. The inner coat of the thoracic aorta was more easily separated than usual from the middle; the cellular tissue there surrounding the artery was inflamed. The abdominal aorta contained some blood and air, as was ascertained before any great vessel had been divided, the abdomen having been first opened. The lining membrane both of the aorta and venæ cavæ was tinged red; the former slightly, the latter strongly; yet in each there was but little blood. Both lungs were generally adhering, and their lobes to each other. The substance of both was unduly red, and contained an excess of blood. The bronchia were of a dark red, as was also the pharynx. The abdominal viscera, with the exception of some adhesions, were of tolerably normal appearance.

The state of the heart and vessels in this case might at first view suggest the idea of their being implicated in the disease; but whether truly so, is questionable, considering the time that had elapsed between the death and the autopsy, and the stoutness of the cadaver, so much the more retentive of heat, and the heat favoring putrefaction, and that favoring discoloration by staining. A like doubt, too, may be entertained regarding the air found in the aorta. Both it, and the redness of the lining membrane of the heart and vessels, being contrary to ordinary experience, it would be illogical to view them as the effects of disease and concerned in its phenomena, unless it were clear that they were not *post mortem* occurrences.

Case 9.—Of cellular inflammation, with hydrops pulmonis.—A. M'Guire, ætat. 28; 28th F.; admitted 28th November, 1821; died 3rd January, 1822.—"Hepatitis chron."—This man had been invalided on account of chronic hepatitis of ten months' duration, for which he had been frequently blistered and bled. On admission he had pain in the right hypochondrium, increased by pressure; decubitus easy on the back only; frequent cough, with mucous expectoration; respiration short and easily hurried; appetite pretty good; no emaciation. Until the 7th December he appeared to be mending; then he experienced a severe rigor, followed by increased heat and sweating. On the following morning he had headache, deep-seated pain of left side; breathing short and quick; pulse 102, full and strong; much thirst. V.S. 28 oz.; the blood was slightly buffed; some relief followed. On the 9th there was erysipelatous inflammation of the left side of face; slight strabismus; headache, skin hot and dry; pulse quick and hard. V.S. 22 oz.; an aperient; the blood more buffed. On the 10th the face was generally swollen, red and painful; the skin less hot; pulse 118, rather hard. V.S. 16 oz.; an aperient. On the 11th, a bad night was reported, and that both eyes were closed. Pulv. Cinchonæ. On the 14th the inflammation was subsiding on the face and extending over the neck and chest; the surface very painful and slightly red. Decoct. Cinchonæ. On the 20th, much inclination to doze; the skin hotter; the pulse more rapid. Desquamation was in progress. On the 23rd there was some diarrhœa. The tongue brown and parched; pulse quick; skin cool; a throbbing of the carotids. On the 25th there was an increase of diarrhœa; great debility; is emaciating. Infus. extract. Hæmatox. Vinum opii. c. Decoct. Cinchonæ. He gradually sank without any marked change of symptoms.

Autopsy 20 hours after death. Sub-emaciated; and yet excess of adeps, especially in the abdomen. The brain not examined. A small collection of pus, about a drachm, was found in the substance of the right sterno-thyroid muscle; another, and about the same quantity, in the cellular membrane investing the aorta just where it penetrates the diaphragm; and a third in the same tissue, just above the bifurcation of the artery in the pelvis. The left lung, except being generally and firmly adhering and unusually red, was tolerably sound. The right lung was absolutely distended with serous fluid, which, on incisions being made, flowed out copiously. The bronchia were very red. Several deep ulcers were found in the upper part of the tongue. The peritoneal coat of the liver, especially of the right lobe, was considerably thickened; it adhered in a few places to the diaphragm. Beneath the thickened membrane the substance of the liver was unusually soft and red, suggesting an inflamed state. The spleen was larger and firmer than natural; it contained several small white tubercles of a cheesy consistence. The small intestines were in parts unduly red. The colon and rectum were thickened. The mucous coat of the latter was smeared with purulent fluid and was red, soft and swollen, as if from inflammation.

In this case there was no suspicion during life of the main organic lesions to which the fatal issue, it may be inferred, was owing. It is true that a slight cough was noticed latterly and a rapid respiration, but the stethoscope not having been used, its cause was not ascertained. Probably whilst the repeated bloodlettings did not arrest the deep-seated inflammation, they may have favored serous effusion into the lung.

The great variety of morbid appearances discovered in these cases is remarkable, as well as the diversity of symptoms witnessed during their progress—the former accounting tolerably for the latter. The remaining cases—those which I keep back—exhibit much the same variety, and equally accord with what I have said of the protean character of the disease.

Of all the varieties of lesion, it is worthy of note that the most common was that which could be ascertained only by dissection—viz., inflammation and suppuration in the mediastina, along the course of the great vessels; in as many as eight of the cases out of the seventeen, such was one of the principal seats of the morbid action. Whether the vessels themselves were implicated in these instances and in the disease generally, seems doubtful. In one of the cases only, No. 8, was the inner coat of the aorta apparently altered. Redness of the vessels and a soft state of the heart were both frequently observed, and occasionally when one would not have expected, calculating merely on the interval of time between the death and the examination of the body: both, however, might have been owing to an undue tendency of the blood and muscle to putrefaction; the one favoring the staining of the vessels with which it came in contact; the other favoring a softening of the muscular fibre. To this cause, on the ground of probability, I would rather refer both, than to inflammatory action.

I have given some particulars of the treatment in several of the cases, with the hope of affording a little aid towards determining the principles on which the treatment of the disease should be conducted—that a most difficult matter, I apprehend, and mainly owing to the disease being so variable as to intensity and tendency to a fatal issue. This is well shown by results, as recorded in the Returns of the General Hospital, thus:—Of 7 treated in 1821, none died; of 7 in 1822, 1 died; of 10 in 1823, 3 died; of 10 in 1839, all recovered.

As debility appears almost invariably to be connected with the disease, and may be considered a predisposing cause, the abstraction of blood seems to be contraindicated either altogether, or if indicated at all, by a fulness and strength of pulse and much pyrexia, only in great moderation. All the cases that have come under my observation, in which much blood was abstracted, have had a fatal termination; on the contrary, I have known several severe cases do well under the use of bark combined with saline medicine, such as the acetate of ammonia, and gentle aperients.

Regarding the use of local applications to the surface I am somewhat doubtful, partly from not having witnessed any marked good effect when they have been employed, and partly from observing that the danger has arisen—judging from the fatal cases—not from superficial, but from deeply seated inflammation. Looking, too, to the event—that often prosperous when vesication had occurred—I have even been led to consider severity of superficial inflammation rather a favorable symptom than the contrary.

There are other questions relating to the disease, two of which only I shall now mention : one, whether it is contagious or not; another, whether in the more formidable examples of it, the blood is not tainted with pus, or with a morbid matter of the nature of pus?

There are high authorities in favor of the opinion of its contagious or infectious nature ; but, when one considers the comparative rareness of the disease, and the difficulty of distinguishing between a contagious and a purely epidemic disease, data at least seem wanting to enable one to arrive at any positive conclusion either *pro* or *contra*.

As to the state of the blood, whilst many circumstances seem to indicate that it is in a vitiated or altered condition, I know of none that are perfectly demonstrative that pus or a matter like pus exists in the circulation. This at least seems certain, that whenever there are purulent collections within the body, a peculiar morbid action is excited, and this mostly, if not invariably, fatal, unless issue be given them, so that they can be drained and carried off.

I shall here offer the results of some trials made so long ago as 1838-39, on the injection of purulent fluids into the pleura of animals, chiefly with the intent of endeavoring to ascertain whether pus can be removed or not by absorption.

Experiment 1.—On the 19th December an ounce of pus from a vomica, homogenous in appearance, consisting, as seen under the microscope, of granules and globules, was injected into the right pleura of a healthy dog. For two or three hours there seemed to be some suffering from the operation. The following day he was lively, and had a good appetite. On the 23rd he was killed. The wound was healed. In the right pleura 2½ oz. of a brownish fluid were found; in the left 5 oz. of a similar fluid. It appeared on examination to consist of serum, of blood corpuscles, and of pus; on rest, the latter subsided.

Experiment 2.—On 11th January, injected 2 oz. of purulent fluid into the right pleura of a dog in health; the lung was not wounded, and none of the fluid escaped. The fluid was obtained from the pleura of a man who had died of empyema. On the 12th the dog refused his food. On the morning of the 13th he was found dead. On opening the thorax, both lungs collapsed; 7 oz. of purulent serum were found in the right pleura, and 4½ oz. in the left. The right lung partially adhered; the substance

24

of the adhesions—coagulable lymph—was soft and weak, and coagulable lymph had been thrown out on the surface of the lung. The lungs themselves were sound.

Experiment 3.—On the 9th March injected about 1 oz. of pus into the right pleura of a spaniel; the pus was from the same body as that used in the preceding experiment; it had been kept in water, and the water occasionally changed. On the 11th the dog was found dead; judging from the temperature of the body (the right ventricle was 66°, the left 70°), he must have died in about a day and a half from the commencement of the experiment. About 6 oz. of reddish turbid serum were found in the right pleura, about 2 oz. in the left*; there were pellicles of lymph on both lungs; the right was compressed; neither was diseased. There was much dark coagulated blood in the right cavities of the heart, without buffy coat or fibrinous concretion. The fluid, it is worthy of remark, was acid, by the test of litmus, and the reddening was not evanescent. As in the other instances, when agitated with common air, this fluid gave off some gas, which was found to be, at least in part, carbonic acid. Its reddish hue it owed to coloring matter, probably of the blood, but no blood corpuscles could be detected in it.

Experiment 4.—On 15th March injected 2 drachms of the purulent sediment of the fluid taken from the pleuræ of the dog, the subject of the last experiment, into the right pleura of a half-grown cat; the lung was punctured; a little air escaped; a suture was applied. The first day she was ailing; after the second she ate bread and milk. She was killed on the 20th. About half an ounce of fluid was found in the right pleura; the pleura was covered with lymph; the fluid was slightly red and turbid, and contained shreds of lymph. Nearly as much was found in the left pleura; this fluid was colorless, and only very slightly turbid. Neither was acid.

The blood in each instance was examined for pus; and globules were found in it somewhat like those of pus, and were supposed at the time to be such, but that they really were I cannot venture to affirm : at the time the observations were made, the white corpuscles of the blood had hardly been recognized.

The results of these experiments, if too few and insufficient in their negative bearing to disprove the possibility of the removal of pus by absorption, at least show its very injurious effects when introduced *ab externo*, especially contrasting it with that of serum, which, in the one or two instances that I have tried it (the serum of the blood of man injected into the pleura of a dog) has been rapidly absorbed, without apparently affecting the health of the animal. *A priori*, I need hardly now remark that the removal by absorption of a pus globule in its integrity, is in

---

* The effusion found in all these instances in the pleura which had not received the injection, and in one in even greater quantity than in the pleura which had, seems remarkable. In regard to it, it may be observed that the relative position of the pleuræ of the dog is somewhat peculiar—the right almost communicating with the left beneath the apex of the heart, where at least the two come in contact, constituting the boundary of the compartment which contains the additamentum of lung, noticed by Haller in his "Adversaria." Such a proximity may conduce to an extension of morbid action.

the highest degree improbable—indeed, may it not be said, to be impossible?

It may be objected to these experiments that the pus used was not what is called "healthy pus"—pus free from air*, free from incipient putrefaction. This objection I cannot but allow: I cannot but admit that had pus of the most untainted kind been employed, and the same results obtained, the inference from them would be more reliable. On the other hand, it may be stated, that in a large number of instances (such as those recorded in this chapter) on cellular inflammation, the pus is not of the benignant kind, and not rarely is rather puruloid than true globular pus.

* From "healthy pus" I have never obtained air by the action of the air-pump. See Res. Phy. and Anat., ii., 462.

CHAPTER XII.

ON ANEURISM AND THE DILATATION AND OCCLUSION OF ARTERIES.

Lesions these in a manner cognate.—Statistics of aneurism in the cavalry and infantry and in different climates.—Varieties of, and their localities.—Cases illustrative, with comments.—The constitution most prone to suffer from the disease. —Remarks on its pathology and symptoms, and the dependency of the latter on the seat of the lesion.—Example of spontaneous cure.

THESE lesions being nearly allied, the dilatation of an artery commonly, it may be inferred, preceding its rupture, and the latter often associated with the occlusion of the adjoining vessels, they naturally come to be considered together, and, it is presumed, that the several changes cannot but aid in elucidating each other.

Reflecting on the strained exertions which soldiers on service are occasionally under the necessity of making, it might be expected that they would be more than ordinarily exposed to aneurism. The following table, formed from the army statistical medical reports, shows its degree of frequency among the Dragoon Guards and Dragoons, and infantry during the periods specified, the former serving at home, the latter in our colonies. The aggregate strength is given on account of the smallness of the numbers of those who have experienced the disease.

		Agg. Strength.	Admitted.	Died.
Dragoon Guards, etc.... { from 1st January, 1830, to 31st March, 1837 }		44,611	9	6
Gibraltar ... ... from 1818 to 1836............		60,269	7	5
Malta ... ... from 1817 to 1836............		40,826	8	2
Ionian Islands ... do. do.		70,293	11	4
Bermudas ... ... do. do.		11,781	—	—
Nova Scotia and New Brunswick ... ... do. do.		46,442	11	2
Canada ... ... do. do.		64,280	5	3
West Indies, Windward and Leeward Command ... ... do. do.		86,661	18	10
Black Troops ... ... do. do.		40,934	7	2
Jamaica ... ... do. do.		51,567	17	7
Black Troops ... ... do. do.		5,729	—	—

			Agg. Strength.	Admitted.	Died
Ceylon	do.	do.	42,978	14	2
1st Ceylon Malays ...	from 1818 to 1836		34,630	1	1
Cape of Good Hope ...	do.	do.	22,714	8	3
Hottentot Troops ...	from 1822 to 1834		4,136	1	1
The Mauritius ...	from 1818 to 1836		30,515	4	1
Black Troops ...	from 1825 to 1836		1,395	1	1

Casting up this account, the general results per 10,000 of deaths from aneurism, are the following :—

Cavalry, infantry and black troops ....,....................	0·77
Cavalry	1·34
Infantry	·73
Black troops	·57

Taking another, a later period, from 1st April, 1837, to 31st March, 1847, inclusive, the results as deducible from the following table are somewhat different.

	Agg. Strength.	Admitted.	Died.
Dragoon Guards, etc.............,....,..,..............,........	54,374	23	17
Gibraltar.....................................,...........	33,131	19	12
Malta	21,172	7	5
Ionian Islands	26,201	3	3
Bermudas	11,224	3	2
Nova Scotia and New Brunswick............,.........,........	26,806	3	2
Canada	90,456	14	7

Showing, taking the general results, the deaths per 10,000, to have been,

Cavalry and infantry	1·7
Cavalry.. ...	3·1
Infantry.........................,....................................	1·4

That the cavalry service should be more productive of aneurism than the infantry is, perhaps, what might be expected, keeping in mind the concussions to which the former are exposed. But that the lesion should vary so much in degree of frequency in similar bodies of men at different periods, seemingly irrespective of station, is not what might have been anticipated. Does it not tend to support a conjecture more than once already alluded to, that there may be influences prevailing at different periods acting on the human constitution and productive of certain effects, such as may be witnessed in sporadic as well as in epidemic cases,

Of the cases (inclusive of those of dilatation) of which I have notes, these 49 in number, the following is an analysis :—30 were examples of false aneurism ; 28 were of the aorta, 2 of the femoral artery. Of these 19 were examples of rupture and of death in consequence; 7 burst into the pericardium; 5 into the trachea; 5 into the cavity of the chest; 2 into the cavity of the abdomen; the remaining 9 terminating without a rupture.

The average age of the total number of men affected was 37 years; that of the oldest was 55 (a general officer), of the youngest 24. The average age of those who died laboring under dilatation of the aorta was as high as 49 years; next was that of those in whom death occurred before rupture—viz., 37 years; and lowest, that of those in whom the fatal event was owing to rupture—viz., 35 years.

Neither the averages of age, nor the greatly predominant seat of the disease were such as might *a priori* have been expected. In the instance of infantry soldiers (and they were all with one exception of this class) men whose extremities are so much tasked in marching and the manual exercise, it might be expected that the arteries, at least of the lower limbs, would have been more frequently the seat of the disease, than in persons in private life, following various occupations; but the contrary appears to be the case, and that in a remarkable degree.* The explanation of this singularity I shall not attempt: I would merely ask, can the inordinate action to which the heart of the soldier is almost daily excited, when exercised in heavy marching order, be concerned in rendering the aorta so unduly subject to the malady? It may be thought perhaps that the peculiarity as to situation is more apparent than real, and that were the cases which may have been operated on for aneurism of the extremities taken into account, the anomaly would disappear. This, however, I cannot admit; for, during the whole period of my service, I have known only two or three operations of the kind; and I am not aware of a single man invalided on account of aneurism admitting of operation. As the soldier has a bad reputation for drunkenness, this his failing may be imagined to predispose him to the disease. Referring to the individual cases, I find that the great majority of them have been temperate men, at least not distinguished as intemperate; consequently drunkenness must be dismissed as a cause. Most of them have been remarkable for robustness of frame, and up to a certain time, for general good health, and that often even up to

* See Traite des Maladies des Artères and des Veins, par J. Hodgson, traduit par G. Breschet, i. 103.

the termination of life from the rupture of the aneurism; this a state of health offering a remarkable contrast to that of persons subject to coagulation of blood in the veins. If there be any aneurismal diathesis, is it not marked by abundance of blood, a richness of that fluid, a powerful muscular development, a tendency not to excess, but to a moderate degree, of fat—in brief, by qualities denoting high vital action, high vascular pressure? In a large proportion of the cases these qualities were conspicuous. The cases I propose to offer are selected from the whole, as most noteworthy and illustrative. The first I shall give is a remarkable one, and may be taken as a kind of connecting link between diseases of the veins and arteries.

Case 1.—Of dilatation of foramen ovale, complicated with great dyspnœa.—M. Coney, ætat. 37; 45th Foot; admitted 14th March, 1823, died 24th March.—This man was sent home invalided from Ceylon, on account of organic disease of the heart of two years' duration, marked by constant dyspnœa, by inordinate action of that organ, visible externally, and by some lividity of lips and countenance, as if from venous congestion. On admission, the pulse was quick and small; there was no throbbing of the jugular veins; no pyrexia; the skin cool. Whilst under treatment he was subject to paroxysms of dyspnœa, mostly at night. These increased in severity, and also the dyspnœa, the pulse becoming quicker, feebler, and intermitting, with suppression of expectoration and great debility; the breathing was laborious; he was unable to lie down. Death was preceded by insensibility, and that, the latter, by delirium. The treatment was chiefly palliative. In Ceylon, according to the abstract of his case, he was always relieved by blood-letting. After his arrival here, it was once employed, without marked benefit. The blood was slightly buffed, but not cupped.

Autopsy 20 hours after death. Body very muscular. The lungs, not collapsed, were both redder and heavier than natural; inferiorly, they were gorged with blood. The trachea and large bronchial tubes were very red; the latter were covered with puruloid exudation. The pericardium contained 4 oz. of fluid, which, after a short exposure to the air, coagulated and formed a thin jelly; 3 oz. of a similar fluid were collected in the left pleura. The heart was somewhat larger than usual. The right auricle and ventricle contained coagulated blood and fibrinous concretion. Both were unusually capacious and thick, as was also the auricular-ventricular passage. What was most remarkable was the absence of the fossa ovalis; the two auricles freely communicated; the opening between them was sufficiently large to admit the four fingers and thumb pressed together, so far as the first joint; the margin of the passage was smooth and rounded; its form nearly circular. The pulmonary artery was unusually large, so too were the pulmonary veins. The left side of the heart was proportionally small; the passage from the auricle into the ventricle small; the parieties of the ventricle very little if at all thicker than those of the right. The aorta was smaller than natural; at its origin it was only just large enough to admit my forefinger with a little distension. The venæ cavæ were much larger than usual. The brain was apparently sound; there was a minute quantity of bloody fluid in its ventricles. There was no obvious disease in any of the abdominal viscera.

I have stated in another work (Res. Anat. and Physiol., i.,

305), that an oblique, a valvular opening in the fossa ovalis is so frequent an occurrence as to give the idea of its being normal. I have found it to vary in size from an aperture barely admitting a probe, to one readily receiving the little finger; and this without any appreciable influence on the respiratory functions. Probably, in the instance just described the aperture was always unduly large, and not valvular, so allowing of the flow of blood from one auricle into the other, which flow itself might gradually have had the effect of enlarging it more and more, until diseased action resulted: the right and left cavities of the heart, the aorta and the pulmonary artery and veins and the venæ cavæ as gradually becoming altered in their proportions; and the balance altogether overturned. Judging from the state of the air-passages and the puruloid exudation on them, may it not be inferred that death in this case was the conjoint result of imperfect oxygenation of the blood and of bronchial inflammation?

The next cases, four in number, are examples of dilatation without rupture, approaching in character to the true aneurism of authors, and not so much fatal by themselves as by the diseases associated with, and, if not engendered, certainly promoted and aggravated by them.

Case 2.—Of hypertrophy of heart, with irregular dilatation of the aorta.—J. Wood, ætat. 40; 36th Foot; admitted 3rd November, 1836; died 3rd December.—This man, of 21 years' service, is reported to have had ague repeatedly, and an attack of " acute pulmonic disease" from which he never perfectly recovered. On admission, sent home invalided, he was laboring under habitual dyspnœa, with general œdema, and some effusion into the abdomen, indicated by slight fluctuation. The pulse was 86, hard and jerking; the heart's action was diffused with bellow's sound, and so strong that the head moved conspicuously with each pulsation. In the recumbent posture percussion on the right side gave a clear sound, on the left a dull one. There was slight cough, with muco-purulent expectoration. The appetite was good; sleep little disturbed. While under treatment he had now and then slight febrile attacks of an ephemeral kind. He thought himself improving, yet the dropsical swelling continued to increase. On the 2nd December, after rising, he experienced a slight rigor; the pulse was 104; the breathing difficult. On the following day his pulse was 80; his breathing easy; the heart's action moderate; no bruit. He died suddenly at the time of the evening visit. The instant he became insensible—and it was in an instant—no pulse could be felt.

Autopsy 36 hours after death. Not emaciated; partial anasarca, especially of the penis and scrotum. A small plate of bone was found in the falciform process of the dura mater. The left vertebral artery was larger than the right, and its coats thickened. The pericardium contained 6 oz. of serous fluid. There were some very small bony concretions in the pulmonary pleura and in the parenchyma of the lungs, which were otherwise pretty sound. The heart was rather more than twice its natural size. All its cavities were large. The walls of the left ventricle were much thickened. The valves of the aorta were thickened and contracted; wart-like excrescences were attached to two of them. The aorta was more or less diseased throughout; its inner surface had lost its smoothness; in two places, these in its ascending portion, small pouches had formed, as if the beginning of aneurism. One of these, when divided, showed the inner coat thickened, the middle coat almost entirely absorbed, the outer condensed. There was coagulated blood in the descending aorta; and a good deal of blood in the body generally. The abdominal cavity contained a pint of serum. The liver weighed 4 lbs., and was rather pale. The gall-bladder and its ducts were œdematous. The spleen was about twice its natural volume, soft and friable; the pancreas large, and also the kidneys; their surface spotted red.

In this instance we witness disease of heart and aorta super-vening on an impaired worn-out constitution, after repeated attacks of ague (these leaving their mark in an enlarged spleen), and occasioning death, may it not be surmised, considering how suddenly it took place, from exhausted cardiac power, the heart ceasing to act.

Case 3.—Of dilatation of aorta, complicated with emphysema and a tuberculated state of lungs.—P. Mullin, ætat. 41; 8th Foot; admitted into regimental hospital, Malta, 22nd August, 1836; died 16th September.—This man, a non-commissioned officer, of 25 years' service in various climates, had for a considerable time been subject to affections of the chest, and for three years to palpitation of heart. His symptoms on admission were those of advanced pulmonary consumption, combined with those of cardiac disease, such as pectoriloquy (this on left side of chest), muco-purulent expectoration tinged with blood, bruit de soufflet, etc. No improvement took place. The expectoration became fetid; the palpitation more severe. He gra-dually sank. During the three last days, when he had become very weak, he had little suffering. The treatment was merely palliative.

Autopsy 36 hours after death. Much emaciated. With the exception of the fornix being rather soft, the brain was of natural appearance. The right lung, adhering at its apex, was exceedingly distended and emphysematous. In its superior lobe there were a few small clusters of granular tubercles. The left lung was very firmly adhering, and this generally; it was very heavy. There were several cavities in its superior lobe, containing a reddish fetid fluid; the largest was capable of holding a walnut. This and the inferior lobe abounded in tubercles in different stages of progress; hardly any part of either was pervious to air, being more or less hepa-tized or indurated by tubercular deposit. Its pleural covering was much thickened. The pericardium contained 4 oz. of serum. The heart was rather large; its structure pretty natural. The pulmonary artery was large; the aorta very large, exceedingly distended, and this from near its origin to where it becomes descending. Just above its valves, it was 4 inches in circumference; where most dilated, $6\frac{1}{2}$ inches; and where its enlargement terminated, $2\frac{1}{2}$ inches. In the most dilated portion, a mass of crassamentum and fibrin adhered to it. The rounded form of the mass conveyed the idea that it must have been formed during life. Underneath the spot to which it was attached there was an elliptical space about the size of a sixpence, rough and fibrous, showing a deficiency of the inner and middle arterial coat. Generally the inner coat was smooth, but much thickened; the middle coat very thin, and in some places deficient. The innominata, the left common carotid and subclavian arteries, were of large size, and their inner surface unequal; the diameter of each (not including the innominata) was about $\frac{1}{2}$ inch; the space between them was less than $\frac{1}{4}$ inch. There was no well marked disease of any of the abdominal viscera; no ulceration of the intestines.

This case is chiefly noteworthy for its unusual complications— viz., granular tubercles and extreme emphysema in one lung, and softening tubercles and tubercular excavations in the other, with a dilated and diseased aorta.

Case 4.—Of dilatation of the aorta, and of incipient aneurism.—J. Davies, ætat. 40; 3rd R.V.B.; admitted 9th July, 1821; died 13th October.—This man's health began to fail in 1813. Four months ago his last illness began. On admission he labored under great dyspnœa; his face was bloated; there was œdema of legs and feet; he could not lie down except his head and shoulders were much raised; the sitting posture, the body bent forward, was easiest. His pulse was quick and strong, but not irregular; there was much thirst; anorexia; scanty urine. He experienced some relief from V.S., the use of purgatives with opiates, and afterwards from diuretics. His complaint advanced, every now and then becoming aggravated, but with little change of symptoms. Vomiting latterly was of frequent occurrence; and occasionally he had paroxysms of pain at scrobiculus cordis, as if from a gall-stone in transitu.

Autopsy (time not specified). Much emaciated; lower extremities much swollen from œdema. Each pleura contained about a quart of serous fluid. There was much œdema of both lungs. The pericardium was adhering, and that generally—on one side to the diaphragm and lungs, on the other to the heart—and so closely as to require for its separation careful dissection. The heart was a little enlarged; the left auricle and ventricle considerably; the right, on the contrary, were rather smaller than natural; the walls and the columnæ carneæ of the former were thickened. The aorta, from its origin to where it becomes descending, was much enlarged and diseased. Where most so, its circumference was about 7·3 inches; where least, about 6 inches. At the upper portion of its arch an additional dilatation was found. This was a lateral one, a pouch capable of holding a lemon. It was lined with a deposit of soft lymph, and was bounded apparently by the external fibrous coat condensed. There were no traces in it of either the inner or middle arterial coat. In other parts of the aorta the inner coat remained, but much thickened, as it was also in the descending trunk, even to its bifurcation; and here and there it was ossified. The abdominal cavity contained a small quantity of serous fluid. There was an adhesion between the right lobe of the liver and the peritoneum. In the parenchyma of this lobe a sac was found, of an oval form, measuring 3·5 inches by 2·5, of cartilaginous appearance and firmness. It contained a thick, white, soft matter, consisting of phosphate and carbonate of lime (the latter in larger proportion than in bone), and of an albuminous matter. The gall-bladder was unusually large, and the ducts much dilated. The other abdominal viscera were apparently sound.

In this instance the principal lesions appear to have been two, œdema of the lungs and dilatation of the aorta, with a morbid state of its coats; the latter, probably by impeding the free circulation of the blood, conducing to the former; and that, the œdema, the cause of death. The state of the right lobe of the liver and the distension of the gall bladder may account for the pain supposed to have been owing to a gall stone.

Case 5.—Of dilatation of the aorta and aneurism, complicated with pneumonia and bronchitis.—P. O'Brien, ætat. 32; 75th Foot; admitted 13th October, 1837; died 25th October.—This man's illness commenced about eighteen months ago at the Cape of Good Hope, from whence he is just returned. Its chief feature was reported to have been inordinate action of heart, with a very rapid pulse, seldom less than 120 in the minute. On admission here, in addition to the palpitation of heart, he had symptoms of acute bronchitis contracted a few days ago, marked by mucous râles. He rapidly became worse. On the 21st he was in a state bordering on suffocation, from effusion into the bronchia; he was then incoherent. On the following day and the next he was easier and a little revived, and took some food. His pulse was 105, and soft. At 3 a.m. of the 25th, he had a fresh accession of dyspnœa, which rapidly ended in death. The treatment consisted of antimonials, blisters, etc.

Autopsy 32 hours after death. Not emaciated. The right lung did not collapse, was closely attached to the spine, and was for most part hepatized: it weighed 3 lbs. Its bronchia were nearly full of thick muco-purulent fluid. In each of its lobes there were a few clusters of granular tubercles. The left lung weighed 1½ lb. Its bronchia, like those of the right, were red, and obstructed with muco-purulent fluid. The trachea also was very red. The left ventricle of the heart was rather thicker than natural. In the ascending aorta there were several aneurismal pouches. The first was just above the semi-lunar valves, and was capable of holding the half of a boy's playing marble. One, at the upper part of the arch, was capable of holding an orange; it was full of coagulated blood, and pressed on the trachea and on the innominata. The great vessels rising from the arch were somewhat contracted at their mouths by a thickening of their inner coat. The ascending aorta was not increased in size generally, but considerably, as it seemed, in length: for whilst its circumference (measured slit open) was 2½ inches, the innominata was 3½ inches distant from the semi-lunar valves. The larger pouch was a false aneurism; the smaller appeared to be destitute of a middle coat, with the inner coat thickened and the outer more or less condensed. There was no distinct lesion of any of the abdominal viscera.

Judging from the contents of the false aneurism, it was probably recent; and from its position it may have been an aggravating if not a predisposing cause of the fatal disease—pneumonia complicated with bronchitis.

The following five cases, examples of false aneurism, more deserving of the name of true, all opened into the pericardium, necessarily occasioning death, and that suddenly, and in all but one almost without any warning or preceding serious ailment.

Case 6.—Of aneurism of the aorta, bursting into the pericardium.—J, Hunt, ætat. 36; 7th R. F.; died suddenly in barracks in Malta, 9th May, 1834.—This man up to the time of his death was considered in good health. During a period of 18 years he had been only twice in hospital, once for continued fever, once for intermittent, both mild. His only known ailment was "fits," for which he had never been under medical treatment; they were said to have been of an epileptic kind, slight and of short duration, and commonly brought on by intemperance. About an hour after dinner, whilst reading, he suddenly fell from his seat and instantly expired. By an order from the coroner, an examination of the body was made by a civil surgeon, a Maltese. In his report, of four pages foolscap, he stated his opinion that death was owing to sanguineous apoplexy, having found much blood in the vessels of the brain and some transparent fluid in the ventricles. The dissection by him was carried no further, indeed it was limited to two incisions laying open the cavities mentioned.

Autopsy 24 hours after death. The body muscular and rather fat; the limbs rigid. The substance of the brain, and especially of the cerebellum, was softer than natural; the fornix was so soft as to be almost pultaceous. The basilar artery contained a loose concretion, which was readily pressed from one part to another; it was spherical, about the size of a large pin's head, hard, of cartilaginous appearance and firmness, smooth and slightly shining.* The right lung was generally adhering, the left partially; both contained a good deal of blood. The bronchia and trachea seemed unduly red. The pericardium was very tense, distended with a large quantity of reddish serum and crassamentum. There was a good deal of blood similarly coagulated in the right ventricle and auricle and vena cava, but none in the left cavities of the heart. The heart was free from disease. The ascending aorta was somewhat enlarged; its inner coat irregularly thickened, its middle coat atrophied; its outer thickened and indurated. About an inch above the coronary arteries a small aneurismal sac was detected; it was of an irregular form, of about the size of a walnut, and had burst into the pericardium. A little higher another pouch was found; it was capable of holding a filbert; the lining membrane of both was rough and continuous with the inner coat of the aorta. The descending aorta was of natural size and was sound. There was much pultaceous food colored by wine in the stomach; portions of its lining membrane were red. Near the cardia and throughout the great arch, this membrane was very soft and easily detached. The duodenum contained some brownish chyme; the jejunum some whitish, approaching to chyle; the ileum some yellowish soft matter; the cœcum some fecal matter. The inner coat of the jejunum was very red, as if injected, and without softening. There was no appearance of Peyer's glands in the ileum. There were many solitary glands in it and in the jejunum. The thoracic duct was empty. The spleen was rather soft; it was gorged with blood which had coagulated. The liver, the pancreas, and kidneys contained a good deal of blood; they too had the appearance of having been injected.

As this man just before death was apparently in perfect health, all his functions seemingly well performed, I have been somewhat particular in describing the appearance and contents of the stomach and intestines, these, it may be inferred, being in their normal condition. The death so sudden, considering its cause, hardly needs a comment. With other facts of the like kind, it seems to prove how very devoid of sensibility are the parts which were the seat of the rupture. May not the moveable concretion in the basilar artery have been concerned in the "fits" of an "epileptic kind," to which this man was subject?

Case 7.—Of hæmorrhage into the pericardium, with aneurism of the aorta, without visible rupture.—J. Hoyle, ætat. 30; R. B.; died suddenly on parade at Malta, 18th February, 1829.—This man on the day of his death was supposed to be in perfect health; he had dined heartily, and was one of a fatigue party employed in carrying the dinners of the men on guard; after which, at 4 p.m., he went on parade for drill. After being in the ranks two minutes, he suddenly staggered forward, wheeled to the

* Before the blow-pipe it burnt like cartilage and yielded no appreciable residual ash.

right, and uttering a low groan, fell down insensible; a few respirations preceded death. The assistant-surgeon was present, and within five minutes he was seen by him. A vein was opened in each arm; only a few drops of blood escaped. It was ascertained that about three months before, when cutting wood, he was struck by a large piece in the left arm and side, and knocked down "stunned." He presently recovered. No report of it was made at the time to the surgeon. He continued to do his duty well; but he occasionally said to his comrades that "he was a gone man," but without explaining why.

Autopsy 17 hours after death. Body stout and muscular. The substance of the brain was healthy. The vessels of the dura mater were much distended with blood, which flowed from them when they were divided. The lungs collapsed the instant the thorax was opened. They were of a dark red hue, especially their inferior portion, where the blood had gravitated. The bronchial tubes were red and "unusually vascular." The thoracic duct was large and distended with chyle, of a slight milky appearance and having suspended in it minute oil-globules, which were distinct to the naked eye. Every part of the body abounded in blood; it flowed from all the vessels divided; was of a dark color, darker than common venous blood. No coagulum was seen except in the pericardium. The pericardium was very much distended; it contained 16 oz. of serum and 8 oz. of crassamentum, this of moderate consistence and quite free from buffy coat. The venæ cavæ nearest the heart and the right sinus venosus were moderately distended with blood; the right ventricle contained little, the left cavities very little. The opening into the pericardium was carefully sought for, but in vain.* Contiguous to the left sinus venosus, an aneurismal sac was detected protruding into it, its parieties thin but entire; it communicated by a large orifice with the aorta, just where it becomes descending. The sac contained some liquid blood and was lined with a very little fibrin; in size it was about equal to an orange; its inner coat was rough and was continuous with the inner coat of the aorta, which was also rough; no middle coat could be found in it. The aorta was diseased throughout; the ascending was a little enlarged as was also the descending so far as the cæliac. The inner coat was irregularly thickened; the middle was yellower than natural and irregularly thinner; in some places it had nearly disappeared, whilst the outer coat had become almost cartilaginous. In the abdomen it was in places œdematous; its vasa vasorum were unusually red, as if injected, and here and there on its cellular sheath there were spots of ecchymosis. The pericardium was stained red, as were also all the parts with which the blood was in contact. The body was cold; the thermometer at the time was about 60°; during the night it might have been so low as 52. The stomach showed the hour-glass contraction. The intestines were all of a reddish hue, of a soft, flabby appearance, and their vessels much injected with red blood.

That in this case there was a tendency to hæmorrhage, however it may be explained, seems to have been indicated by the partial ecchymosis on the aorta; and, may it not be added, by the abundance of blood in the body and the fulness of the vessels.

* Emptied of blood, it was washed; and although there was some blood and that liquid in the heart and great vessels, none could be seen oozing into the pericardium. The auricles were inflated and the coronary veins and arteries were followed, but equally without success, leading to the inference that the blood which had collected had come from minute vessels.
A man of the Rifle Brigade died suddenly in Malta in 1827. The pericardium was found distended with coagulated blood, about 12 oz.; a large coronary vein was ruptured; the portion of vein, anterior to the ulcerated opening into the pericardium, contained shreddy lymph.

As the blood in the pericardium was coagulated and like healthy blood, its quality probably was not in fault.

Case 8.—Of aneurism of aorta, bursting into the pericardium.—M. M'Innes, ætat. 34; 42nd Foot; found dead in bed in barrack in Malta, October 14, 1833.—This man for many years had had uninterrupted good health. The day before his death he made a good dinner. About 6 p.m. he complained to a comrade of pain in the region of the stomach; it soon ceased. At tatoo-beat he was seen cleaning his appointments for the following morning. After going to bed, he spoke to the soldier in the adjoining bed on some indifferent matter. At 6 a.m. the next day he was found dead and cold; the limbs in natural position, the countenance tranquil.

Autopsy at 11 a.m. The body very stout. The vessels of the brain were generally very turgid with blood. The arachnoid was slightly opaque, and was raised in some places by a little fluid effused between it and the pia mater. There was a good deal of serosity in the lateral ventricles and at the base of the brain. The lungs did not collapse. Some blood was contained in their inferior portions, and some frothy fluid in the bronchia. The pericardium was distended with serum and crassamentum, together about two pints. The blood was found to have entered by a very minute aperture, barely admitting a bristle, in the sack of an aneurism of the aorta, situated just above its origin. The heart was normal; there was no blood in its cavities. The jugular veins were distended with blood. The aneurismal sac was capable of holding a small orange, and was lined unequally with layers of reddish fibrin. It pressed on the pulmonary artery, and that artery seemed to form a part of its boundary; where they were in contact the inner coat of the artery was discolored greyish. At the spot where the sac had penetrated into the pericardium, there was an appearance of ulceration, limited to a space that might be covered with the nail of the little finger. The opening into the aneurism from the aorta was circular, and about $\frac{1}{2}$ inch in diameter. The aorta generally was not enlarged. Its inner coat to a small extent, two or three inches above the semi-lunar valves, was partially thickened and opaque. The abdominal viscera were sound.

It may, perhaps, be asked—Was the pain of stomach that was complained of some hours before death any wise connected with the approaching rupture of the aneurism? Considering how short was its duration, and how well the man felt after, may it not be inferred that it was merely casual, and independent of the lesion in progress?

Case 9.—Of aneurism of aorta, penetrating into the pericardium.—J. Stars, ætat 29; 38th Regiment; admitted into regimental hospital, Canterbury, 23rd October, 1836; died 1st November.—According to the report made by the regimental surgeon, this man was considered healthy, "always *marching* and doing his duty without complaint." When admitted into hospital, he had slight pain of back, and acute pains referred to the shoulders and arms; the pulse 76. On the 1st November the surgeon, called suddenly to see him, found him in *articulo mortis;* he expired a few minutes after. There had been no previous alarm.

Autopsy 6 hours after death. Body stout. The lungs were healthy. The pericardium was distended with dark fluid blood and some coagula, together about two pints. The aorta was a little enlarged; the inner coat of the ascending vessels was irregularly thickened; the middle coat was unduly thin. A small aneurism was found close to the aortic valves, between them and the mouths of the coronary arteries. It was rather larger than a chestnut; it projected, pressing on the left auricle, and partially obstructing the auricular-ventricular passage. The opening into it from the aorta was about ¼ inch in diameter; it contained a little adhering fibrin. About half an inch higher, a larger aneurism was detected, one about the size of an orange, but nearly pear-shaped. It communicated with the aorta by a circular opening, barely large enough to admit a goose-quill, and with the pericardium by an aperture in its side little larger than the one described. This aperture, judging from its appearance, was chiefly formed by the ulcerative process. The sac was of cartilaginous firmness, and, where thickest, as much as a quarter of an inch thick. It contained some buff-colored fibrin of firm consistence, closely adhering to its base, and some black coagulated blood. This second aneurism was detected at Fort Pitt, where the parts above described were sent to be prepared for the Museum.

As regards the pains experienced in this case, the same question as in the preceding may be asked, as to their being premonitory, or casual and independent of the aneurism.

Case 10.—Of aneurism of aorta, opening into the pericardium.—J. Sellars, ætat. 40; 18th Foot; admitted 19th May, 1836; died 22nd May.—This man, of 20 years' service, had, it is stated, good health till about two years ago, since when he had been almost constantly suffering from various ailments, such as rheumatism acute and chronic, acute catarrh, and lastly anasarca. On admission here on return from India, his breathing was oppressed, preventing his sleeping at night; the legs œdematous; urine scanty; pulse 100 and small; none at the right wrist—according to report it had ceased there about a year ago. Using mild diuretic medicine he experienced some relief. He died suddenly.

Autopsy 33 hours after death. Body robust. The pericardium was found distended with serum and crassamentum, together about two pints. The heart was large. The mitral and semi-lunar valves of the aorta were thickened. A little above the latter, an aneurism was detected, about the size of a small orange, nearly filled with fibrinous matter. Another, and greatly larger, was found above it, including the great arch. Its sac was very large, and descending, it had burst into the pericardium. It was nearly filled with firm fibrin. An included fibrinous mass, about the size of the fist, pressed on the sternum. The innominata and left carotid, rising from the sac, were impervious, closed by lymph. The left subclavian and right carotid and subclavian were unobstructed. The coats of the aorta throughout its whole extent were more or less diseased—the inner coat rough and thickened, the middle coat wasted. The left pleura contained about 3 pints of serum; the right about 2 pints. The left lung was very small and condensed, partly from the pressure of the aneurismal tumor, and partly from the fluid effused. It weighed less than a pound, was destitute of air, and consequently sank in water; its parenchyma seemed sound. The right lung was but little compressed; portions of it were slightly œdematous. The bronchia, trachea, and larynx were redder than natural. The liver weighed 3½ lbs; its section was nutmeg-like. The other abdominal viscera were tolerably sound.

This case offers a great contrast compared with the preceding, and this chiefly owing to the bulk of the aneurism, and its pressure on important parts, nerves and vessels, occasioning probably the pains experienced, and doubtlessly the effusions into the pleuræ.

The four following are examples of the same kind as the last, but opening into the air-passages, accompanied during life with more derangement of health, especially of the respiratory organs, and yet almost as sudden in their fatal effect.

Case 11.—Of aneurism of aorta, perforating the left bronchus.—J. Clarke, ætat. 28; 44th Regiment; admitted into regimental hospital, Malta, 23rd March, 1834; died 9th April.—This man was in good health until the 1st March. He then came under treatment for slight catarrh, with some uneasiness of chest. The digestive organs were at the same time deranged, and he had pain of left side of head. There was no pyrexia and his pulse was moderate. On the 19th he was discharged to duty. On the 23rd he was re-admitted with nearly the same ailments, excepting that he had no headache, and that the pectoral symptoms were more marked, having cough with wheezing asthmatic breathing, and also great derangement of stomach and pain in the left hypochondrium. His pulse was 74 and soft. He was blooded and blistered without relief. About the 6th April his respiration became more difficult, and from time to time he experienced severe paroxysms of dyspnœa and cough. On the 8th, in the evening, there was a great aggravation of all the symptoms, with orthopnœa and ineffectual attempts to expectorate. Life was protracted with much suffering until next day, when he died at 6 a.m., as if suffocated. About a minute before, he brought up about 4 ounces of dark blood.

Autopsy 17 hours after death. Not emaciated. A coagulum of blood was found in the trachea completely plugging it up; it extended into both lungs through some of the principal bronchial tubes. In the right lung it reached even the minute branches, so that when a section was made, it had the appearance of extravasated blood, but with this difference, that the cell-structure was distended with air; the blood was confined to the bronchia. This lung, free from any adhesion, was unusually distended with air; there was no collapse of it, as if the blood had been poured out during inspiration, and had stopped the egress of air. The left lung was very generally adhering; its structure was pretty natural. In the trachea, about midway, a small spiculum of bony matter projected from the cartilage through the mucous membrane. In the left bronchus, in its upper portion, there were two fungus-like growths, of a soft, spongy consistence, through which it was found that blood had oozed from the sac of an aneurism. In one of them, after 24 hours' maceration, an opening was detected capable of admitting a crow-quill. The heart was normal. The aorta at its origin, and until it became descending, was rather larger than natural; its inner coat in one or two places was thickened. The first portion of the descending aorta was much diseased. Just below the origin of the left subclavian, a false aneurism was found; it was about the size of a small orange, with a circular aperture of about an inch in diameter, and was nearly full of a firm grey mass of fibrin; at its fundus, its sac was very thin, and there it was ruptured opening into the bronchus; below this aneurism there were two very small ones, the largest about the size of half a boy's playing marble. Where they were situated the inner coat of the aorta adjoining was thickened, the middle absorbed, or nearly so, the outer rather condensed; beyond, the appearance of the vessel was pretty natural. The stomach and intestines were much distended; the intestines chiefly with air; the stomach with a large quantity of blackish fluid, which derived its color probably from some blood swallowed and darkened by acid; the great arch was dark red, as if stained by blood. The aorta and vessels generally were stained red, though the body had not been kept by five hours so long as one that had died of phthisis, in which the vessels in contact with blood were free from stain. The 8th nerve could be only followed a little way;

where it had been subjected to the pressure of the aneurismal tumor, it could not be found, as if obliterated, and where it first came in contact with the tumor, it was flattened. The abdominal viscera generally were of natural appearance.

This case is very noteworthy for its symptoms in connection with their cause, an aneurismal tumor pressing on the windpipe, and finally bursting into it, and pressing also on the 8th nerve, occasioning its absorption; and thus, may it not be said, giving rise to two trains of morbid actions, one of the respiratory, the other of the digestive organs? It is remarkable how little the heart was affected and how the local disease advanced without emaciation, or pyrexia.

Case 12.—Aneurism of the aorta opening into the trachea.—P. Langan, ætat. 39; 88th F.; admitted into regimental hospital, Corfu, 17th June, 1827; died 26th August.—This man when admitted complained of pain of chest, of three weeks' duration, accompanied with cough and some pyrexia. Between the 17th June and the 29th he had been twice blooded copiously to the amount of 150 oz. on account of exacerbations. Between the last date and the 4th August there was an increase of pyrexia with pain of head and nausea. On the 4th, when there was some abatement of these symptoms, he experienced pain in the inferior part of the trachea. 40 leeches; relief. On the 8th the cough and dyspnœa were more severe, especially when lying on his back. The skin was hot; the pulse 106. Little change occurred until the 14th, when there was a great aggravation of the pectoral symptoms, suffocation threatening from mucus collecting copiously in the air-passages. On the 18th the expectoration was abundant and was tinged with blood; and so on to the 26th, when he was startled out of his sleep by a violent fit of coughing. He expectorated two clots of blood; a gush of fluid blood followed, about half a pint, and instantly he expired.

Autopsy 6 hours after death. Muscular; sub-emaciated. There were bubbles of air in the veins of the pia mater. The arachnoid was slightly opaque. The large blood-vessels were rather turgid. There was a good deal of fluid in the ventricles and at the base of the brain. The lungs did not collapse. The left was sound; so too was the greater part of the right; the exception was at its upper portion, where it was pressed on by an aneurismal tumor; its principal bronchial branches were full of coagulated blood. In the trachea, just above its bifurcation, three small perforations were detected communicating with an aneurismal sac; two were large enough to admit a surgeon's probe. The mucous surface adjoining was rough, as if from ulcerative absorption. The heart was normal, except that the corpora Aurantii were slightly ossified. Both auricles and ventricles were empty. In the aorta, a few lines from its origin, a small pouch was found, equal in size to about the half of a boy's playing marble. An inch higher there was a false aneurism, that which had burst into the trachea; it was equal in bulk to a large orange; its orifice admitted the little finger; and it was full of laminated coagulum. The whole of the ascending, and a portion of the descending aorta were larger than natural, and where most dilated, as in the instance of the smaller pouch, the inner coat was thickened, the middle atrophied. The left carotid and subclavian arteries and the innominata were rather contracted, and their inner coat was slightly rough. The stomach exhibited the hour-glass contraction. The transverse and ascending colon were distended with air; other portions of this intestine were contracted. The urinary bladder was empty and contracted; on its inner surface there were patches of redness and of œdema approaching to vesication. There was strangury during the last two or three days, probably from a little lytta in an ointment used to keep up a discharge from an old blistered surface.

Though this case in its lesions so much resembled the last, yet there was a marked difference in their symptoms. Was the pyrexia in this, and its absence in the other, connected with a difference as to the mode of penetration between the aneurism and the trachea; in the one seemingly proceeding from the sac by an ulcerative process; in the other, with more of ulceration, proceeding from the trachea to the sac?

Case 13.—Of aneurism of aorta, opening into the left bronchus.—G. Darcey, ætat. 24; 73rd Foot; died suddenly at Malta, 28th September, 1832.—This man, an hospital orderly, was somewhat delicate and short-winded, and in consequence was considered hardly equal to any severe duty. After making a good dinner, and when tired with running about the yard in sport with his comrades, he lay down on a form in the kitchen. There, whilst smoking a cigar, a stream of blood suddenly gushed from his mouth. He ran towards the hospital with his hand to his mouth, the blood continuing to flow, and in the act dropped down and expired.

Autopsy 12 hours after death. Tolerably stout and muscular. The lungs did not collapse. With the exception of being spotted dark red, which was found to be from coagulated blood, they appeared healthy in structure. There was a little reddish fluid in the bronchia, and a good deal of liquid blood in the trachea. In the left bronchus a small ulcerated opening was detected which communicated with the aorta. It was just large enough to admit the end of a blunt probe. By its side there was a minute papilla, little larger than a pin's head. It was covered with coagulable lymph, which yielding to the gentle pressure of the probe, exposed another opening into the aorta. The pericardium contained about half an ounce of serum. The heart was normal; all its cavities empty. The aorta, immediately below its arch, was dilated, forming a shallow pouch or sinus where the communication with the bronchus had taken place. Both at the arch and a little way below the aneurism, as well as immediately round it, the coats of the artery were diseased; the inner generally very much thickened, and also the outer, and condensed, whilst the middle was very thin or entirely deficient. The stomach contained some coagulated blood of a dark brownish hue. Its mucous coat was red. In the duodenum there were some small softened masses of beef. There was about half a tea-spoonful of dilute yellow bile in the gall-bladder. There was a little milk-like chyle in the lacteals. With the exception of some adhesions, the abdominal viscera appeared sound.

Was the aneurismal pouch in this instance a true aneurism, *i.e.* merely a dilatation of the aorta? It seems doubtful; and yet its lining membrane was continuous with the inner coat of that vessel. But, it may be asked, were it of the character of a false aneurism, would not its lining membrane be similar? So far as I have been able to ascertain such is always the case. Comparing this case with the two preceding, though there is a certain similarity in the lesions, yet how great is the difference, as regards symptoms, in the effects! In this last instance no uneasiness seems even to have been produced. Was this owing to the smallness of the dilatation, and to its exercising very little pressure on any important organ? May it not be inferred, considering how little blood was found in the lungs, that the sudden and great gush of blood was simultaneous with an act of expiration?

Case 14.—Aneurism of aorta, opening into the trachea.—W. Kirkwood, ætat. 33; 92nd Foot; admitted 15th February, 1839; died 27th February.—This man was sent home invalided from Malta, on account of dyspnœa, with pain of chest, which began in July, 1827. On admission he complained chiefly of difficulty of breathing, and of pain in the left side of chest. The action of the heart was inordinate; there was a distinct bruit de soufflet; the pulse of the left radial artery was much stronger than that of the right, and the pulsation on the left side of the neck was unusually strong and high up. There were sonorous râles over the greater part of the chest. His countenance was sallow; the lips occasionally livid. He was unable to sleep in the recumbent posture. After ten days, as he felt easier, he was allowed to go out of hospital. On the morning of the 27th, when standing in the open air, in conversation, he experienced a sudden fit of coughing, which was followed by profuse hæmorrhage from the mouth, and that in a very few minutes by death.

Autopsy 3 hours after death. Body of spare habit, but not emaciated. The calvaria was very thick and heavy. The inner table of the frontal and of the right parietal bone exhibited several small depressions, as if from absorption; the corresponding spots in the dura mater were unusually thin. The inner coat of the internal carotids was very soft and easily detached. A strong transverse band was found in the basilar artery.* The lungs did not collapse. They were distended with air in part, and in part were injected with blood. There was a good deal of blood in the bronchia. The left pleura contained 6 oz. of bloody serum; the pericardium 2 oz. of serum. The heart was large; the left ventricle was considerably thickened; it contained a little coagulated blood; the right ventricle was empty; its cavity was not enlarged like that of the left, but rather, it seemed, diminished. The ascending aorta was very much dilated, so much so that at its origin it pressed on the pulmonary artery; where this pressure was, there the inner coat of this vessel had become of an opaque white. A very small false aneurism was detected, which had opened into the trachea close to its bifurcation. The perforation was barely large enough to admit a probe. The minute sac contained no clot or adhering fibrin. The arch of the aorta was greatly dilated, especially at its summit; it reached nearly the thyroid gland. The right subclavian and the right carotid rose directly from the aorta. At their origin they were a little contracted, as was also the left carotid. The left subclavian, for the space of an inch, was so much dilated as to admit the thumb. The aortic coats were exceedingly irregular; the inner coat thickened in many places, the middle thinned, the outer thickened.

In this instance again the symptoms were somewhat different, and, may it not be inferred, not so much owing to the minute size of the aneurism as to the generally dilated state of the aorta.

---

* See my Res. Anat. and Physiol. vol. i., p. 301, for some remarks on this peculiarity.

388 DISEASES OF THE ARMY.

Had not the perforation taken place, life probably might have been protracted many years. An hour and half after death the jugular vein and carotid artery were examined for air; none was found in either. The blood that flowed was liquid; it presently coagulated. Mixed with potassa, fumes were produced on the approach of properly diluted muriatic acid. The following day the mixture of the blood and alkali gave off a strong *pure* smell of ammonia, suggestive of the one favoring not only the evolution but also the formation of the other.

Of the next three cases, two are examples of aneurism bursting into the cavity of the chest, one of a rupture into the cavity of the abdomen.

Case 15.—Of aneurism of aorta, opening into the lung.—R. Walker, ætat. 28; 28th F.; admitted into regimental hospital, Corfu, 25th December, 1827; died 11th January, 1828.—This man for two years had been subject to pulmonary ailments gradually increasing in severity, with the addition latterly of pain in the left side of chest and of muco-purulent expectoration tinged with blood. When last admitted into hospital, on the 25th December, there was much febrile excitement; with urgent dyspnœa, bloody expectoration, a hard pulse. V.S. 24 oz.; antiphlogistic treatment; relief. On the 30th there was an increase of all the symptoms; more blood was expectorated; pulse 94. V.S. 20 oz.; T. Digitalis, etc. On the 3rd January there was an increase of pyrexia and more blood was coughed up. V.S. 24 oz.; relieved. On the 10th there was another exacerbation. V.S. 16 oz.; relief. On the following day, when at close stool, he died suddenly, suffocated by hæmorrhage.

Autopsy 18 hours after death. Body not emaciated. There was pretty much fluid in the tissue of the pia mater and at the base of the brain. The right lung was sound. The left was generally adhering and in part hepatized. Many of its bronchia contained a reddish brown sanies; the larger branches were full of coagulated blood. That part of the inferior lobe corresponding nearly to the 7th rib contained a mass of fibrin of about the size of a large walnut; it was easily removed from the lung in which it was imbedded; it was found to belong to an aneurism of the aorta, of about the same size; and that the hæmorrhage which proved fatal had taken place through a minute aperture in its sac. The pericardium contained 3 oz. of serum. The heart was normal. The aorta was much diseased; slightly at its origin where it was a little changed, more at its arch; just below the latter there was a small false aneurism; a little below that another; and lower still a third, just above the cæliac artery. All three were little larger than walnuts; all pressed on the vertebræ, the substance of which was partially absorbed; the first and third were not ruptured; the second was that which had opened into the lung; it was nearly filled with fibrin; the mouth of each was proportionally large, large enough to admit the tips of three fingers. The aorta where diseased had its inner coat rough and friable, and in some places ossified; its middle coat discolored yellow and more or less atrophied; the outer coat thickened. The pulmonary artery transversely divided, was found of unequal thickness; a portion of it was extremely thin. The lower part of the inferior vena cava was slightly diseased; in two places its inner coat was thickened and hardened. There were several concretions in the situation of the bronchial glands, and also close to the minor pancreas; the largest were about the size of a small chesnut; they consisted of phosphate of lime, with a little carbonate of lime and animal matter. The thoracic duct was large, especially its receptaculum, and was full of milky fluid. There was much chyme in the small intestines and chyle in the lacteals. The abdominal viscera were of healthy appearance.

In this instance the distressing symptoms appear to have been occasioned by the pressure of the small aneurismal tumors on important parts, in the lung probably exciting inflammation. It is remarkable how well the large and repeated blood-lettings were borne, as well as the relief they afforded. The chylopoietic viscera being sound, and there being probably no cachectic taint, blood, it may be inferred, was rapidly formed, emaciation prevented and strength sustained.

Case 16.—Of aneurism of the aorta, burst into the pleura.—P. M'Gregor, ætat. 41 ; 72nd Foot; admitted into hospital, December 3rd, 1837; died December 4th.—This man, a non-commissioned officer of excellent character, had come home after 21 years' service, for discharge on modified pension. Shortly after landing he was taken into hospital for rheumatism, as it was supposed, affecting the loins and shoulders. On the 29th October he was discharged relieved. On the 3rd December he was re-admitted, complaining of pain in his left side "which caught his breathing." A blister was applied and some antimonial medicine prescribed. No apprehension was entertained, the symptoms were so mild. At the evening visit, he spoke of being faint, which was attributed to the effect of the antimony ; he complained of nothing more, with the exception of pain across the lumbar region. He died at 3 a.m. of the following day.

Autopsy 33 hours after death. Body very robust. The right arteria Sylvii was closed by a firm deposit. There was no septum lucidum; no velum interpositum. The cerebral substance was natural. The left pleura contained 3½ pints of serum and 5½ pints of crassamentum. There was no fluid in the pericardium. The heart was of moderate size and free from disease ; its cavities were almost empty; their lining membrane and that of the aorta were stained red by blood. The left lung was greatly compressed; in its superior lobe there were some granular tubercles and a few small putty-like concretions; the inferior portion of the right lung contained some bloody serum. The aorta, from its origin to its bifurcation, was more or less diseased; its inner coat irregularly thickened, its middle coat softened in patches, as it were converted into a yellow, pultaceous, atheromatous matter, corresponding to which there was a bony deposit on, or in the inner coat. Under the heart, and pressing on the lung and spine, an aneurism was detected, which had burst into the pleura. It was about the size of an ordinary orange; its mouth large and circular, rather more than an inch in diameter. Where it came in contact with the spine two of the vertebræ had suffered, the bone had experienced loss of substance more than the intervertebral medium ; there was a loss of substance also of the lung where it had been subjected to pressure. There was nothing peculiar found in any of the abdominal viscera.

In this case we have a striking example of an aneurism making progress without affecting the general health, and for a time without producing any symptoms.

Case 17.—Of aneurism bursting into the abdominal cavity.—J. Fairweather, ætat. 34 ; 72nd Foot; admitted into hospital 20th January, 1838 ; died 21st July.—This

man, of ten years' service, had recently returned invalided from the Cape of Good
Hope. It was stated that in December last he experienced dyspepsia, with spasmodic
pains in the stomach and bowels, and that about the same time a pulsation was
detected about an inch above the umbilicus. There was much irritability of stomach,
hiccough, and severe pain of loins, resisting treatment. On admission here he complained of "a beating" in the abdomen, between the ensiform cartilage and the
umbilicus; there was tenderness there on pressure. His breathing was difficult, and
was increased by the slightest exertion; he was unable to lie on his back; vomiting
commonly occurred about an hour after taking food. His symptoms continued much
the same until the morning of the day he died. At 5 a.m. he suddenly experienced
a violent dragging pain in the right hypochondrium; the stomach rejected whatever
he swallowed. He continued conscious, gradually sinking till 10 a.m. when he
expired.

Autopsy 26 hours after death. Body robust. Rather more fluid than usual in the
ventricles of the brain. The lungs, with slight exceptions, were of normal appearance.
The right pleura contained 6 oz. of thin liquid cruor, with a small portion of coagulum
about the size of a bean. The posterior mediastinum was distended with coagulated
blood. A little coagulated blood was found in the inferior lobe of each lung, immediately under its pleural covering. The mediastinum was ruptured close to the
diaphragm, allowing the flow of blood into the pleura on the right side. The heart,
excepting that its mitral valves were somewhat thickened, was pretty natural, as was
also the ascending and thoracic aorta. A large quantity of coagulated blood was
found in the great and small omentum. The small intestines adhered together, and
the large to the adjoining parts, as did also the liver, requiring careful dissection to
expose the aorta. A large aneurism was found close to the cæliac artery, with two
circular openings, each capable of admitting the little finger. The aneurismal sac
was full of coagulum and fibrinous concretion in layers, not softening; it pressed on
the pancreas, the left lobe of the liver, the spleen, and left kidney; there was an
opening in its fundus produced by its bursting. The viscera were pretty natural.
The vesiculæ seminales were distended with fluid of the appearance of whey, abounding
in spermatozoa. There was healthy chyle in the duodenum. The cartilages of the
patellæ were softened and fissured.

This case is as much noteworthy for its distressing symptoms
as many of the preceding were for the contrary, and evidently
owing to the situation of the aneurism and its volume, and the
pressure it made on the adjoining parts.

The two following and last are given as instances of false
aneurism proving fatal, not so much *per se*, as by their disturbing influence, chiefly referrible to pressure on the parts
adjoining—gradually and slowly taking effect—increasing with
the increase of the tumor.

Case 18.—Of aneurism of the aorta, proving fatal without rupture; complicated
with bronchitis.—J. Irwin, ætat. 46; 11th Foot; admitted into hospital 8th Sept.,
1836; died 13th September.—This man, of 23 years' service, had good health until
three years ago, when he began to have rheumatic pains with some difficulty of
breathing, from which ever since he has never been free. Before embarking at Corfu
to return home to be invalided, he performed such easy duties as did not require much
exertion. On arrival at Fort Pitt he was in tolerable health, and was not taken into

hospital; there was no suspicion of the existence of an aneurism. When at last admitted, it was on account of a sudden accession of catarrh. Besides the ordinary symptoms of this ailment, he had pains in his shoulders, much dyspnœa, increasing to orthopnœa, with wheezing and puriform expectoration, most severe at night. The pulse was quick; there was a feeling of much and of increasing weakness, with little appetite. Sonorous râles were perceived over the chest generally, and at some points mucous râles. Using emetics, etc., some relief was afforded until the 11th Sept. Then the cough became incessant, expectoration more difficult, with increased irritability and diminution of strength, and without abatement or material change of symptoms up to the time of his death.

Autopsy 38 hours after death. Body slightly emaciated. The vessels of the brain were much congested. On removing the sternum, a tumor was brought into view, which, by pressure on the upper and inner surface of that bone, had produced a large, deep, and nearly circular cavity—a portion of bone having been absorbed, the periostum remaining. The tumor was found to be a false aneurism of the aorta, rising from within half an inch of the semi-lunar valves, and ascending beyond the innominata and the left common carotid and subclavian arteries, these vessels remaining pervious. It pressed on the left bronchus, the cartilages of which on the side of the sac were laid bare. In circumference it was 11 inches; and except allowing passage to the blood, it was completely filled with pale laminated fibrin. The canals through the fibrinous mass leading to the great vessels, including the descending aorta (for at the arch there was a deposition of lymph on its lower surface), were smooth, lined with a false membrane not unlike the inner coat of the aorta itself. When turned out of its sac, the fibrinous mass was a complete cast. No traces could be detected in the sac of the proper arterial coats. The heart was of usual size, free from disease, as was also the aorta, except near the portion involved in the aneurism. The circumference of the aorta at its origin was 3½ inches; there its inner coat was a little thickened and rough. The innominata was about an inch and a half from the left carotid; and the latter half an inch from the subclavian. Both lungs were free from adhesions. The bronchia and trachea were red; the former smeared with purulent fluid, the latter granular. An ulcer was found in the cœcum, about the size of a sixpence, close to the appendicula vermiformis; it was partially healed. The appendicula was clogged with fæcal matter. The abdominal viscera generally were healthy.

What seems most noteworthy in this case is—first, that the aneurism escaped detection during life; this probably owing to its sac being completely filled up, and to there being a free passage of blood through the canals formed in the fibrinous mass: and, secondly, that the death was the result not so much of the aneurism as of the bronchitis, which the aneurism had probably excited, and certainly aggravated.

Case 19.—Of aneurism of the innominata, proving fatal, without rupture or marked complication.—D. Sillete, a Maltese; died in the civil hospital, Valetta, December 25th, 1832.—This man's disease was of many years' duration, and had been slowly gradually increasing. During the last few days of his life he had been under the care of Dr. Portelli, surgeon of the civil hospital, from whom, when I was present at the *post mortem* examination, I had a brief account of the case. When admitted he was feeble; had no appetite; no pain; occasional palpitation of heart; occasional confusion of intellect; no cough; no considerable dyspnœa. He died suddenly.

The autopsy was on the day following. The body much emaciated. The pericardium contained 3 oz. of serum. The heart and its valves were free from disease. The aorta throughout its whole course was rather larger than usual, and more or less diseased; its inner coat was opaque in several places and of different degrees of thickness, from a line to a quarter of an inch; its middle coat corresponding also varied in thickness, from nearly its natural degree to the greatest possible thinness, generally it was very thin; where the inner coat was thick, there the outer was indurated and yellow. In the innominata, just above its commencement, a circular opening was found, about half an inch in diameter, abrupt, with rounded edges, without any dilatation of the artery. Within the opening was an enormous aneurismal sac; it occupied the whole of the right side of the neck, extending upwards to the submaxillary glands, downwards to the first rib, laterally to the trachea and to a line a little beyond the outer edge of the sterno-clydo-mastoideus muscle; it was everywhere entire; but in several places it was almost in a state to burst, especially about two inches below the jaw; there its coat consisted merely of the skin, which to the extent of a crown-piece was black, as if gangrenous, and from which before death there had oozed a reddish sanies. The muscles subjected to its pressure seemed to have been absorbed. The right pneumo-gastric nerve could be traced with difficulty; only a slight vestige of it remained. The internal jugular vein was partially obstructed by fibrin which firmly adhered to its inner coat. Where in contact with the clavicle and the first rib, there the periosteum constituted the wall of the sac; the bone underneath was rough from absorption. The sac contained pretty much coagulated blood, but not nearly sufficient to distend it; none of the coagulum was firmly adhering, nor was there any appearance of fibrous concretion of long standing. The inference was that most of the coagulum had formed after death. The inside of the sac presented an unequal surface, opaque and slightly shreddy, formed, as it seemed, of false membrane and very like the diseased inner coat of the artery, and continuous with it. There was no minute examination made of the thoracic and abdominal viscera, the attention having been chiefly directed to the aneurism. The abdominal blood-vessels appeared to be large generally, especially the arteries. The stomach was small and contracted. The thoracic duct was large and empty. The left pneumo-gastric nerve seemed larger than usual, and especially its semilunar ganglion.

This case, from what was known of it, seems remarkable for the little suffering attending so large an aneurism, and for the comparative mildness of its morbid phenomena. Exhaustion, as it were, from functional debility, rather than acute disease, appeared to have been mainly the cause of the fatal issue.

These foregoing cases accord generally with the remark I have made in introducing them, that the aneurismal diathesis, if there be one, is of the sthenic kind: the abundance of blood in the cadaver in most of these cases, the chyle detected in one or two of them in the lacteals and the thoracic duct, the spermatozoa in the vesiculæ seminales of others, are circumstances all in favor of the same view.* Yet, this condition does not appear

---

* It is worthy of remark, that in the many instances recorded of sudden death from aneurism of individuals at the time seemingly in perfect health, their digestive organs

to be absolutely essential, as in more than one instance the aneurism has been associated with tubercles in the lungs : Cases 3, 5, 16, are examples of the occurrence, unless, indeed, it be maintained, that inasmuch as tubercles in their early stage are not incompatible with apparent vigorous health, these cases hardly come under the head of exceptions.

As in the individual cases the condition of the diseased artery has been commonly stated, I have little to add on that matter. The subject of the structure of aneurism, is an acknowledged difficult one. That the outer cellular coat commonly constitutes the sac of a false aneurism, is now I believe universally admitted, also, that the middle coat is deficient, and probably the inner likewise, its place supplied by a false membrane. Even in true aneurism, I have not been able to satisfy myself that the inner coat is the original coat merely thickened, and not a false membrane altogether; it is so like the inner lining membrane of a large aneurismal sac, which may be traced in continuity with the thickened lining of the artery where the rupture has taken place.

In only a few of the cases given, was there any atheromatous matter, or bony matter deposited in the diseased coats, so as to be conspicuous. Had microscopic examination been employed, I have no doubt that both would have been frequently detected. We have assurance of the fact by Mr. Gulliver, in the paper I have more than once quoted, "on fatty degeneration of the arteries." In that paper, he has given the results of some analyses which I made at his request of atheromatous deposits, showing that they are composed chiefly of various fatty substances, such as oleine, margarine and cholestric acid, with which cholesterine is commonly mixed. Whether these matters are to be considered as a materies morbi, is open to question, inasmuch as there does not appear to be any accordance between the amount of them present and the amount of arterial disease. I am more inclined to view them commonly as accidental or incidental precipitates, or deposits like the fibrin. In passive

in an active state, some food in the stomach, and chyme in the small intestines, yet no solution of the stomach has been witnessed, merely a softening of its mucous coat. May this have been owing to the presence of food, which, as during life, may have been subjected to the action of the gastric juice, and thus may have protected the membrane ? If this be admitted as probable, it will apply to the cases of accidental deaths, described in a preceding chapter, in no one instance of which was there, as already observed, any solution of the stomach.

dilatation of the heart's cavities, we have an instance of what can be effected by an expansive force constantly acting. But, commonly, though such depositions may not be concerned as the causa mali, sometimes they may be so concerned, as in the instances in which an aneurism results from a sudden rupture of a very limited spot, that spot being in a state of disorganization connected with an atheromatous infiltration, the calibre of the artery elsewhere remaining unaltered; of which some of the preceding cases may be considered examples.

I have mentioned one or two cases in which shortly after death, three or four hours, the blood-vessels were examined for air, and the blood for ammonia: the trials were many more in number than those described; of all of them, the results were pretty uniform; no air was detected in the internal jugular vein or carotid artery, but a trace of ammonia was always detected in the blood, slight indeed, at the time specified after death, but strong a few hours later. This rapid increase suggests that even when first detected, it may have been owing to incipient putrefaction: and, I am more disposed to this conclusion from experiments I have made tending to show that ammonia is not a constituent part of healthy blood, and consequently, nowise concerned in its coagulation;* indeed, if it were present, and its escape were essential to that phenomenon, it would be difficult to imagine how coagula could form during life in the veins and arteries.

Whilst noticing the blood, I may briefly advert to the abundance in which it is commonly found in the bodies of those who have died of aneurism, before any wasting disease has set in, and how when the fatal event has been most sudden, the viscera performing their functions at the time, many of them have had their vessels in a plethoric state, so injected, as it were, as to convey the idea of inflammation, prompting the necessity of caution in judging of inflammation of a part merely by its apparent vascularity.

As to the symptoms of aneurism, we can hardly be surprised that they should be so various, and differ so much in kind and degree, in some instances the disease affording no manifestations of its existence; in others attended with a complication of dis-

---

* See Transact. Roy. Soc. of Ed., vol. xxii. p. 51.
In note to case 14, I have offered another conjecture—viz., that the ammonia might have been formed by the action of potassa on the blood.

tressing ailments. The locality of the lesion in each case and the degree of pressure exerted on the adjoining organs may, I believe, tolerably suffice to account for the phenomena in all their diversity, especially if it be admitted, that *per se*, an aneurism does not vitiate or taint the organism, or affect the general health.

Of the occlusion of arteries, the cases given are less remarkable than some I have not introduced, especially two, which have been already published, and to which I beg to refer.* In commenting on those cases and on the occlusion of arteries generally, I expressed my belief " that whenever the middle coat of an artery becomes diseased, whether from atrophy, or change of structure, or deposition in it of atheromatous or other matter, then invariably, an effort is, as it were, made to strengthen the part by the deposition of lymph on both sides, and that according to the rate of progress of the two processes, there is either a closure of the vessel, or an aneurism established : if the lymph be deposited copiously and rapidly, the former ; if the atheromatous matter, the latter ; and also the latter, if the absorption, or weakening of the middle coat, from diseased alteration in its texture, proceed with more speed than the deposition of lymph." This view, at the same time, I designated as hypothesis, and as I then ventured to offer it, for the sake of calling attention to the subject, I must rest now on the same excuse for re-introducing it. It might perhaps be well for medical science, were etiological speculations, for the most part, to be similarly considered.

In enumerating, at the beginning, the kinds of aneurism, two only out of the 40 cases, were of the femoral artery, One of these, which occurred in a private soldier at Barbadoes, at the time I was stationed there, was operated on by ligature and proved fatal in consequence of secondary hæmorrhage, and after suppuration. The other, at home, was an example of spontaneous cure ; the subject of it a pensioner, aged 39, objected to be operated on ; one night in bed, he suddenly experienced much pain in the groin, the seat of the aneurism, with, at the same time, very uneasy sensations in the abdomen above, followed shortly after by the subsidence of the pulsating tumor ; of the aneurismal character of which there could be no question. The cure no doubt was owing to the occlusion of the artery by lymph, happily for the sufferer, in the right place.

* Anatom. and Physiol. Res. vol. i. p. 426.

CHAPTER XIII.

ON DEATHS FROM ALCOHOLIC INTOXICATION.

The subject still open for inquiry.—Evils of intemperance.—Statistics of *delirium tremens*.— Suggestions for checking drunkenness in the army.—Fatal cases of alcoholic poisoning.— Remarks on the action of alcohol, and on its morbid effects.—Pneumonia one of its most common sequences.—The lungs the chief emunctory of alcohol.

FEW subjects have been more studied than the action of alcohol on the animal system, yet, I believe, it must be confessed that the inquiries instituted have not yet attained an exhaustive length, and that there is still scope for further research. My intention at present is to do little more than describe the cases I have witnessed which have ended fatally, after the drinking of a large quantity of ardent spirits, and in which an examination of the body was made after death: they were eight in number. I shall first detail them individually, and in conclusion offer a few comments chiefly as regards their pathological bearing. Incidentally I may remark, that the loss of life amongst our troops, sad as that is, is not the least of the evils the result of intemperance; greater far, it must be admitted, are those which are slowly engendered by continued habits of indulgence, enfeebling the body, and not less the mind, conducing to loss of health, the production of organic disease, to loss of character and of self-respect. As might be expected, the greater the facility in procuring spirits the more is their use abused: thus, in the West India Command, it would appear from the Army Medical Returns, that the number of cases of *delirium tremens* per 10,000 men in those colonies, is 154, with a mortality of 20; whilst for the same number of men at home, in the Mediterranean, in Canada and Ceylon altogether, the number of cases is no more than 21, and the deaths from the disease only 2. The Mauritius is another example in point. Of that island, as of the West Indies, the great staples are sugar and rum; and in the one as in the other, there being the same facility to commit excess, and with the same kind of spirit—new rum—the cases of *delirium tremens* and the deaths from it, are in about the same proportions ; the former rather greater—viz., 169 per 10,000 ; the latter somewhat less, 16 per 10,000.*

Now that the health of the army is beginning to have attention paid to it by the higher authorities, we may, I trust, indulge in hope that drunkenness will be checked, and not as heretofore too often in a manner encouraged. It is to be hoped we shall never again hear of such disasters as befell the starving force in the earlier part of the siege of Sebastopol, where, during the winter, for many weeks rum was the only article of the soldiers' rations that was regularly and unstintedly supplied. It should be laid down as a first maxim, founded equally on common sense and all experience, that we can never have an efficient army unless it be sober and healthy, for the attainment of which not a few things are requisite—such as good provisions in sufficient quantity—the quantity varying with climate—well ventilated and not crowded barracks—a dress suitable to the duties to be performed, and also to the climate and season—and sufficient recreation, such as may be needed to render military life during peace not terribly irksome and oppressive to the mind. Were good tea and coffee supplied, there would be a greatly lessened temptation to drink and get drunk. Were any fermented liquors to be allowed, the least noxious should be selected for use—such as light wine or bitter beer, or light punch ; this last compounded of old rum, lemon or lime juice, and good Muscovado sugar. In some situations, especially where salt provisions are issued and vegetables are scarce, a small allowance of such a beverage, taken with or after dinner, might be wholesome and a preventive of scurvy. Some of the cases I am now about to record could hardly have taken place had not intemperance been encouraged.

Case 1.—Isaac Rohiti, a Jew, ætat. 25, residing in Vathi, Ithaca, when in perfect health, for a wager of half a dollar, in four minutes drank the whole of a bottle of rum (not quite a pint and half), eating at the same time some figs. This was in the morning of the 25th January, 1825, just twenty minutes after ten o'clock. Immediately after, it is said, he did not appear to be affected ; he walked out apparently well. At about 11 a.m. he was met by two Jews his acquaintances at the Sanita Office, to whom he spoke distinctly. Whilst conversing with them he became

* Amongst the black troops in the West India Command, the number of cases of *delirium tremens* per 10,000 men is only 13, and the deaths only 2. These troops are peculiarly suitable to the climate ; their general mortality is only about one-half that of our countrymen, to whom the climate with all its accessories is so unfit.

confused, and could not end his story. He walked between them a little way, then becoming unable to stand, they carried him home to his bed. When laid there, he said he should soon be well after some sleep. He continued from noon till 3 p.m. sleeping, his breathing noisy, without exciting alarm. At three o'clock his friends looked, and found that he had vomited a little. Now his appearance frightened them. A physician was sent for, who came immediately and found him moribund. He died between 3 and 4 p.m.

The examination of the body was made 19 hours after. Being at the time in Ithaca, I assisted Dr. Monato, the physician who had been called in, in conducting it. He had seen him just before he expired. The limbs were rigid. The vessels of the dura and pia mater, and of the plexus choroides, were unusually turgid with blood. No fluid was found in the ventricles, or at the base of brain. The lungs, slightly red, contained rather more blood than natural. The tract of the great vessels in the posterior mediastinum was reddish, as if from blood-stain. There was no fluid in the pericardium, and very little blood in either side of heart. The thoracic duct was empty. On opening into the abdomen, the stomach and colon were seen very much distended. The omentum and large intestines externally were slightly red; the duodenum and other small intestines were redder, especially some portions of the latter. The stomach was found to contain, besides air, a considerable quantity, perhaps a quart, of fluid, of a dark brownish hue, as if discolored by blood, with a good deal of glairy mucus, and some masticated figs. The contents smelt pretty strongly of rum. The mucous coat was redder than natural in patches, especially towards the pylorus. Fluid of the same kind was found in the duodenum; its villous coat was bright red with patches of ecchymosis, and was smeared with a bloody exudation. The upper part of the jejunum was less red, and the ileum still less; yet in particular spots the redness of its mucous coat was well marked. A slight blush of red was seen here and there in the mucous coat of the large intestines. The pancreas generally was very red, as if gorged with blood, and unusually soft. The liver contained a great deal of blood, as did also the kidneys, which were very red. There was much pale, clear urine in the bladder; it had no smell of rum. This man previously had been temperate, was strongly built, and had excellent health. All the viscera, with the exception of indications of inflammation in certain of them, were remarkably sound.

Case 2.—M. Fennelly, ætat. 28, 36th Regiment, stationed at Corfu, was found dead in his bed, on the morning of the 28th April, 1825. He was notoriously intemperate, but never was in hospital, except after punishment. After dinner on the 27th, in company with another soldier, his comrade, he drank about a pint of aqua vitæ and some wine. He was carried drunk to his barrack between 3 and 4 p.m. and laid in bed. No notice was taken of him till 5 a.m. the following day, when life was extinct.

The examination of the body was made about 18 hours after. The face, neck, and upper part of chest were livid from congestion of venous blood. The longitudinal sinus was turgid, and when opened a great deal of black blood flowed from it. The vessels of the dura and pia mater and plexus choroides were turgid with the same kind of blood. Numerous red spots were seen in the sections made of the brain. Its substance generally was softer than natural. The lungs were unduly red, as was the whole of the aspera arteria. A small piece of meat was found in the rima glottidis, and minute portions of the same in the trachea. There was a little blood in the right auricle; the other cavities were nearly empty. The thoracic duct contained a very little limpid fluid. A large quantity of masticated food, without any fluid, was found in the stomach, and portions of meat also in the gullet. The stomach internally was very red, mostly in streaks and patches. The duodenum exhibited a redness of the same kind. The upper portion of the jejunum was unduly red. The remainder of the small and the whole of the large intestines had no marked appearance of disease. The kidneys were red, and rather gorged with blood. The spleen was small; it and the liver appeared sound; both contained little blood. The pancreas was soft and red. The urinary bladder was much distended with fluid. The inference at the time was that death was owing to suffocation. His comrade, who, it was said, had committed the same excess, had drank nearly the same quantity of spirits, and was equally drunk after, was pretty well the following day.

Case 3.—W. Smith, a boy, ætat. 14, at Corfu, in August, 1827, for a wager drank a large quantity of spirits, it is supposed at least a pint. He was brought to the hospital of the 88th Regiment in a comatose state. Symptoms of inflammation of the lungs almost immediately appeared, which resisted V.S. and the usual antiphlogistic treatment actively employed. Several days before death his breath became very fetid, and his body generally emitted an offensive odor.

The examination of the body was made 17 hours after death. The left lung partially adhered to the costal pleura. It was generally inflamed and hepatized; its inferior lobe contained several irregular sinuses in a gangrenous state. The right lung was redder than natural, and contained a good deal of blood and serum. There was much serum in the pericardium, and several ounces of bloody serum in each pleura. The thymus was large. The thoracic duct was large. The inner membrane of the heart and veins was stained strongly red by blood. The stomach and intestines were much distended with flatus. The cardiac portion of the former was œdematous, distended by bloody serum effused under its mucous coat. The bile in gall-bladder was in large quantity, pale and dilute. The brain was not examined.

Case 4.—J. Brown, ætat 28; R.B.; admitted into regimental hospital, Malta, 22nd January, 1832; died 29th January.—This man, in perfect health, had three days' leave from his commanding officer, having received his bounty-money (£3) on re-enlisting after the expiration of his period of limited service. On the 21st Jan., after hard drinking, and when under its influence at the canteen, he drank off a pint and half of ardent spirits in the space of a few minutes, at five successive draughts. At 2 p.m. he was carried to his barrack room in a state of insensibility, where he remained in bed neglected till the following morning. When brought to hospital at 9 a.m. on the 22nd, he was laboring under great prostration of strength, hurried and labored respiration, with mucous râle; acute pain in right side; extremely rapid pulse; much anxiety of countenance and collapse of features; his breath smelt of spirits. An emetic of sulphate of zinc and ipecacuanha (drachm of each) was given, and the throat irritated; he threw up some brownish fluid, which did not smell of spirits. A vein had previously been opened; he became faint when only a small quantity of blood had been abstracted. Some leeches were applied to the pained side, and he had a purgative enema with croton-oil. The treatment had no marked effect; the pulse continued small and rapid; the respiration quick and labored; there was occasional delirium; not much pyrexia; little or no cough. He died on the 8th day from admission.

Autopsy 16 hours after death. The arachnoid was in many places opaque. There was pretty much fluid under it and between the convolutions of the brain, and in the ventricles, and at the base of the brain. 3 oz. of serum in the pericardium. The heart normal. The right pleura contained 39 oz. of serum and purulent fluid; the latter inferior. The lung partially adhered. The pleura was covered with a thick layer of coagulable lymph, under which the membrane was of a dark red. The inferior lobe was so condensed by pressure that it sank in water; the middle lobe was less condensed; the superior was tolerably crepitous. The bronchial vessels were unduly red. The left lung was generally adhering. Its parenchyma was redder than natural and heavier, and in places hepatized in a slight degree. The bronchia were red; the larger branches contained a good deal of fluid. The liver was rather large; its section nutmeg-like. The stomach showed remarkably towards the pylorus the hour-glass contraction; its inner coat generally was perhaps a little softer than natural, but not distinctly diseased. A portion of the jejunum was redder than natural. The large intestines, in parts, were distended with air.

Case 5.—J. Edwards, ætat. 24; 94th Regiment, Malta; found dead in his bed, 26th September, 1832.—This man was discharged from hospital in the afternoon of the 25th September, where he had been about a fortnight under treatment for boils in his feet; his general health good. According to the report of his comrades, between half-past five and eight o'clock, he drank a pint of common red wine, half a pint of white wine, four glasses of gin and two glasses of brandy. At 8 o'clock he was so stupidly drunk that he required to be carried to his barrack-room, be undressed and put to bed by his comrade. Early on the following morning he was found dead, lying on the floor, having fallen out of bed.

The autopsy at 11 a.m. The vessels of the brain were rather turgid with blood. There was pretty much fluid between the membranes, in the ventricles and at the base of brain; no blood was effused; there was no softening, or any other change discoverable. In the right cavities of the heart there was a good deal of fluid blood and some air-bubbles. Half an ounce of serum in the pericardium. Neither lung collapsed. A little reddish serum was found in both pleuræ. Both lungs throughout were œdematous; their inferior parts were loaded with a reddish serosity, which, on an incision being made, flowed out copiously; their parenchyma was redder than natural, and in some places slightly hepatized. The bronchia were full of a frothy fluid; the whole of the air-passages were unduly red, especially the larynx and trachea. Some transparent lymph in the thoracic duct. A large quantity of food, like minced meat, in the stomach; it had a strong smell of spirits. The abdominal viscera generally were of healthy appearance.

Case 6.—A. Fraser, ætat. 32; 94th Regiment; admitted into regimental hospital, Malta, August 6th, 1833; died August 8th.—This man was conveyed to hospital in a state of insensibility, with stertorous breathing and contracted pupils. It was said that he had drunk about 2½ pints of gin, nearly at one draught, for a wager. Tepid water was introduced into the stomach and removed by the stomach-pump. In about an hour he recovered sensibility. He was pretty well until the following morning, when he had a short cough, pain of right breast, hurried and oppressed respiration, with "general disturbance." He was cupped and had calomel and opium. In the evening V.S., 30 oz., and was blistered; relief followed. He appeared to be doing well till the evening of the 7th, when the cough and dyspnœa became much aggravated, pulse very frequent and irregular and easily compressed; great restlessness; extremities cold and clammy. These symptoms increased with low delirium, till 1½ p.m. the next day, when he died.

Autopsy 22 hours after. Body remarkably robust. The lungs did not collapse; the right lung was very generally adhering, weakly to the pericardium, by soft coagulable lymph, firmly to the ribs by strong adhesions. This lung, with the exception of its superior lobe, which was crepitous, was generally hepatized and impervious to air. Its parenchyma in some places was red, in others fawn-colored; when pressed, a dirty yellow fluid came from its cut surface. The left lung was free from adhesions; its marginal air cells were very large; its pendent parts contained a good deal of blood and serum. The bronchia, indeed the aspera arteria generally, was dark red and covered with a thin exudation, resembling coagulable lymph. Blood firmly coagulated and fibrinous concretions were found in all the cavities of the heart. In the right ventricle, the concretion there was so firmly adhering, that it was broken in removing it; it had the *appearance* of being vascular, as if formed before death, and was in process of organization. There were bloody spots, like petechiæ, in the outer surface of the heart, and some ecchymosis on that of the right ventricle. The valves in contact with blood were hardly perceptibly stained. Some adhesions between the liver and duodenum and the liver and colon. The stomach was large; much mucus adhered to it; there were some red patches, but no softening. The abdominal viscera generally healthy. The temperature of the room 80°; under the liver 86°. The brain was not examined.

Case 7.—J. Pocock, ætat. 23; 72nd Regiment; admitted into regimental hospital, Barbadoes, March 16th, 1848.—This man, of intemperate habits, was brought to hospital at 6 a.m., in a state of stupor; respiration hurried and laborious; lips livid; pulse almost imperceptible; skin clammy; feet cold; pupils contracted and not affected by light. The stomach-pump was used and some spirituous fluid was extracted; a vein was opened, but little blood could be procured, and that of a very dark color; other means were used, but without effect in restoring him. He died at 11 a.m. He was one of a large party of the 72nd Regiment, which on the preceding evening had been entertained by the Grenadier company of the 88th Regiment. Great excesses were committed. Six men were brought to hospital on the following morning, all in a dangerous state—including this fatal case—and one of the same company was found dead in his bed; of the five who recovered one had a severe attack of pneumonia, commencing on the 16th, which was subdued by V.S.

The body of Pocock was examined 7 hours after death. The face pale; the abdomen not distended; slight suggilation of shoulders. The brain was normal, of firm consistence; there was no well-marked congestion of its vessels; very little fluid in the lateral ventricles. The lungs were not collapsed, nor crepitous; they were heavy and in the first stage of hepatization; they contained a good deal of sero-purulent fluid, which flowed from the cut portions. The bronchia very red, contained a frothy fluid. There was little difference between the upper and under surface of either lung. The heart was normal; its valves pale; some coagulated blood was found in the right auricle and ventricle. The mucous coat of the stomach was generally pale. The urinary bladder was distended with urine. The body exhibited no marks of putrefaction; the brain was not quite cold.

Case 8.—Wm. M'Killigan, ætat. 28; 72nd Regiment, the case referred to above, found dead in his bed.—The body was cold when found at gun-fire, denoting that death must have taken place shortly after the carouse, which ended at midnight. By his bedside there was no appearance of his having vomited.

The examination was made at 5 p.m., probably 18 hours after death. The abdomen was greatly distended. The face, neck, scalp, shoulders, and back were quite livid from exudation, suggilation, and blood injected in the cutaneous vessels. A reddish fluid flowed in small quantity from the nose and mouth. Much blood flowed from the divided scalp. The vessels of the brain were distended with blood. Its substance generally was soft; the fornix and septum lucidum pultaceous; the ventricles contained a little fluid, which had a distinct smell of garlic. The lungs were very red and congested, but crepitous. The valves of the heart were stained dark red, as was also the substance of the kidneys. The stomach and intestines were distended with air. Putrefaction had commenced.

If we reason on these cases, what are the inferences deducible from them? I shall take them *seriatim*. In the 1st case, the

manner of death, the time at which it took place—about five
hours after swallowing the spirits—the state of the vessels of the
brain, so turgid with blood, favor the idea that this organ was
the part which bore the brunt of the poisonous effect, and that
the fatal termination was of the nature of apoplexy.   How far
other parts were under the deleterious influence of the alcohol,
and might have contributed to the result, it is difficult to say.
Probably in most cases of the kind, as all parts of the system
are more or less acted on through the medium of the poisoned
blood, so the effect is not a simple but a compound one.

In the 2nd case, the inference already given—formed after
the examination of the body, and the discovery of the obstructed
state of the air-passages—that death was owing to suffocation,
seems most probable : the cause being quite adequate to the
effect.   In this instance, too, the state of the brain, under the
noxious alcoholic action, might have contributed to the fatal
result by lessening the sensibility and the regulating power of
the larynx, especially of the epiglottis and glottis.

In the 3rd case, the first and immediate morbid effect of the
alcohol appears to have been on the brain, judging from the
state of coma ensuing ; and the second, and that rapidly following, seems to have been inflammation of the lungs, ending in
gangrene.

In the 4th case, one bearing a considerable resemblance to
the last, the fatal result was clearly owing to inflammation of
the pleura and lungs, especially of the right pleura, in which so
large a quantity of serum and puruloid fluid was effused.   The
low state in this instance, marked by the slight pyrexia, and
perhaps also by the little cough, is noteworthy.

In the 5th case, the indications as to the immediate cause of
death are less clear than in the preceding.   Was it the combined
effect of the gorged state of the vessels of the brain, of the effusion
into the parenchyma of the lungs, and of the presence of air in
the right cavities of the heart ?

In the 6th case there was no room for doubt that death was
owing to inflammation of the lungs, chiefly the right, rapidly
lighted up by the alcoholic poison.   The condition of the blood
in this instance, firmly coagulated, with fibrinous concretions in
all the cavities of the heart, and in the right ventricle apparently
becoming organized, is worthy of note, especially as it is sup-

posed that alcoholic poisoning induces a contrary state of the blood—a loose coagulation, or a privation or destruction of the coagulating quality of the fibrin.

In the last two cases is not the presumptive evidence in favor of the conclusion, that death was the effect of the poison acting chiefly on the respiratory organs? The absence of congestion in the blood-vessels of the brain in the 7th, the general paleness of that organ, the paleness of the stomach, the effusion into the lungs, all seem to point to this inference. And the circumstance that one of the five men who were brought to the hospital at the same time had a severe attack of pneumonia, I cannot but think strengthens the inference. Respecting the precise cause of death in the 8th case, the conclusion necessarily must be more uncertain, owing to the obscurity, as regards the *post mortem* appearances, from the putrefactive change which had commenced from the delayed examination of the body.

These cases, taken altogether, seem to show that the lungs are most liable to suffer from large poisonous doses of alcohol. And is not this what might be expected, taking into account certain well ascertained facts, those, namely, tending to prove that these, the respiratory organs, are the true emunctories of alcohol;—in moderate doses, perhaps, consuming it in part as fuel for the production of animal heat,* and in part exhaling it, as is indicated by the odor of the breath; in excess, on the contrary, diminishing the amount of carbonic acid formed in the act of respiration,† and at the same time diminishing the temperature of the body,‡ and consequently, not being consumed, liable to accumulate in the parenchyma, and give rise to inflammation. Next to the lungs, the brain and the liver appear to be most subject to the deleterious action of alcohol. Both these organs contain substances soluble in alcohol, and so far consequently may be considered as having an affinity for it, and an aptitude to retain it, and in danger of suffering from its action. On the same ground of reasoning, as the stomach, the spleen,

---

* From the most recent researches, especially those of Dr. Edward Smith, the consumption of any alcohol in respiration seems to be very doubtful. See his paper "On the Detection and Use of Alcohol," in British Med. Journal, Nov. 2nd and 16th, 1861, where other papers of his on the same subject are referred to.

† As proved by Dr. Prout's experiments (Annals of Phil., vol. ii. and iv.)

‡ As shown by the experiments of the author, "On the Temperature of Man within the Tropics."—Phil. Trans. for 1850.

the kidneys have little or no affinity for it, should not these organs suffer from it in a less degree? Experience seems to justify the conclusion.

The experimental facts on which this reasoning is founded are chiefly those of Dr. Percy, who found alcohol to lodge in the brain and liver longer than in any of the other organs in which he sought for it, whether in man or animals, after death resulting from its poisonous effects. He could detect it rarely in the urine, indeed he found it only in one instance of the many in which he sought for it in that of dogs, and in one only of that of man,* tending to show that the kidneys are not the eliminating organs of this poison; a conclusion I had a long time ago arrived at, having when a student in Edinburgh similarly failed in detecting it, but the trial I made by the distillation of the urine of a man who had been very drunk was a solitary one.

That other parts of the nervous system suffer in common with the brain from the abuse of spirits, seems an almost unavoidable conclusion, though but little insisted on. As their composition is so similar, it may be inferred that had the spinal chord and the nerves been tested for it, after alcoholic poisoning, in the same careful manner as the encephalon, it would have been detected in them. In *delirium tremens* the nature of the symptoms are sufficiently indicative of a morbid condition of the nerves and spinal chord from the cause in question: and that they are as much immediately affected as the brain, the tottering gait and the impaired or lost power of the extremities of the drunkard sufficiently show.

The treatment of these sad cases, in which life is so eminently endangered by alcoholic poisoning, is difficult indeed. No rules that I am aware of can be laid down with any confidence for the guidance of the medical man, excepting a very few of unquestionable propriety—such as as soon as possible the use of the stomach-pump, coupled with the injection of tepid water, and the disuse, or very sparing use, of the lancet. Should the stomach-pump not be at hand, there can hardly be a question of the propriety of employing an active emetic, such as ipecacuanha or the sulphate of zinc, or a mixture of the two. Some caution, however, should be observed in administering the latter.

* Dr. Percy "On the Physiological Influence of Alcohol," p. 104.

I find appended to my account of Case No. 2, an extract from a letter of the late Dr. M'Arthur, dated Zante, 18th May, 1825, where he was then stationed with his regiment, the 90th, of which he was surgeon, as bearing on the caution I have suggested, and as otherwise interesting in relation to the subject.   I venture to give it in the subjoined foot-note.*

Further, as regards the treatment, I need not insist on the propriety of watching the patient carefully, so as to be prompt in encountering the diseased action that may be excited—the predominant one, whether it be inflammation of the brain or its membranes, or of the lungs or pleuræ, or of any of the abdominal viscera. Apart from inflammation, if life be not overpowered by the first impression made by the alcohol on the nervous system, there seems little to apprehend as regards recovery : a few hours sleep and little more seem sufficient in most instances to remove the anesthesia of the drunkard.   The lasting organic lesions to which the brain and liver appear to be most subject, are of a chronic kind, very slowly forming, and the results of habitual intemperance.

---

* "I have lately had what I consider rather an interesting case of poisoning by ardent spirits : a young man was carried into hospital in a state of apoplexy, three hours and a half after swallowing at one draught a buck (about a small wine-glass more than a pint) of aqua'dente.   Vomiting was excited by the exhibition of 6 grs. of tartar emetic, followed in an hour by 25 grs. of sulphate of zinc, and tickling the fauces with a feather, but not without great difficulty. The apoplectic symptoms gradually subsided, and were followed by enteritis of so obstinate and severe a nature as to require copious V.S. and the application of many leeches for its cure.   The stomach apparently was not affected ; and I am at a loss whether to attribute the abdominal inflammation to the spirit or to the sulphate of zinc, which I once remember to have produced a similar effect."   He adds :—" This is the third case of the kind which has occurred in the regiment within the last three years. The two former were fatal.   One was treated by the late Mr. Morrison, who unfortunately did not see the man until about seven hours after he had taken, for a trifling bet, a buck of aqua'dente at a draught : on dissection, the stomach was found to be highly inflamed."

CHAPTER XIV.

CASES OF SUICIDE AND OF DEATHS FROM ACCIDENT.

Motives for introducing such cases.—Suggestions for recording them in the public service.—
Detailed cases ; one of which remarkable for extensive solution of the stomach and diaphragm.
—Remarks on the tendency of suicide from ennui in the instance of the soldier.—Expression of
hope of the opprobium ceasing with increased attention to the comfort and health of the men.
—Suggestive remarks as to how the *post mortem* appearances of organs suddenly arrested in
action by death, may serve as checks in necroscopic research, and be of service in medical
jurisprudence.

THE following are some of the principal cases of the kind
which have come under my notice. I am induced to give them
with the hope that they may yield some useful information in
relation both to pathology and medical jurisprudence.

The number of cases is comparatively small, for it is only at
times of leisure, and not after a battle, when the wounded
engross entirely the attention of the medical officer, that inquiries
of the kind can be made. To be of any worth the examinations
must be minute, their value indeed depending very much on the
degree of minuteness attained.

If I might offer a suggestion it would be that a special necro-
logical register should be kept for cases of the kind amongst the
records of the medical department in the office of the Director-
General, and that medical officers should be invited to give their
special attention to the subject, and in the description of the
autopsies which they may have to make, to be as minute and
accurate as possible.

Case 1.—Of death from fracture of cranium, with solution of stomach and diaphragm.—Henry Smith, ætat. 34 ; 85th Regiment; admitted into regimental
hospital, Malta, Nov. 1, 1830; died Nov. 4th.—This man was admitted into
hospital after a fall down stairs the preceding night, when drunk. He was rational,
but somewhat confused, as if not quite sober. All the injury that could be discovered
was a contusion of the integuments over the right parietal bone. On the 2nd, he had
some headache, chiefly frontal, without pyrexia. 18 oz. of blood were taken by
cupping from the back of the neck. Croton oil 1 drop. In the evening he felt
better; bowels constipated. A cathartic enema. At 4 a.m. of the 3rd, the assistant-
surgeon was called to see him. He had excruciating pain of head, and was much
excited, and extremely anxious; the pulse "bounding." V.S. 40 oz. ; 32 leeches to

head; oil and enema repeated. At 10 a.m. there was little change of symptoms; pupils dilated; bowels but slightly moved. V.S. 30 oz.; blister to nape of neck; jalap, with cream of tartar. The report at the evening visit was, that the bowels had been freely opened; that there was a disposition to coma, and that when roused he was incoherent. The following morning he was comatose; the pupils "closely contracted;" pulse more natural; bowels open; occasional vomiting; extremities rather cold. He died at 6 p.m.

Autopsy 17 hours after death. The body extremely well formed, stout and muscular, exhibited no particular appearance. There was some ecchymosis over the right parietal bone, and a good deal of coagulated blood between this bone and the dura mater, and some also similarly situated on the opposite side. There were spots of ecchymosis likewise scattered over the surface of the cerebrum, with some coagulable lymph, and in a less degree on the cerebellum. The substance of the brain generally seemed sound, with the exception of the fornix and the surface of the fissura Sylvii, which was unusually soft. A fracture, without depression, was detected in the right parietal bone, which extended from the middle of it to the sella turciqua; it passed across the groove of the maningeal artery and some of its branches, from which probably the hæmorrhage was derived. Only the right lung was adhering. The inferior portion of each was very red, as were also the bronchia. There were fibrinous concretions in the heart, and a good deal of blood in its right cavities. The thoracic duct contained a little reddish fluid. The liver was firm, yellowish and granular. The bladder was very much distended with urine. A large portion of the great curvature of the stomach, that between the cardia and the part resting on the spleen, was "dissolved." The breach exceeded the open hand in size. Portions also of the diaphragm were "dissolved," and in consequence the contents of the stomach were found in the left pleura. The appearance of the margin of the stomach and diaphragm was, as if they had been immersed in a fluid of a purely solvent quality. A portion also of the omentum was "dissolved." There was some oil in the fluid in the chest and in that in the left hypochondrium. The fluid was brownish; it was thrown away before it could be examined. The portion of the stomach not "dissolved" appeared to be perfectly healthy, as did also the intestines and the other abdominal viscera.

This case is very much the counterpart of Case 3, in the chapter on cellular inflammation, and like that is chiefly remarkable for the solution of so large a portion of the stomach and diaphragm. There is the same obscurity about both. As in that instance so in this, it seems to me more probable that the solution was effected chiefly before death than after; but whether before or after that event, the phenomenon seems almost equally mysterious.

Case 2.—Edward Cuthbert, ætat. 22; killed by a fall from the Castle rock, Edinburgh, as described in p. 160.—The face was black and swollen from extravasated blood. The chin was deeply cut, and beneath the cut the lower jaw was fractured. No fracture of the cranium was detected. A small quantity of blood was effused under the dura mater on the right hemisphere of the cerebrum, cerebellum, and medulla oblongata. The vessels of the brain were generally turgid; but no rupture of any one was found. There was much blood effused into the cellular tissue of the thyroid gland. The pericardium contained only a few drops of serum. The heart was firm and contracted, and all its cavities empty. In each pleura there was a good deal of blood—about two pints in each; and some in the trachea and bronchia. The right lung adhered here and there by pretty long bands. Its middle lobe was rent to the depth of about a quarter of an inch, and its pleural covering torn, exposing a bony concretion of irregular form, little larger than a cherry-stone. The vena azygos on the right side of the spine, corresponding to about the second rib, was ruptured. Where ruptured, it communicated with the pleura. There was some dark ecchymosis in the course of the posterior mediastinum. The left lung posteriorly adhered pretty firmly. The source of the blood effused into the pleura of this side escaped detection. There was some coagulated blood, about two or three ounces, in the cavity of the abdomen, amongst the convolutions of the intestines; and the peritoneal investment of all the abdominal viscera was stained with blood. The left lobe of the liver, near the suspensory ligament, was lacerated in two places deeply and irregularly. In the right lobe, there were a few rents in its convex surface to the depth of a few lines. There were similar rents in the corresponding part of the right lobe; and internally, as exposed by section, a considerable laceration was found in the substance of this lobe, contiguous to the gall-bladder. There was much ecchymosis about the pancreas and in its substance; also about the left kidney, and its infundibula. The bladder contained a good deal of limpid urine; its inner coat was colorless. There was a little ecchymosis in the loose cellular membrane between the bladder and pubes. The stomach, of small size, contained a very little chymous fluid; its mucous surface was contracted into rugæ.

Case 3.—Wm. Hamilton, ætat. 25, the comrade of the preceding, and who was killed by a similar fall, as mentioned p. 161.—There was a wound in the back part of the head, about two inches long, penetrating to the bone—the occipital—corresponding to a fracture of that bone in an oblique direction. A good deal of blood was effused under the dura mater on the left cerebral hemisphere, but none on the right. The base of the cerebrum was just stained with blood; and there was a little coagulated blood contiguous to the cerebellum and medulla oblongata. A small blood-clot was found in the left ventricle. The fornix in the same lateral ventricle was slightly rent. No ruptured vessels could be discovered. About the thyroid gland there was some ecchymosis. The left lung adhered very generally and closely; the right partially. There was some blood in the trachea and bronchia. The right pleura contained between two and three pints of blood; and there was a little in the pericardium. The pericardium communicated by a lacerated opening with the right pleura, under the ascending vena cava. The heart was firm and contracted, and contained very little blood. The fourth, fifth, sixth, and seventh ribs were fractured, and all but the fourth in two places, one near the spine, the other close to the cartilages. The fractured ends of the latter had deeply wounded the middle lobe of right lung, and had occasioned probably the rent in the pericardium. In the cellular membrane between the ribs and the costal pleura, there was a slight degree of emphysema round the spot where the fractured ends of the ribs had penetrated the pleura, seeming to indicate that respiration was not instantly arrested by the fall. The liver was lacerated in a manner very similar to the preceding. The spleen was slightly lacerated. The pancreas exhibited much the same appearance as in Cuthbert, as did also the urinary bladder and the right kidney. There was a good deal of chymous fluid in the œsophagus, and pretty much in the stomach, the inner coat of which also was contracted into healthy rugæ.

Case 4.—A man, a Maltese, ætat. 65, was instantaneously killed by lightning on the 15th November, 1832.—The body was brought to the civil hospital in Valetta, and was examined about 24 hours after the event. The hair on the left side of the chest was slightly singed. There were no other external well defined marks of injury. The cutaneous vessels generally were much distended with blood; the face and neck were purplish red; the inferior surfaces purplish. The fingers were contracted and rigid. The abdomen was very much distended, tympanitic, and hard. There was froth at the mouth, mixed with some of the contents of the stomach. On opening into the abdomen, the stomach and intestines were found to be immensely distended with air. There was much air in the cellular structure generally, and especially in that of the gall-bladder. The blood-vessels were of a dark red, as was also the lining membrane of the heart and bronchia, and indeed all structures were more or less similarly stained. The right cavities of the heart contained a little soft coagulum and some frothy blood. In the veins there was frothy blood in a liquid state. The lungs were red and distended with air; the brain generally was soft.

The remark made at the time was, that I had rarely, in the hottest weather, witnessed such advanced putrefaction. This advanced state was indicated not only by the quantity of gas disengaged, and by the offensive odor, but also by the discoloration of the vessels and membranes stained by blood, and by the softening of the muscular fibre, especially of the heart. This softening may appear incompatible with the *rigor mortis* as exhibited by the fingers; yet such was the fact, however it may be explained. The temperature of the air at the time of the fatal event was low for Malta, probably not above 55°. On the following day, when the autopsy was made, and this within doors, it did not exceed 608

Case 5.—A young officer, ætat. 22; stationed in Malta; on the 13th March, 1832, was killed by a fall from the ledge of a house, about 47 feet in height. The accident occurred a little after midnight; the autopsy was made about 12 hours later. The body was well formed and muscular. The right side of the chest was very livid; the same side of the abdomen was livid, but in a less degree. The skin of the elbow was broken. The os humeri was fractured a little above the joint, as was also the thigh-bone of the same side at its neck. There was a cut over the right eyebrow, but not deep. 51 oz. of blood were found in the right pleura. The right side of the pericardium was ruptured, as was also the right lung to a small extent, close to the great vessels. Some blood was effused into the parenchyma of this lung, which was collapsed and compressed (compressed by the blood in the pleura), and also into the bronchia. The right side of the diaphragm was ruptured across from its crus to its very insertion, and the liver was projecting through the opening into the cavity of the chest. This viscus was ruptured in several places; the fissures about three or four lines deep. There was a little blood in the cavity of the abdomen. The stomach was nearly empty. The spleen was small and not apparently injured. The intestines were distended with some flatus, especially the large. When the skull-cap was removed, pretty much blood flowed out of the divided sinuses. There was an undue quantity of serosity between the membranes, in the ventricles, and at the base of the brain; the fornix was soft and lacerated. No large blood-vessel was found ruptured. The hæmorrhage, it may be inferred, came from the ruptured parts.

The individual was previously considered to be in good health. During the preceding summer, after great intemperance, he had

a severe attack of *delirium tremens,* which may account for the
fluid effused in the brain. The temperature of the air at the
time is not stated; the average temperature of March in Malta
is a little higher, about one or two degrees, than that of February.
This I mention, in aid of the comparison between the state of
this body, and that of the preceding, one so great that it may
well excite reflection.

Case 6.—A private soldier, ætat. 42, stationed in Malta, was found dead, lying on
his face, below a flight of steps, about 20 feet high, from the top of which, there is
reason to suppose he fell perpendicularly, when returning from Valetta to his barracks
in Floriana. The face and the superior part of the trunk were very livid. No external
injury could be detected. When the skull-cap was removed and the great vessels
were divided, although the head was a little raised, yet the blood flowed freely from
them and in considerable quantity, especially from the vertebral arteries. A flow of
serum was observed from the carotids, the blood probably having coagulated in these
vessels. The cerebral vessels were turgid with blood, but no blood was effused within
the cranium. There was some red serum in the ventricles. The substance of the
brain was natural. Both lungs were adhering; they both contained much blood. A
good deal of blood was found effused into the cavity of the abdomen, which, it was
inferred, came from the liver. This organ was ruptured in several places, both in the
left and right side, and both in the convex and concave surfaces; the fissures where
deepest little exceeded a few lines. No other internal injury was discovered. From
the position of the body, it was conjectured that he fell on his chest and belly and
was killed instantly by the shock.

The day of the month has been omitted in my too brief notes
of the case, and the hour of the autopsy. The body was found
in the morning, and the examination, it is stated, was made on
the same day.

Case 7.—A private soldier of the 94th Regiment, ætat. 26, stationed in Malta, was
on the 15th December, 1832, early in the morning, found dead, beneath a rampart of
St. Elmo, between 30 and 40 feet high. It was supposed that in returning to his
barrack in the evening after drinking, a little after 8 o'clock, he had walked through
an embrasure.

The examination was made on the 16th at 2 p.m. There was no fracture of the
cranium or laceration of the brain. There was an extensive fracture and laceration
of the left elbow-joint, and a fracture of the os humeri of the same side, near the
shoulder-joint. There was no apparent injury of any of the thoracic viscera. The
abdominal integuments were not discolored. On opening into the cavity of the
abdomen, a large quantity of blood was found effused and in part coagulated. The
spleen was deeply ruptured. The liver was ruptured in two places. The left kidney
also was ruptured. The cellular tissue adjoining the ruptured organs was in a state
of ecchymosis.

The individual previously had been in good health. The
average temperature of the air in Malta in December is about
55°.

Case 8.—A Maltese lad, ætat. about 14 or 15, on the 14th February, 1834, was killed by an explosion of gunpowder, the exact quantity not known. It took place in a schooner at anchor in the harbour. Eleven men were killed—the master was one of them—and eight were wounded. The examination of the body was made three quarters of an hour after. The bones of the cranium were broken in, and the brain crushed. No other material injury was discovered. The temperature under the liver was 94°-95°; in the cavity of the pelvis and under the left ventricle of the heart it was 97°. The lungs were collapsed; each weighed 8 oz. The thymus gland was large, as if it had increased since birth, it was so large. The larynx was small, like that of a girl of the same age. The testes were small; there was no hair on the pubes, or indeed any indications of the development peculiar to puberty. A large quantity of food was found in the stomach, consisting chiefly of oranges and hard-boiled egg. There was no liquid, and no gaseous distension. The contents of the stomach were removed, and, after the lining membrane had been slightly washed, some milk was introduced. In a few seconds it was coagulated; the coagulum was soft, like that produced by rennet. There were round worms (A. lumbricoides) in the duodenum. With the exception of the liver and spleen adhering to the adjoining parts, they showed no marks of disease. The muscular fibre had entirely lost its irritability. In another body killed at the same time, that of an English sailor, ætat. about 22, who was blown up, and fell in the water, from which he was taken by dragging about half an hour after, the fibres of the pectoralis major muscle contracted when punctured.

Case 9.—A non-commissioned officer, ætat. 46, was shot through the head by a private soldier in Malta, in 1831. He was previously in good health, and had been remarkable during a long period of service—23 years—for excellent health, and for good conduct. The ball entered at the left side of the occiput, and passed in a straight line out at the right os unguis. Death was immediate. There was an effusion of much blood from the wound.

Autopsy 18 hours after. The body was well formed, muscular, and fat; the chest very hairy; the countenance tranquil. The lungs were free from adhesions, were collapsed, and very crepitous. A little blood was found collected in their inferior parts. Both together weighed 1 lb. 11 oz. Each pleura contained about 2 oz. of serum. The thoracic duct was empty. The heart, in comparison with the bulk of the body, was rather small. There was an oblique opening in the fossa ovalis sufficiently large to admit the little finger. The Eustachian valve was connected with the valve of the coronary vein by two or three long tendinous fibres. The heart contained very little blood; that in the ventricles was coagulated and broken up, showing that its coagulation had taken place before the heart had ceased to act. The abdominal viscera were very healthy. The omentum was loaded with fat. About 1 oz. of serum was found in the cavity of the abdomen. There was a large quantity of chyme or half-digested pultaceous food in the stomach. There was also half-digested food in the ileum, cœcum, and transverse colon; it was of a darker color than that in the stomach, and was without fæcal smell. In the sigmoid flexure and rectum there was soft fæcal matter. The spleen was of moderate size; when squeezed, after incision, there exuded from it a chocolate-colored pultaceous matter. The mesenteric glands were distinct, ovoid; the largest hardly ¼ inch in length.

Case 10.—A private soldier, ætat. 38, was drowned at Malta on the 6th June, 1830.—He had dined with his wife at about half-past one, eating heartily. He seemed in excellent health, but a little under the influence of the wine he had drank at the meal. Shortly after he went with two of his comrades to bathe, saying the "waves would sober him." After swimming some time he called out for aid. One of his companions made the attempt; but not being able to support him, and in danger of sinking himself, he let him go.   He sank, and was brought up by a diver about an hour after.

Autopsy at 3 p.m. of the following day.   The body was well formed, muscular, and fat; the limbs rigid.   There was slight lividity of the skin of the neck, deepest in the back part.   The arachnoid was of a milky whiteness.   The cerebral vessels were turgid with blood; the minute vessels injected, producing an appearance commonly called inflammatory.   There was a good deal of fluid in the ventricles, at the base of the brain, and in the spinal canal.   The fornix was soft, softer than natural.   The substance of brain generally normal.   The liver was adhering throughout; its substance natural.   There was a moderate quantity of bile in the gall-bladder.   The stomach contained a considerable quantity of food, partially colored with red wine, and but little changed.   The inner membrane of the organ was generally redder than is considered natural, with many patches of dark red, nearly the appearance of ecchymosis.   The duodenum was very red; the other small intestines were of the same color in a less degree; their inner coat was most colored; thick mucus was adhering to it.   There were no glandulæ aggregatæ in the lower portion of the ileum; the solitary glands were many and distinct.   There was a good deal of blood in the right cavities of the heart, and pretty much in the aorta.   The blood, wherever found, was liquid.   The aortic valves were rigid from incipient ossification.   The aorta at its origin was a little larger than common; its inner coat irregularly thickened; in some places three or four lines; in others not at all; the middle coat also exhibited inequalities as to thickness, but not always corresponding to those of the inner; it was of an orange yellow hue; the outer cellular was generally thickened.   Each pleura contained about 3 oz. of reddish fluid—a dilute serum, yielding some coagulum when heated or when acted on by nitric acid.

Case 11.—A private, ætat. 33 ; 2nd B.R.B. ; stationed in Malta; shot himself on the 14th June, 1830.—He was in confinement at the time for a slight offence.   His temper was bad, but he had exhibited no marks of insanity ; had shortly before been drinking.   He told a comrade, who was bantering him about further punishment, that he would not give the colonel an opportunity to inflict it.   He shot himself in the recumbent posture, and his lower limbs were found in the attitude in which he had placed them for pulling the trigger.

The examination was made 21 hours after death.   The body was short, but muscular and well formed.   The limbs were rigid.   The fingers were livid, and there was lividity of the shoulders.   The loss of blood from the wound amounted to about three quarts.   The ball entered under the right jaw, fractured and dislocated the bones of right side of the face and cranium, so that the brain could be examined without the use of the saw or hammer, and passing out nearly in a straight line, its course was marked by an altered state of the brain, which had a soft mashed appearance, and a greyish hue.   There was blood in both the lateral ventricles.   The left side of the brain had sustained little injury.   There was a little serum in the pericardium, and about an ounce in each pleura.   The posterior mediastinum was slightly œdematous.   No blood was found in the left cavities of the heart, and very little in the right.   The lungs were of natural appearance; anteriorly, pale and crepitous ; posteriorly, rather red, and containing a little blood and serum.   There was pretty much coagulated blood in the trachea derived from the wound, and in the large bronchial branches; their inner, the mucous membrane, though in contact with blood, was not stained, contrary to what might have been expected.   There was a great deal of masticated food, chiefly ham and bread, in the stomach ; its inner coat was unusually pale, without any softening.   The duodenum was pale; in its lower portion there was some chyme in a state of fermentation.   There was no redness of any part of the small or large intestines. The liver was of natural color. The gall-bladder contained pretty much bile, dilute and of a light orange color. The spleen was small and soft, and when broken by the pressure of the fingers, a pultaceous matter exuded from it, not unlike corrupted crassamentum, similar to what is often witnessed in this organ in cases of remittent fever in the Ionian Islands. The kidneys were pale and soft. There was about a pint of serous fluid in the cavity of the abdomen. The health of the man had always been good. The temperature of the air during the twenty-four hours was between 70° and 78°.

Was the absence of staining in the trachea and larger bronchia owing to a coating of mucus? That was a conjecture made at the time. The sudden and great loss of blood might also have been concerned in the prevention; that loss would favor a rapid cooling of the body, and the rapid cooling would retard putrefaction.

Case 12.—A private, ætat. 30; 2nd B.R.B.; shot himself in his barrack-room in Malta, on 5th August, 1830, at 5 a.m.; he died about an hour after.—He appears to have committed the act in the sitting posture. Two balls were used. They entered the mouth, passed through the anterior part of the palate, shattered the anterior portion of the spheroidal bone, the parietal, and a portion of the occipital, especially of the left side. A considerable portion of the left hemisphere of the cerebrum was carried away, and the whole of the upper part of the cerebrum was lacerated, so that it was not possible to distinguish its regions. A good deal of blood was mingled with the mangled mass. There was a good deal of bloody fluid at the base of brain. Below the tentorium the brain had sustained little or no injury; the cerebellum, medulla oblongata, pons Varolii and crura appeared to be sound. Hence, no doubt, is to be explained his not dying immediately. According to the assistant-surgeon who saw him, he lived an hour; his breathing slow and laborious; the respirations about five in a minute. He was in an unconscious state.

The examination was made 8 hours after death. The body was stout and muscular; the limbs were rigid. The pericardium contained about an ounce of serum. There was very little blood in the cavities of the heart. In the aorta there was some, and that florid. The thoracic duct was large, and contained a very little transparent lymph. There were ossific spots about the size of mustard-seed on the inner coat of the aorta, just above the coronary arteries, as if deposited from the blood, not being covered by the membrane. The right lung adhered very generally; it weighed about half a pound; the left was free; it contained some blood; it weighed about three quarters of a pound. Both were crepitous and sound. There was a good deal of bloody fluid in the large bronchial tubes, suggesting death from suffocation— the blood flowing in from the wound above. There was some bloody fluid also in the stomach, derived no doubt from the same source. The inner surface of the stomach was of a pinkish hue, as seen after the removal of some thick adhering mucus. There was no softening of the organ. The liver was of a light brown color, and rather soft. The gall-bladder contained pretty much bile, of a brighter yellow than ordinary. The spleen was rather small and firm. The kidneys small and pale. There was a good deal of pale urine in the bladder. The duodenum and upper part of the jejunum contained some chyme-like fluid, colored by bile. In the inferior part of the jejunum and the upper part of the ileum there was pretty much semi-fluid, which adhered to their sides; it was of a pasty consistence, and nearly white. In the inferior portion of the ileum and in the cœcum there was some soft dark matter, with which were mixed small fragments of undigested food. It had a fæcal smell in the colon, but not in the ileum; there its smell was peculiar. The contents were partly colored by bile, yellowish, and partly nearly colorless. There were small projecting granules scattered over the inferior ileum, cœcum, and ascending colon, probably the relics of a dysenteric attack which he had experienced in 1825. In 1826 he experienced a contusion of the thigh, from a fall when drunk from a height of about twelve feet. It was followed by a slight shortening of the limb, and by some awkwardness in marching. On examining the bone, some exostosis was found below its neck; the neck itself was nearly at right angles to the shaft; the round ligament appeared to have been broken, and the broken part to have become attached by adhesions to the acetabulum. The capsule did not appear to have been injured, nor were there any traces discoverable of a fracture.

Since 1825, except for the hurt of thigh, he had never been in hospital. He had been observed in an excited state from drink the evening before he shot himself.

Case 13.—A private, ætat. 28; shot himself about 2 p.m. on the 26th Jan. 1832; he died at 10 p.m. of the same day.—The ball entered about half an inch above the umbilicus; it passed through the stomach, then distended with food, entering close to the small arch, two or three inches above the pylorus, making a perforation just sufficient for its entrance, it made its exit through the middle of the large curvature, carrying away a portion of an irregular form, nearly the size of the hand. The boundary of the opening was red and ragged. Much of the contents of the stomach was found in the cavity of the small and great omentum. The spleen was not injured nor the kidney; but the descending colon was wounded, and a portion of it, about 2 inches in length and 1 in width, was carried away. The muscles of the flank beneath the intestines were mangled and comminuted and blackened to a considerable depth. In the left region there was a pretty large hole in the integuments just above the kidney, through which four or five fingers might have been introduced, and through which when first seen the intestines were protruding. A considerable quantity of blood was effused into the cavity of the abdomen and some fæcal matter, as well as some of the contents of the stomach. The intestines generally were stained red, as was also the peritoneal lining, and there was some coagulated blood in the colon. The thoracic viscera were healthy; the brain was not examined. The surgeon of the regiment saw him two minutes after the commission of the act. He looked faint, but was sensible, and he continued so, his mind clear, till a few minutes before he expired, when there was a slight delirium. His pulse immediately after the vast injury received was very feeble, and so it continued, only just perceptible, until the extinction of life. The skin was of moderate temperature. He vomited more than once and had hiccough. He complained of little pain, and that little he referred chiefly to the region of the bladder and to the penis. The catheter was introduced several times; the first quantity of urine drawn off was large; the latter small. There was no other treatment, except the returning of the protruding intestines and the giving a draught of T. opii. (thirty drops), twice repeated. He shot himself bending over his rifle, pretending to be oiling the lock. He was in the guard-house at the time, and was about to be taken away to be punished for theft, a crime he had committed and had been punished for three or four times before, whilst stationed in Malta. He had never shown any marks of insanity.

In reading this case, it may be well to keep in mind two effects, that of the ball passing through the stomach, and that of the explosion acting more widely on the left lumbar region. The peculiarities of the case,—the vomiting, the continuance of life so long, etc., need not be dwelt on.

Case 14.—A private, ætat. 26, stationed in Malta, shot himself on the 3rd July, 1833.—The ball entered under the chin, passed through the brain, rending the cranium and carrying before it a portion of brain. There was profuse hæmorrhage and immediate death.

The examination was made about 5 hours after. The body was well made and stout, with a healthy proportion of fat. His health had been good. The left lung was collapsed and very sound; it weighed 8½ oz.; there was no blood in its vessels; its bronchia were pale. The right lung was also healthy, but adhering; it weighed 9 oz. The pericardium contained about 2 drachms of serosity. The heart was empty. The liver and kidneys, and indeed all the abdominal viscera, were, with the exception of being unusually pale, of natural appearance. The gall-bladder was distended with thin, light-colored, yellow bile. There was some chyle in the thoracic duct. The temperature of the body was low; the heart did not feel warm; the intestines and concave surface of liver felt only slightly warm. There were no indications of putrefaction. The thermometer was about 82°; the wind N.W. The man was considered perfectly sane. Lately he had lived irregularly, had been often drunk, and had exposed himself to censure and punishment.

The occurrence of three suicides in the same regiment—the 2nd B. Rifle Brigade—in so short a time may appear surprising to those not acquainted with the army, and with the depressing mental effect of garrison duty, the same from day to day all the year round. Such is the monotony and tedium, that a portion at least of the drunkenness of the soldier may be attributed to it; and that reacting and aggravating may create such an indifference to, such a disgust of, life as to lead to the crime in question.

It is mostly on foreign stations in the infantry that these suicides are committed, and chiefly in islands from which there is no escape, and after a tedious residence prolonged to three or four years. In other stations where there are opportunities for desertion, as at Gibraltar and the Canadas, desertion is the prevailing offence rather than suicide.

Let us hope that as the condition of the soldier is improved, and as his comforts and amusements are more attended to and increased, both these great evils, the opprobria of our army, will be checked.*

In introducing these cases I have expressed the hope that they

* To endeavour to put a stop to the crime of suicide at Malta, the body of the last suicide was disgraced: it was dragged round the barrack-yard by an ass, and buried in unconsecrated ground. The effect was not known, as the regiment shortly after was removed to the Ionian isles.

may prove of some use to pathology and to medical jurisprudence. As regards the first, do they not teach us to attach but little importance to the following conditions—viz., fluid effused between the membranes of the brain, in the ventricles, at the base of the organ, and in the spinal canal; in the pericardium, the pleuræ, and peritoneal sac, in somewhat abnormal quantity; adhesions of the different viscera, especially the lungs and liver to their parieties; a softened state of the spleen; partial ossification of blood-vessels;—all these having been found in bodies which, up to the time of their sudden death, were considered in perfect health. And, extending the induction to aneurisms, have we not good reason to believe that there may be much disease of blood-vessels, even up to the moment of a rupture, without the general health being materially affected?

As regards the second, medical jurisprudence, do they not show that no just inference can be drawn from the external appearance of the cadaver that has owed its death to a blow or a fall, as to the internal injuries received, the integuments often being sound when bónes are broken and viscera ruptured? And, further, that only a very wide guess can be made from the temperature of the body, or from the degree of putrefaction it exhibits when found, of the time that has elapsed between its death and its discovery.

In another relation some of these cases are noteworthy, especially the second and third, as showing the multiplicity and variety of lesions which may be produced by a fall from a certain height—fracture of bones, laceration and rupture of organs, hæmorrhagic effusions, etc. Even the slighter lesions, such as the laceration of the fornix, the fissured state of the liver, etc., are not without interest. Are they not fairly suggestive of the probability of the occurrence of the like injuries from concussion in certain cases, and that the morbid effects, whether followed by recovery or death, may often be owing as much to the positive lesion of organs as to the mere shock of the system?

It is worthy of special mention that, as in the instances of death from aneurism, so in none of these cases, with the exception of the first very remarkable one, many of them seemingly more favorable than that to the result, no solution of the stomach took place.

CHAPTER XV.

ON URINARY AND BILIARY CALCULI, AND ON ENTOZOA.

Unfrequency of calculi in the army.—Conjectures why so.—Cases in which found noticed.—
Instances given of calculi in brute animals.—A peculiar kind of biliary calculus (indigo and
copper detected in it) described. Remarks on entozoa. Their unfrequency in the army.—
Frequency of them, owing to peculiar circumstances, amongst the inhabitants of Malta.

1. OF URINARY CALCULI.—These concretions are comparatively rarely met with in the *post mortem* examination of the
bodies of soldiers. And is not this what might be expected,
keeping in mind the age and conditions of military life?—the
age commonly between twenty and forty ; the conditions such
as are little conducive to repletion and congestion, the diet being
rather spare than full, the bodily exercise, if erring in degree,
being rather in excess than deficiency. A corpulent soldier
accordingly is rarely met with in the ranks, and arthritis does
not enter into the list of the recognized diseases of troops.

In recording the few cases in which I have found the concretions in question, I shall, as in the preceding chapter, briefly
notice those in which they occurred, premising that in the great
majority of instances the urinary bladder and kidneys were
examined.

1.—In a man, ætat. 27, who had died of chronic dysentery, a small calculus
weighing one grain was found in the pelvis of the left kidney. It was composed
chiefly of oxalate of lime, with a little animal matter. A larger calculus was found
in the pelvis of the right kidney. It weighed 26 grs., and consisted of oxalate of
lime and uric acid, with a trace of phosphate of lime and of ammoniaco-magnesian
phosphate.

2.—In a man, ætat. 23, who had died of pulmonary consumption, three minute
calculi, about the size of millet-seed, were found in the pelvis of one kidney. They
were semi-transparent, of a light greyish brown, and were composed of oxalate of
lime, with a trace of animal matter. In the pelvis of the other kidney there was a
small rough calculus of irregular form, its weight 3 grs., and of the same color and
composition as the preceding. Lithic acid was sought for in vain.

3.—In a man, ætat. 18, who had died of pneumonia, the urinary bladder was
found incrusted partially with calculous matter. It occurred in patches ; it consisted
of lithate of ammonia.

4.—In a man, ætat. 35, who had died of chronic dysentery, a small calculus, formed
of lithate of ammonia, was found in the pelvis of the left kidney.

5.—In a young man who had died of inflammation of the kidneys, three calculi were found in one kidney, each about the size of a walnut, with a good deal of gravel. The larger were of irregular form; the smaller were spherical, or a near approach to that form. They were impacted in part in the infundibula, and in part were lodged in the pelvis of the organ. The substance of the kidney was very much wasted; the ureter greatly enlarged; the bladder thickened. It bore marks of old inflammation, and perhaps of ulceration. There was, moreover, a great enlargement—a pouch—anterior to the verumontanum, which extended more than an inch between the mucous and muscular coat of the bladder. The other kidney contained no calculi, but was in substance very much wasted, and its cavity and ureter were much enlarged, as if from the influence of calculi at a former period. He had been operated on for stone some time previously, and a rough calculus had been extracted. The calculi and sand from the kidney were all of the fusible kind, formed of ammoniaco-magnesian phosphate. In none that were examined could I detect any lithic acid.

6.—In a man, ætat. 44, who had died of pneumonia, many small calculi were found in the pelvis of the left kidney. The ureter was enlarged and thickened; it was large enough to admit the little finger. The urinary bladder was thickened and contracted. The kidneys were both of them very pale and flaccid. There was no suspicion that I could learn of stone during life. The calculi were not examined.

7.—In a man, ætat. 31, who had died of pulmonary consumption, a small calculus was found in the pelvis of one of the kidneys. Its composition was not ascertained.

8.—In a man, ætat. 24, who died of pulmonary consumption, the left kidney was smaller than natural; its pelvis large. It contained, partially sacculated, a calculus of an irregular form, weighing 60 grs.; also a good deal of loose gritty matter. The right kidney was abnormally large; there was a little sand in its pelvis. Near its surface, embedded in the parenchyma, was a cyst, closed, apparently fibrous, of about the thickness of writing paper. It contained 105 minute calculi; the largest weighed 6 gr.; the smallest, ·2 gr. They were different forms; some ovoid, some trihedral, some polyhedral; those analyzed were found to consist of oxalate of lime. There was no distinct disease of the substance of either organ. No calculus was found either in the ureters or in the urinary bladder.

9.—In a man, ætat. 38, who had died laboring under epilepsy, two calculi, both of an extremely irregular form, were found in the pelvis of one of the kidneys.

10.—A calculus, extracted from the bladder of a soldier, ætat. 30, by Mr. Gulliver, was found to consist of phosphate of lime, of ammoniaco-magnesian phosphate and of carbonate of lime, the phosphate of lime greatly preponderating, with some animal matter and a trace of lithic acid. As soon as taken out, it had a putrid urinous ammoniacal odor, and the urine of the patient when voided was offensive, denoting a putrescent fermentation in the bladder.

11.—A calculus taken from the ureter of a man who died at Fort Pitt, weighed 80 grs.; its surface was smooth and polished, with the exception of a few dull protuberances; it was formed of concentric layers enveloping a dark brown, almost black nucleus; the outer layers were some of a fawn color, some white and of a granular structure; the middle layers were of a light brown and firmly radiated. The dark nucleus was finely granular and crystalline; it consisted of oxalate of lime with a trace of phosphate of lime and a considerable proportion of dark-colored animal matter, probably blood, which in drying, after having been acted on by an acid, separated like a pellicle, leaving the nucleus of a grey color. The enveloping layers were composed of phosphate of lime, ammoniaco-magnesian phosphate, and of a lithic acid, with a little carbonate of lime and animal matter.*

* A calculus given me by Dr. Marshall Hall, of about the size of a walnut and

These are the only instances in which I have detected urinary calculi during the whole of my army experience. In addition to the reasons already assigned when attempting to account for their rareness in men leading a military life, there is another deserving, perhaps, of some consideration—I mean a warm climate, especially a tropical climate. That calculous complaints are uncommon in these climates, is pretty certain. In a note, bearing the date of Ceylon, 1817, I find it stated, that to all the inquiries I there made on the subject, the invariable reply from medical practitioners who had been many years in the island, was that calculous affections were unknown amongst the native population.* And in the West Indies the information I received was similar.† I also find from my notes that I was impressed by the circumstance of the absence of lithic deposit in the urine, comparing my experience there with my experience at home. There it appeared to me that there was greater functional activity of the surface of the body than in a cooler climate, as denoted by a more rapid growth of the beard and of the hair generally, and of the nails, accompanied probably by a quicker waste and renewal of the cuticle. Now, as the hair, the nails, and the cuticle contain a large proportion of nitrogen, the nitrogen so thrown off may possibly be one of the causes of a lessening of the calculous and arthritic diatheses; and if so, would be applicable to British soldiers, who, taking with their regiments their turn of duty, unavoidably spend not an inconsiderable portion of their period of service either in the East or West Indies, Ceylon or the Mauritius, or in the Mediterranean and other warm climates.

As allied to the preceding, I may notice a gouty concretion which I analysed, remarkable for the many parts in which it was deposited, and I shall add a brief account of two or three

nearly of the same form, was remarkable for being studded with bright trapezoidal crystals apparent to the naked eye. A section of it showed it to be composed of compact hard concentric layers. Its principal ingredient was oxalate of lime, with which was mixed a little carbonate of lime and animal matter.

* This recalls a somewhat ludicrous incident. A zealous Staff Surgeon, after assiduous search for a case to operate on, was directed to a Moorman, whom, to my friend's disgust, he found not laboring under stone, but a dealer in precious stones.

† With one exception—viz., at St. Kitt's, where I heard of a case of stone—a patient of Dr. Rawling's, who by an operation extracted it from the bladder ; it was small, of a cylindrical shape, as if formed in a ureter, and rounded at its ends. On examination, I found it to be of the lithic acid kind.

calculi taken from the urinary bladder of animals, and of one from the stomach.

In the pathological museum at Fort Pitt is the hand of an officer deceased, who had suffered much from gout. It abounded in concretions. The chief seat of the deposit was the cellular tissue, especially the subcutaneous. In some of the joints there was a very slight incrustation on the cartilages; in others none, nor in the sheaths of the tendons. In the substance of two of the tendons there was a concretion of about the size of a small pea. None was visible on the bones, nerves, or blood-vessels. A little was to be seen in the very substance of the cutis; this was towards the extremity of the little finger, of which a section had been made. The deposited matter resembled chalk, being opaque, white and soft. From an analysis I made of it, it appeared to be composed of

94·5 Superlithate of soda,
4·5 Phosphate and carbonate of lime,
1·0 Animal matter, chiefly cellular tissue.

That animals, at least of the higher orders, are subject to nearly the same diseases as man, is now an acknowledged fact. Yet a work on comparative pathology is still a desideratum. I shall add here a very small contribution, in a brief notice of the few calculi which I have examined, found in brutes.

1.—In the bladder of a rabbit some very fine sand was found; it was of a fawn color, effervesced strongly with an acid, and was composed chiefly of carbonate of lime, with a little animal matter. My friend, Mr. Gulliver, from whom I received it, informed me that he had often met with a deposit of the same kind in the urinary bladder of this animal.

2.—In the bladder of a fox-hound minute crystals were found which were presented by Mr. Gulliver to the pathological museum at Fort Pitt. Under the microscope they were seen to be of different forms, some prismatic, some tabular. Subjected to analysis they were found to be composed of phosphate of lime and of ammoniaco-magnesian phosphate with a little animal matter.

3.—In the urinary bladder of an old rat, opened at Fort Pitt, a calculus was detected, about the size of a pea; it adhered slightly to a small soft excrescence from the inner coat at the fundus; it was of a light brown color, nearly spherical, and was formed of a congeries of low four-sided prisms, bevilled at the edges, radiating from a central point. The crystals were of a size visible to the naked eye. They were composed of oxalate of lime with a trace of animal matter.

4.—In the urinary bladder of a pig four calculi were found. The largest weighed 4½ grains; the smallest 3 grains. They were polyhedral, of a greyish hue, very compact, hard and tough; they consisted of carbonate of lime, with a trace of phosphate of lime and animal matter.

5.—In the large intestine of a horse a calculus was found of about the size of a man's fist; it was of a globular form and consisted of brown fibrinous matter included in a hard crust of the same color. The fibres were of vegetable matter matted together irregularly and cemented by phosphate of lime with a little carbonate of lime and a trace of magnesia; intermixed were some grains of siliceous sand. The crust contained but a small proportion of vegetable matter.

6.—A calculus, rather less than a hen's egg, was found in the large intestine of another horse; of an oval form, it was composed of concentric layers, with an iron nail for a nucleus. Phosphate of lime, with a little phosphate of magnesia and a little animal matter were its chief ingredients.

7.—In the bladder of an ox 50 small calculi were detected. The largest was very little larger than a grape seed; it weighed 8 grain; the smallest were not larger than the finest mustard-seed and weighed less than $\frac{1}{100}$th of a grain; they were all of a pearly lustre, of a yellowish brown hue externally, and of silvery white internally. The smallest were spherical; the larger irregularly globular. When heated, they decrepitated, breaking up into fine concentric laminæ. They were composed, like pearls, of carbonate of lime and of animal matter, probably albumen, but whether, as in the instance of pearls, in alternate layers, was not ascertained. After the removal of the carbonate of lime by an acid, the remaining animal matter, which was diaphanous, retained the form of the concretion.

8.—In the water-cells of the pacho's stomach (Auchenia Paco) many black mulberry-like concretions were found; hardly a cell was without one. One of them, sent to me by Mr. Gulliver, weighed 25·3 grs. Broken, it was seen to consist of a mixture of black and fawn-colored matter, distributed somewhat irregularly in layers. From the analysis I made of it, it appeared to be composed of

82·9 Phosphate of lime, with a trace of peroxide of iron and a little silica,
·4 Two bits of siliceous gravel,
17·7 Brown combustible matter, chiefly vegetable.

The bits of gravel were in the middle of the concretion and may be considered its nuclei.

2. OF BILIARY CALCULI.—The proportional frequency of calculi of this kind in the same class of men seems to differ but little from that of the urinary, and probably for like reasons, as to diet and regimen. The following instances are all those of which I have notes. Almost in every fatal case the gall-bladder was examined, so their rareness of occurrence cannot justly be attributed to oversight.

1.—In a man, ætat. 26, who died of remittent fever, three small biliary calculi were found in the gall-bladder. They were of an unusual form, being flat; were almost black, but imparted a bright yellow streak to paper; they gave the same color to alcohol, but were not sensibly diminished in bulk by its action; of a soft consistence, they had a slightly bitter taste. No cholesterine was found in them; they were formed chiefly of dark coloring matter, with a little inspissated bile.

2.—In an officer, ætat. 56, who had died of apoplexy and was very corpulent, three large concretions were found, all three of the cholesterine kind.

3.—In a man, ætat. 46, who had died of chronic dysentery, two small calculi of the black kind were found in his bladder.

4.—In a man, ætat. 26, who had died laboring under diarrhœa, several small calculi were found; they consisted of cholesterine.

5.—In a man laboring under acute rheumatism, ætat. 36, a concretion was found, of about the size of an almond, composed partly of cholesterine, and partly of black matter.

6.—In a man, ætat. 33, who had died of pulmonary consumption, many small calculi were found in the gall-bladder; they were of the black kind. Two of the same kind were impacted in and obstructed the cystic duct.

7.—In a man, ætat. 56, who had died dropsical and laboring under disease of the heart, a calculus was found, nearly the size of an almond, and composed of cholesterine.

8.—In a man, ætat. 57, who had died of chronic dysentery, a calculus was found of moderate size, composed of dark brown insoluble matter, and of inspissated bile.

9.—In a man, ætat. 28, who had died of chronic dysentery, complicated with pulmonary consumption, five small calculi were found in the gall-bladder, all of the black kind.

In none of these cases had there been, that I am aware of, any symptoms of the presence of these concretions during life.

Of the several kinds of biliary concretions, the black kind is perhaps the rarest. Its composition is peculiar. It is not, as described by an eminent pathologist, " chiefly carbonaceous," * but is a mixture of two or three or more proximate principles, one of them indigo, or a substance nearly allied to indigo. A small specimen—and the smallest are commonly the purest— which at my request was analyzed by Dr. Edmund Davy, in the Laboratory of the Royal Dublin Society, was found to consist of

$$53 \cdot 38 \text{ Carbon,}$$
$$6 \cdot 77 \text{ Hydrogen,}$$
$$7 \cdot 62 \text{ Nitrogen,}$$
$$25 \cdot 34 \text{ Oxygen,}$$
$$6 \cdot 89 \text{ Ash.}$$

The ash I have found to be composed chiefly of phosphate of lime, with magnesia and a trace of lime and peroxide of iron. In the ash of two specimens with which I was supplied by the late Mr. Quikett, from the collection of the Royal College of Surgeons, an unmistakeable trace of copper was also detected.† These specimens—they were a small portion of the whole—were marked in the College Museum Catalogue B.B. 10 and 12.

3. OF ENTOZOA.—Probably in no class of men are entozoa less frequent than in men of the British army. This may be owing to the quality of their diet, and to the circumstance that few soldiers restrict themselves to water as a beverage; and also

---

* Dr. Bennett, Clin. Lect., etc., Ed. 3rd, p. 256.

† In five other specimens I have sought for copper, but without success, proving that this metal is not an essential constituent part of the concretion.

in part to the fact that the water with which they are supplied is commonly the best that can be obtained in the neighbourhood of their barracks, and is mostly spring or pump water.

The following are the few instances in which I have detected entozoa—at least of which I have made a note :—

1.—In a man, ætat. 45, a private of the Malta Fencibles, and a native of Malta, who had died of fever, a tape-worm was found in the jejunum.

2.—In a man, ætat. 28, who had died of aneurism, a tape-worm was found in the upper part of the small intestines. He had been ten years in the Mediterranean, and was just returned from Malta.

3.—In a man, ætat. 27, who had died of peritonitis in Corfu, a living ascaris lumbricoides was found in the right iliac fossa, close to a perforation of the intestine.*

4.—In a man, ætat. 28, who had died of continued fever, an hydatid, included in its sac, about the size of a large orange, was found in the liver. The hydatid was dead, and was in process of change.

5.—In a boy, a Maltese, ætat. 2 years, who had died laboring under dysentery, a very large quantity of round worms (A. lumbricoides) was found in the stomach, the liver, and the small intestines, and of ascarides (A. vermicularis) in the large intestines. The common duct was very large, about the size of the thumb, and was full of worms to distension, as was also the hepatic duct. The liver was large; it contained several abscesses, in each of which was one or more round worms—these probably the cause of the suppuration. The boy was an orphan, and a charity-child, the mother having died shortly after his birth ; he had been taken in at the Ospizio, and was probably ill-fed and neglected.

It is worthy of remark, in relation to the etiology of entozoa, that the Maltese are peculiarly subject to these parasites. Whilst stationed there, I was in the habit of attending the *post mortem* examinations in the large civil hospital of Valetta, and rarely a body was opened there in which worms were not found. The round worm was most common. The cause of this prevalency, I am induced to think, is not connected with the climate of the Island, that on the whole being very dry and warm, but with the diet of the laboring class, consisting largely of crude vegetables and fruits ; and, even more than the diet, with the water used for drinking, most of it being rain-water, collected in tanks from surfaces exposed to the air, with little attention to their cleanliness—especially in the instance of field-tanks, which during the rainy season receive water from the public roads, these abounding in impurities, and in the excrements of man and animals.

* See Case 3, p. 336.

CHAPTER XVI.

ON PECULIARITIES OF ORGANS AS TO FORM AND POSITION.

Notice restricted to such peculiarities as met with in ordinary *post mortem* examinations.— Examples described; 1st, Of the alimentary canal; 2ndly, Of the liver, spleen and pancreas; 3rdly, Of the kidneys and generative organs; 4thly, Of the lungs and some adjoining parts; 5thly, Of the mammæ; 6thly, Of the heart and blood-vessels; 7thly, Of the brain and nerves. —Questions as to the correlation of the abnormal; of their influence in relation to health, and their approximation to the normal in other animals.

THE peculiarities which I am about to describe were noticed in the ordinary *post mortem* examinations, made not for the purpose of seeking what is abnormal in structure or form, but in search of pathological changes, lesions connected with the fatal disease. Had the search been special, no doubt more would have been discovered, and, also more, had all the examinations been made leisurely with the requisite attention, and not—and this unavoidably—often conducted either hastily for want of time, or under the further disadvantage of unfit place, want of good light and the other favorable circumstances which the dissecting-room should be provided with. I make these remarks, calling to mind the wretched state of some of the " dead-houses" attached to military hospitals on foreign stations, and how occasionally the autopsy was conducted even in churches, the Latin and Greek. If there were one exception it was at Malta, where the old laboratory belonging to the great hospital of the knights, that in which Dolomieu had worked, was used for the purpose. I make this statement with the intent of conveying my impression that peculiarities of structure are more common than is generally believed, and that the more they are sought for, the less rare they will appear. In accordance with this, it may be remarked, that they have been noticed most in those parts in which they are most easily seen and requiring least scrutiny for their detection, such as the intestines as regards position, the larger viscera as regards form, the arteries as regards origin and distribution. And, might not this have been anticipated when we consider how subject to variation are the parts which are external, especially the features of the face and the forms of the hands and feet.

The observations being altogether of a miscellaneous kind I shall give them without much attention to order, and nearly in the words in which they were described at the time.   When the contrary is not stated, it is to be understood that the subjects were the bodies of soldiers.

1. Of the Alimentary Canal :—

1.—In a man, ætat. 26, who had died of acute dysentery, the colon passed from the left side across the spine to the right, and the rectum descended on the right side.   No other peculiarity was observed in conducting the autopsy.   And, here I may remark that in the cases in which more than one organ was found abnormal, the complication will be given, and that if only one is specified, only one was detected.

2.—In a man, ætat. 25, who had died of acute dysentery, an unusual convolution of the colon was found in the cavity of the pelvis.   This during life might have led to the inference—an inference actually formed—of there being an obstruction in the upper portion of the rectum, impeding an attempted introduction of a probang.

3.—In a man, ætat. 20, who had died of pulmonary consumption, the cœcum lay loose over the brim of the pelvis.   There was an unusual fold of the colon parallel to the sigmoid flexure, and the rectum was on the right side.   The right lung had only two lobes.

4.—In a man who had died of chronic dysentery, a very unusual convolution of the colon was found in the cavity of the pelvis.

5.—In a man, ætat. 27, who had died of acute dysentery, the cœcum was found resting anteriorly on the urinary bladder and posteriorly on the sacrum.   During health he had been subject to great irregularity of bowels.

6.—In a man, ætat. 34, who had died laboring under ascites, there was an unusual turn of the colon over the brim of the pelvis from the left to the right side and back to the median line.   The liver was small; in the place of its left lobe there was a substance more like the pancreas in structure than the liver, very little larger than the suprarenal gland and much of the same form, firm, pale and yellow.

7.—In a man, ætat. 72 (a Maltese), who had died of pleurisy and pericarditis, the cœcum was found surrounded by convolutions of the small intestines.   The large intestines were loaded with hardened scybala.

8.—In a man, ætat. 56, who had died of pneumonia and pleurisy, the colon was about twice its natural length, unusually large and making very unusual turns; it was distended with fæces.   He was a Maltese, a common beggar.

9.—In a man, ætat. 23, who had died of remittent fever, the descending colon in the left lumbar region ascended from the brim of the pelvis to the middle lumbar vertebra, and from thence descended in a line with the spine into the pelvis, in the cavity of which it lay in two or three loose convolutions.

10.—In a man, ætat. 20, who had died of remittent fever, there was an unusual convolution of the colon in the pelvis, between the sigmoid flexure and the rectum.

11.—In a man, ætat. 30, who had died of remittent fever, there was a considerable portion of the large intestine lying loose in folds in the cavity of the pelvis.

12.—In a man, ætat. 32, who had died of remittent fever, an unusual quantity of colon was found in the cavity of the pelvis.

13.—In a man, ætat. 31, who had died of remittent fever, the course of the colon was irregular; on the left side it ascended nearly to the diaphragm, and an unusual quantity of it was collected in the cavity of the pelvis.

14.—In a man, ætat. 31, who had died of the same disease, an unusual fold of the intestine was found in the cavity of the pelvis.

15.—In a man, ætat. 34, who had died of pneumonia, the colon descended and re-ascended on the right side before becoming transverse.

16.—In a man, ætat. 36, who had died of pneumonia, the cœcum was unattached to the lumbar region, but a portion of the colon about eight inches from it, was so attached. The cœcum was loose and large and lay incumbent on the right portion of the transverse colon.

17.—In a man, ætat. 29, who had died of pneumonia, the lower part of the colon, between the sigmoid flexure and the rectum, made an unusual turn towards the right side of two or three inches, folding on itself.

18.—In a man, ætat. 31, who had died laboring under empyema, the colon was unusually long and of irregular course; both its ascending and transverse portion were convoluted; the latter was so high as to lie beneath the stomach; it was loaded with hardened scybala.

19.—In a man, ætat. 27, who had died of empyema, the cœcum was only very slightly attached to the lumbar region; it was almost floating. The transverse colon dipped up and down.

20.—In a man, ætat. 41, who had died of diarrhœa, the colon, instead of going transversely across from the right to the left, descended obliquely to the symphysis pubis, where it was attached to the peritoneum, and from thence it re-ascended obliquely to the left hypochondrium, descending in the usual manner. There were several convolutions of the small intestines in the cavity of the pelvis.

21.—In a man, ætat. 28, who had died of chronic dysentery, the colon where it began to ascend was bent back; it crossed just under the umbilicus, leaving a space of about four fingers' width between it and the duodenum: in this space there were three folds of the jejunum.

22.—In a man, ætat. 38, who had died of pulmonary consumption, there was an unusual curvature of the colon from the left iliac fossa over the spine, before descending into the pelvis.

23.—In a man, ætat. 25, who had died of pulmonary consumption, there was a considerable length of the colon in the cavity of the pelvis; it was there convoluted two or three times.

24.—In a man, ætat. 24, who had died of peritonitis, the cœcum was situated higher than usual; the end of the ileum occupying the ordinary place of the cœcum, and there firmly adhering.

25.—In a man, ætat. 32, who had died of pulmonary consumption, the rectum was tortuous.

26.—In a man, ætat. 38, who had died of paralysis, laboring under amentia, the lower part of the ileum crossed over to the lower part of the right psoas muscle, from whence it ascended straight to the cœcum. The cœcum was unusually high up. There were several folds of the colon in the cavity of the pelvis.

27.—In a man, ætat. 58, who had died of pulmonary consumption, laboring under amentia, the transverse colon was exceedingly tortuous. The testes, etc., were very small; no albuginea could be detected.*

28.—In a man, ætat. 60, who had died laboring under mania, the cœcum was found lying loose in the cavity of the pelvis.

---

* See Case 9, chap. viii., where the case is described.

29.—In a man, ætat. 27, who had died laboring under epilepsy, the appendicula vermiformis was lying over the right kidney and adhering to it. The cœcum was loose. The ileum joined the cœcum from below, and was bound down where the latter is usually attached.

30.—In a man, ætat. 38, who had died of peritonitis, the inferior portion of the ileum was found deep in the cavity of the pelvis; thence it ascended into the right iliac fossa, the usual situation of the cœcum, and joined the latter higher up.

31.—In a man, ætat. 18, who had died of peritonitis, a large portion of the ileum was found in the cavity of the pelvis.

32.—In a man, ætat. 39, who had died of chronic hepatitis, a large quantity of the small intestines was found in the cavity of the pelvis.

33.—In a man, ætat. 27, who had died of pulmonary consumption, a pouch, a blind sac, projected from the ileum about a foot from its termination, a vestige probably of the omphalo-mesenteric duct. There was an unusual turn of the colon in the cavity of the pelvis.

34.—In a man, ætat. 25, who had died of pulmonary consumption, a similar sac proceeded from the lower part of the ileum.

35.—In a man, ætat. 41, who committed suicide laboring under melancholia, the transverse colon descended obliquely nearly to the brim of the pelvis; a large portion of the small intestines lay in the cavity of the pelvis; the jejunum was situated above the small arch of the stomach; the spleen was large, composed of two globular masses, as if double; the two were connected by a ligamentous band.

36.—In a man, ætat. 23, who had died of rubeola, the stomach, with the liver, were situated very high up; the superior portion of each reached the fourth rib. They were completely hid by the ribs. The pancreas, duodenum, spleen, etc., were proportionally higher than usual. The capacity of the chest was consequently small. There was no flatulent distension, or obvious cause of this unusual position of the viscera.

37.—In a male child, a few days old, a portion of the duodenum was deficient. The infant otherwise, so far as was ascertained, was well organized, and of full size. It had died of starvation. It sucked at first vigorously, and cried lustily.

38.—In three men, one ætat. 27, who had died of chronic dysentery; another, ætat. 37; and a third who had died of pneumonia (and some other instances were met with) the stomach exhibited the hour-glass form—this commonly attributed to abnormal contraction, but which I am more inclined to consider as an abnormal form and, when occurring, permanent.

2. OF THE LIVER, SPLEEN, AND PANCREAS:—

1.—In a man, ætat. 26, who had died of pulmonary consumption, the liver was of unusual form; the left lobe was about the size of a hen's egg. The weight of the whole was 4 lbs.

2.—In a man, ætat. 40, who had died laboring under paralysis, the lobulus Spigelii was nearly of a globular form, and was attached to the body of the liver by a narrow band only. The left lobe was very small, and the part of it connected with the lateral ligament tapered gradually to a point. The descending colon made an unusual turn.

3.—In a man, ætat. 31, who had died laboring under paralysis, the liver in form resembled the heart; it was small, consisting almost entirely of the right lobe. The left was represented by a small mass, not larger than the lobulus Spigelii of its ordinary size. The lobulus Spigelii was deficient. The structure of the organ was normal; its weight 2½ lbs.

4.—In a man, ætat. 36, who had died of remittent fever, the liver was of very irregular form, and had several lobes. The situation of the omentum was unusual; it was reflected over the transverse colon, and was lying on the stomach and gall-bladder, to the latter of which it was attached.

5.—In a man, ætat. 32, who had died of remittent fever, the liver, of a globular form, was composed almost entirely of the right lobe. In place of the left there was a small triangular body, firm, yellowish, and granular, in substance more like a pancreas. A very minute lobule was attached to it, hardly the size of a hazel-nut, of the color and appearance of the right lobe. The testicle (the left) could not be felt. On laying open the scrotum, it was found very much wasted; hardly a vestige of it remained attached to the chord. A small calculus accompanied it, which, on cutting through the tunica vaginalis (also much wasted), came out. It was enveloped in a pretty firm membrane.* The vesiculæ seminales were both small; both contained a brownish fluid. There was no appearance of the caput galinaginis. The left epigastric artery was nearly obliterated; its mouth was so contracted as to admit only a hog's bristle; and it soon dwindled away in a part of the peritoneum where there was an unusual degree of roughness.

6.—In a man, ætat. 33, who had died of pulmonary consumption, the left lobe of the liver was about twice the length of the right. Imbedded in it was a spherical cyst, nearly the size of a billiard ball; it contained what seemed dead hydatids, somewhat altered, matted confusedly together, greyish, soft, and membranous. Flakes and grains of cholesterine were conspicuous amongst them.

7.—In a man, ætat. 48, who had died of chronic hepatitis, there were two hepatic ducts of nearly the same size; the cystic duct communicated with the nearest to it.

8.—In a man, ætat. 24, who had died of pulmonary consumption, the liver was of an unusual form. There was a vestige only of the left lobe, and that was not continuous with the right. The lobulus Spigelii was very small; two small lobules were attached to it. The ligamentum rotundum was apart from the broad ligament.

9.—In a man, ætat. 23, who had died of pulmonary consumption, the lobulus Spigelii was larger than common, and was attached to the right lobe only by a narrow neck. An unusual fold of the peritoneum formed a sac capable of holding all the small intestines. The descending colon was attached to its upper surface.

10.—In a man, ætat. 23, who had died of dysentery, a small mass about the size of a hazel-nut, the structure of which appeared to be the same as that of the liver, was attached to the concave surface of that organ by a delicate ligament.

11.—In a man, ætat. 25, who had died of pulmonary consumption, the spleen was lobulated and large, in figure resembling the liver.

12.—In a man, ætat. 27, who had died of pneumonia, there were two supernume-rary spleens, about the size of cherries, connected with the spleen by vessels and cellular tissue.

13.—In a man, ætat. 44, who died of peritonitis, the pancreatic duct terminated in the duodenum, about an inch apart from the common biliary duct.

14.—In a man who had died of pulmonary consumption, the pancreatic duct opened into the intestine, about half an inch from the common biliary duct.

15.—In a man, ætat. 33, who died asthmatic, the pancreatic duct, just before joining the common biliary duct, was largely dilated, resembling a ranula. The sac it formed contained little masses of a greyish hue, moderately firm, but compressible. They consisted, it may be conjectured, either of albuminous matter, or of inspissated mucus. The pancreas was large.

---

* It was slightly diaphanous, and of a finely crystalline structure. It effervesced slightly with nitric acid, and was composed of albuminous matter and of phosphate and carbonate of lime.

3. Of the Kidneys and Generative Organs :—

1.—In a man, ætat. 32, who had died of pulmonary consumption, laboring under amentia, the kidneys were joined; the line of junction was not perceptible. The ureters were large, and passed over the anterior surface of the renal mass.

2.—In a man, ætat. 33, who had died of pulmonary consumption, the left kidney gave off two ureters, each from the opposite end of the pelvis; they joined about three inches above the bladder; each was larger than an ordinary ureter.

3.—In a man, ætat. 27, who had died of peritonitis, the left kidney lay over the aorta, just at its bifurcation.

4.—In a man, ætat. 32, who had died of pulmonary consumption, the left vesicula seminalis consisted of one compartment—that is, it was without cells. It communicated with the vas deferens about half an inch from the abrupt termination of the latter. The vesicula had its own duct, which terminated at the verumontanum. The other vesicula was formed of cells as usual, and was no wise peculiar.

5.—In a man, ætat. 39, who had died of chronic dysentery, one testicle was deficient; the chord, tunica vaginalis and tunica albuginea were found in the scrotum. There was a small hernia of the jejunum, the villous coat protruding through the muscular, about the size of a filbert. It was formed of the peritoneal and mucous coat, without the muscular, as if the muscular had been ruptured, or had been deficient *ab origine*.

6.—In a man, ætat. 27, who died of chronic dysentery, the left testicle had not descended into the scrotum. It was small and soft, as was also the other.

4. Of the Lungs and some Adjoining Parts :—

1.—In a man, ætat. 28, who had died of pulmonary consumption, the right lung consisted of two large lobes and of three lobules, the left of two lobes and one lobule.

2.—In a man, ætat. 26, who had died of hæmoptysis, both lobes were very much lobulated.

3.—In another, the left lung consisted of three lobes.

4.—In another, the right lung consisted of two lobes.

5.—In a man, ætat. 28, who had died of chronic dysentery, the right lung had five lobes, the left three. There was an unusual convolution of the colon in the cavity of the pelvis, below the sigmoid flexure.

6.—In a man, ætat. 41, who had died of pulmonary consumption, the right lung had no middle lobe.

7.—In a man, ætat. 34, who had died of remittent fever, a large bronchial tube terminated abruptly. There was no appearance of disease in the part.

8.—In a man, ætat. 33, the thyroid gland consisted of one lobe only, the right, which was of moderate size. In the situation opposite, on the left, there was a small vesicle, about the size of a cherry, distended with a transparent fluid. The thyroid arteries on this side were very small, disappearing in the cellular tissue. The thyroid cartilages were ossified.

9.—In a man, ætat. 37, who died asthmatic, there was a small additional uvula in the form of a fleshy excrescence.

5. Of the Mammæ.—Amongst the cases already given there is more than one instance of these organs being developed in men judging merely from size and appearance. Whilst I was in Barbadoes, a colored woman came under my notice, with the peculiarity of having what might be called a third mamma. In

her left axilla, about an inch from its deepest part, a faint areola
was observable, distinguishable by its darker hue from the adjoining skin. The part included was slightly protuberant, but
without a papilla. On pressure a milky fluid exuded from it by
two minute orifices. A small portion of this fluid was collected,
also a little milk from the right breast. The examination satisfied
me that the fluid was of the nature of milk, differing no more
from ordinary human milk than might have been expected,
taking into account that it had not been regularly drawn.* The
woman when I saw her was about 30 years of age, in good
health and robust, the mother of eight children, the two youngest
twins. When nursing her other children, she experienced, she
said, a sense of fulness in the axilla, and an uneasy sensation
there, but without any flow of milk from the part. When she
had twins, and not before, the exudation took place. Sometimes
when the infants were at the breast, so copiously was it secreted
as to flow down and wet her clothes.

6. Of the Heart and Blood-vessels :—

1.—In a man, ætat. 20, who had died of continued fever, there were only two
semilunar valves to the aorta; these were large; one of them extended upwards
obliquely, and nearly hid the mouth of one of the coronary arteries. The spleen
was large and fissured. There were twelve supernumerary spleens attached to
it, the largest about the size of a boy's playing marble; their structure was like that
of the spleen. The larynx was small, as before puberty; so too was the thyroid
gland. There was only one kidney; it was of a somewhat irregular form, and about
one-third larger than usual; it was situated on the brim of the pelvis, resting on the
vena cava and in part on the aorta and common right iliac artery, dipping into the
pelvic cavity nearly in contact with the bladder; it had two emulgent arteries, one
emulgent vein, one ureter.

2.—In a man, ætat. 33, who had died of pneumonia, the aorta took its rise from
the left side of the ventricle, behind a portion of the mitral valve, instead of to the
right of it. Part of the mitral valve was attached to the septum of the ventricles.

3.—In a man, ætat. 36, who had died of hæmoptysis, the aorta took its rise from
the side opposite to that from which it usually has its origin.

4.—In a man who had died of diarrhœa there were four coronary arteries.

5.—In a man, ætat. 35, who had died of pulmonary consumption, the arteria innominata rose from the arch of the aorta, a little to the left of the median line under the
trachea. The descending aorta was small.

* The milk from the axilla had the whiteness of cow's or goat's milk; that from
the breast was of a pale greyish hue; the former was much thicker than the latter,
and when the vessel holding it was inclined it did not flow so readily as the other
similarly placed. Under the microscope, it was seen to abound more in globular
particles and granules. By evaporation the former yielded 23·8 per cent. solid
residue; the latter 10·3 per cent. After a rest of four days the former fluid had
thrown up a thicker oleaginous film than the latter.

6.—In a man, ætat. 40, who had died laboring under *delirium tremens*, the left vertebral artery rose immediately from the aorta between the carotid and subclavian; it was unusually long before entering the spine. The right as usual rose from the subclavian.

7.—In a man, ætat. 58, who died of apoplexy, there was no right vertebral artery, the left was unusually large.

8.—In a man, ætat. 52, who had died of *delirium tremens*, the left carotid artery rose from the innominata.

9.—In a man, ætat. 27, who had died of pulmonary consumption, the superior thyroid artery was given off unusually low from the carotid, and descended tortuous over that artery before entering the gland, so as to be in the way were the carotid to be tied. The colon in descending passed from the left iliac fossa, across the spine, under and close to the caput cœcum.

10.—In a man, ætat. 20, who died of pulmonary consumption, a delicate filamentous chord stretched across the basilar artery, its interior, close to the mouth of the right vertebral artery.

11.—In a man, ætat. 29, who died of pulmonary consumption, a band crossed the basilar artery close to the junction of the vertebral arteries; it supported a small concretion about the size of a grape-stone, firm, white and nearly oval.

12.—In a man, ætat. 35, who died of pulmonary consumption, the Eustachian valve was large. A similar valve was found in the left auricle between the mouths of the pulmonary veins and the auricular ventricular opening; it was larger even than the Eustachian.

13.—In a man, ætat. 26, who had died of remittent fever, the Eustachian valve was connected with the side of the auricle by a lace-work of fibres.

14.—In a man, ætat. 30, who had died laboring under hœmaturia, the Eustachian valve was connected with the adjoining surface, the vena cava, etc., by very long fibrous chords.

15.—In a man, ætat. 32, who had died of dysentery, the Eustachian valve was indistinct.

16.—In a man, ætat. 19, who had died of abscess in the liver, etc., a valve was found in the vena cava superior, very like the Eustachian valve; it was connected with the Eustachian valve by a curious network of "tendinous fibres." The mouth of the coronary vein was immediately under the Eustachian valve, and was without its proper valve, the Eustachian supplying its place.

17.—In a man, ætat. 24, who had died of remittent fever, the foramen ovale was sufficiently open to admit the little finger, and without, what is more common, a lapping over of the sides; so in this instance there was no impediment in the way of the blood passing from one auricle into the other.

18.—In a man, ætat. 20, who had died anasarcous, there was a direct opening in the fossa ovalis, sufficiently large to admit the little finger; there were also four other small openings in the septum of the fossa, admitting bristles.

19.—In a man, ætat. 33, who had died of diffuse cellular inflammation, there were several small openings in the fossa ovalis; two were large enough to admit a goose-quill. The membrane was very thin.

20.—In a man, ætat. 25, who had died of dysentery, there was an oblique opening in the fossa ovalis large enough to admit the little finger, but from its valvular overlapping structure the passage of blood from the left auricle into the right was completely prevented.*

* In a large number of cases there has been a vestige of the foramen ovale; indeed in a moiety at least of the whole there has been an opening in the fossa ovalis varying

21.—In a man, ætat. 24, who had died of pulmonary consumption, the ascending vena cava was situated on the left side of the spine; it crossed to the right close to the cæliac artery under the aorta.

22.—In a fœtus, of about 5 months, which had died *in utero*, a large opening was found between the right and left ventricle, situated in the septum, just below the origin of the pulmonary artery and of the aorta. The heart was pretty large; the foramen ovale small; the Eustachian valve indistinct; the left auricle small; the right large; the ductus arteriosus large—so large that the pulmonary artery appeared to form a part of the aorta.

The mother three years before gave birth to a child at its full period, which lived several days: its color was that of a person with morbus cœruleus.

23.—In a man, ætat. 21, who had died of dysentery, the thoracic duct gave off a large branch in the thorax, which re-united with the trunk about an inch higher, forming a semicircle.

7. OF THE BRAIN AND NERVES:—

1.—In a man, ætat. 38, who had died of apoplexy, there was in the brain, besides the common posterior cornua, an additional one adjoining, which as to position and relative length, might be compared to the thumb and index finger. It was in the right lateral ventricle.

2.—In a man who had died of peritonitis there was no distinct septum lucidum.

3.—In a man, ætat. 22, who had died of pulmonary consumption, a thread of medullary matter was found in the right lateral ventricle, extending from the upper margin of the septum lucidum to the surface of the corpus striatum; it was about a quarter of an inch long, and about a line thick; it passed from the substance of the one into that of the other. The pancreas was large, and there were several small bodies between its head and the pylorus, in structure very like the pancreas; the largest was nearly the size of a common hazel-nut.

4.—In a Maltese child, ætat. 2 years, who had died of complicated disease of lungs and brain, and was blind of the left eye, the cornea of this eye was found opaque, the pupil closed, the lens deficient, its capsule remaining, the vitreous humor much shrunk and firmer than usual; behind it was a fluid like the aqueous humor; the retina apparently was unaltered. The optic nerve was smaller than that of the right, and this both before and after decussation, as if there had been no interruption in the chiasma. No mention is made of any preceding disease of the eye bearing on the question whether the peculiarities were congenital or not.

5.—In a man, ætat. 58, who had died of gangrene of lung, laboring under amentia, the pineal gland was deficient; not a trace of it was discernible.

6.—In a man, ætat. 35, who had died of pulmonary consumption, the great sympathetic nerve in the neck on the right side was unusually large; it terminated in delicate filaments a little above the clavicle, these vanishing without entering into the ganglion just under that bone. This ganglion was rather larger than usual, whilst the thoracic ganglia were rather smaller. On the left side the union of the parts was complete; both nerves were of a light yellowish wine hue.

7.—In a man, ætat. 41, who had died of hæmorrhage from the rupture of an aneurism, there was no septum lucidum, no velum interpositum, and a free communi-

in size from an aperture admitting a surgeon's probe to one admitting a bougie of the largest size, or the end of the little finger.

cation consequently between the lateral ventricles and the third ventricle. He was remarkable for good sense and good conduct.

A child of Maltese parents, dead-born at full time, had six fingers on each hand, and six toes on each foot.* The mother and grandmother had the same peculiarity. The additional finger in each was next to the little finger. The mother had the perfect use of all her fingers, as well as of her toes. A child that preceded this had hands and feet like its father's.

It is not my intention to offer any speculative conjectures on the preceding observations, with the exception of proposing a very few queries :—

1. Considering the many cases of pulmonary consumption in which some peculiarity of structure was noticed, is it not probable that a certain constitutional debility may be connected both with the disease as to its origin, and the abnormal state of organ or organs?

2. Does there not seem to be some correlation of the abnormal, inasmuch as in a certain number of instances the abnormal form was not single and solitary?

3. Is there a sufficiency of data for the induction that irregularity of position of the intestines, especially of the large intestines, is etiologically connected with insanity?

4. Is there not a special interest attached to an inquiry of this kind into abnormal forms, and the irregular position of parts in man in connection with organic development in other animals; as tending to show how in the abnormal of the one there is a certain agreement with, and approximation to the normal in the other; and thus continuing, in a partial degree and in a limited number of instances in the fully-formed adult, a similarity of organization so remarkably witnessed in embryonic life, with so little distinction of species?

---

* In this child the Eustachian valve was found distinct, and so situated—as indeed it usually is—as to direct the blood from the vena cava ascendens towards the foramen ovale, and prevent its falling into the right ventricle, serving, as Bichat conjectured, the part of a bridge to convey the blood over the auricular-ventricular opening. The ductus arteriosus was becoming obliterated by coagulable lymph in the form of fine cellular tissue. The valve of the foramen ovale was large and delicate, sufficiently large to cover the foramen completely, and on its adhesion taking place, to form the fossa ovalis.

INDEX.

Air, expired in cholera, quality of, 119.
„ in lungs after death, composition of, 91, 196, 175, 326, 327.
„ in intestine, 102.
Alcoholic fatal intoxication, remarks on, 396.
„ cases of, 397.
„ comments on, 402.
Allan, Dr., referred to on the fevers of Madagascar, 56.
Ammonia in the blood, *post mortem?* 14, 394.
Anæmia, remarkable example of, 105.
Aneurism, statistics of, 372.
„ cases of, 375–392.
„ etiology of, 393.
„ fatal, without rupture, cases of, 390–392.
„ spontaneous cure, instance of, 395.
Appendicula vermiformis, closure of, 273; „ communicating with ileum, 276.
Arteries, occlusion of, remarks on, 395.
Arthritic diathesis, remarks on, 419.
Ascaris lumbricoides in liver, 423.

Barracks, remarks on, 60.
Blair, his view of yellow fever, 62.
Blood, *post mortem* observations on, 13.
„ effect of pressure on its flow, 222.
„ corpuscles of in yellow fever, 62.
„ ammonia in, question respecting, 14.
„ clot in heart, broken up, 185, 208, 257, 271, 272.
„ carbonic acid in, in excess in cholera, 119; after death in other diseases, 243, 249.
„ coagulation of, in vessels during life, examples of, 286.
„ remarks on, 287.
„ coagulation of, after alcoholic poisoning, 400.
Brain, flattened appearance of from pressure, 41.

Calculi, urinary, remarks on, 417.
„ instances of, 417.
„ biliary, 421.
„ black kind, analysis of, 422; copper in, 422.
Cholera morbus, common and spasmodic, „ statistics of, 111.
„ report of epidemic in Ceylon in 1819, 113, 122.
„ extracts of reports on ordinary cholera, 122, 127.
Chyme, fermenting, a check to softening, 10.
Constitution of man, question concerning, 330.
Concretion, peculiar bony, 280.
„ gouty, analysis of, 420.

Diaphragm, partial ossification of, 107.
Diabetes, remarkable case of, 220.
Delirium tremens, statistics of, 397.
„ influence of, in other diseases, 402.
Diet, remarks on, 60.
Diagnosis, mistaken, anecdotes of, 175.
Discoloration of organs, remarks on, 6.
Dissipation, instance of, 210.
Dowler, Dr., on *post mortem* temperature, commented on, 362.
Dress, soldiers', 212.
Dormatories, defects of, 211.
Duodenum, rupture of, 345.
Dysentery, chief causes of, 66.
„ statistics of, 67.
„ complications of, 71, 76.
„ acute, cases of, 72, 84.
„ chronic, 89, 107; treatment of, 37.
„ suggestions prophylactic, 110.
Ductus arteriosus, vestige of ossified, 103.
Duct, common biliary, distended state of, 95.

Duct, cystic, peculiar state of, 81.
  „ mouth of obstructed by mucus, 36, 38.

Elephantiasis, remarkable case of, 172.
Embolus in basilar artery, associated with epilepsy ? 380.
  ,. in heart, peculiar state of, 284.
Empyema, remarks on, 245.
  „ cases of, 246, 255.
  „ treatment of, 265.
Entozoa, remarks on, instances of, 423.
Euthanasia, favoured by excess of carbonic acid in the blood, 243.
Exercise, carriage, effect of, 64.

Fatality of disease, variability of, instances of, 368.
Fevers, not distinct entities, 17.
  „ prevalency of in connection with climate, 19.
  „ intermittent, statistics of, 22; cases of, 23, 24.
  „ remittent, statistics of, 26; cases of Ionian Islands, 28, 32; in Malta, 33, 38; continued statistics of, 39; cases of, 40, 41.
  „ yellow fever, statistics of, 42; cases of, 44, 46; etiology of, remarks on, 47; pathology of, 61.
  „ acclimation, influence of, 63.
  „ treatment of, 64; Sydenham's caution respecting, 65.
Fibrin, deliquescence of in air, with production of heat, 267.
  „ liquefaction in vacuo, 215.
  „ puruloid softening by coction, 267.
  „ absorption of, 290.
Finlayson, George, mention of, 119.
Fingers and toes, supernumerary case of, 375.
Fistula in ano rare in phthisis, 209.
Flannel, properties of, 57.
Folchi, Dr., referred to on the agues of the Roman Compagna, 55.
Foramen ovale, remarkable case of, 375.

Gall-bladder, peculiar state of, 81.
  „ its mucous changed into a serous membrane, 81.

Gall-bladder, inflamed state of, 83.
  „ peculiar contents of, 315.
Gardens, companies', mention of, 216.
Gangrene of lungs, instance of recovery from, 282.
Glands, Payer's, apparent absence of, 106.
Gulliver, Mr., experiments of on the softening of fibrin, 288.
  „ on fatty degeneration of arteries, 393.

Hæmatemisis, illustration of, 339.
Heart, weight of, 5.
  „ softening of in cholera, 117.
  „ air in, composition of, 40.
Hiccough, one cause of, 85.
Hepatitis, acute and chronic, and icterus, statistics of, 130.
  „ predisposing causes of, 130.
  „ cases of, 132, 154.
  „ treatment of, 156.
  „ abscess, whether connected with dysentery, 155.
Hepatization of lung, remarks on, 329.
Hospital, Turkish, maladministration of, 84.
Hydrogen, sulphuretted, not the cause of malaria, 48.
Hydrothorax, cases of, 255.

Icterus, with pale hepatic blood-vessels, 41.
Ileum, abnormal formation in, 342.
Indigo in biliary calculi, 422.
Inflammation, cellular, statistics of, 354.
  „ cases of, 356, 366.
  „ treatment of, 368.
  „ question as to contagion, 369.
Intestines, perforation of, remarks on, 354.
  „ abnormal position of, 425-427.
Ipecacuanha, use of in dysentery, 37.

Jackson, Dr., recommendation of gestation in fevers, 64.

Kidneys, weight of, 5.
Kit, soldiers', 58.
Knee, healed state of after a gun-shot wound, 149.

Lithic acid in joints, 317, 318.

„ deposit of in urinary bladder, 80, 324.

Lightning, death from and state of body, 409.

Lungs, weight of, 2.

„ chief emunctory of alcohol, 403.

Liver, weight of, 4.

„ diseases of, statistics, 129.

„ influence of climate and diet, etc., 131.

„ greasy feel of, sometimes deceptive as to presence of oil, 100.

M'Arthur, Dr., cases of alcoholic poisoning, 405.

Malaria, remarks on, 48.

„ facts respecting, 50.

„ means of protection from, 54, 61.

„ different kinds of? 53.

Mamilla, instances of, 180, 277.

Mammæ, supernumerary case of, 429.

Maltese subject to intestinal worms, 423.

Meals, soldiers', 58.

Meat, salted, bad effects of, 69.

Military service, wear of on the constitution, 294.

Mercury, abuse of, 109.

Muscle, rectus abdominis, laceration of, 195.

„ abdominal, contraction of, four hours post mortem, 101.

Nerve, optic, wasted state of, 204.

Opium, use of in dysentery, 87.

Organs, weight of, 1.

„ sexual, arrested growth of, 278.

„ rupture of from falls, 407–409.

„ peculiarities of form of, 424.

„ „ alimentary canal, 425.

„ liver, spleen, and pancreas, 427.

„ kidneys and generative organs, 429.

„ lungs, 429.

„ heart and blood-vessels, 430.

„ brain and nerves, 432.

Oxygen, noxious effects of, 265.

Pancreas, peculiar lesion of, 258.

Paracentesis by perforation of rib, 248.

Peritonitis, statistics of, 258.

„ cases of, 259–263.

Pericardium, dry state of, 298.

„ retentive power of, 317.

Periodicity of diseases, remarks on, 258–355.

Pneumonia, statistics of, 291.

„ its relation to climate, etc., 293.

„ cases of, 297.

„ complicated with cellular inflammation, 303.

„ „ with cardiac disease, 308.

„ „ with cerebral disease, 310.

„ „ with peritonitis, 312.

„ „ with pulmonary abscess, 315.

„ „ with rheumatism, 316.

„ „ with tubercles, 319.

„ chronic cases of, 325.

„ general treatment of, 329.

Pneumathorax, degree of frequency of, 218.

„ cases of, 219, 241.

„ composition of the air and its indications, 243.

„ perforation of pleura, remarks on, 243.

„ general treatment of, 244.

Prison dieteries referred to, 60.

Privies, remarks on, 70, 212.

Ptyalism, peculiar instances of, 109.

Pulmonary consumption, mortality of at different stations, 157.

„ statistics of, 159.

„ latent, cases of, 160–163.

„ latent, from insanity, cases of, 164–173.

„ from other diseases, cases of, 174.

„ not latent, analysis of cases of, 187.

„ acute, cases of, 201–209.

„ question of curability, 215.

„ treatment of, 216.

„ prevention of, remarks on, 217.

Pus, healthy, destitute of air, 371.
  „ experiments on injection of, 369.

Quinine, use of in fevers, 64.
Quarantine, the cause, amongst other evils, of falsification of nomenclature, 42.

Rations, soldiers', 210.
Races of men, how affected by fever, 63.
Recruits, examination of, 193.
Rigor mortis, remarks on, 14.
Rokitansky, Professor, remark of, 333.

Sash, salutary use of, 110.
Serum, injected, absorption of, 370.
  „ variable specific gravity of, 225.
Softening of organs, remarks on, 9.
Stomach, solution of, remarkable examples of, 359, 407.
  „ apparent absence of softening, remarks on, 392, 416.
Strangury from lytta, and its relief, 8.
Spleen, weight of, 4.
  „ abnormal state of, 41.
  „ ammonia in, 46.
Spermatozoa, presence of, active *post mortem*, 194.
Sydenham, caution from, on the treatment of fevers, 65.
  „ his idea of malaria, 48.
Suicides, proportional frequency of, 210.
  „ cases of, 407, 415.

Tank-water, occasional bad quality of, 70.
Temperature *post mortem*, remarks on, 11.
  „ notes of, 73, 96, 152, 344, 370.
  „ remarkable instance of, with comment, 361.
Tenesmus, cause of, 85.
Thrombosis, remarks on, 267.
  „ vessels in which found, 269.
  „ cases of, 269, 286.
  „ comments on, 287.
Thoracic duct, peculiar lesion of, 273.
Tubercle, prevalency of, 159.

Tubercle, prevalency of in sheep, 164.
  „ „ in various organs, 191.
  „ chemical composition of, 214.
Tuberculosis, etiology of, 209.
  „ diathesis, 210.
  „ disposing causes of, 211.
  „ influence of on intellect? 186.
  „ „ on procreative power? 200.
Tubercular cavity in process of healing, instances of, 172–185.

Ulcers, intestinal, not commonly painful, 86.
  „ dysenteric, healing, 91.
Urea in blood, 38, 144.
Urine, quality of in fevers, 63.

Valve of aorta, rupture of, 286.
  „ ileo-cœcal, destruction of, 342.
Vena portæ, peculiar lesions of, 93, 274.
Vein, hæmorrhoidal, rupture of, 286.
  „ mesenteric, rupture of, 270.
Vessels, air in, remarks on, 12.
Vomit, black, composition of, 42–46.
  „ notice of, in fever of Malta, 37.

Water, impure, a cause of dysentery, 69.
  „ iced, good effects of, 87.
  „ of ponds in Barbadoes, sometimes poisonous, 70.
Winds, etesian and sirocco contrasted, 11.
  „ temperature of, 57.

Yellow fever, question of its contagion, 44–61.
  „ „ blood-corpuscles in, 62.
  „ „ blood-vessels, peculiar state of, 62.
  „ „ microscopical preparations illustrative of its pathology, 62.

Young, Dr., optical test of pus, 168.

CORRIGENDA.

Page 11 line 12 *for* tower   *read* town.

,, 30 ,, 25 ,, portion   ,, portions.

,, 34 ,, 20 ,, ichteric   ,, icteric.

,, 36 ,, 22 ,, tissues   ,, tissue.

,, 40 ,, 14 ,, cornea   ,, cornua.

,, 54 ,, 35 ,, or   ,, on.

,, 64 (note) 8 ,, of   ,, and.

,, 66 ,, 19 ,, cachetic   ,, cachectic.

,, 155 ,, 29 ,, epithenomena   ,, epiphenomena.

,, ,, ,, 40 ,, cachetic   ,, cachectic.

,, 177 ,, 10 ,, periostum   ,, periosteum.

,, 180 ,, 33 ,, mammillæ   ,, mamillæ.

,, 204 ,, 15 ,, never   ,, nerve.

,, 209 ,, 23 ,, villous   ,, inner.

,, 311 ,, 28 ,, typanitic   ,, tympanitic.

www.ingramcontent.com/pod-product-compliance
Ingram Content Group UK Ltd.
Pitfield, Milton Keynes, MK11 3LW, UK
UKHW040659180125
453697UK00010B/285